Stephens' Detection of New Adverse Drug Reactions

Fifth Edition

Stephens' Detection of New Adverse Drug Reactions

Fifth Edition

Edited by

John Talbot
*Director, Global Drug Safety, AstraZeneca R&D Charnwood, Loughborough,
Leicestershire, UK*

Patrick Waller
Consultant in Pharmacovigilance and Pharmacoepidemiology, Southampton, UK

John Wiley & Sons, Ltd

Copyright © 2004   John Wiley & Sons Ltd, The Atrium, Sourthern Gate, Chichester,
West Sussex PO19 8SQ, England

Telephone (+44) 1243 779777

Email (for orders and customer service enquiries): cs-books@wiley.co.uk
Visit our Home Page on www.wileyeurope.com or www.wiley.com

This publication is designed to provide accurate and authoritative information in regard to the subject matter
covered. It is sold on the understanding that the Publisher is not engaged in rendering professional services. If
professional advice or other expert assistance is required, the services of a competent professional should be sought.

Other Wiley Editorial Offices

John Wiley and Sons Inc., 111 River Street, Hoboken, NJ 07030, USA

Jossey-Bass, 989 Market Street, San Francisco, CA 94103-1741, USA

Wiley-VCH Verlag GmbH, Boschstr. 12, D-69469 Weinhein, Germany

John WIley & Sons Australia Ltd, 33 Park Road, Milton, Queensland 4064, Australia

John WIley & Sons (Asia) Pte Ltd, 2 Clementi Loop #02-01, Jin Xing Distripark, Singapore 129809

John Wiley & Sons Canada Ltd, 22 Worcester Road, Etobicoke, Ontario, Canada M9W 1LI

Wiley also publishes its books in a variety of electronic formats. Some content that appears in print may not be
available in electronic books.

British Library Cataloguing in Publication Data

A catalogue record for this book is available from the British Library

ISBN 0 470 84552 X hardback

Typeset in 10/12 Times by Keytec Typesetting Ltd, Bridport, Dorset, England
Printed and bound in Great Britain by TJ International Ltd., Padstow
This book is printed in acid-free paper responsibly manufactured from sustainable forestry
in which at least two trees are planted for each one used for paper production.

Contents

Stephens' Detection of New Adverse Drug Reactions Fifth Edition edited by John Talbot and Patrick Waller
© 2004 John Wiley & Sons, Ltd   ISBN: 0 470 84552 X

Foreword

When does a book become a classic? The fact that Stephens' Detection of New Adverse Drug Reactions is now in its fifth edition speaks volumes for its value to a multiplicity of readers. The science of pharmacovigilance has grown in breadth and depth over the eighteen years of the book's existence and the present edition shows not only how the scope of the field has increased, with chapters on the safety of biotechnology products and vaccine safety surveillance, but also how the operating techniques of statistical analysis, legal aspects and ethical issues now form important areas for debate in the field of drug safety.

The history of drug safety is a roll call of the practice of medicine and of the science of pharmacology and toxicology which underpin it. Even the nomenclature of adverse drug reactions has evolved as we understand more of the underlying scientific basis. Nowhere is this better illustrated than in the area of drug interactions. Two examples serve to illustrate this. The broad division into pharmacokinetic and pharmacodynamic interactions has been further complicated by new understanding of how cellular transporter mechanisms are utilised to transfer drugs across tissue boundaries in the gut, liver, kidney and brain, and how this now forms the basis of a new set of ways in which one drug can alter the disposition and response to another. Secondly, as our knowledge of the human genome has evolved, the science of pharamacogenomics has increased our ability to select patients who will respond to specific drugs, and this response may be beneficial or adverse. Again, such information must be factored into our appreciation of the basis of drug interactions.

As well as considering how we have reached our present position in considering adverse drug reactions, this book looks to the future. The chapter by Patrick Waller and Stephen Evans is particularly important in this respect, showing how the prediction of drug safety will form the future of pharmacovigilance, whereas in the past this depended more on the demonstration of harm. Medicinal chemists who design drug molecules appreciate the toxicity potential of various chemical groupings in a molecule, and are increasingly able to design out the offending entity without impairing efficacy. The clinical pharmacologist and the drug regulator, always aiming to reconcile possible risk with benefit, appreciate how critical is appropriate dose selection in achieving this balance. The clinician will always play an important role by his careful documentation and reporting of patient harm on systems such as the Yellow Card. Such spontaneous reporting systems will always serve the public health by creating signals of drug safety which can be augmented and further analysed in other more sophisticated ways.

The concept of balancing risk with benefit, a theme to which the book correctly repeatedly returns, remains the bedrock of drug therapy. It is not an idea which either the public or the

Stephens' Detection of New Adverse Drug Reactions Fifth Edition edited by John Talbot and Patrick Waller
© 2004 John Wiley & Sons, Ltd ISBN: 0 470 84552 X

media wish to embrace, preferring to regard medicines as magic bullets. The achievement of this latest edition of Stephens' Detection of New Adverse Drug Reactions is to demonstrate very clearly that as science moves forward, so must our appreciation of this balance. We can safely predict, I think, that this Fifth Edition will not be the last.

Alasdair Breckenridge

Preface to the fifth edition

This is the fifth edition of a book first published in 1985. The aims of the book have changed little over the nearly 20 years since the preface to the first edition was written, but the scope of the book, the accumulated knowledge, international regulations and number of people working in the field of pharmacovigilance have grown enormously. This book is intended for all those working in pharmacovigilance and pharmaceutical medicine, whether they be in drug regulatory authorities, the pharmaceutical industry or academia, and in all continents.

This is the first edition where Dr Myles Stephens has not been the principal author and editor. The editors of this edition gratefully accepted the task from him, but Myles has still made a significant contribution to this fifth edition in the form of two large chapters and the co-authoring of another chapter. In fitting recognition of his immense contribution to previous editions and the discipline of pharmacovigilance over many years, the book has been re-titled 'Stephens' Detection of New Adverse Drug Reactions'. We were very pleased at Wiley's positive response to our proposal for this change and with their enthusiasm and support for the new edition generally.

The book covers the issues and problems involved in the detection of new adverse drug reactions throughout the life cycle of a medicine from animal studies through to clinical trials, its introduction to the market, followed by wide clinical use and eventual decline in use or withdrawal. This theme is supported by topics that reach across the life cycle, such as causality assessment, regulations, legal aspects, dictionaries and coding and ethical issues. Chapters from the fourth edition have either been extensively revised or replaced. We are grateful to those authors who updated their work and welcome several new authors. Some topics have new authors and there are some completely new chapters, for instance those looking at particular types of medicine that present special safety problems such as vaccines and biotechnology products. As before, chapters are extensively referenced and there is a bibliography and list of websites to direct readers to a wealth of other resources.

John Talbot

Patrick Waller

Stephens' Detection of New Adverse Drug Reactions Fifth Edition edited by John Talbot and Patrick Waller
© 2004 John Wiley & Sons, Ltd   ISBN: 0 470 84552 X

List of Contributors

Dr BDC Arnold, Vice President, Global Drug Safety, AstraZeneca, 11F133, Alderley Park, Macclesfield, SK10 4TG, UK
Email: barry.arnold@astrazeneca.com

Christine Bendall, Arnold & Porter, 25 Old Broad Street, London EC2N 1HQ, UK
Email: christine_bendall@aporter.com

Professor Alasdair M. Breckenridge, Department of Pharmacology and Therapeutics, University of Liverpool, Liverpool, L69 3BX, UK
Email: ambreck@liv.ac.uk

Dr Benton Brown, 4641 Calle San Juan, Newbury Park, CA 91320, USA
Email: bentonmd@yahoo.com

Dr Elliot Brown, Managing Director, Elliot Brown Consulting Ltd, Rowan House, 7 Woodfall Avenue, Barnet, Herts EN5 2EZ, UK
Email: eb@ebconsulting.co.uk

Dr Alan Craig – (general correspondence), 13 Court Close, Princes Risborough, Bucks HP27 9BG, UK
Email: alan+craig@lineone.net

Dr Alan Craig – (publication details), Consultant Clinical Scientist, Pivotal Laboratories Ltd, Pivotal House, Aviator Court, Clifton Moorgate, York YO30 4UT, UK
Email: a.craig@pivotal-labs.com

Professor Stephen Evans, Professor of Pharmacoepidemiology, Medical Statistics Unit, London School of Hygiene & Tropical Medicine, Keppel Street, London WC1 7HT, UK
Email: Stephen.Evans@lshtm.ac.uk

Dr Elizabeth Miller, Head of Immunisation Division, PHLS Communicable Disease Surveillance Centre, 61 Colindale Avenue, London NW9 5EQ, UK
Email: liz.miller@phls.org.uk

Professor Phil Routledge, Department of Pharmacology, Therapeutics & Toxicology, University of Wales College of Medicine, Health Park, Cardiff CF14 4XN, UK
Email: proutledg@compuserve.com

Professor Saad Shakir, Drug Safety Research Unit, Bursledon Hall, Blundell Lane, Southampton SO31 1AA, UK
Email: saad.shakir@dsru.org

Dr David Snodin, Principal Consultant, PAREXEL International, River Court, 50 Oxford Road, Denham, Uxbridge, Middlesex UB9 4DN, UK
Email: david.snodin@parexel.com

Stephens' Detection of New Adverse Drug Reactions Fifth Edition edited by John Talbot and Patrick Waller
© 2004 John Wiley & Sons, Ltd   ISBN: 0 470 84552 X

Professor Janet Steiner, Director, Safety Strategy, US Drug Safety, AstraZeneca LP, FOC-2W, 1800 Concord Pike, PO Box 15437, Wilmington DE 19850-5437, USA
Email: janet.steiner@astrazeneca.com

Dr Myles Stephens, 49 Kings Court, Bishop's Stortford, Hertfordshire CM23 2AB, UK
Email: stephmdb@onetel.net.uk

Dr John Talbot, Director, Global Drug Safety, AstraZeneca R & D Charnwood, Bakewell Road, Loughborough, Leicestershire LE11 5RH, UK
Email: John.Talbot@astrazeneca.com

Dr Hugh H. Tilson, Senior Advisor to the Dean, Public Health Leadership Programme, Rosenau Hall Room 260, University of North Carolina, School of Public Health, Chapel Hill, NC 27599-7400, USA
Email: hugh_tilson@unc.edu

Dr Patrick Waller, Patrick Waller Limited, Consultancy in Pharmacovigilance and Pharmacoepidemiology, 15 Tamella Road, Botley, Southhampton SO30 2NY, UK
Email: patrick.waller@btinternet.com

Dr Margaret M. Westland, Fellow of American College of Preventative Medicine (ACPM) Recently retired from a career in Pharmacovigilance
Email: riofish@aol.com

1
Introduction

Myles Stephens

Mercury

'Were we to believe all that has been said about this drug, we should welcome in it a cure for all the ills that afflict humanity, the veritable panacea of the old dreamers. Unfortunately we cannot do this. But it is an agent of wondrous properties, a remedy of vast and varied power; perhaps, altogether, the most useful in our Pharmacopoeia. It is the very prince of that class of remedies, unfortunately too few, that are capable of entering the system, of grappling with a disease in the blood, and coming off victorious in the struggle (Headland, 1859).

Introduction to pharmacovigilance

Definition

The word 'pharmacovigilance' was coined by the French as the 'study of the undesirable effects of drugs'. It is derived from the Greek '*pharmakon*', a drug or medicine, and from the Latin '*vigilans*' watchful or careful. Pharmacovigilance has been defined as being 'All methods of assessment and prevention of adverse drug reactions. The framework of pharmacovigilance is broader than that of post-marketing surveillance and includes clinical and even pre-clinical development of drugs' (Bégaud, 1993). An alternative, fuller, description is given in an EEC directive: 'System set up to collect information useful in the surveillance of medicinal products, in particular with regard to adverse reactions in human beings. The system contributes to ensuring the adoption of appropriate regulatory decisions concerning the medicinal products authorised within the Community, having regard to information obtained about adverse reactions to medicinal products under normal conditions of use' (Directive 75/319/EEC. Article 29A), with the latter phrase implying that it applies to the post-marketing period. The proposed World Health Organization (WHO) definition is the science and activities relating to the detection, evaluation, understanding and prevention of adverse drug reactions or any other drug-related problems (Edwards, 2002). The International Society of Pharmacoepidemiology defines it as 'a type of continual monitoring for unwanted effects and other safety-related aspects of drugs that

Stephens' Detection of New Adverse Drug Reactions Fifth Edition edited by John Talbot and Patrick Waller
© 2004 John Wiley & Sons, Ltd   ISBN: 0 470 84552 X

are already on the market. In practice, pharmacovigilance refers almost exclusively to the spontaneous reporting systems which allow health care professionals and others to report adverse drug reactions to a central agency' (www.pharmacoepi.org/aboutpe.htm). One of the most recent definition is 'Pharmacovigilance involves the monitoring, detection, evaluation and responding to drug safety hazards in humans during premarketing development and post marketing' (Shakir and Layton, 2002). However, Mann and Andrews (2002), in *Pharmacovigilance* look upon it as being 'the study of the safety of marketed drugs under the practical conditions of clinical usage in large populations; the MCA, meanwhile, defines it as 'the process of evaluating and improving the safety of marketed products, (Waller *et al*, 1996). The National Audit Office (UK) defines it as 'The science of medicines safety monitoring'. Confusion reigns. Let us hope that the WHO definition prevails.

Aims

The aims of pharmacovigilance are:

- The identification and quantification of previously unrecognized adverse drug reactions (ADR)s.

- The identification of sub-groups of patients at particular risk of ADRs (the risk relating to dose, age, gender and underlying disease).

- The continued monitoring of the safety of a product, throughout the duration of its use, to ensure that its risks and benefits remain acceptable. This includes safety monitoring following significant newly approved indications.

- The comparative ADR profile of products within the same therapeutic class.

- The detection of inappropriate prescription and administration.

- The further elucidation of a product's pharmacological/toxicological properties and the mechanism by which it produces ADRs.

- The detection of significant drug–drug interactions between new products and co-therapy with agents already established on the market, which may only be detected during widespread use.

- The communication of appropriate information to health-care professionals (Rawlins *et al.*, 1992).

- The refutation of 'false positive' ADR signals arising in the professional or lay media, or from spontaneous reports (Rawlins and Payne, 1997).

The history of pharmacovigilance

ADRs must have started at the dawn of time, when man first used plants as medication and learned to brew alcohol. The history of ADRs is sparse until this century, when it slowly gathered pace until the end of World War II, since when there has been an explosion of new drugs and the consequent increase in ADRs.

c. 4000 BC   Sumeria recorded euphoric effect of the poppy.

c. 2000 BC   The Babylonian code: a physician who caused the death of a patient should lose his hands.

2000 BC   Emperor Shin Nong. Ma Huang – ephedra sinica (ephedrine, pseudoephedrine) causing tachycardia and hypertension.

c.1700 BC   The use of inhaled smoke (opium) to reduce pain, belladonna and colchicine were mentioned in Ebers Papyrus (Atkins, 1995).

c. 1500 BC   Dried myrtle leaves containing salicylates were rubbed on for relief from rheumatism.

c. 950 BC   Homer said 'Many drugs were excellent when mingled and many were fatal'.

c. 500 BC   Hippocrates said '*Primum non nocere*'. His oath includes 'I will neither give a deadly drug to anybody if asked for it nor will I make a suggestion to that effect. Similarly I will not give to a women an abortive remedy'.

c. 450 BC   Hippocrates speaks of scurvy (Jaramillo-Arango, 1953).

c. 400 BC   Extract of poplar (salicylic acid) used to alleviate pain of childbirth.

120 BC   Mithridates VI, King of Pontus, concocted 'Mithridatium', a panacea for almost all ills (Shah, 2001).

AD 230   Hoa-Tho (Wei dynasty) administered fumes of aconite, datura and hyoscyamus (Atkins, 1995).

361   Licensing system for practising physicians was established in Constantinople.

c. 994   'New remedies should first be tried in animals' (Half Abbas).

980–1037   Avicenna (Abu 'Ali al-Husayn 'Abd Allah ibn Sina) wrote '*Al-Qanun fi al-Tibb*' describing 760 medicinal plants and drugs. Also laid out the basic rules of clinical drug trials. (http://users.erols.com/gmqm/euromed1.html).

1123   St Bartholomew's Hospital (London) founded.

1386   Chaucer depicted a man called 'placebo' in *Canterbury Tales* and defines him as a sycophant or servile flatterer (De Deyn, 2000).

1460   Mercurial ointment used for syphilis.

1498   College of Physicians of Florence published a pharmacopoeia (Ricetario).

1538   Paracelsus (Teofrasto Bombasto di Hoenheim) said 'All things are a poison and none is without poison, only the dose makes that a thing is a poison'. Obviously, he did not know about type B reactions.

1540   Discovery of digitalis by Leonhard Fuchs of Tubingen.

1541   *Dispensatorium Pharmacopoearum* published at Lyon.

1640   Introduction of cinchona bark (containing quinine) from Peru (Sneader, 2000).

1617   Establishment of The Worshipful Society of the Art and Mistery of Apothecaries from the Guild of Grocers (Mann, 1988).

1618   First edition of *London Pharmacopoeia* by Royal College of Physicians.

1634   First reference to rickets in London Bills of Mortality.

1658   'Remedies often make disease worse … It takes a wise doctor to know when not to prescribe'. Baltasar Gacian 1601–58, *The Art of Worldly Wisdom*.

1662   The original randomized clinical trial (Rose, 1982.).

1665–66   Great plague of London caused approximately 56 000 deaths.

Late 1600s Friedrich Hoffman (1660–1742) described adverse effects of ergot (Borghi and Canti, 1986) and its use was prohibited in some European countries (the first official drug withdrawal).

17th century Voltaire 'They poured drugs of which they knew little into bodies of which they knew less'.

1709   Dover's powder: potassium sulphate and nitrate, each 40 parts, plus dry opium powder and ipecacuanha powder, each 10 parts. Thomas Dover 1660–1742.

1712   *A Compleat History of Drugs*, written in French by Monsieur Pomet, 'chief druggist to the present French King; done into English from the originals'.

1714   Short report on variolation using purulent matter to prevent smallpox (Emanuele Timoni).

'Cur'd yesterday of my disease, I died last night of my physician' (Matthew Prior).

1721   Nathanel Bailey's *Universal Etymological Dictionary* lists several English words to describe the mis-prescribing of amateur doctors:

Empirick, a physician by bare practice;

Mountebank, a pretender to Physick (from *montimbanco*, Italian, i.e. soapbox salesman);

Quack or Quacksalver, a bold and ignorant Pretender to the Art Of Physick. Quack-salver possibly from Old Dutch 'Quacker' (to prattle and 'salf' (healing ointment).

1753   Lind JA. described a comparative study in scurvy ($N = 12$) with six different groups: a quart of cider daily, 25 drops of elixir vitriol (dilute sulphuric acid) tds, two spoonfuls of vinegar, half pint of sea water, two oranges and one lemon daily, electuary of herbs (Lind, 1753).

1763   Rev. Edmund Stone published 'An account of the success of the bark of willow in the cure of the agues', i.e. use of salicylic acid.

1785   William Withering wrote 'Account of the foxglove and some of its medical uses', including 'Foxglove when given in large and quickly repeated doses occasions sickness, vomiting, giddiness, confused vision, objects appearing green or yellow'.
            The *New Medical Dictionary* described placebo as 'a commonplace method or medicine (De Craen *et al.*, 1999).

1796   Jenner first 'vaccinates' against smallpox.

1799   Introduction of nitrous oxide.

1801   Possibly the first placebo-controlled trial (De Craen *et al.*, 1999).

1810   Hahnemann introduced homeopathy.

1820   First US Pharmacopoeia. Pierre Joseph Pelletier isolated colchicine from autumn crocus for gout.

1839   First observation of anaphylaxis in rabbits by Magenta (Borghi and Canti, 1986).

1845   On 12 March Francis Rynd gave the first hypodermic injection at Dublin's Meath Hospital.

1846   First use of ether (16 October 1846) at Massachusetts General Hospital by dentist William Morton.

1847   First use of chloroform (Turk, 1994), invented by Samuel Guthrie in 1831. Used by James Young Simpson on 5 November 1847.

1864   First British Pharmacopoeia.

1869   Chloral hydrate first used.

1877   British Medical Association (BMA) met to investigate the sudden deaths associated with chloroform (Royal, 1973).

1880   Toxicology of anaesthetics reported (Anon., 1880).

1883   First use of paracetamol.

1884   Introduction of phenacetin.

1896   First injection of anti-typhoid serum by Almroth Wright.

1898   Anaphylaxis 'discovered' by Richet.
        First randomised clinical trial: diphtheria treated with serum and standard treatment versus standard treatment alone (Hróbjartsson *et al.*, 1998).

1899   Introduction of acetylsalicylic acid (Aspirin) by F. Bayer and Co.

1902   Biologics Control Act passed following deaths in 10 children in St Louis, USA, caused by diphtheria antitoxin contaminated with live tetanus bacilli (Roberts, 1996).

1903   Introduction of barbital.

1905   Discovery of arsphenamine for spirochaetal disease (replacing mercury for the treatment of syphilis) by Paul Erlich (1854–1915).

1906   Pure Food and Drugs Act (USA) concerned labelling and adulteration.
        Clemens Von Pirquet coined the term 'allergy'.

1916   First placebo-controlled clinical trial (Delay and Pichol, 1973); see 1801.

1922   Insulin discovered.

1925   Therapeutic Substances Act (USA) regulated the manufacture and sale of substances requiring biological testing.

1926   Insulin was produced.

1927   Thyroxine synthesized.

1928   Fleming discovered penicillin.

1933   Dinitrophenol found to cause weight reduction but caused sclerosing cataracts, leading to blindness, and fatal hyperthermia. Forced off the market by the Food and Drugs Administration (FDA) in 1935 (Hecht, 1987).

1935   First use of prontosil red (sulphamidochrysoidine) (Turk, 1994).
            Cortisone and ergometrine isolated.

1937   Elixir Sulfonamide containing 72 per cent diethylene glycol (DEG) given to 353 patients during the period of a week. There were 105 deaths, including 34 children, due to renal failure caused by the DEG (Geiling and Cannon, 1938). In 1969, in South Africa, seven children died of renal failure due to DEG. In 1986 there were 14 deaths in Bombay. In 1990, 47 children died similarly in Nigeria (Wax, 1995). In 1995 there were 51 deaths due to DEG (Hamif et al., 1995). In Haiti, 88 children died as a result of paracetamol syrup being contaminated with 14.4 per cent DEG (O'Brien et al., 1998). In 1998, a cough syrup containing DEG was implicated in 33 deaths in India (WHO, 2001). And so it goes on.

1938   Federal Food, Drug and Cosmetics Act (USA) as a result of the DEG 'epidemic'.

1941   First patient (a policeman with septicaemia) treated with penicillin, but he died because they ran out of penicillin (Ellis, 1997).

1947   Recognition that mercury in teething and worming powders caused Pink disease (Black, 1990).

1948   Introduction of chloramphenicol. It was found to cause aplastic anaemia in between 1 in 58 000 and 1 in 75 000 patients and was removed from the French market in 1987, but it remains in other markets for very restricted use.
            Vitamin B$_{12}$ isolated.

1948   First modern randomized clinical trial of Streptomycin by the Medical Research Council (MRC).
            Creation of UK National Health Service.

1952   First book on ADRs: Meyler's Side Effects of Drugs.

1953   Renal damage by phenacetin suspected.
            DNA structure proposed by Watson and Crick.

1954   'Stalinon' an organic compound of tin (diethyltin di-iodide + vitamin K) used in the treatment of boils, had impurities that were alleged to have killed 102 patients in France (British Medical Journal 1958; Gruner, 1958).

1961   McBride and Lenz reported phocomelia due to thalidomide (Distillers Company, 1961; McBride, 1961; Lenz, 1962, 1966, 1989; Lenz and Knapp, 1962; Mellin and Katzenstein, 1962; Burley, 1988). The FDA delayed marketing approval of thalidomide because its toxicity in acute animal studies was questioned by Dr Frances Oldham Kelsey in view of clinical reports of polyneuritis (D'Arcy and Griffin, 1994). It had not been tested in pregnant animals, but the same effect was found in mice, rats, hamsters, rabbits, macaques, marmosets, baboons and rhesus monkeys. The first case was born on 25 December 1956.

1961–67   Asthma deaths due to high isoprenaline nebulizer usage (Inman and Adelstein, 1969).

1962   Kefauver–Harris Amendments (USA). All clinical testing of investigational drugs to be reviewed and subject to veto by the FDA. New drugs to be effective as well as safe before marketing. This was as a result of the thalidomide disaster.
            Medicines Act (UK). Both the Committee on Safety of Drugs (CSD) and the Medicines Act were delayed responses to the thalidomide disaster.
            MER/29 (Triparanol) cataract disaster. The FDA found falsified laboratory data concerning cataracts in rats and dogs (Rheingold, 1968).

1963   CSD formed in the UK 'to advise whether a new drug should be submitted for clinical trials, to advise whether a drug should be released for marketing and to study adverse reactions to drugs already in use' (Mann, 1988).
            Epidemiology of adverse drug reactions first mentioned (Cluff *et al.*, 1964). Finney (1963) called for a detailed study of persons given a specific drug to detect any untoward development even though apparently unassociated with the drug given.

1966   First description of 'torsades de pointes' (Dessertenne, 1966).

1967   WHO resolution 20.51 laid basis for international system of monitoring ADRs (Venulet, 1993).

1968   Professor Jan Venulet, one of the founders of pharmacovigilance, becomes head of the WHO pilot research project for international drug monitoring set up in Alexandria, VA, USA.

1970   Thromboembolic disease with high dose oestrogen oral contraceptives discovered (Inman *et al.*, 1970).
            Sub-acute myelo-optic neuropathy (SMON) due to halogenated hydroxyquinolones, clioquinol or enterovioform, given for non-specific gastro-enteritis (Tsubaki *et al.*, 1971; Kono, 1980). There were more than 11 000 Japanese victims between 1955 and 1969. It had been produced in Switzerland by Ciba-Geigy in 1900 and used since 1930. There had been two case reports published in Argentina in 1935 (Barros, 1935; Grawitz, 1935). At first Ciba-

Geigy said that it could not cause SMON as it was essentially insoluble and, therefore, not absorbed. This was incorrect. Finally removed from the market in 1985.

1971   Diethylstilboestrol given for threatened abortion produced vaginal carcinoma in the daughters of the recipients 10–20 years later (Herbst *et al.*, 1971).
Committee on Safety of Medicines (CSM) replaced the CSD to advise the licensing authority on the safety, efficacy and quality of the medicinal products on which advice was needed.

1973   The French pharmacovigilance system was implemented.

1974   Pertussis vaccine and encephalopathy (see p. ●).
The first use of the term 'epidemiological pharmacology' (pharmacoepidemiology) with a description of objectives and methods of work of the new discipline (Venulet, 1974, 1978, 1999).

1975   European Committee for Proprietary Medicinal Products (CPMP) set up.
Practolol caused the oculomucocutaneous syndrome (Wright, 1975; Nicholls, 1977; Tierny, 1977).

1976   First attempt at gene replacement therapy (Rogers, 1976; Nevin, 1998).

1978   WHO ADR monitoring moved to Uppsala, Sweden.
Halcion (triazolam) fiasco. Dr C. Van der Kroef gave details of four patients with severe psychiatric symptoms, including anxiety, derealization and paranoid ideas (Van der Kroef, 1979; Lasagna, 1980). Subsequent studies showed that it could cause anxiety (Oswald, 1989) and next-day memory impairment (Bixler, *et al.*, 1991).

1981   Recognition of AIDS – pneumocystic pneumonia.
Benoxaprofen Opren/Oraflex disaster (Abraham, 1995). It caused cholestatic jaundice, photosensitivity, Stevens–Johnson syndrome, erythema multiforme, renal failure and thrombocytopenia. Lilly pleaded guilty to criminal charges for not reporting ADR occurring overseas. Lilly were fined US$25 000 and Dr William I. Shedden, the former chief medical officer, fined US$15 000.
Deaths in premature neonates due to benzyl alcohol, used as a preservative for injectable drugs, not being metabolized by the immature liver (Roberts, 1996). Fatalities in neonates due to untested parenteral vitamin E preparation containing benzyl alcohol (Martone, *et al.*, 1986) and also benzyl alcohol in saline and water used for irrigating through intravenous (IV) catheters (Hiller *et al.*, 1986). Its toxicity had been reported earlier (Brown *et al.*, 1982; Gershanik *et al.*, 1982).

1983   HIV identified.

1988   European Rapid Alert system started (Wood, 1992).

1989   Fenoterol – beta agonists linked to deaths in asthmatics in case-control study (Pearce, *et al.*, 1995; McEwan, 1999).

1993   Fialuridine caused hepatic deaths in patients with chronic hepatitis B in pre-marketing trial (FDA Task Force, 1993; Anon, 1994; Horton, 1994; Manning and Swartz, 1995; McKenzie *et al.*, 1995; Nickas, 1997).
            Soruvidine, an anti-viral agent for shingles, interacted with 5-fluorouracil causing severe neutropenia, killing 15 patients (Ross, 1994; Hirokawa, 1996). Nippon Shoji charged with failing to report two deaths out of three in Phase III studies.
            Professor Duilio Poggiolini, Chairman of the CPMP, accepted bribes from more than 12 Italian companies and was jailed for 12 years; his wife was jailed for 6 years.
            UK Medicines Information Bill sabotaged by Pharma Group (Glaxo, ICI, Fisons, Smith Kline Beecham, Boots, Wellcome) despite the bill's backing from the BMA and Patients' Association.
            The European Society of Pharmacovigilance was founded.

1995   Establishment of the European Medicines Evaluation Agency (EMEA).
            Third-generation oral contraceptives and venous thromboembolism controversy (McPherson, 1996; McEwan, 1999).

1997   The Erice Declaration on communicating drug safety information (www.who-umc.org/publ.html). Unfortunately, those who had the power to effect the proposals were not there 1998–2002.
            Mumps, measles and rubella (MMR) vaccine: autism controversy.

2000   Formation of the International Society of Pharmacovigilance.

2002   The concern about MMR does not die away, but yet another paper denies any association with autism (Mäkelä *et al.*, 2002).

Under-reporting of adverse drug reactions

One might expect that reporting of adverse events (AEs) during clinical trials would be complete; but some investigators are prone to fail to document and report AEs, and there have been cases where the investigator chose not to report AEs because it was too much effort or they were deliberately attempting to defraud. In addition, some investigators are confused as to what constitutes an AE (Mackintosh and Zepp, 1996). 'Both Japanese and US published reports of drug clinical trials are inadequate for assessing drug safety' (Hayashi and Walker, 1996); see Chapter 4.

It has been suggested that once a drug is marketed only about 10 per cent of its ADRs are reported (Inman, 1972). This estimate was based on the pertussis vaccine ADRs and the thromboses with the oral contraceptive. There is evidence that the deaths attributable to excessive use of bronchodilating aerosols were under-reported (Inman and Adelstein, 1969), as were the thromboembolic deaths due to the oral contraceptive (Beral, 1977; Crooks,

1977) and the practolol eye problems (Tierny, 1977). Poor reporting is not confined to the UK. The USA (Hemminki, 1980), France (Bader, 1981), Spain (Alvarez-Requejo *et al.*, 1994), Italy (Conforti *et al.*, 1995), Denmark (Hallas *et al.*, 1992) and Germany (Schonhofer, 1981) have reported similar experiences. Reporting of ADRs is compulsory in Sweden and France.

Studies on under-reporting

It is only rarely that the number of cases of a reaction that really occurred, as opposed to reported, can be known; but with certain diseases it is possible:

- In aplastic anaemia with phenylbutazone/oxyphenbutazone only five out of 44 (11 per cent) deaths were reported (Inman, 1986). Of the 32 fatal blood dyscrasias with phenylbutazone only four (12.5 per cent) were reported (Inman, 1977).

- Practolol. Only one case of conjunctivitis was reported in clinical trials, but it was soon followed by nearly 200 cases within 5 weeks of the first publication of a series of cases.

In Uppsala, Sweden. All known cases of cytopenias were collected from hospital discharge notes. Only 33 per cent of thrombocytopenias, 34 per cent of aplastic anaemias, and 25 per cent of agranulocytoses in the years 1966–70 were reported. Several assumptions had to be made in order to derive these figures (Bottiger and Westerholm, 1973). Of the 84 hospitalized cases of drug-associated neutropenias only 29 (35 per cent) had been reported (Arneborn and Palmbled, 1982).

- Oral contraceptives and fatal thromboembolism. Only 15 per cent were reported. (Beral *et al.*, 1977; Crooks, 1977).

- A Rhode Island (USA) survey, cited in a recent report, suggests that the average physician sees one serious ADR and seven moderate ADRs per year. The FDA only receive 12 reports of any type for every 100 US physicians involved in patient care (Baum *et al.*, 1988).

- Sweden. Eighty per cent of all children who developed osteitis after BCG vaccination were reported. This was derived from the number of positive *Mycobacterium bovis* BCG cultures in bacteriology laboratories (Bottiger *et al.*, 1982).

- The use of protamine in patients undergoing cardiopulmonary bypass was monitored in a US hospital during 1990–91:

  the incidence of serious ADR was 6.6 per cent (confidence interval (CI 5.1 to 8.4 per cent)

  the chart records showed was 1.7 per cent (CI 1.0 to 2.8 per cent)

  the incidence of ADRs reported to the hospital ADR program was 0.3 per cent (CI 0.07 to 0.9 per cent) (Kimmel *et al.*, 1995).

- Monitoring an Italian 72-bed ward for a year disclosed 89 AEs (7.4 per cent of patients), none of which had been reported to the official national drug surveillance system in the previous year. Of 120 randomly chosen patients, 22 had AEs that were considered as constituting expected AEs but only nine were actually reported (Maistrello *et al.*, 1995).

- In the UK, 14 cases of fibrosing colonopathy with high-strength pancreatic enzyme preparation were all reported on 'yellow cards' (Smyth *et al.*, 1995).

- Three studies in France gave figures for serious reactions actually reported as 5.26 per cent, 4.16 per cent and 4.75 per cent (Bégaud *et al.*, 2002).

- All patients commenced on a black triangle drug in a Division of Psychiatry at Manchester Royal Infirmary over the previous month were investigated. Of the 22 patients, 16 (60 per cent) suffered an ADR, two of which were serious. No yellow cards were completed (Brown and Faloon, 2001).

- In the USA 27 cases of haemorrhagic stroke associated with phenylpropanolamine were found in a 5 year project, but none had been reported to the FDA (La Grenade *et al.*, 2001).

Under-reporting in general practice

There may be under-reporting by the patient to their doctor.

- A study in the Netherlands compared the responses from a questionnaire that had been sent to all dispensing GPs and to all their patients who had been prescribed sumatriptan. (Ottervanger *et al.*, 1995):

	Doctors	Patients
Dizziness	30 (1.7%)	96 (8.1%)
Nausea/vomiting	26 (1.5%)	
Drowsiness/sedation	25 (1.4%)	
Chest pain	23 (1.3%)	94 (7.9%)
Paraesthesia		139 (11.7%)
Feeling of heaviness		95 (8.0%)

The doctor response was 86 per cent and the patient response was 70 per cent.

- Patients in general practice were asked 'Have any medicines or tablets ever disagreed with you or caused an allergy?' and 'Are you able to take aspirin or penicillin?' These questions identified 97 reactions. Of these, 76 per cent were likely to be related to the drug. The doctors only recorded half of them and did not preferentially record well-established reactions (Cook and Ferner, 1993).

- In order to discover the degree of under-reporting in UK general practice, a survey was undertaken in 1986 of 24 training practices. Only 6 per cent of AEs were reported (Lumley *et al.*, 1986). It is not possible to extrapolate from training practices to all practices, and even this figure is doubtful since the GPs knew that they were being monitored and were asking the patients leading questions. It also depended on the GP's diagnosis of a suspected ADR.

- A random sample of 100 French GPs was surveyed to obtain data on AEs observed. Overall, 81 GPs agreed to enter data during three consecutive days and these were compared with the spontaneous reports received from GPs at the Bordeaux pharmacovigilance centre during the reference period. The average number of AEs observed per day was 1.99. The under-reporting coefficient was 24 433 (95 per cent CI 20 702–28 837). This was equivalent to only one out of every 24 433 ADRs being reported to the centre (Moride *et al.*, 1997).

- A survey of hospital records in five English districts showed that five times more cases of idiopathic thrombocytopenic purpura occurred following the MMR vaccination than were reported to the UK CSM (Farrington *et al.*, 1995).

- When the reporting on 10 new drugs subject to Prescription Event Monitoring (PEM) was compared with reporting to the CSM only 9 per cent had been reported to the CSM and it was highest (31.1 per cent) for serious/unlabelled reactions and lowest (6.5 per cent) for non-serious/labelled reactions (Martin *et al.*, 1998).

- In the Netherlands, a survey showed the following reasons for not reporting:

  72 per cent were uncertain whether the reaction was caused by the drug

  75 per cent thought the ADR too trivial

  93 per cent thought the ADR too well known

  18 per cent were not aware that they should report it

  22 per cent did not know how to report it

  38 per cent did not have enough time

  36 per cent thought reporting was too bureaucratic

  26 per cent knew which ADR to report (Eland *et al.*, 1999).

- Of 188 hepatic ADRs reported in northeastern England almost half were almost certainly unrelated (Guruprasad *et al.*, 1999).

- In the UK, 9 per cent (CI 8.0–9.8 per cent) of the reports received by PEM were reported to the CSM, but for serious reactions the figure was 53 per cent (CI 39–67 per cent) (Heeley *et al.*, 2001). However, this figure is biased by the fact that only 59.4 per cent of doctors who prescribed the drug sent reports to PEM and that the doctors were reporting adverse events to PEM but ADRs to the CSM.

Factors affecting reporting

The following factors have been suggested as affecting direct reporting:

- Severity of the reaction. Too trivial (Hasford *et al.*, 2002).

- The length of time that the drug has been on the market (Tubert-Bitter *et al.*, 1998).

- Attribution by the patient. One in four outpatients did not discuss their symptoms with their providers (Klein *et al.*, 1984). A patient survey showed that 42.9 per cent would not consult their GP for a serious ADR associated either with a conventional drug or a herbal preparation (Barnes *et al.*, 1998). Those with poorer self-assessed health status reported ADR experience at a higher rate than others. Choice of contact regarding ADR: physician, 93 per cent; pharmacist, 45 per cent; nurse, 21 per cent; emergency room, 5 per cent; friends, 3.8 per cent; family members, 3.8 per cent and nobody, 2 per cent (DeWitt and Sorofman, 1999). Patients of 65 years and older who reported ADRs, with the name of the medication, had their report confirmed by documentation in 94 per cent of cases (Chrischilles *et al.*, 1992).

- Whether the reaction has previously been seen by the doctor.

- Legal implications.

- Unusual nature of the event (Milstein *et al.*, 1986). However, 90 per cent of reports to the FDA come from the pharmaceutical companies, and there is considerable variation between them (Baum *et al.*, 1987).

- The religion of the area. Countries with a predominant Catholic population report less than those with a predominant Protestant population (Dukes and Lunde, 1979). This may be related to the greater literacy of the Protestants due to increased study of the Bible.

- The regulations of the country (Griffin and Weber, 1986).

- The year of the reporting (Sachs and Bortnichak, 1986). Dr J. C. P. Weber plotted the mean number of ADR reports for seven non-steroidal anti-inflammatory drugs (NSAIDs) over the first 5 years of marketing and showed that they peaked at 2 years and then declined rapidly. This has been called the Weber curve (Weber, 1984). It cannot be presumed that it will apply in all circumstances; but it did apply to anti-infective, endocrine, pulmonary and cardiovascular drugs (Brodovicz *et al.*, 2001). When 10 drugs on the French market, which gave rise to approximately 100 sponta-neous reports each during the first 4 years of marketing, were examined the reports peaked at 1 year and then decreased (Haramburu *et al.*, 1997).

- The physician's age, specialty and years qualified (Spiers *et al.*, 1984; McGettigan *et al.*, 1996).

- Whether in hospital practice (more ADRs, cancer and haematology) or not (newer drugs, metabolism and nutrition) (Vega *et al.*, 1996). From four hospitals in Lombardy, Italy, 40.5 per cent female doctors had reported an ADR compared with 29.4 per cent for males. Those graduating after 1985 reported half the amount of those graduating before then (Cosentino *et al.*, 1999).

- Nationality (Sachs and Bortnichak, 1986; Belton and European Pharmacovigilance Research Group, 1997). For one Pfizer product the relative reporting rate (patients per 10^6 patient-months) was one in Germany, 9.8 in Sweden, six in the UK, and three in the USA (Gordon, 1985). In clinical trials, Australia, Canada, Sweden and the UK had reporting rates of more than 50 per cent, whereas Denmark, Finland, France, Hong Kong, the Netherlands and Norway had between 35 and 45 per cent. Belgium, Germany and Italy were below 30 per cent (Joelson *et al.*, 1997). France seems to be refuting the religious trend. In Germany, 75–85 per cent of physicians never reported to the health authorities (Hasford *et al.*, 2002).

- Media publicity (Rawlins, 1988a, b). Following publicity of the neuropsychiatric effects of mefloquine (Lariam) the reporting increased six- to seven-fold (Bhasin *et al.*, 1997).

- The seriousness of the ADR (Griffin and Weber, 1986; McGettigan *et al.*, 1996).

- The ADR mechanism (Milstein *et al.*, 1986).

- The cumulative total of prescriptions (Rawlins, 1988a, b).

- Doctor's lack of familiarity with the regulations (Scott *et al.*, 1990) in Ireland (McGettigan and Feely, 1995), Belgium (Kurz *et al.*, 1996), Netherlands (Eland *et al.*, 1998) and the UK (NAO, 2003).

- Local health district, in the UK (Bateman *et al.*, 1991).

- Notoriety of the ADR in France (Tubert-Bitter *et al.*, 1998);
  ADR well known (Hasford *et al.*, 2002).

- Availability of report form in Ireland (McGettigan and Feely, 1995; McGettigan *et al.*, 1996), Belgium (Kurz *et al.*, 1996) and the UK (NAO, 2003).

- Misconception that confidence in diagnosis was important in Belgium (Kurz *et al.*, 1996).

- Lack of time in Belgium (Kurz *et al.*, 1996), the Netherlands (Eland *et al.*, 1998) and Ireland (McGettigan *et al.*, 1996); PEM (Key *et al.*, 2002).

- Uncertainty about the causal relationship between a suspected drug and an ADR in Germany (Göttler *et al.*, 1998) and the Netherlands (Eland *et al.*, 1998).

In 1986, the relatively large number of reports for Piroxicam produced a defensive report from Pfizer in which they gave evidence that there were reporting biases present for drugs that are:

- in the first few years of marketing

- launched after 1980 in the USA or 1976 in the UK

- vigorously marketed by the sales force

- subject to publicity

- distributed by one manufacturer worldwide

- used on a long-term basis

- used in a population with a high background risk

- used in conjunction with other therapy (Sachs and Bortnichak, 1986).

Calculation of the degree of under-reporting

Under-reporting was quantified by the under-reporting coefficient U, calculated as the ration between the number of effects actually observed by physicians and those spontaneously reported to the pharmacovigilance system, according to the following formula:

$$U = \frac{m}{k \times n/N}$$

where m is the number of AEs observed in the survey, n/N is the sampling fraction (n is the number of GP days in the sample, N is the total GP days in the catchment area), and k is the number of AEs spontaneously reported to the pharmacovigilance centre during the reference period.

Recommended reading: 'Analyse d'incidence en Pharmacovigilance-application á la notification spontanée' Second edition. Published by ARME-Pharmacovigilance in 1992. The 'comité de redaction' is headed by Professor B. Bégaud, Hôpital Pellegrin, 33076 Bordeaux, Cédex, France.

In Bordeaux the number of cases of cough with ACE inhibitors was estimated at 3925 for the region based on a pilot study of 60 practitioners, but only three cases were reported to the pharmacovigilance centre. The under-reporting coefficient U was 1305 (Bégaud *et al.*, 1994), but when the Bordeaux team looked at a sample of ADRs seen by 81 GPs during three non-consecutive days the under-reporting coefficient was 24 433, i.e. only one case out of every 24 433 ADRs was reported to the local pharmacovigilance centre. The figure for serious and unlabelled effects was 4610 and for recently marketed drugs it was 12 802 (Moride *et al.*, 1994, 1997), whereas the *U* figure for Spain was 1144 (95% CI: 941–1347) (Alvarez-Requejo *et al.*, 1994).

Conclusion

It is clear that no general figure can be given for under-reporting and that the best estimate can be obtained by a study in a sample of the relevant population.

Incidence of adverse drug reactions

There are many factors that will affect any incidence figure:

- National prescribing habits.

- Definition used for ADR and the causality method.

- Method used to detect AEs.

- Locality, type of institution, specialty.

- The under-reporting of the numerator (see above) and the extrapolation of the denominator from: amount of drug produced, sales figures, defined daily dose, prescribed daily dosage, market research audits (St George, 1996). However, all these are open to many biases which may be exploited.

The latter calculation has been described as 'more of an art than a science' (CIOMS V 2001). The problem is well described by Bégaud *et al*. (1993: 51–70) and (CIOMS V: 163–185).

National prescribing habits

In France, 90 per cent of consultations will be followed by a prescription for 4.2 products (average), compared with the European average of 0.8 (Dawalibi, 2002). The total sales in France and in Germany are approximately twice as high as those in the UK or USA and are nearly three times as high as in New Zealand (Figure 1.1). Presumably, these last three countries do not suffer from under-medication; presumably, the increased levels in France

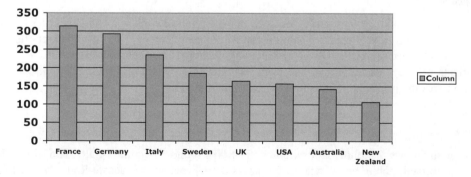

Figure 1.1 Total sales of pharmaceutical products per inhabitant, in US dollars (After Dawalibi, 2002). Reproduced by permission of Le Figaro Economie

and Germany are due to non-essential drugs. Non-essential drugs are less likely to cause type-A ADRs, since they are likely to be less efficacious. This implies that the increase in ADRs due to the increased prescribing will not be in proportion to the sales figures.

UK

- A survey of a Yorkshire general practice showed that 1 in 40 (2.6 per cent) consultations were 'iatrogenic consultations'; these included surgical adverse events. The figure for ADR consultations was 1.5 per cent. Some ADRs required more than one consultation, so this is not an ADR rate (Mulroy, 1973).

- Another survey, this time in Derbyshire (UK), showed that 25 per cent of the practice population may have had an ADR of some kind and that 41 per cent of the patients receiving drugs had a certain or probable ADR, 90 per cent occurring by the fourth day. Patients completed a questionnaire (Martys, 1979).

- A survey of a single practice in Scotland over 6 months showed a consultation rate of 1.7 per cent for ADRs (probables, 72 per cent; possibles, 28 per cent), 272 in 16 253 consultations for a practice size of 11 201 patients, i.e. 1 in 60 consultations (Millar, 2001).

- A study of 36 470 consultations showed that 1.7 per cent (1 in 59) of consultations were for suspected ADRs: 0.6 per cent in the 0–20 year olds, 1.3 per cent for 21–50 year olds and 2.7 per cent for the over 50s. The responses were to the question 'Is the medicine suiting you?' (Lumley *et al.*, 1986).

Netherlands

Extrapolating from a Dutch study, in general practice approximately 2.6 per cent (1 in 38) of the population were seen with an ADR, with only 4.8 per cent being serious. Almost all the ADRs were known (Hoek *et al.*, 1995).

Sweden

Between 1994 and 1999, a survey of 2018 patients, between the ages of 20 and 85 years, from 16 of Sweden's 24 counties showed that 32 per cent ($n = 651$; 1 in 3.1) had reported a total of 882 specific ADRs. Of the patients with ADRs, 15 per cent were hospitalized. The patients had been asked if they had ever experienced an ADR regardless of confirmation from a treating physician (Sundström *et al.*, 1998, 2000a, b).

France

- A study over 2 months in a sample of 254 GPs found 13 *serious* ADRs, two of which were fatal, giving an average of 2.6 cases per GP per year (Lacoste-Roussillon *et al.*, 2001). The figure given by a group of French GPs was two ADRs per day, per doctor (Moride *et al.*, 1997).

- A 3 month study by three urban physicians found 20 ADRs from 2094 patients seen. Prevalence rate was 1 per cent of visits (2.2 ADRs per GP per month) (Montastruc *et al.*, 1995).

- Over 1 year there were 37 suspected side effects from 3341 consultations in a single practice: 1.07 per 100 consultations (Grange, 1990).

Italy

Active monitoring by volunteer family paediatricians (29) over 1 year found 388 ADRs (1.6 per cent, or 1 in 61) out of a list total of 24 000 children (Menniti-Ippolito *et al.*, 2000).

Germany

A survey of all the paediatric practices in Brandenberg over 3 months found a 1.2 per cent (or 1 in 83) incidence of mild to moderate ADRs (Lewis *et al.*, 1998).

USA

In Olmsted County, 0.4 per cent of the elderly were hospitalized for ADRs over a 5 year period (Silverstein *et al.*, 1994).

Conclusion

There are many different factors which may be responsible for the variation in these figures; but somewhere between 1 in 30 to 60 of consultations and 1 in 30 to 40 patients seems the core range, with the Martys (1979) study being the odd one out. The ADR incidence in children is between 1 in 60 and 1 in 83.

Adverse drug reactions responsible for hospital admission

ADRs requiring hospital admission are, by definition, serious and more expensive, since the entire hospital costs are attributable to the ADR. The problems with all these surveys are the variations in admission policy from one hospital to another and different criteria for drug-relatedness (Atkin and Shenfield, 1995). ADRs have been reported to cause 3 to 6 per cent of all hospital medical admissions (Davies, 1985).

USA

- ADRs result in 300 000 admissions per annum in the USA (Atkin and Shenfield, 1995).

- A study in two US tertiary care hospitals over 6 months in 1993 gave a figure for adverse drug events of 6.5 per cent, of which 28 per cent were judged to be preventable (Leape *et al.*, 1991, 1995; Bates *et al.*, 1997). A repeat study in 1994–95 in one of these hospitals using a computer-based monitor gave a figure of 2.3 per cent (1.4 per cent after adjusting for sampling) (Jha *et al.*, 2001).

- In a Salt Lake City hospital with 520 beds (1989–90), 0.153 per cent of the admissions were due to ADRs. This study targeted ADRs requiring change in therapy and/or prolonged patient hospitalization, not to screen for mild and self-limited ADRs (Classen *et al.*, 1991).

- The latest figure (based on 25 original studies between 1972 and 1996, with 90 per cent from the USA) is that 5.8 per cent (4.2–6.0 per cent) of all admissions to medical wards were due to ADRs, including relative overdosing. The length of hospital stay ranged from 5.8 to 13 days, with a median of 8.7 days (Muehlberger *et al.*, 1997).

- The figure for admission of children is 2 per cent from a survey of five hospitals in the USA (Mitchell *et al.*, 1988).

- Approximately 1.5 per cent of all hospitalizations in the elderly (65 and over) from Olmsted County were due to ADRs (Silverstein *et al.*, 1994).

Canada

- A survey of patients aged 50 or over in a Winnipeg hospital showed that 12 per cent of admissions were for drug-related events (Grymonpre *et al.*, 1988).

- ADRs in Ontario increased from 104 per 10 000 hospital admissions or day surgeries in 1992 to 162 per 10 000 in 1997 (Hunter and Bains, 1999).

UK

- In seven wards of the John Radcliffe Hospital, Oxford, over the period 1990–93, 6.87 per cent of admissions were for suspected ADRs (Smith *et al.*, 1996).

- Over a 1 year period in 1965–66 in two Belfast hospitals the ADR rate was 10.2 per cent (Hurwitz and Wade, 1969).

- Over a 6 month period at City Hospital, Nottingham, preliminary analysis suggests that 10 per cent of admissions will be judged as being drug related (Avery *et al.*, 2001).

- Over a nine week period in 1999, 10.1 per cent of the admission at Addenbrooke's hospital were identified as drug-related; 18 per cent were therapy failures; 30 per cent were related to overdose or abuse and 6.3 per cent were ADRs (Bhalla *et al.*, 2003).

Netherlands

- One in six (16.6 per cent) of elderly (70 and over) patients had an ADR on admission and 24 per cent of these were severe (potentially life-threatening or led to admission). A comparison of patients, with a severe ADR with those without, showed that the significant factors were: a fall before admission; the presence of gastrointestinal (GI) bleeding or haematuria; the use of three or more drugs (Mannesse *et al.*, 1997).

Germany

- St Elisabeth Hospital, Cologne–Hohenlind, in the Medical and Intensive Care Unit: 2.4 per cent (Shoenemann *et al.*, 1998).

- The eight hospitals in three German towns (Dresden, Jena and Rostock) undertook intensified pharmacovigilance from October 1997 to December 1998. There were 435 cases for drug-related admissions; an incidence of between 1.5 per 10 000 and 24 per 10 000 for each three months for treated patients in their catchment areas (Schneeweiss *et al.*, 2001a, b). A further study in the latter two towns from October 1997 to March 2000 gave 9.4 (CI 9.0–9.9) admissions per 10 000 (Schneeweiss *et al.*, 2002).

- A neurological department reported that 2.7 per cent of admissions were caused by ADRs (Thuermann *et al.*, 2002).

France

- A study over 7 weeks in 1998 in 33 hospitals showed that 3.19 per cent (CI 2.37–4.01 per cent) of patients were admitted for ADRs (Pouyanne *et al.*, 2000).

- Excluding attempted suicides, 3 per cent of admissions were drug related and 6.6 per cent of inpatients had significant ADRs, i.e. necessitated changes in drug treatment or prolonged hospitalization (Moore *et al.*, 1995a).

- At another French hospital the figures were 6 per cent of admissions (Moore *et al.*, 1995b).

- At Lille cardiological hospital the ADR rate was 0.5 per cent of admissions (Bordet *et al.*, 2001).

- At a cancer institute, 5 per cent of admissions were due to ADRs (Lapeyre-Mestre *et al.*, 1997).

- At Tours, over a period of a week, 1.53 per cent of paediatric admissions were for ADRs (Jonville-Béra *et al.*, 2002).

- At Toulouse University Hospital, over four separate weeks, the incidence rate was 6.1 per cent (Olivier *et al.*, 2001).

- At Rouen University hospital, 16 per cent of patients over 70 years had probable ADRs on admission (Doucet *et al.*, 2002), though this was not necessarily the cause of admission.

India

Admissions via a medical emergency department caused by ADRs were 6.7 per cent of the total 578 elderly patients admitted (Malhota *et al.*, 2001).

Spain

- Of the admissions via an emergency ward at La Paz Hospital over 5 months, 4.8 per cent were due to ADRs or acute drug intoxication, with ADRs alone being 3.9 per cent (Garijo *et al.*, 1991).

- The figure for a cardiology department was 1.1 per cent (Vargas *et al.*, 1996).

Israel

Over a 2 month period, a 34-bed medical ward, using automatic computerized laboratory signals, found that a quarter to one-third of admissions had ADRs (Levy *et al.*, 1998).

Switzerland

- A 6 month survey of admissions to an emergency department showed that 7 per cent were mainly caused by ADRs (Wasserfallen *et al.*, 2001).

- At the university hospital in Zurich, 3 per cent of admissions were due to an ADR (Fattinger *et al.*, 1998).

Australia

- The ADR figure was between 2.4 per cent and 3.6 per cent (Roughead *et al.*, 1998).

- Of admissions through the emergency department to Royal Melbourne Hospital over a month in 1994, 5.7 per cent were drug related (16 per cent were definite, 46 per cent were probable, 38 per cent were possible). The drug-related reactions were classified as being 26% prescribing factors, 27 per cent, patient non-compliance and 47 per cent ADRs. This gives an ADR rate of 2.35 per cent (Dartnell *et al.*, 1996).

Hong Kong

Drug-related problems were responsible for 9.5 per cent of admissions; 6.2 per cent were ADRs (Chan and Critchley, 1994).

Sweden

- Five per cent of a 2000 control-pool population were hospitalized for ADRs (Sundström *et al.*, 2000b).

- In the university hospital of Umeå, 12 per cent of admissions were suspected ADRs and for certain and probable ADRs the figure was 3 per cent of admissions (Mjörndal *et al.*, 2002).

Denmark

In Odense University, the ADR admission rate was 8.4 per cent (Hallas *et al.*, 1992).

Worldwide

- A review of 36 articles covering 49 hospitals (30 from North America, 10 from Europe and nine from the remainder of the world), between 1964 and 1989, gave a prevalence for ADRs ranging from 0.2 to 21.7 per cent, median 4.9 per cent, mean 5.5 per cent. However, these covered all specialties, and those with rates over 10 per cent were: UK geriatric 10.5 per cent, Canadian 19.4 per cent; psychiatric, 12.2 per cent; paediatric cancer, 21.7 per cent; cardiology, 11.5 per cent. For 'general/medical', or 'medical', then the overall figure is 4 per cent – 1051 cases out of 26 075 admissions (Einarson, 1993).

- A review of 17 studies from seven different countries, mainly USA, UK and Spain, showed that the overall rate for children was 2.09 per cent (CI 1.02–3.77 per cent) (Impicciatore *et al.*, 2001).

- A further review of 13 publications from Hong Kong (one), Denmark (six), Spain (one), UK (one), USA (two), Taiwan (one) from the period 1990–93 covering geriatrics, pneumonology, cardiology, gastroenterology, and internal medicine gave a figure of 5.5 per cent (2–17 per cent) (Moore *et al.*, 1998).

- In six Western countries there were 25 studies with an average admission rate to medical wards of 5.8 per cent (Schneeweiss *et al.*, 1997).

- A multicentre study of geriatric hospitals found that 15.5 per cent of admissions were due to ADRs (Williamson and Chopin, 1980).

- A survey of 25 studies (90 per cent USA) between 1972 and 1996 gave a figure for admissions to medical departments of 4.2 per cent to 6.0 per cent (lower and upper quartiles repectively) with a median of 5.8 per cent (Muehlberger *et al.*, 1997).

- A survey of studies since 1975 in geriatric patients found 27 studies with 15 087 patients and 8.1 per cent of elderly patients that had been admitted with ADRs (Göttler, 2000).

Conclusion

There are too many factors involved to give an accurate overall figure; but it varies between 4.2 and 6 per cent with a median of 5.8 per cent (Muehlberges *et al.*, 1997).

Adverse drug reactions during hospitalization

USA

- Of 1024 patients in the medical wards of a 350-bed hospital 23 per cent had ADRs and 29.6 per cent of elderly patients had ADRs. The independent factors in the elderly were female gender, decline in renal function and polymedicine. The paper by Bowman *et al.*, (1996) also has a table giving results from 24 surveys from 1964 until 1991.

- A survey of 1000 patients in the USA showed that 15 per cent indicated that they had had a side effect on medication (Brown *et al.*, 1983). Almost 4 per cent of patients hospitalized in Massachusetts (Boston) in 1984 suffered an AE due to medical treatment (Brennan *et al.*, 1991) and 19.4 per cent of these were due to drugs (Leape *et al.*, 1991).

- A survey of two large US hospitals (Boston) showed that there were 6.5 adverse drug events per 100 admissions during their hospital stay (Bates *et al.*, 1995).

- In a Salt Lake City hospital (LDS; 1989–90), 36 653 patients were monitored for AEs. There were 731 AEs in 648 patients (1.67 per cent). Of the AEs, 96 per cent were moderate or severe and 91 per cent were type-A reactions. Over 76 per cent of verified ADRs did not have the causal agent stopped until the study personnel informed the physician of the ongoing ADR. This study quotes that 30 per cent of hospitalized patients will have an ADR and that 0.31 per cent of all admissions will have a fatal ADR (Classen *et al.*, 1991). In the same hospital during the following period, 1990–93, the ADR rate had increased to 2.43 per 100 admissions with an increased stay of 1.91 days. There was an almost twofold increase in deaths (Classen *et al.*, 1997).

- A review of 39 studies of ADRs in hospitals in the USA has shown an incidence of 10.9 per cent (CI 7.9–13.9 per cent) in hospitalized patients with a total of 3607 patients suffering ADRs and of these 63 (0.19 per cent) died. The figure for both those on admission plus those during admission was 62 480 patients (15.1 per cent; CI 12.0–18.1 per cent), with 46 625 deaths (0.32 per cent; CI 0.23–0.41 per cent). When extrapolated to the whole of the USA the figure was 106 000 deaths. This represented 4.6 per cent of all deaths and was ranked the fourth to sixth most common cause of death (Lazarou *et al.*, 1998). A critique of this meta-analysis said 'Meta-analysis was invalid because of heterogeneity of the studies. Most of these studies did not report the data needed for incidence calculations. The methodology used was seriously flawed, and no conclusions regarding ADR incidence rates in the hospitalized population in the United States should be made on the basis of the original meta-analysis' (Kvasz *et al.*, 2000).

- A survey of geriatric nursing facilities found that two-thirds had an average of two probable ADRs over a 4 year period (Cooper, 1996).

- The risk of hospitalization secondary to adverse medication outcomes in elderly patients is estimated at 17 per cent, which is almost six times greater than that for the general population (Nanda *et al.*, 1990).

- The rate of preventable adverse drug events (ADEs), i.e. an injury resulting from medical intervention related to a drug, and potential (incidents with potential for injury related to the use of the drug). ADEs in intensive-care units (ICUs) was 19 events per 1000 patient days, nearly twice the rate of non-ICUs (Cullen *et al.*, 1997).

UK

- A survey of 437 patients in a Birmingham hospital found 97 AEs (22 per cent) and most were due to a drug (76 per cent) i.e. 16.9 per cent of the total admissions; but the doctors had only recorded half of these reactions in the patients' notes (Cook and Ferner, 1993).

- In an analysis of inpatient ADRs 23 per cent of patients had an ADR and 37.5 per cent of these were elderly – 30 per cent of the elderly admissions had an ADR (Bowman *et al.*, 1996). This paper also gave the results from 23 similar studies carried out between 1964 and 1991, which showed the average ADR rate was 15.6 per cent and the range 1.5 to 35 per cent.

- In an ICU for children the incidence was 7 per cent (Gill *et al.*, 1995).

France

- In an internal medicine unit over a 4 month period, 4.7 per cent of all admissions, during hospitalization, had an ADR (Lagnaoui *et al.*, 2000).

- In Lille Cardiological hospital the ADR rate was 1.7 per cent (Bordet *et al.*, 2001). Another cardiological centre at Angers had an incidence of 2.3 per cent (Jamaa *et al.*, 1993).

- At the Remiremont Hospital cardiology and internal medicine departments the incidence of ADRs was 4.7 per cent over 4 months (Curien-Chevrier *et al.*, 1997).

- In a cancer institute, ADRs accounted for 3.5 per cent of the hospital stays in 1993 (Lapeyre-Mestre *et al.*, 1997).

- At Tours, 2.64 per cent of paediatric patients had an ADR (Jonville-Béra *et al.*, 2002).

- At another French hospital the ADR rate was 8.4 per cent of inpatients (Moore *et al.*, 1995b).

- A multicentre survey of geriatrics found that 63.6 per cent had side effects over a year (Ferry and Piette, 1993).

- On a single day, in a sample of French hospitals the prevalence rate was 10.3 (CI 8.7–11.9), of which 33 per cent were serious and gave an estimate of 1 300 000 patients per year in hospital (Imbs *et al.*, 1999).

Germany

- In a medical ward of a university hospital over a period of 6 months, using a computer-based monitoring system, 12 per cent had ADRs, with an average increase in stay of 3.5 days (Dormann *et al.*, 2000).

- In a neurological department, 18.7 per cent of patients had at least one ADR (Thuermann *et al.*, 2002).

Norway

Ulleval hospital had 25 per cent of children with one or more ADRs (Buajordet *et al.*, 1998).

Netherlands

Over a 2 month period, a prospective study in the paediatric and internal medicine wards of two hospitals found that 29 per cent of patients had an ADR (Van den Bremt *et al.*, 1998).

Spain

- Over an 8 year period, 12.9 per cent of patients in a cardiology ward had an ADR (Vargas *et al.*, 1996).

- Over a 2 year period, the incidence in hospitalized children was 16.6 per cent (Martinez-Mir *et al.*, 1996, 1999).

Switzerland

A clinically relevant ADR occurred in 9 per cent of inpatients of the university hospital in Zurich (Fattinger *et al.*, 1998).

India

Intensive surveillance over 6 months found an incidence of 1.73 per cent (Dharnidharka *et al.*, 1993).

Chile

- Intensive and prospective surveillance revealed an incidence of 13.7 per cent (Gonza-lez-Martin *et al.*, 1998).

Seven-country survey in children

A review of 17 studies showed an overall incidence of 9.53 per cent (CI 8.43–16.17 per cent) (Impicciatore *et al.*, 2001).

Conclusion

There is a large range, from 1.7 to 29 per cent, due to the many variables. In the elderly it varies from 17 to 30 per cent with a figure of 60 per cent over a 4 year period. For children it varies from 1.73 to 25 per cent. Many of the factors influencing admission rates also affect inpatient rates. Whereas all ADRs causing admission are 'serious' by definition, those involving inpatients may be quite trivial and will depend on the illness for which they were admitted. The paper by Lazarou *et al.* (1998) covers the largest number of patients and, therefore, gives the most reliable figure, but it only applies to the USA; the quotable figure is 11 per cent, which is approximately double the admission's figure.

Adverse drug reactions reported at outpatient visits

- Drug-related visits to an Italian multidisciplinary hospital emergency department in Milan over a 3 month period were 4.7 per cent for drug-related illnesses (Raschetti *et al.*, 1997).

- Drug-related visits to three emergency departments in Italy over 10 days caused 5.52 per cent of visits (36 ADRs from 2800 visits); hospital admissions represented 2 per cent of visits (Calogero *et al.*, 2001).

- A review of 17 paediatric studies showed that the overall incidence rate was 1.46 per cent (CI 0.7–3.03 per cent) (Impicciatore *et al.*, 2001).

- In an internal medicine group practice, 5 per cent of ambulatory outpatients had a probable or definite ADR (Hutchinson, 1986).

- Of 299 outpatients, 30 per cent identified at least one medication causing an ADR (Klein *et al.*, 1984).

- At a French paediatric hospital emergency department, 0.93 per cent of attendances were for an ADR (Jonville-Béra *et al.*, 2002).

- A Spanish paediatric emergency room detected 0.96 per cent of ADR cases; this compares with 1.03 per cent reported for adults (Munoz *et al.*, 1998).

- A US tertiary care emergency department identified 1.7 per cent of visits as due to ADRs (Hafner, 2002).

Conclusion

About 5 per cent of general outpatients have an ADR, but for paediatrics the figure is lower at about 1 per cent; but no large study has been identified. The figure of Klein *et al.* (1984) was probably due to it representing the patient's opinion.

Deaths due to adverse drug reactions

It is difficult to determine the incidence of deaths due to ADRs, but it has been estimated as being less than 0.01 per cent of people taking drugs (Jick, 1974). The figure given for the USA for 1995 was 206 deaths according to death certificates, but 6894 according to MedWatch (Chyka, 2000). These figures should be compared with the specific studies below. In the Boston Collaborative Drug Surveillance Programme (BCDSP), 0.9 patients per 1000 were considered to have died as a result of drugs. The rates varied from zero in Israel and Italy to 1.4 per 1000 in New Zealand (Porter and Jick, 1977).

USA

- There were 160 000 deaths each year in US hospitals (Shapiro *et al.*, 1971).

- A figure of 199 000 deaths per year in the USA due to medication-related problems has been calculated (Johnson and Bootman, 1995).

- Inpatient hospital deaths have been estimated as 140 000 per year in the USA, which would make it the third leading cause of death (Kelly, 2001).

- A survey of 39 hospitals showed that 0.32 per cent (CI 0.23–0.41 per cent) of hospitalized patients had a fatal ADR. Estimated deaths of hospital patients, in the USA in 1994 due to ADRs, was 106 000 (CI 76 000–137 000) (Lazarou *et al.*, 1998). Others have said that this is an overestimate (Fremont-Smith, 1998; Kravitz, 1998).

- It is expected that 0.31 per cent of hospitalized patients in the USA die of ADRs (Classen *et al.*, 1991).

- In Olmsted County, 2.9 per cent of patients admitted died of ADRs (Silverstein *et al.*, 1994).

- In a New Jersey hospital the death rate due to ADRs was 3.2 per cent (Suh *et al.*, 2000).

- In seven US hospitals from 1974 to 1985 there was a 0.03 per cent death rate amongst children (Mitchell *et al.*, 1988).

- At a Salt Lake City hospital (LDS) the increased risk of death due to ADRs was 1.88 (CI 1.54–2.22) (Classen *et al.*, 1997).

Canada

It was estimated that 0.05 per cent of in-hospital mortality is associated with coded ADRs. Extrapolating from this figure, drugs are the 19th leading cause of death in Canada (Bains and Hunter, 1999).

UK

The number of deaths due to unforeseen adverse effects of drugs has increased from approximately 200 in 1990 to 1044 in 2000 (Figure 1.2) in England and Wales (Audit Commission, 2001; Eaton, 2002).

Norway

Akershus Central Hospital: over a 2 year period, of the 732 patients who died, 18.2 per cent (CI 15.4–21 per cent) were classified as being directly (48.1 per cent) or indirectly (51.9 per cent) associated with one or more drugs (Ebbesen *et al.*, 2001; Gottlieb, 2001).

Number of deaths

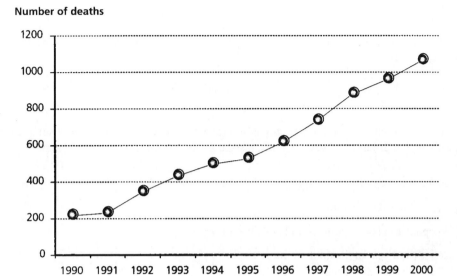

Figure 1.2   The number of deaths in England and Wales from adverse effects 1990 to 2000, amended from Audit Commission (2001). Reproduced by permission of Audit Commission

Finland

Helsinki University Central Hospital: in 2000, 5 per cent of deaths were associated with a medication (Juntti-Patinen and Neuvonen, 2002).

France

- The mortality in hospital admissions in a French survey was 0.12 per cent (CI 0.034–0.33 per cent) (Pouyanne *et al.*, 2000).

- In Le Havre, 13 per cent of those admitted with an ADR died, which was 40 per cent of the total deaths in the ward; but 28.3 per cent of the total admissions were for alcohol-related problems (Moore *et al.*, 1998).

- In Lille cardiological hospital the death rate due to ADRs was 5 per cent (Bordet *et al.*, 2001).

- In a cancer institute, 2.2 per cent of ADRs were fatal (Lapeyre-Mestre *et al.*, 1997).

Germany

Of those admitted with an ADR, 1.6 per cent died of it (Riethling *et al.*, 2000).

Worldwide

A review of 36 articles indicated that 3.7 per cent of patients admitted with ADRs died (Einarson, 1993).

Conclusion

This enormous variation in hospital admission rates for ADRs and rates after hospitalization is partly due to different survey methods, but the following were also probable factors:

- causality assessment methods
- ADR/ADE/AE definitions
- hospital admission policies and bed availability
- length and year of hospital admission
- type of hospital (mixture of wards)
- country (most surveys are from the USA)
- number of new chemical entities used
- whether ADRs were on admission or developed during admission
- aim, type, intensity of survey.

The following were found to be risk factors in some of these studies: age, number of drugs, sex, previous medical history, race, country, weight, alcohol intake, renal function, length of stay and infections.

The financial cost of adverse drug reactions

The science of pharmacoeconomics has grown rapidly in the last few years. The financial cost of a disease (hospitalization, etc.) is balanced against the cost of intervention, e.g. cost of drugs or operations. One factor in the cost of drugs is the cost of dealing with ADRs. In general terms the following problems occur:

- Definition of the AE for search purposes.
- Causality assessment of the AE. Few AEs are definitely ADRs or definitely not ADRs.
- If they occur in hospitalized patients there is difficulty in judging the prolongation of hospitalization due to the ADR or additional hospital costs.
- The hospitalized patient is not representative of the general population.
- Frequently, there is no satisfactory control group (Abadie and Souetre, 1993).

There are costs to the patient, the physician, the manufacturer and the nation.

Cost to the patient

This cost will vary from nil for a mild transitory ADR, lost earnings for a temporarily incapacitating ADR, to many thousands of pounds for a permanently incapacitating ADR. Unfortunately, the patient's future depends on whether they can sue somebody successfully.

Cost to the physician

Depending on the circumstances, the additional cost of diagnosis and management may be claimed from a private patient or be considered part of a health service commitment and, therefore, has to be absorbed by the practice/partnership. There may be additional costs either in trying to avoid ADRs or in insuring against those caused by negligence.

Cost to the manufacturer

This will include the cost of pharmacovigilance and the additional costs of detecting ADRs in clinical trials, as well as insurance and/or possible litigation and compensation costs. If there is evidence that may affect the share price then the evidence must be reported to the stock exchange, and thence to the press, whereupon there may be a large fall in share price (Richman, 1996; Senard et al., 1996).

Cost to the nation

This will include part of the social insurance costs and a proportion of the cost of a nationalized health service, as well as the cost of pharmacovigilance. We now move from generalizations to more specific costs in individual countries.

France

- Stenoses and gut perforations due to potassium chloride in Nancy over a period of 42 months amounted to 14 perforations and three stenoses at a direct cost of 2 160 530 (Royer, 1990).

- At a general hospital in Le Havre over a 16 day period in 1992, non-suicide drug-related admissions represented 2.5 per cent of all admissions and 6.4 per cent of medical admissions. The cost overall was FR6600 and the per ADR-patient cost was FR500 (Moore et al., 1995a).

- In France, in a 36-bed ward over 2 months, 52 patients were admitted with an ADR, 27 patients developed an ADR whilst in hospital and five patients fell into both categories. Total costs were FR695 134 (GB£89 810; US$136 512; DM206 114) (Moore et al., 1995c).

- The yearly cost of the excess duration related to ADRs in a French 29-bed ward was FR758 016 (GB£94 752 or €113 136). This represents around FR37 400 (€5589 or GB£4700) per hospital bed per year (Moore et al., 1998).

- In a cardiological hospital in Lille over 18 months there were 2.2 ADRs detected per 100 admissions at a cost of €4150 per ADR; the average stay was 11 days for those with an ADR versus 7 days for those without (Bordet *et al.*, 2001).

- In a Bordeaux hospital in 1996–97, in a 23-bed internal medicine unit over a 4 month period 26.1 per cent (116) of patients had an ADR. For 7 per cent (32) of admissions it was the reason for admission, 22 per cent (26) had an ADR during admission and 50 per cent (58) had an ADR on admission but this was not the reason for admission. For the 4 month period the total cost was €87 073 (Lagnaoui *et al.*, 2000).

- In a cancer institute the average cost of an ADR was FR33 037 at 1993 rates. This was 1.8 per cent of the global budget for the hospital (Lapeyre-Mestre *et al.*, 1997).

- An evaluation of 62 hospital departments over 14 days found that 3137 patients were hospitalized for ADRs, for a mean of 9 days; this gives a total number for the year of 130 000 (CI 100 916–156 620). The mean cost for an ADR related hospitalization was estimated at FF 16 000. (Detournay *et al.*, 2000).

USA

- In a US hospital over a 2 year period 109 patients suffered clinical consequences due to ADRs or medication-related errors at a cost of US$1.5 million in 1994 (Reactions No. 578, 1995; Schneider *et al.*, 1995).

- A two-hospital (Boston) study in 1993 gave an estimated figure of US$2595 per event for 1 year and the patient stay was prolonged by 2.2 days; the actual costs increased by US$3244 per ADR. The estimated annual cost for a 700-bed hospital was US$5.6 million or GB£3.45 million. The national costs of the preventable in-hospital events have been estimated to be US$2 billion (Bates *et al.*, 1997).

- In a further study in the USA (1990–93) the excess cost of hospitalization attributable to an ADR occurring in the LDS hospital was US$2013 (GB£1266, DM3279, FR11 027) and their stay in hospital was prolonged by 1.74 days (Classen *et al.*, 1997).

- In a New Jersey hospital over a 5 month period, 131 patients who had an ADR were compared with those without an ADR. The mean length of stay was 10.6 days versus 6.8 days and the cost US$22 775 versus US$17 292, which they said supported the Bates *et al.* (1997) and Classen *et al.* (1997) figures for increased stay of 2.2–3.2 days and a cost increase of US$3244–$4655 (Suh *et al.*, 2000). The difference between the Bates *et al.* (1997) and Suh *et al.* (2000) figures arises because the calculations were based on post-event costs and the total cost of hospitalization respectively.

- Drug-related morbidity and mortality have been estimated to cost more than US$136 billion a year in the USA and a major component of these costs is ADRs (Classen *et al.*, 1997).

- At the LDS hospital in Salt Lake City in 1992, it was found that those with ADRs stayed 8.19 days compared with matched controls staying 4.36 days and cost US$10 584 compared with US$5350 – attributable difference 1.94 days and US$1939 – (Evans *et al.*, 1994).

Spain

The cost of ADRs in a Spanish emergency ward was 42 732 ecus in 1 month (Ayani *et al.*, 1999).

Germany

- Over 14 months, there were 151 admissions to a university clinic in Germany. There was one death. The length of stay for those who had an ADR on admission or during their stay had a mean of 10.4 days versus 9.4 days at an additional cost of DM630 000 (Hippius *et al.*, 1999).

- The total direct charges for *severe* ADRs leading to hospital admission in Germany totalled US$656 million (GB£409 million/FR3785 million/DM1124 million) in 1965 (Schneeweiss *et al.*, 1997).

- An estimate of the direct costs of hospital admissions due to ADRs in Germany is DM1050 million per year (GB£374 million or US$619 million). Another figure is DM1300 million per year (Göttler, 1998). The median length of stay for ADR admissions was 8.7 days at a cost of DM465 per day (Göttler *et al.*, 1997). For elderly patients the direct cost of hospital admissions for Germany was US$815 million (Göttler, 2000).

- The 2001 figure for Germany was €400 million ppp adjusted (Schneeweiss *et al.*, 2002).

Switzerland

The cost per case for ADR admissions to an emergency department was €4121 ± 39 or US$6404 ± 57 (Wasserfallen *et al.*, 2001).

Canada

The mean direct cost of severe cutaneous or hypersensitivity reactions to anti-epileptic drugs was CA$3128 (range CA$1149–21 293) (Schlienger *et al.*, 1998).

Australia

For the Royal Melbourne Hospital the estimated annual cost for all drug-related admissions was AU$3 496 956 and for unavoidable reactions AU$1 629 494 (Dartnell *et al.*, 1996).

UK

The cost of errors in drug prescribing plus ADRs cost the NHS as much as GB£1.1 billion (US$1.5 billion or €1.8 billion) (Eaton, 2002).

Summary

The increased costs per ADR patient (2001 values in parentheses) are as follows.

Evans *et al.* (1994)	US$1939 (US$2389/€2714/GB£1658); increased stay 1.94 days
Classen *et al.* (1997)	US$2013/€1357 (US$5135.4/€5833.4/GB£3566.6); increased stay 1.74 days
Bordet *et al.* (2001)	US$3800/€4150/GB£2535, increased stay 4 days (2001)
Bates *et al.* (1997)	US$2595/€2900 (US$2862.8/€3252/GB£1987.7); increased stay 2.2 days
Suh *et al.* (2000)	US$5483 (US$5557/€6312.7/GB£3859); increased stay 3.8 days
Hippius *et al.* (1999)	DM4172, (GB£1502.95/€2460/$2165.5); increased stay 1 day
Lagnaoui *et al.* (2000)	€2721 (US$2395/GB£1662); increased stay 1.8 days
Moore *et al.* (1995)	FR17 488/GB£2186/€2610 (£2326/$2297.5), or FR500 (GB£74.50/€121.9) per patient; increased stay 6.8 days
Lapeyre-Mestre *et al.* (1997)	FR30 037 (GB£4463.9/€7306.5/US$6429.8)
Detournay *et al.* (2000)	FR16 000
Wasserfallen *et al.* (2001)	€4121 ± 39, US$6404 ± 57, GB£2718 ± 24 (2001)

Computerized ADR detection reduced the numbers of ADRs by 30 per cent and reduced one US hospital's costs by US$300 000 per year (US$330 960/GB£229 857/€375 970.5) (James, 1997).

Conclusions

It is important that figures for drug-related costs are broken down into their various constituents, since they may include drug under-dosage, suicides, untreated indications, failure to receive drugs and drug use without indication. Bearing in mind all the variables mentioned above, studies cannot be compared unless they have used the same definitions and methods.

Preventability of adverse drug reactions and adverse drug events

In France, 80 per cent were avoidable (Lagnaoui *et al.*, 2000). At Toulouse University hospital it was estimated that 65 per cent of ADRs were definitely unpreventable, 25 per cent were potentially preventable and 9 per cent were definitely preventable (Olivier *et al.*, 2001).

A study of 2814 patients over 70 years of age found that 40.2 per cent of probable ADRs/ADEs were considered preventable (Doucet *et al.*, 2002).

In the USA, 28 per cent of ADRS were preventable (Bates *et al.*, 1995); 60.5 per cent of ADEs were preventable, and when appropriate steps were taken the ADE rate dropped by more than 30 per cent (James, 1997).

Another survey gave a figure of 62.3 per cent of ADR-related hospital admissions as being preventable (McDonnell *et al.*, 2002).

In Australia, 5.5 per cent were definitely avoidable and 60 per cent possibly avoidable (Dartnell *et al.*, 1996).

In Italy, 1.4 per cent of the total admissions were due to avoidable ADEs, but 35.5 per cent of admissions due to ADEs were potentially preventable (Raschetti *et al.*, 1997).

In Germany, 28.5 per cent were considered to be preventable (Hippius *et al.*, 1999).

Another figure is 30 per cent, which means DM400 million could be saved (Göttler, 1998). In elderly patients the estimate was 41.5 per cent, leading to a potential saving of US$340 million (Göttler, 2000).

Conclusion

Again, there is a wide variation with several different factors, with causality and personal opinion of the assessor among them. The figure varies from 28 to 80 per cent. King Edward VII, when introduced to patients with TB as 'a preventable disease', said 'if preventable then why don't you prevent them?'.

Risk–benefit ratio

This is a poor term, in that it should be either 'the risk of harm/risk of benefit ratio' or 'harm benefit ratio' (Veatch, 1993); but the commonest term used is risk/benefit ratio (Ernst and Resch, 1995, 1996). The use of the word 'ratio' implies the use of figures and exact measurement. Better words would be analysis, assessment or evaluation.

Risk–benefit analysis

There are three methods that can be used:

- formal analysis

- comparative analysis

- comprehensive analysis (Rawlins, 1989).

Formal analysis

A randomized well-controlled clinical trial of sufficient power will give an exact answer. This can be expressed as the number of AEs caused for each case of disease successfully treated or prevented. For example, the MRC trial of treatment of mild hypertension showed that, for each cardiovascular event prevented, 33 men experienced ADRs (mostly impotence and fatigue) and 20 stopped treatment (Anon., 1985; Robson, 1997).

Comparative analysis (so-called 'bootstrapping')

Drugs used for similar purposes are compared. Rawlins (1989) describes its limitations as:

- assumption of similar efficacy in the drugs compared
- it is insensitive to changing standards over time.

Judgement analysis

This is the intuitive integration of all known factors. Its equivalent in causality assessment is clinical judgement or 'global introspection'. The main problem with clinical judgement is that it is not usually possible to say which factors have been included and which have not, nor what weight has been given to each factor. It will depend on training, clinical experience, subjective bias, degree of investigation of the literature, time available, etc. This is an inadequate précis of Professor Rawlins's chapter in *Risk and consent to risk in medicine* (Rawlins, 1989). This is the commonest method used, but an attempt should be made to explain the factors responsible for the decision.

Trade offs

These remaining methods have been outlined by Rawlins (1989) as follows.

Human capital   This is an economic assessment where the financial costs of goods and services diverted from other areas are set against the output costs by premature death or retirement through ill health. It is not adequate for dealing with human parameters.

Willingness-to-pay   Again, in financial terms (proportion of the patients income in exchange for degrees of cure).

Standard gamble   What risk of death would patients take for a complete cure (see p. •).

Other methods

Utility analysis   This is not too dissimilar to the use of Bayes theorem for causality assessment, in that the risks and benefits can be broken down into their constituents and the alternative possibilities expressed numerically. The numerous probabilities can be calculated (Lane *et al.*, 1987). This method, like BARDI (Bayesian Adverse Reaction Diagnostic Instrument), requires a lot of data and, therefore, would be too complicated to use except for very important decisions.

Merit analysis This uses a general 'principle of threes structure': seriousness, duration and incidence of the disease; level of improvement produced by the drug; and adverse effects of the drug; each is graded as high, medium or low (Edwards *et al.*, 1996). This is too crude a method to use for important decisions.

A quantitative method has been put forward using the 'number needed to be treated to prevent one additional event (NTT)' and the 'number needed to harm (NTH)'. To these is added a term 'minimum clinical efficacy' (MCE) evaluating the benefits and risk of available treatments (Holden *et al.*, 2003).

The benefits: measurement of efficacy

The efficacy of a drug in the treatment of a disease needs to be considered compared with three alternatives:

1. No treatment and, therefore, the natural progress of the disease.

2. Placebo, which is the same as the above plus a psychological effect and a non-specific trial effect, which may produce objective benefits or costs.

3. The standard treatment for that disease. If there is more than one standard treatment, then a comparison with each may be necessary.

If it is presumed that the healing rate for the standard therapy is greater than the natural healing rate or that induced by placebo, and if we take as an example a healing rate of 60 per cent for the standard therapy, then the number of patients required in the trial can be calculated. In order to be approximately 95 per cent certain of detecting a 5 per cent difference between the standard therapy (60 per cent) and the new therapy (55 or 65 per cent), 500 patients would be required (Bulpitt, 1983). If the results are accepted as an adequate indication of the drug's efficacy, then would this number of patients give an adequate indication of the safety of the drug? It should be able to establish the incidence of very common side effects, but what chance would one have of detecting a more rare serious side effect? There would be a 95 per cent chance of finding a side effect with a true incidence of 1 per cent if the background rate of the AE is 1 in 1000.

The risk

Perception of risk

Humans are not necessarily logical creatures when it comes to balancing risks and benefits: 'a bird in the hand is worth two in the bush', a benefit or gratification of a desire now is worth more than the distant probability of retribution or payment. How else can we explain the number of youngsters taking up smoking or other addictive drugs? Many human decisions are made emotionally and justified intellectually. Professor Lee has tabled the factors that distinguish between objective risk and perceived risk (Lee, 1987):

1. Voluntary risks – involuntary risks.
    The 3000 embryopathies per year due to alcohol abuse in pregnancy compared with the thalidomide disaster.

2. Familiar – unknown.
    AIDS deaths have a lot of publicity, but tobacco-related cardiovascular deaths are rarely publicized.

3. Immediate – delayed effect.
    The explosion of the TWA, flight 800, Boeing 747 on the 17th July 1996 killed 230 people and produced a world wide reaction, whereas nearly five times that number die in the USA each day (1096 in 1990) due to tobacco (Longo et al., 1996). That is about 20 per cent of the total deaths in the USA. In China, the Ministry of Health estimates that smoking may be responsible for killing 50 million children and youths currently alive in the country (Goldsmith, 1996).

4. Threat to self – threat to society.
    The unexpected death of a contemporary reminds one of one's own mortality, whereas the 12.2 million children under 5 years of age dying due to famine in the world produces little reaction (Kevany, 1996).

5. Catastrophic – chronic.
    The Chernobyl nuclear explosion caused far more alarm than the world total of 500 deaths due to mining per year (Heilman, 1988). There are 42 000 fatalities due to road traffic accidents each year in the EU. The circumstances of the catastrophe make a great deal of difference. The aftermath of the 11th September 2001 destruction of the twin towers in New York with the death of 2830 people will echo around the world for a long time to come. The *New Internationalist* (No. 340, November 2001) estimated that worldwide 24 000 people also died of hunger on 11th September; 6020 children were also killed by diarrhoea and 2700 children died of measles. On 1st July 1916, some 20 000 British soldiers died on the first day of the battle of the Somme. The deaths of approximately 7000 East German refugees on the German ship 'Wilhelm Gustloff' sunk by Russian torpedoes in the icy Baltic Sea on 31 January 1945 scarcely caused a ripple against the background of war. The media constantly distort our idea of risk by their repetitious portrayal of the dramatic and the emotional events of life.

6. Fates worse than death – clean sharp death.

Different viewpoints of risk

Patients will have a different view from their physician, and both of them will differ from those with a broader perspective, i.e. the regulatory authorities and the pharmaceutical industry.

The patient   The sources of information will include the patients' information leaflet, the prescribing physician, the pharmacist, the media and the patient's friends. None of these is satisfactory from the point of view of making a valid cost/benefit judgement. The patient's judgement will also depend on their knowledge of alternative treatments and their cost/ benefit ratio for their particular circumstances. There are major differences in the perception of risk of ADRs between health professionals and non-health professionals, i.e. the general population (Bongard *et al.*, 2002).

The patient information leaflet, although mentioning possible ADRs, may give no guide as to the severity or frequency, nor was it the intention that the patient would be able to make a cost/benefit judgement from it. The prime reason was to improve patient understanding of the use of their medicines. In the UK, only 30 per cent of patients read all of the leaflet, 8–12 per cent never read any of it, 40 per cent said that too little information was provided, and 20 per cent would like to see more information on the likelihood of the listed side effects (NAO, 2003). The patient will rarely have the knowledge and background to be able to make an adequate assessment of the cost/benefit ratio. However, that does not mean that they will not attempt to make that judgement on whatever information is available. Their assessment may be expressed in non-compliance, e.g. 14.5 per cent of patients failed to have their prescription dispensed in a UK general practice (Beardon *et al.*, 1993). However, when verbal and written information about side effects of antidepressant medication was given it did not reduce compliance or increase the reporting of side effects by the patients treated with the drug (Myers *et al.*, 1987).

When patients with rheumatoid arthritis (RA) were asked what risk they were prepared to take for a cure of their disease they said that they would accept a 27 per cent risk of death for a guaranteed cure (Thompson, 1986). Another paper mentions that patients would accept a median risk of death of no more than 1 in 10 000 000 for a 90 per cent probability of a complete cure. Their physicians would accept a risk of 1 in 10 000. The risk of death for NSAIDs is between 1 in 260 and 1 in 360 over a course of a patient's treatment for RA (Pullar *et al.*, 1990). It seems that the answer depends on how you word the question.

'Well tolerated'

This term is used frequently to describe the response to a drug.

The Concise Oxford dictionary defines '*tolerate*' as:

1. Allow the existence or occurrence of without authoritative intervention.

2. Leave unmolested.

3. Endure or permit, especially with forbearance.

4. Sustain or endure (suffering etc).

5. Be capable of continued subjection to (a drug, radiation, etc) without harm.

6. Find or treat as endurable.

From the Latin '*tolerare*' to endure.

The 'well' implies 'in a satisfactory or right way',

The passive form 'well tolerated' indicates that it is the recipient of a drug who is doing the tolerating but without quantifying or qualifying what it is they are tolerating. There is the presumption that what they are tolerating is caused by the drug and that it is not pleasant. If a patient does not tolerate a drug there are several courses open:

1.   Reduce the dose.

2.   Stop the drug.

3.   Add or remove some other causal factor or add a drug that mitigates the problem.

4.   Complain to the prescriber who, having decided on the balance of probabilities that the event was caused by the drug, may indicate that the benefit-risk balance is favourable and, therefore, that the patient should continue with the drug despite its adverse effect.

Analysis of the study data should reveal the number of adverse events due to the drug that have been tolerated using these criteria. The word 'well' could apply to single patients and, if so, would be impossible to define: in that the patient; who was very reluctant to tolerate the drug, but did so by persuasion; could be said to have tolerated the drug badly, but still tolerated it. On the other hand the 'well' could apply to the population taking the drug and therefore would need to be quantified with a percentage or proportion. The next question is what should be the threshold for 'well'? Should the threshold be the same for a life-saving drug for a life-threatening disease as for a sleeping tablet? The answer might be to abandon the 'well' and give the percentage of patients who tolerated the adverse effects of the drug. At the moment it is a meaningless phrase that implies lack of adverse effects without any duty to demonstrate it.

The prescribing physician   The prescribing physician will not discuss with the patient all the elements necessary to make a judgement; they simply do not have the time and they very rarely have enough information. There is a presumption that the physician knows all the relevant factors and has weighed up the probability of ADRs and the probability of benefit before prescribing a drug for that particular patient. However, there is evidence that doctors are not necessarily any better at judging probabilities than are their patients (Kee, 1996; Ashworth, 1997). The UK NHS physician will usually have available MIMS, ABPI Medicines compendium, British National Formulary and Current Problems. Other countries will have their equivalent texts. There are other specific journals that are not supplied free of charge as are the above. One example is *Préscrire International*, which deals specifically with cost/benefit ratios of new drugs.

The benefit half of the equation consists of the chance that the patient in question will be cured or relieved by the drug. This would involve extrapolating from all the clinical trial patients to the individual patient or, more likely, extrapolating from the drug company representative's spiel to the individual patient. The cost half of the equation can be assessed from the drug's ADR profile (see p. ●), but comparative data on drugs of the same class are rarely available. Unfortunately, the necessary information is not available to the average prescriber and the Summary of Product Characteristics (SPC) is totally inadequate for this purpose. In a study of the factors that influence GPs' decisions on whether or not to prescribe, 51 per cent mentioned side effects as a source of concern (Bradley, 1992). Almost half of the prescribing changes (48.6 per cent) initiated by a random sample of 340 physicians in 15 American and Canadian metropolitan areas were as a result of information supplied by pharmaceutical manufacturers (Putnam, 1990).

The regulatory authority   They have a continuous responsibility to the public to monitor the risk/benefit ratio throughout the life of a product. They have the ability and authority to obtain any relevant data. Many regulatory authorities are under-staffed and, therefore, are unable to fulfil their mandate.

Before allowing marketing of a new drug, consumers can expect regulatory authorities to use six types of assessment of the supporting data submitted by the manufacturers in balancing risk and benefit:

• Regulatory authorities should establish that the product is of satisfactory quality and that this will be maintained during post-marketing manufacture.

• Regulatory authorities should ensure that the product is efficacious in all the clinical indications that the manufacturer wishes to promote. With a combination product each ingredient should contribute to its overall therapeutic activity and they should be pharmaceutically and pharmacokinetically compatible.

• Regulatory authorities will expect the animal and clinical studies to have rigorously explored the likely toxicological hazards to man during therapeutic use. Regulatory authorities, prescribers and consumers should be aware, however, that at the time a new drug is marketed only rough estimates of risk can be made because of the relatively short duration of treatment and limited numbers of patients involved in clinical trials.

• Consumers expect the regulatory authorities to carry out an objective and impartial risk/benefit assessment from the evidence of safety and efficacy. With non-narcotic analgesics, used in symptomatic relief of pain, formal analysis is impossible and regulators must use their professional judgement in making their assessment. The subjective nature of this form of risk/benefit evaluation, however, makes it inevitable that no decision will go unchallenged.

• Regulatory authorities should ensure that prescribers are provided with sufficient objective, unbiased information to enable them to exercise proper professional judge-ment on when and how to use the product. Prescribers will also wish to know how the product compares with others in the same therapeutic class; such information is not usually provided, either by the regulatory authorities or by the manufacturers, and may more appropriately be the responsibility of professional organizations (e.g. National Drug or Formulary Committees) or consumer groups (e.g. Drug and Therapeutics Bulletin).

• Regulators should also have sufficient legal and executive powers to ensure that they can enforce actions against a manufacturer who makes exaggerated claims of efficacy or safety for their product (Rawlins, 1986).

Before treating a patient, a doctor must balance the expected benefits of a drug against its potential risks, i.e. evaluate the risk/benefit ratio. The situation is similar for the licensing authority, in that their decision as to whether to allow a drug to be marketed must depend on the risk/benefit ratio for the whole population at risk.

The CSM, in their assessment, consider the following issues:

• Quality

- Efficacy

  a)   new evidence for lack of efficacy

  b)   uniqueness of therapeutic properties

  c)   uniqueness of efficacy in small sub-groups

- Safety

  a)   spontaneous reports

  b)   cohort studies

  c)   case-control studies

  d)   animal carcinogenicity.

But the CSM do not consider:

- Impact on company or competitors

- Unknown/unsuspected benefits

- Decisions by other regulatory authorities

- Misuse – potential or actual

- Pressure – parliamentary, media or from pressure groups (Rawlins, 1985).

The question then arises as to whether the regulator should consider the alternative therapies. 'Before regulatory action is taken, the risk associated with available alternative therapies should ideally be evaluated and compared with the risk at issue. Moreover, the benefits of the actual and alternative therapies should be evaluated and weighed in the final evaluation of the situation' (Wiholm, 1991). 'Furthermore the substances being evaluated must be compared with the alternatives' (benefit/benefit and risk/risk evaluation) (Bass, 1987). Is this synonymous with 'uniqueness of therapeutic properties'? Presuming that alternative therapy is considered in the final analysis, does a new drug have to be as good as or better than current alternatives? Direct comparative studies, of sufficient size, with the main competitors are unlikely to have been performed before a drug is approved. Like the prescribing physician, a regulatory authority must make their decision on inadequate evidence.

The pharmaceutical company   'Scientists who work for the pharmaceutical industry get steeped in corporate culture and slip into biases in favour of their own drugs' (Jasanoff, 1993). In the same way that mothers think that their baby is the most beautiful, so the people in clinical research tend to consider that the drug that they are working on is more unique than it is. This is a good reason for separating drug safety from efficacy clinical research, but it tends to pervade the whole of the staff at all levels.

Although all the relevant information will be, or should be, available to the research company it will rarely have been analysed or assembled into a readable package for the marketing company to pass onto enquiring prescribers.

It should be the pharmaceutical industry's aim to provide the information necessary such that these decisions can be made, i.e. undertake the first five assessments mentioned above.

Calculation of the risk

With a sample size of 5000 patients there is a greater than 99 per cent certainty of finding one case of an ADR with a true incidence rate of 1 in 1000. If more than one case is required on which to base a decision as to whether this drug was safe to market, then the chances of finding them diminish rapidly, there being only a 73 per cent chance of finding four such cases in the sample of 5000 patients. However, the proviso mentioned earlier, that the AE is identified as being due to the drug, is important. If the ADR cannot be clearly differentiated from naturally occurring disease, then the problem is formidable. For instance, consider a drug that produces a 10 per cent increase in disease symptoms with a natural incidence of 1 in 1000. Now, to be 95 per cent certain of detecting this we would require some 1 100 000 patients, and for doubling in the incidence of the disease symptoms we would need approximately 16 000 patients. Hence, for a given number of patients there will be far more certainty about a drug's efficacy than its safety.

The reason for this situation is that a standard treatment nearly always means that it is efficacious in 10 per cent or more of the population ($p_1 = 0.1$) and may even be effective in 50 per cent of the population ($p_1 = 0.5$). With a new treatment, an increase from 10 to 11 per cent ($p_2 = 0.11$) or a doubling to 20 per cent ($p_2 = 0.2$) in the first instance and from 50 to 55 per cent ($p_2 = 0.55$) and doubling to 100 per cent healing ($p_2 = 1.00$) in the second instance are relatively large figures compared with the figure for ADR that would be of interest, e.g. a background death rate of approximately 1 in 10 000 ($p_1 = 0.0001$) doubling due to treatment to 2 in 10 000 ($p_2 = 0.002$); see Table 1.1 (Lewis, 1981). To show an increase from 50 per cent efficacy to 55 per cent efficacy would need a total of 3280 patients in the study, whereas if it was necessary to detect a doubling of the rate of 1 in 10 000 of an ADR the figure required would be 474 000 patients. To identify a rarity like the aplastic

Table 1.1 Number of observations needed in each group (populations p_1 and p_2) to detect given change in proportion (power 80%, significance level 5%). Reprinted from *Trends in Pharmacological Science*, **2**, Lewis JA, Post-marketing surveillance: how many patients?, pp. 93–94, copyright (1981), with permission from Elsevier Science

p_1	p_2	N
0.5	0.55	1640
	1.00	20
0.4	0.44	2490
	0.80	30
0.3	0.33	3890
	0.60	50
0.1	0.11	15 130
	0.20	240
0.01	0.011	168 000
	0.020	2700
0.001	0.0011	1 684 000
	0.0020	23 000
0.0001	0.00011	11 860 000
	0.0002	237 000

anaemia caused by chloramphenicol, 1 500 000 observations would be needed (Melmon and Nierenberg, 1981). At the other end of the spectrum, if a comparison of a new hypertensive drug with a placebo was planned and an 80 per cent certainty of finding a difference of 20 mmHg in blood pressure (significance level 5 per cent) was required, then only 16 patients would be needed (see Table 1.2). It will be obvious that absolute safety is unobtainable, even in the relatively short term. The problem of the changing risk–benefit ratio in the longer term is even more difficult: practolol introduced a medium-term ADR problem with a mean time to onset of eye signs of 23 months (Wright, 1974), and the delay between the use of diethylstilboestrol and the appearance of vaginal adenocarcinoma in the daughters of its recipients was at least 21 years (Herbst *et al.*, 1971) and is representative of the long-term problem. The problem of long-term evaluation of the risk/benefit ratio has been illustrated by clofibrate, where ultimately the risk exceeded the benefits but the reasons were unknown (Committee of Principal Investigators, 1978, 1980). It is essential that maximum advantage be taken of clinical trials to establish the side-effect burden of a drug; great effort must also be made to collect side effects presenting after marketing, and these must then be correctly assessed.

Table 1.2 Number of observations needed in each group to detect a given difference in the group means in a parallel group trial (power 80%, significance level 5%, SD ≈ 14). Reprinted from *Trends in Pharmacological Science*, **2**, Lewis JA, Post-marketing surveillance: how many patients?, pp. 93–94, copyright (1981), with permission from Elsevier Science

Difference in means	Number of observations
2	700
5	120
10	30
15	15
20	8

The changing risks with new drugs

There is no way of establishing the complete safety of a new drug before it comes into widespread use. As the number of patients increases, so the risks can be defined with greater accuracy. This will continue until the drug is marketed, after which there is no longer a 100 per cent reporting on the fate of each patient treated. The decision as to how many patients should be treated before allowing a drug onto the market will depend on several factors. A relatively small number may be required for a new drug for a rare fatal disease for which there is no treatment; however, several thousands may be required for a drug that needs to be taken on a long-term basis for a common chronic disease, or for an antibiotic for an infection that is rarely fatal and for which there are already acceptable treatments. For the UK, for the years 1987–89, the median number in licence applications was 1528 patients, with 95 per cent CI of 1194–1748 and a range from 43 to 15 962 (Rawlins and Jefferys, 1993).

The regulatory authority will be influenced by the government, who in turn will be influenced by the general opinion within parliament, which should reflect public opinion.

There have been several occasions when the reaction to the publication of an ADR has resulted in the unjustified condemnation of a medication.

Drug withdrawals

There have been four major surveys of drugs withdrawn from the market:

- Bakke *et al.* (1984) covered 24 drugs from the USA and UK over the period 1964 to 1983.

- The second covered 126 drugs from the UK, Germany and France over a 30 year period (Spriet-Pourra and Auriche, 1988, 1994).

- The third covered 29 drugs from the USA, UK and Spain from 1974 to 1993 (Bakke *et al.*, 1995). See Appendix 1 for further details.

- The fourth covered 121 drugs from around the world from 1960 to 1999 (Fung *et al.*, 2001).

The median period of market life for 97 products was 8 years, with 25 drugs equal to or less than 2 years, 23 more than 2 years but less than 8 years and 49 more than 8 years. Most of the reactions were of type B, involving hepatic (26.6 per cent), haematological (10.5 per cent), cardiovascular (8.7 per cent), dermatological (6.3 per cent) and carcinogenic reactions (6.3 per cent) (Fung *et al.*, 2001). The commonest drugs were NSAIDS (13.2 per cent), which accounted for double the number of withdrawals compared with antibiotics/anti-infectives, analgesics/antipyretics, and antidepressants (Spriet-Pourra and Auriche, 1994). The results of these surveys have formed the basis of the table in Appendix 1. The decision to take a drug off the market for safety reasons is frequently very difficult, with different countries taking different decisions at different times. Both the manufacturers and the regulatory bodies collect data on suspected ADRs, but with varying success.

It would be naïve to believe that the sole consideration for drug withdrawal was for the patients' welfare. There are several other factors that probably play a part. A drug may be withdrawn for safety reasons or commercial reasons:

- By the pharmaceutical company.

  (a) Purely because of concern for patients.

  (b) Because the benefit/risk to the company is no longer favourable. A company may choose to withdraw a drug ostensibly for commercial reasons, but also because of the fear that admitting a safety reason might make them liable to legal action.

  (c) Because they have been leant on by the regulatory authority to withdraw the drug 'voluntarily'.

- By the regulatory authority.

(a) 'Drug withdrawals do not reflect a judgement concerning the absolute safety of a drug but reflect a judgement about the risks and rewards of a drug in the context of alternative treatments' (Heinrich, 2001). 'Drug withdrawals may occur because the drugs are used incorrectly by health professionals and patients not because the drugs are inherently dangerous' (Heinrich, 2001).

(b) After a series of warnings of adverse effects: restrictions on dose, dosage forms, indications, incipients or prescription (from over-the-counter (OTC) to prescription or change of schedule), monitoring of liver function tests (LFTs) or white blood cells (WBC), 'black box' warnings, Dear Physician (Health Professional) letters. These are frequently ignored by prescribers. Dear Healthcare Professional letters and a press release for Cisapride had very little effect (Smalley, 2001); prescribing Cisapride with an interacting medicine only fell from 11.9 to 10.7 per cent (NAO, 2003); withdrawal then becomes the only solution.

(c) When a new drug with presumed absence of a particular problem is marketed; e.g. COX 2 inhibitors, where there was a presumption of few GI problems. The term 'withdrawal' is difficult to define in this context, and the list in Appendix 1 includes drugs where an indication or formulation has been removed and where a drug has been suspended or withdrawn and then subsequently reintroduced. The four surveys mentioned have analyses of the results. The amazing diversity of opinions as to withdrawal suggests that there are local differences of occurrence, attitude and usage; but some are incomprehensible.

False alarms

Oxygen and retrolental fibroplasia

The discovery in 1953 that 100 per cent oxygen, when given to neonates, could cause retrolental fibroplasia produced a change in practice that caused a large number of neonatal deaths from hypoxia. Cross, 1973; Bolton and Cross, 1974) suggested that there were about 200 000 deaths in England and Wales and over 180 000 deaths in the USA over the subsequent two decades. These numbers were 16 times larger than the estimated number of babies who would have been blinded by a more liberal oxygen policy.

Pertussis vaccine and encephalopathy

The reports of neurological illness following the use of pertussis vaccine resulted in the immunization figures for the UK dropping from 80 per cent of neonates to 31 per cent (Miller *et al.*, 1981), and produced the largest epidemic of pertussis for 20 years (Meade, 1981); 3.5 per cent of children in the encephalopathy study had had triple vaccine within 7 days, compared with 1.7 per cent of controls. The relative risk was 2.4; if the child had previously been neurologically normal then the relative risk was 3.3, but there was no significant risk if the child had diphtheria and tetanus vaccine alone. The risk of serious impairment within 7 days was 1 in 110 000 and the risk of permanent impairment was 1 in 310 000 (Anon., 1981a).

Teratogenicity of Debendox (Bendectin)

There remain some controversies concerning ADRs where publicity has not helped to resolve the problem. Although on three occasions the CSM has carefully examined all the available data on the issue of whether Debendox for the treatment of morning sickness in pregnancy has produced an increased incidence of congenital abnormalities in the offspring of mothers treated with the drug, they found no evidence that there was an increased risk of foetal damage with the use of this agent (Fleming *et al.*, 1981; Orme, 1985). The adverse publicity produced such a large fall in sales that it was no longer viable commercially and it was withdrawn from the market. It was the first drug victim of trial by the media (Austrian, 1996). It has subsequently reappeared in Canada and Spain (Einarson *et al.*, 1996).

Cancer in children following vitamin K administration

A case-control study in 1992 reported an increase in cancer and leukaemia in children given intramuscular vitamin K for prevention of haemorrhagic disease of the newborn (Golding *et al.*, 1990, 1992). The British Paediatric Association then recommended oral vitamin K, but in 1993 there were five reports of late haemorrhagic disease in infants receiving the oral form. Two later studies could find no association between intramuscular vitamin K and cancer (Klebanoff *et al.*, 1993; Von Kries *et al.*, 1996) or leukaemia (Ansell *et al.*, 1996). It was suggested that there were design flaws in the Golding *et al.* study (Zipursky, 1996). A further four studies have confirmed that there is no link between vitamin K and solid tumours, but a small risk of leukaemia cannot be ruled out (Von Kries, 1998).

Cancer and depression caused by reserpine

These findings originated from a study by the BCDSP (Cohen, 1974; Jick, 1984); later, there was contrary evidence (Fraser, 1996).

Mumps, measles and rubella vaccination and autism, 1998–2003

In a study of 12 children with bowel abnormalities and serious developmental regression, nine were found to have autism; eight of these nine children developed the disease after receiving MMR vaccine and it was hypothesized that there was a causal relationship (Wakefield *et al.*, 1998). This causal relationship was subsequently denied (Nicholls *et al.*, 1998; Kaye *et al.*, 2001; Dales *et al.*, 2001; Farrington *et al.*, 2001). This is a case where emotionalism fanned by the media has overwhelmed logic.

Expression of risk

There are various methods for expressing risks. They may be in absolute terms or relative terms; (Table 1.3).

Relative risk is the probability of an event in the active group divided by the probability of the event in the control group. i.e. (Incidence among exposed)/(Incidence among not exposed). It is good for establishing associations (Kaufman and Shapiro, 2000). This 'has been shown to give a more favourable impression of the effectiveness of a drug than absolute risk estimates' (Bucher *et al.*, 1994). Consider the Bristol–Myers–Squibb adver-

Table 1.3 Comparison of absolute and relative risk. From Skolbeldeen (1998), *British Medical Journal*. Reproduced with permission of BMJ Publishing Group

Treatment Group		Placebo Group		Relative risk Reduction (%)	Absolute risk Reduction (%)
Survivals	Mortalities	Survivals	Mortalities		
9000	1000	8000	2000	50	10
9900	100	9800	200	50	1
9990	10	9980	20	50	0.1
9999	1	9998	2	50	0.01

tisement: 'People with high cholesterol can rapidly reduce their risk of having a first-time heart attack by 31% and their risk of death by 22% by taking a widely prescribed drug called pravastatin' (Skolbekken, 1998).

Absolute risk is the (Incidence among exposed) − (incidence among non-exposed). It is the best measure of the importance of associations (Kaufman and Shapiro, 2000). The Bristol–Myers–Squibb advertisement can be expressed in absolute risk terms: 'People with high cholesterol can rapidly reduce their (absolute) risk of having a first-time heart attack by 1.9% and their (absolute) risk of death by 0.9% by taking a widely prescribed drug called pravastatin' (Skolbekken, 1998).

Study results should give both relative and absolute risks, since exclusive emphasis on the reduction in relative risk may overstate the effectiveness of a treatment (Bucher *et al.*, 1994). It is likely that the furore over the original announcement concerning the dangers of the third generation of oral contraceptive was due to the undue emphasis, by the media, on the relative risk and the lack of emphasis on the absolute risk (Mills and Edwards, 1999).

The number of patients that need to be treated for one additional patient to be harmed (Bjerre and LeLorier, 1997, 2000) is as follows:

$$\text{NNTH} = \frac{1}{(\text{Odds ratio} - 1) \times \text{Unexposed event rate}}$$

Language

The 1992 US National Adult Literacy Survey showed that 21 per cent of Americans could not read the front page of a newspaper and 48 per cent could not decipher messages with words or numbers, such as a bus schedule (Schwartzberg, 2001). The problem is that individuals have great difficulty comprehending extremely low-probability events, such as differentiating a risk of 10^{-7} from 10^{-5}, a risk 100 times as large (Zeckhauser and Viscusi, 1990). There is a tendency to overestimate rare causes of death and underestimate common causes (Lichenstein, 1978).

When asked to choose between two treatments, A and B, a group consisting of patients, students and physicians were told that with treatment A the 1-year survival rate was 90 per cent, whereas for treatment B there was a 10 per cent mortality rate; otherwise, the drugs were the same. Most respondents showed a preference for treatment A (McNeil *et al.*, 1982). When failure rates were displayed there was double the frequency (93 per cent versus

47 per cent) of correct decisions compared with when response rates were displayed (Elting *et al.*, 1999). It would appear that we like to hear the 'good' news but not the 'bad'. Unfortunately, the interpretation of verbal terms for risk varies. The CIOMS Working Group III (1995) proposed a scale that has been accepted for the European Commission Pharmaceutical Committee guidelines and is used below. This scale was tested on students, patients and doctors (not using identical protocols; see Table 1.4).

Table 1.4   Interpretation of verbal risk terms by various groups; after Berry *et al.* (2003)

Student estimate ($N = 268$) Verbal term	CIOMS (EC) definition	General population ($N = 360$)	Doctors
Very common 65% (SD 24.2)	>10%		46 (%)
Common 45% (SD 22.3)	>1% but <10%	50% (SD 24.4)	
Uncommon18% (SD 13.3)	>0.1% but <1%		
Rare 8% (SD 7.5)	>0.01% but <0.1%	21% (SD 17.7).	2%
Very rare 4% (SD 6.7)	<0.01%		

So, people significantly overestimate the likelihood of adverse effects given specific verbal describers. Doctors do the same, but not to such a large extent. If patients or doctors misperceive the risk then their decision to prescribe or take the drug may be affected (Berry *et al.*, 2002, 2003).

This does not encourage compliance. In reply to four specific questions: 76.2 per cent of patients said that they wanted to know all possible adverse effects; 13.3 per cent only if an adverse effect occurred 1 in 100 000 times; 10.2 per cent only if such an occurrence was 1 in 100 times; and 0.4 per cent were not interested in any information (Ziegler *et al.*, 2001). The phrases commonly used to express risk are: possible, probable, etc.; low, high, negligible, etc., common, uncommon.

Physicians

The terms used by physicians and their equivalent numerical risk vary with different authors. Two groups of physicians (one American and the other Canadian) gave their estimates of probability; see Table 1.5.

Table 1.5   Estimates of probability by US (Kong *et al.*, 1986) and Canadian (Bryant and Norman, 1980) hospital staff

American Hospital Staff (Kong *et al.* 1986)	Canadian Hospital Staff (Bryant and Norman 1980)
Almost certain 82% Interquartile range 12	
Probable 65% Interquartile range 21	Probable 81% SD 68–94, range 36–97
Possible 27% Interquartile range 23	Possible 48% SD 27–68 range 3–85
Unlikely 14% Interquartile range 11	Unlikely 25% SD 5–47 range 2–97

The pharmacovigilance team from Bordeaux inquired of 300 French GPs and found that 'frequent' corresponded to a frequency of 1 in 10, 'rare' to 1 in 200 and 'very rare' to 1 in 3300; however, only 19 per cent of the doctors replied, so that these figures may not represent true opinion (Péré *et al.*, 1984).

A Canadian paper (Toogood, 1980) has reported on the use of everyday adjectives to describe medical events:

'Rarely' ranges (95 per cent confidence limits) 0–17 per cent, mean 5 per cent.

'Occasionally' (95 per cent confidence limits) 0–43 per cent, mean 21 per cent.

'Often' (95 per cent confidence limits) 27–91 per cent, mean 59 per cent.

Two American authors (Roberts and Gupta, 1987) did their own survey comparing the undertanding of terminology by house staff (Juniors) and full-time attending physicians (Seniors):

'Frequently' – the house staff had a mean of 72.4 per cent and a range of 35–90 per cent; the physicians had a mean of 65.7 per cent and a range of 40–90 per cent.

'Often' – the house staff had a mean of 71 per cent and a range 61–85 per cent; the physicians had a mean of 59 per cent and a range of 30–80 per cent.

'Occasionally' – the house staff had a mean of 21 per cent and a range of 5–40 per cent; the physicians had a mean of 17 per cent and a range of 5–30 per cent.

'Rarely' – the house staff had a mean of 5.2 per cent and a range of 3–15 per cent; the physicians had a mean of 8.7 per cent and a range of 1–30 per cent.

Two French clinical pharmacologists have attempted the same exercise (Marion and Simon, 1984), with the following results:

'Rarement' range 2.3–6.1 per cent (95 per cent confidence limits).

'Souvent' 37.5–56.9 per cent (95 per cent confidence limits).

The German regulatory authority (Bundesgesundheitsamtes), in their 1986 guidelines (Enstellung, 1986) on how to express established or estimated incidences of AEs, gave:

Incidence over 10 per cent – may occur frequently.

Incidence between 1 and 10 per cent – has been observed occasionally.

Incidence below 1 per cent – may occur rarely.

The Swiss classification   is:

frequent, >5 per cent

occasional, 5–10 per cent

rare, <0.1 per cent.

In Sweden, the classification for entry into the Swedish pharmaceutical drug handbook (FASS) is:

frequent, >1 per cent

less frequent, 0.1–1 per cent

rare, <0.1 per cent.

In Japan they use the *Japanese Pharmaceutical Reference* (second edition), 1991–1992:

Rarely, <0.1 per cent

Infrequently, 0.1 to ⩽ 5 per cent

Greater than 5%, 'no specific designation'.

CIOMS definitions 1995 (Table 1.6), adopted by the European Commission (Notice to Applicants, volume 2C: A Guideline on Summary of Product Characteristics, December 1999). This system did not base its selection of verbal descriptors on systematic empirical evidence (Berry *et al.*, 2003).

Table 1.6   CIOMS and EEC verbal definitions of probability

CIOMS		EEC	
Verbal description	Quantification	Verbal description	Quantification
Very common (optional category)	>10%	Very common	>1/10
Common (frequent)	>1% but <10%	Common	>1/100 but <1/10
Uncommon (infrequent)	>0.1% but <1%	Uncommon	>1/1000 but <1/100
Rare	>0.01% but <0.1%	Rare	>1/10 000 but <1/1000
Very rare (optional category)	<0.01%	Very rare	<1/10 000

In 1996, the Chief Medical Officer at the UK Department of Health, when discussing risk, suggested the following terminology:

Negligible   less than one AE per million (*cf.* death due to being struck by lightning or death due to release of radiation by nuclear power)

Minimal   one in a million to 1/100 000 (*cf.* death due to a railway accident or vaccination-associated polio)

Very low   1/100 000 to 1/10 000 (*cf.* death at football, at home or at work or death due to homicide or leukaemia)

Low   1/10 000 to 1/1000 (*cf.* death from 'flu or road traffic accident or all kinds of violence and poisoning)

Moderate   1/1000 to 1/100 (*cf.* death from smoking 10 cigarettes daily or from all natural causes at the age of 40 years)

High   >1/100 (*cf.* transmission of measles/varicella or risk of GI effects of antibiotics; (Calman, 1996).

Numerical

When told of death rates of 1286 out of 10 000 some Japanese rated these as more risky than rates of 24.14 out of 100 (Yamagishi, 1997). The interpretation of numerical information is problematic (Edwards *et al.*, 2002).

Most authors use a scale of frequencies: 1 in 1000, etc. This is the basic method; but even when given quantitative data people interpret it differently. A value of 2 per cent was perceived by a sample of the general population as a risk of 9.5 per cent (SD 14.2 per cent) and a value of 0.02 per cent as a 7 per cent risk (SD 15.4 per cent) (Berry *et al.*, 2002). The numerical measures adopted include the following:

1. Scale of frequencies: 1 in 10, 1 in 100, 1 in 1000, etc.

2. Percentages. Best used for risks between 1/100 and 100/100.

3. Number needed to harm one (NNTH). The statistical or epidemiological expressions of frequency, e.g. odds ratio (OR), are not easily understood by the average physician or layman. It has been suggested that NNTH should be used instead: NNTH $+ 1/[(OR - 1) \times$ referent event rate] (Bjerre and LeLorier, 1997).

4. Logarithmic scale: $0 = 1$ in 10 000 000 000; $10 = 1$ in 1, etc.

5. Distance analogue scale: 1 m $= 1$ in 1; 100 km $= 1$ in 100 000; etc. (Calman and Royston, 1997).

6. Community risk scale: individual $= 1$ in 1; family $= 1$ in 10; street $= 1$ in 100; village $= 1$ in 1000, etc. (Calman and Royston, 1997).

7. Safety degree units (the number of noughts in the unicohort size, i.e. $5 = $ in 100 000 (Urquhart and Heilmann, 1983). Logically sound, but has not become popular.

8. Relative risk, absolute risk or odds ratio with 95 per cent confidence limits or excessive risk.

9. *p* values.

10. Number of ADRs per event prevented. Used by the MRC for a hypertension trial (Anon., 1985; Robson, 1997).

11. Lottery-based score (Barclay *et al.*, 1998; Berry *et al.*, 2003).

Graphical

Tables, histograms (bar graphs), graphs, survival curves, pie charts and icons (Edwards *et al.*, 2002). There is some evidence that icons are more likely to produce correct decisions than bar graphs, tables or pie charts, but they are disliked by physicians (Elting *et al.*, 1999).

Conclusion

The fact that patients and physicians have different perceptions of risk terms to the 'experts' means that patients are making decisions on 'incorrect' information and that further work is needed to find appropriate risk terms.

The risks we are prepared to take

It is very difficult to find out what risks the general public would be prepared to run for an effective drug, but one can study the risks they are prepared to take in everyday life and with certain common social drugs (see Table 1.7). The actions that various risks have provoked will give an idea as to whether the public considers them acceptable or not.

1. Fatal accidents presenting risks of 1:1000/person/year are infrequent. That immediate action is taken to reduce such hazards suggests that this level of risk is socially unacceptable.

2. At lethal accident levels of 1 in 10 000/person/year public money is spent to control their causes.

3. Mortality risks of 1:100 000/person/year are still considered candidates for some action but Knox (1975) argues that if the probability from a procedure is less than 1 in 100 000 the public concern ceases and it can be regarded as 'safe' and, therefore, acceptable.

4. Fatal accidents with a probability of 1:1 000 000/person/year are not of concern to most people. Just to put this figure into context, the incidence of fatal ADRs to prescription-only drugs is just less than one per million prescriptions dispensed (O'Brien, 1986).

These figures show the boundaries of acceptable risk to lie between 1:1 000 000 (those associated with natural hazards) and 1:1000, i.e. the annual *per capita* illness and disease

Table 1.7 The risks of common voluntary activities (Pochin, 1975; Dinman 1980a, b; Daily Telegraph, 1987)

Voluntary risk	Deaths/persons/year (odds)
Smoking (20 cigarettes per day)	1 in 200
Drinking (bottle of wine per day)	1 in 13 300
Soccer[a]	1 in 25 000
Cart racing	1 in 10 000
Car driving[a] (UK)	1 in 5900
Motorcycling[b]	1 in 50
Rock climbing[c]	1 in 7150
Taking contraceptive pills	1 in 50 000
Power boating	1 in 5900
Canoeing	1 in 100 000
Horse racing[a]	1 in 740
Amateur boxing[a]	1 in 2 000 000
Professional boxing[c]	1 in 14 300
Skiing	1 in 1 430 000
Pregnancy (UK)	1 in 4380
Abortion (legal less than 12 weeks)[d]	1 in 50 000
Abortion (legal more than 14 weeks)[d]	1 in 5900

[a] Based upon death/per million participants/year.
[b] A figure of one death per 1056 registered motorcyclists is quoted by Urquhart and Heilmann in *Risk Watch*.
[c] Based upon deaths/per million hours/year spent in sport.
[d] Based upon deaths/per million pregnancies per year.

risks. Society appears to accept voluntary risks with orders of magnitude greater than involuntary risks (Dinman, 1980a) (see Tables 1.7 and 1.8). Dinman (1980b) points out that the USA accepts 200 000 excess deaths a year associated with smoking (the figure given in 1996 is 400 000) and 20 000 excess deaths from not buckling seat belts will not pursue extreme risks posed by environmental contaminants. The number of premature deaths caused or accelerated by cigarette smoking in the USA as the equivalent of three fully loaded Boeing 747s (over 1500 people) crashing every day. There was considerable opposition in the UK to the parliamentary bill that made the fastening of front seat belts mandatory, a move that the BMA suggested would save more than 700 lives per annum and 11 000 seriously injured per annum (Daily Telegraph, 1981).

The risks we take with drugs

To compare these death rates with those of deaths caused by drugs is extremely difficult, since there is gross under-reporting of the latter. Therefore, the following figures must be considered in that light and also bearing in mind the source of the figures (i.e. seriously ill patients). In the BCDSP, 0.9 patients per 1000 were considered to have died as a result of drugs. The rates varied from zero in Israel and Italy to 1.4 per 1000 in New Zealand (Porter and Jick, 1977). Tables 1.7 and 1.8 have shown the involuntary risks that patients have to run and those voluntary risks they are prepared to exchange for various pleasurable pursuits. At lethal accident rates of 1:10 000/person/year public money is spent to control their causes and at 1:100 000/person/year mothers warn children of the dangers of playing with fire, of

Table 1.8   Rare (involuntary) risks in life (Dinman, 1980b)

Involuntary risks[a]	Risk of death/persons/year (odds)
Struck by auto (USA)	1 in 20 000
Struck by car (UK)	1 in 16 600
Floods (USA)	1 in 455 000
Earthquakes (California)	1 in 588 000
Tornados (Mid West)	1 in 455 000
Lightning (UK)	1 in 10 000 000
Falling aircraft (USA)	1 in 10 000 000
Falling aircraft (UK)	1 in 50 000 000
Explosion pressure vessel (USA)	1 in 20 000 000
Release from atomic power station:	
at site boundary (USA)	1 in 10 000 000
at 1 km (UK)	1 in 10 000 000
Flooding by dikes (Holland)	1 in 10 000 000
Bites of venomous creatures (UK)	1 in 5 000 000
Leukaemia	1 in 12 500
Influenza	1 in 9 000
Meteorite	1 in 100 billion

[a] These figures are only approximate and may have been calculated using different assumptions. Any individual figure should be treated with reserve.

drowning and of poison, and some people accept inconvenience, such as avoiding air travel (Dinman, 1980a). Where should we draw the line as acceptable risk with, say, a treatment with a new antihypertensive drug? It has been suggested (Anon., 1981b) that, at the time of marketing, risks of 1 in 100 should be known; but this figure is not the risk of deaths, only of ADRs. It would seem that a similar figure for post-marketing surveillance of 1 in 1000 (Inman, 1981) and 1 in 10 000 is acceptable (Shapiro, 1977) which would require a cohort of 10 000 to 20 000 individuals. If a side effect is exceedingly rare, say 1 in 50 000, then no formal system will be sufficiently cost effective to discover it.

The number of patients needed to assess risks

The description of a risk of 1 in 100 needs clarification. It probably refers to those distinct drug reactions for which there is no background incidence. There are two classifications of ADR from the statistical point of view:

1. The adverse reaction that is clearly an ADR and for which there is no naturally occurring background, e.g. the oculomucocutaneous syndrome with practolol (see Table 1.9).

2. The adverse reaction that either simulates disease or produces, in fact, an increase in a naturally occurring disease, e.g. dry eyes caused by beta-blockers (see Table 1.10).

All these tables are based on a 95 per cent probability of success, so that our 10 000

Table 1.9 Number of patients required with no background incidence of adverse reactions. Reprinted from *Trends in Pharmacological Science*, **2**, Lewis JA, Post-marketing surveillance: how many patients?, pp. 93–94, copyright (1981), with permission from Elsevier Science

Expected incidence of ADR	Required number of adverse reactions:		
	1	2	3
1 in 100	300	480	650
1 in 200	600	900	1,300
1 in 1000	3 000	4,800	6,500
1 in 2000	6 000	9,600	13 000
1 in 10 000	30 000	48 000	65 000

Table 1.10 Number of patients required in drug-treated group when background exists. Reprinted from *Trends in Pharmacological Science*, **2**, Lewis JA, Post-marketing surveillance: how many patients?, pp. 93–94, copyright (1981), with permission from Elsevier Science

Size of control	Background incidence of ADR	Required number of adverse reactions		
		1 in 100	1 in 1000	1 in 10 000
Infinite (background	1 in 10	10 000	980 000	98 000 000
incidence known)	1 in 100	1600	110 000	11 000 000
	1 in 1000	500	16 000	1 000 000
5 times as big as	1 in 10	12 000	1,200 000	120 000 000
treated group	1 in 100	9000	130 000	13 000 000
	1in 1000	700	19 000	1,400 000
Equal to treated group	1 in 10	20 000	2 000 000	200 000 000
	1 in 100	3200	220 000	22 000 000
	1 in 1000	1300	32 000	2,300 000

population will give a greater than 95 per cent chance of having at least three recognizable ADRs with an incidence of 1:1000 and a 95 per cent chance of discovering two recognizable ADRs with an incidence of 1:2000.

So, 10 000 patients will give a 95 per cent chance of discovering an additional incidence of 1 in 100 where the background incidence is 1 in 10, but there will be a less than 95 per cent chance of discovering an additional incidence of 1 in 1000 when the background incidence is 1 in 1000 (see Table 1.11).

The rule of three

If no AEs occur in N patients then the upper limit of the 95% CI for the frequency of events is approximately $3/N$. The numerators for the 95% CI upper limits for observed numerators of 0, 1, 2, 3 and 4 are about 3, 5, 7, 9 and 10 respectively (Newman, 1995).

Table 1.11 Number of patients required in drug-treated group to allow for examination of 100 adverse reactions (significance $p < 0.05$). Reprinted from *Trends in Pharmacological Science*, **2**, Lewis JA, Post-marketing surveillance: how many patients?, pp. 93–94, copyright (1981), with permission from Elsevier Science

Size of control	Background incidence of ADR	Additional incidence of adverse reaction		
		1 in 100	1 in 1000	1 in 10 000
Infinite (background incidence known)	1 in 100	23 000	2 000 000	220 000 000
	1 in 1000	3,100	250 000	24 000 000
	1 in 10 000	800	32 000	2,500 000
5 times as big as treated group	1 in 100	27 000	2,600 000	260 000 000
	1 in 1000	4000	300 000	29 000 000
	1 in 10 000	1300	40 000	3 000 000
Equal to treated group	1 in 100	46 000	4,400 000	440 000 000
	1 in 1000	7200	510 000	48 000 000
	1 in 10 000	2900	73 000	5,100 000

Monitoring for multiple adverse drug reactions

The figures above presume that one is only monitoring for one type of ADR, whereas in most cases we will be monitoring for an unknown number of ADRs; and since the 5 per cent level of significance is used, then of every 100 possible ADRs examined there could be five adverse reactions expected by chance (see Table 1.7). It must be realized that this type of post-marketing surveillance, i.e. without concurrent randomized controls, is searching for hypotheses and not testing them; and if it is accepted that nothing will be published until a hypothesis testing study is finished, then this risk is not important, except from the point of view of cost. However, if, as it seems, possible hypotheses are published, then the level of significance must be increased if we are to prevent more widespread apprehension (see Table 1.9). These figures presume that the drug is given to the same population as has the known background incidence of the disease. It is very unlikely that the background incidence will be known in the particular subset of the population who will be prescribed the drug. Another presumption is that there will be no dropout of patients over the monitoring period.

Conclusions

Very many fewer patients are required to detect an ADR that has no background incidence compared with one that mimics or increases a known disease. Nearly all ADRs mimic known diseases, and the means of differentiating between them often does not develop until several years have passed. If a new drug causes a modest increase (10 per cent) in the incidence of a common disease (1 in 100 per annum), then the number of patients needed for monitoring to discover this (250 000) is prohibitively large (Spriet-Pourra *et al.*, 1982).

Definitions

This excludes regulatory authority definitions where their meanings differ from the normal English meaning; for those see Chapter 9. The first three of these definitions should be used when addressing practising physicians or lay people.

Adverse drug reaction   A reaction is a response to a stimulus and, as such, implies certainty as to cause and effect. If anything less than certainty needs to be conveyed then an adjective must precede the phrase, e.g. possible (see FDA definition, p.•)

Adverse event   This covers all types of event not necessarily medical. It has been defined in the medical context as 'unintended injuries caused by medical management rather than disease process (Vincent *et al.*, 2001) or 'an injury caused by medical management (rather than the disease process) that resulted in either prolonged hospital stay or disability at discharge' and its corollary 'adverse drug event' (Leape *et al.*, 1991; Thomas and Brennan, 2000). It is important to realize that since it is caused by 'medical management' it refers to all types of mistake, including preventable type-A ADRs. An ADR may be due to: error in dose or method of use, failure to recognize possible antagonistic or complementary drug–drug interactions, inadequate follow-up of therapy, inappropriate drug, avoidable delay in treatment, physician practising outside area of expertise (Leape *et al.*, 1991).

Expect   The *Concise Oxford Dictionary* 1995 (COD): 'assume as a future event or occurrence'; implies that what is expected will *probably* occur (Brown *et al.*, 2001).

Side effect   Any unintended effect of a pharmaceutical product occurring at doses normally used in man that is related to the pharmacological properties of the drug (http://www.who-umc.org) as adopted by National centres participating in The WHO International Drug Monitary Programme, September 1991. COD: 'a secondary, usually undesirable effect'.

Signal   Reported information on a possible causal relationship between an AE and a drug, the relationship being unknown or incompletely documented previously. Usually more than a single report is required to generate a signal, depending upon the seriousness of the event and the quality of the information (WHO, 1991; Delamothe, 1992).

Associated   Associated with the use of the drug means that there is a reasonable possibility that the experience may have been caused by the drug (21CFR312.32). This differs from the COD meaning of 'A thing connected to another'. The glossary in the third edition of *Pharmacoepidemiology* states: 'An association is when two events occur together more often than one would expect by chance'. Types of association:

- none (independent)
- artifactual (spurious or false)
- chance (unsystematic variation)
- bias (systematic variation)
- indirect (confounded)

- causal (direct or true) (Strom, 1994, 2000).

Most of the associations occurring in pharmacovigilance are temporal in nature, and our task is to decide in which of the six groups a particular association belongs.

Idiosyncrasy   Implies an inherent qualitatively abnormal reaction to a drug (Hoigné, 1997).

Clinically significant   Individual physicians will differ in their interpretation as to what is clinically significant. For the sake of uniformity, within the clinical trial field I would suggest that, for the individual patient, it should be 'any event that requires a change in the medical management of a patient'; for groups of adverse events, clinical or laboratory, it should be 'any group of events that requires a change in management for future patients taking that drug'.

ADR incidence   A numerator may be much smaller when a specific definition is used compared with a term written by the clinician; e.g. the CIOMS definition of pancytopenia (anaemia: Hb level <100 g/l; neutropenia: polymorphonuclear count $<1.5 \times 10^9$/l; thrombocytopenia: platelets $<100 \times 10^9$/l) (Benichou and Solal-Celigny, 1991) compared with the clinician's term 'pancytopenia' which may reflect the normal ranges (Hb $\male$ <130 g/l, $\female$ <120 g/l; neutrophils $<2.0 \times 10^9$/l; platelets $<130 \times 10^9$/l. A denominator derived from the meta-analysis of publications of all the clinical trials with a drug may underestimate it due to the exclusion of unpublished studies or overestimate it by duplication of publications (Tramèr *et al.*, 1997). It is important when calculating incidence rates of ADRs that any provisos are made clear. Frequently, there will be a genuine difference of opinion as to the most appropriate way to calculate or illustrate data; when in doubt, an independent point of view should be sought.

Classification of adverse drug reactions

Severity classification

Severity, which is the quantification of the reaction symptoms, mild, moderate or severe, and are best used as grades of discomfort. These are subjective symptoms and, as such, will vary from person to person. These have been defined by Tangrea *et al.* (1991):

Mild   Slightly bothersome; relieved with symptomatic treatment.

Moderate   Bothersome, interferes with activities; only partially relieved with symptomatic treatment.

Severe   Prevents regular activities; not relieved with symptomatic treatment.

The Early Clinical Drug Evaluation Program (ECDEU) classification is:

Mild   Symptoms do not alter patient's normal functioning.

Moderate   Symptom produces some degree of impairment to function but not hazardous, uncomfortable or embarrassing to patient.

Severe   Symptom definitely hazardous to well-being, significant impairment of functioning or incapacitation (Assenzo and Sho, 1982).

A classification used in German psychiatric hospitals is:

Grade 1   ADR did not lead to any change in medication.

Grade 2   ADR led to a change in medication in the form of dose reduction and/or additional treatment to counteract the ADR.

Grade 3   ADR led to discontinuation of the medication suspected of causing the ADR (including cases where the drug would have been discontinued had it not been vital) (Grohmann et al., 1989).

Adverse event classification

This classification accounts for the source of the reported data, the potential clinical importance and the role of the report in defining the safety profile of the drug.

Class I   Machine findings or findings made by humans using machines.

Class II   Findings of study observers related to the patient's physical condition.

Class III Reports by the subject or patient.

Each of these may be subclassified by somebody with clinical knowledge as:

Subclass A May lead to morbidity or mortality, either acutely or in the near term.

Subclass B May have historically been associated with the class of drug and have expected benign outcomes.

Subclass C Have undetermined significance at the time of reporting (Alexandra, 1991).

Pharmacological classification

Type A (augmented)   Reactions that result from an exaggeration of a drug's normal pharmacological actions when given in the usual therapeutic dose; normally dose dependent. Sometimes referred to as Type 1.

Type B (bizarre)   Those that represent a novel response not expected from known pharmacological action (Rawlins and Thompson, 1977). Sometimes referred to as Type 2.

Type C (chronic)   Adaptive changes, rebound phenomena, other long-term effects.

Type D (delayed)   Carcinogenesis, effects concerned with reproduction (impaired ferti-
                          lity), teratogenesis (adverse effects on the foetus during the early
                          stages of pregnancy), adverse effects on the foetus during the later
                          stages of pregnancy, drugs in breast milk (Aronson and White,
                          1996; Brodie, 1996).

The characteristics for types A and B are listed in Table 1.12. An excellent review of the
ADR mechanisms and their relationship to these classifications has been published by Royer
(1997).

Table 1.12   Characteristics of type A and B drug reactions; after Rawlins and Thompson (1977)

Type A (augmented)	Type B (bizarre)
Pharmacological	Hypersensitivity or idiosyncratic
Dose related	Not dose related
Predictable	Unpredictable
Common	Rare
Usually not serious	Usually serious
Majority discovered before marketing	Majority discovered after marketing
Relatively low mortality	Relatively high mortality

Reaction time classification

Reaction time is defined as the time between the last drug exposure and the appearance of
the first symptom (Hoigné *et al.*, 1990):

   Acute, 0–60 min – this includes 4.3 per cent of reactions.

   Sub-acute, 1–24 h – this includes 86.5 per cent of reactions.

   Latent, 1 day–several weeks – this includes 3.5 per cent of reactions.

Adverse reaction profile

Ideally, an adverse reaction of a drug should have a profile that consists of the following
elements:

* Manifestation (clinical or laboratory), both subjective and/or objective.

* Graded, both for severity and seriousness.

* Frequency or incidence, both absolute and relative to similar drugs, with CIs.

* Mechanism of action.

* Causality.

* Predisposing factors, i.e. renal function, pharmacokinetic factors, etc.

- Treatment and its effect.

- Reversibility or sequelae.

It will be apparent that the present SPCs and the proposed modifications in the CIOMS III report do not provide this data.

Adverse events in a patient's life

The AE must be discussed in the context of the many AEs in the patient's life:

1. The AE is one of the many minor abnormalities that occur to normal persons (Reidenberg and Lowenthal, 1968) – see next section.

2. The AE is part of a disease or is a complication of a disease, which is either that for which the drug was prescribed or another disease.

3. The AE may be caused by a man-made chemical. These may include environmental chemicals. Systemic toxicity can be caused by 220 environmental chemicals, of which 149 are neurotoxins. The signs and symptoms are usually non-specific (Grandjean *et al.*, 1991).

4. Effect of illegal drugs.

5. OTC drugs. Many countries are encouraging the transfer of drugs from prescription-only medicines (POMs) to OTC to relieve the costs of their health services, so we must expect a large increase in their usage.

6. Abuse of prescription drugs, OTCs and alcohol and herbs.

7. Herbal medicines (see below). In a Hong Kong hospital, three out of 1701 patients admitted had reactions to Chinese herbal drugs (Ernst, 1998). Patients may not tell their doctor that they are taking them. In the USA, 70 per cent of patients did not tell their physician or pharmacist (Miller, 1998). Many herbal remedies are not labelled with their ingredients.

8. Food allergies. Peanut and other nut allergies are probably the leading cause of fatal food allergy (Sampson, 1996); shellfish and eggs can cause acute allergic reactions (Finn, 1992).

9. Food additives:

    - Sulphiting agents can cause flushing, itching of the mouth and skin, and asthma. About 5 per cent of asthmatics are susceptible. They may be present in wines, other drinks, shrimps and processed potatoes.

- Nitrates (E249–E252) can cause flushing and giddiness. They give preserved meats their pink colour.

- Colouring agents.

- Flavouring agents may exacerbate eczema.

Adverse reactions to common foods occur in 1.4–1.9 per cent of the population (Lessof, 1992).

10. Complementary medicine. The exponential rise in use of therapies that have no logical explanation over the last few years has produced AEs. Even homeopathy can produce ADRs, e.g. anaphylactic shock, measles-like rash, erythroderma (Aberer, 1991); see Bibliography.

Symptoms in healthy persons

Reidenberg and Lowenthal (1968) investigated 414 healthy students and hospital staff of Temple University, USA, taking no medication, and surveyed their symptoms retrospectively using a questionnaire. Only 19 per cent stated that during the previous 72 hours they had experienced none of the 25 symptoms listed. The median number of symptoms experienced per person was two. Thirty people experienced six or more symptoms. The symptoms listed varied from pains in muscles and joints, headaches, skin rashes and urticaria to mental symptoms and changes in bowel function, all of which have been described as ADRs. Their order of frequency was: fatigue, inability to concentrate, excessive sleepiness, bleeding from the gums after brushing teeth, irritability, headache, nasal congestion, pain in the muscles, insomnia, lack of appetite, pain in joints, faintness on first standing up, skin rash, bad dreams, dry mouth, constipation, palpitations, bleeding or bruising, giddiness or weakness, diarrhoea, nausea, fever and urticaria. These findings were repeated in a further study in Germany 30 years later. Here, there were two personality groups: the first were not nervous, were emotionally stable and were success motivated and these had fewer AEs. The second group were nervous, emotionally unstable and had lack of motivation and these had more AEs (Meyer et al., 1996). Only 26.3 per cent of healthy volunteers denied having had symptoms similar to side effects in the 3 days before a study (Khosla et al., 1992).

The variety of symptoms that can be caused by a disease or any of its complications is vast; but, taking the specific area of hypertension, an AE questionnaire (Bulpitt, 1974) has been used in a survey of normal subjects, untreated hypertensives and treated hypertensives (Bulpitt et al., 1976). So. The normal patients were randomly selected from a local general practice register and the untreated patients were newly referred hypertensives at the Hammersmith Hospital. Although the survey showed that headaches, unsteadiness, light-headedness or faintness and nocturia could actually be caused by raised blood pressure, this was so in only a proportion of those patients complaining of these symptoms (see Table 1.13). It can be seen how common many of these symptoms are in all three groups. Consequently, for person complaining of a symptom, and who was on treatment, there is a difficulty in allocating that symptom to a particular group (Joubert et al., 1977).

Table 1.13 Symptoms in normal persons, untreated hypertensives and treated hypertensives. From Bulpitt *et al.* (1976), *British Heart Journal*. Reproduced by permission of BMJ Publishing Group

Symptom	Normal (%)	Untreated hypertensives (%)	Treated hypertensives (%)
Sleepiness	**31.4**	**43.2**	51.3**
Dry mouth	20.5	**23.7**	**40.2****
Unsteadiness on standing or in the morning	7.9***	**35.4**	33.5
Nocturia	**45.3****	**68.4**	73.2
Diarrhoea	**15.5**	25.8	**30.4**
Depression	**34.3**	44.7**	**29.4**
Blurred vision	14.7	29.8*	20.6
Weak limbs	**18.4**	34.0	**26.4** ns
Nasal stuffiness	**26.8**	**29.7** ns	– ns
Poor concentration	**4.0**	**12.8** ns	– ns
Vivid dreams	25.3	27.8 ns	– ns
Nausea	12.0	19.8 ns	– ns
Impotence	6.9	17.1	24.6***
Slow walking pace	9.5***	24.2***	**37.0****
Waking headache	15.1	**31.3****	15.5
Failure of ejaculation	0	7.3	25.6***

Asterisks within table refer to χ^2 comparisons between one result and the result in bold in other columns: $^*p < 0.05$; $^{**}p < 0.01$; $^{***}p < 0.001$; ns not significant.

Adverse reactions to placebo

A placebo can be defined as 'any component of a therapy (or control in experimental studies) that is without specific activity for the condition being treated or being evaluated' (Joyce, 1982) or 'any therapeutic procedure (or that component of any therapeutic procedure) which is given deliberately to have an effect, or unknowingly has an effect, on a patient, symptom, syndrome, or disease but which is objectively without specific activity on the condition being treated' (Shapiro, 1961). It originates from the Latin *piacere* and translates as 'I shall please'.

Symptoms that are, in some part, caused by treatment must be divided into those effects caused by the chemical constituents and those caused by the giving of a 'medication', even though the 'medication' is known not to cause side effects by its chemical nature. The latter are referred to as 'placebo responses or effects' and have specific characteristics that resemble those of active chemicals. In clinical trials with a placebo group the 'placebo response' is made up of several factors:

1. The natural course of the underlying disease (indication for treatment).

2. Any other incidental medical event unconnected with either the underlying indication or the placebo medication, e.g. a cold.

3. Regression towards the mean. This phenomenon is due to the probability that the patient

on presentation to the doctor is likely to be at the peak of their problems and, since there is fluctuation of all biological variables, the odds will be on the problem not being so intense at the next visit. This has been put forward as a cause of the placebo effect on efficacy, but with an AE it may be a factor in a positive dechallenge – see p. • for further details (McDonald *et al.*, 1989).

4. The effects of being in a clinical trial. These may be mental, e.g. increased anxiety, or physical, e.g. the wearing off of the 'white coat hypertension' as they become used to the trial circumstances, i.e. their blood pressure is lower on the second occasion. In hospitalized volunteers there was a 10 per cent increase in heart rate, the blood pressure remained unchanged but there were increases in the time to sleep iniation and asthenia self-rating suggesting poor neuropsychiatric tolerability (Rosenzweig *et al.*, 1995). The general beneficial effect of being the object of special attention, as in a clinical trial, is known as the 'Hawthorne effect'. It was named after the town in Illinois where work studies at the Western Electric plant, Hawthorne, noted the effect (Mayo, 1933).

5. The true additional affect of adding the placebo medication (Ernst and Resch, 1995).

The first four of these types of event are those of the untreated disease, and only factor five is the true placebo factor. It is extremely unusual to have a placebo control group and an untreated control group in clinical trials. This is because the difference between the active drug group and the placebo group represents the effect of the active drug. The other factors should be equally distributed in both the active drug group and the placebo group (Ernst and Resch, 1995).

Patients are easily prejudiced by past experience, friends, physicians, consent forms and the media; and these prejudices may be manifest in the effects of placebos: consent form and GI symptoms (Myers *et al.*, 1987); patients with food allergies having the same symptoms with saline as well as with the allergen (Jewett *et al.,* 1990); headaches with non-existent electric currents when warned that electric currents passed across the head could cause headaches (Schweiger and Parducci, 1981); asthma with plastic roses (Dekker and Groen, 1956; Luparello *et al.*, 1968).

Commonest complaints

A review of 67 publications for unwanted or toxic side effects that occurred during the administration of a placebo showed that drowsiness was the most common side effect, followed by headache. Stimulation of the central nervous system, manifested as daytime nervousness or insomnia, was the third most common effect, followed by nausea and constipation (Pogge, 1963). In 80 healthy volunteers, taking a single dose of placebo, control for a drug when first used in man, there were 50 AEs. In order of frequency they were (Kitchener *et al.*, 1996): headache 17.6 per cent, rhinitis 7.1 per cent, bruising at injection site 4.7 per cent, pharyngitis 3.5 per cent and coughing 2.4 per cent.

The numbers and types of AE will depend on all the factors previously mentioned plus those due to the physical circumstances of the study. The adverse effects of placebo were called 'nocebo' effects by Kennedy (1961). Nocebo comes from the Latin *nocere*, to harm, hence *nocebo* I will harm; however, *placebo* indicates the intention to help the patient. Nobody prescribes with the intention of harming. It is, therefore, not an appropriate word.

Physical changes

Although the symptoms are activated via the mind they can produce physical changes to the nose, skin, bladder, oesophagus, stomach, colon, heart and blood vessels, and kidneys (Wolf, 1950, 1959a; Wolf and Pinsky, 1954) and effects such as vomiting, sweating, diarrhoea, constipation, eosinophilia, hyperacidity and skin rashes (Joyce, 1982). One case has been reported of a patient meeting the definition of being 'dependent' upon a placebo (Vinar, 1969). Other effects caused by placebo include dermatitis medicamentosa, anaphylactoid reaction, urticaria and angioneurotic oedema and hallucinations (Thompson, 1982).

Frequency of placebo reactions

The placebo tends to increase the severity of symptoms that pre-exist and females tend to have more frequent and severe placebo reactions than males (Domecq *et al.*, 1980). When placebos were administered to professional people, 58 per cent complained of one or more side effects and, contrary to expectations, some symptoms decreased in the institutionalized aged when they were given placebo (Wolf, 1950).

Variation with age and sex

On the whole, the incidence of placebo reaction rises linearly with age (Green, 1964). However, it is not known whether adjustment had been made for the number of drugs taken in addition to placebo, since with active drugs the same rise with age was found to disappear when adjusted for the number of drugs taken (Weber and Griffin, 1986). Occurrence is higher in females than in males (Green, 1964); again, could this be due to the females taking more drugs?

Variability in types of effect

Placebo side effects, when the placebo is used as a control for an active drug, are often similar in type to the side effects of the active drug itself (Letemendia and Harris, 1959), throbbing headaches after placebo in a hydralazine study; 'closed' nose after reserpine placebo (Wolf, 1959b); diminished perception of high tones after streptomycin placebo (Tucker, 1954). Once a patient on placebo or active drug has complained of an AE, an observer will note that these patients have more symptoms than those who did not complain of the AE, suggesting that there is an increased interest in those patients who show change (Thompson, 1982).

Psychological differences in placebo reactors

Lasagna *et al.* (1954) were able to show differences of attitude, habits, educational background and personality structure between the persons who consistently responded to placebo and those who did not, but that reactors were not 'whiners' or 'nuisances', not typically male or female, not younger or old and had the same average intelligence as the non-responders. In volunteers, placebos can cause effects in 66 per cent of subjects (Knowles and Lucas, 1960) and 35 per cent of patients (Beecher, 1955).

When healthy French volunteers were tested with the Bortner rating scale the majority were found to have type-A personalities, i.e. they were 'hurried, hard-driving, competitive and aggressive' and 50 per cent of type A had AEs on placebo compared with 17 per cent of type-B volunteers (Drici et al., 1995).

Placebo pharmacology

It has also been shown that the placebo has its own pharmacology with peak effects, cumulative effects, carry-over effects and a varying efficacy, depending on the severity of the complaint being treated (Lasagna et al., 1958). Symptoms generally become more frequent and severe with an increase in the number of placebo tablets (Green, 1964). Placebos can relieve post-operative dental pain and naloxone blocks this effect, suggesting that the placebo acts through endorphin release (Levine et al., 1978; Fields and Levine, 1981). However, a leader in The Lancet (Anon., 1983), quotes that there is no evidence for an opioid component in placebo analgesia and goes on to say that there is no reason to believe that the placebo effect has a single specific mechanism. The former statement is supported by a study using naloxone with dipipanone and placebo analgesia for tourniquet pain (Posner and Burke, 1985). Placebo treatment for pain was associated with 'increased activity in rostral anterior cingulate cortex', as were opioids (Petrovic et al., 2002).

It has been argued that most improvements attributed to the placebo effect are actually instances of statistical regression, i.e. a tendency of extreme measures to move closer to the mean when repeated (McDonald et al., 1983).

Severity of placebo reactions

The fact that placebo reactions can be severe has been noted by several authors (Wolf and Pinsky, 1954; Green, 1964). In a Norwegian multicentre study (Norwegian Multicenter Study Group, 1981) on the comparison of timolol and placebo in inducing reduction of morbidity and reinfarction in patients surviving acute myocardial infarction, many patients were withdrawn due to an adverse reaction and were subsequently found to be on placebo.

Range of placebo reactions

In a study of more than 1000 cases of side effects of placebo there were 35 different symptoms. The most important are given in Table 1.14 (Schindel, 1972).

It will be apparent that it may well be impossible to tell whether a side effect, which has occurred whilst on active treatment, is due to that treatment or might have occurred if a placebo had been given instead.

The influence of the placebo administrator

After extraction of teeth, under a local anaesthetic, patients assessed their pain using a McGill pain questionnaire at 1 h and 10 min before and after an IV injection or no treatment. Clinicians knew that one group had placebo or analgesic antagonist (Group PN) and the

Table 1.14   Important side effects of placebo; after Schindel (1972)

Symptom	Number with symptom	Total number of treated patients	Percentage of treated patients (%)
Numbness	36	72	50
Headache	23	92	25
Fatigue	10	57	18
Sensation of heaviness	14	77	18
Inability to concentrate	14	92	15
Drowsiness	7	72	10
Nausea	9	92	10
Dryness of the mouth	7	77	9
General weakness	5	57	9
Flushes	6	77	8

other group (Group PNF) would receive placebo plus analgesic or analgesic antagonist. The trial was double-blind. The two placebo groups differed only in the clinicians' knowledge that the possible double-blind had been prescribed or where there had been product substitution. This may also give rise to false positive and negative rechallenge tests (Napke and Stevens, 1984).

Infectiousness of adverse drug reactions

A trial in 28 chronic psychotics, who had been shown to be stable over a period of 5 months, compared placebo and nicotinic acid, 100 mg. The latter produces flushing of the skin with a sensation of heat and sometimes skin irritation, which appears within 30 min and disappearing within a further 30 min. The patients had either schizophrenia or depression and had had no recent psychiatric treatment. The nurses were told that it was a trial of a new preparation. They were questioned about each patient before, during and after the 9 week trial with particular reference to changes in habit, amount of activity and occupation. They were also asked to report at once any unusual signs or symptoms and a number of likely ones were listed, including: giddiness, nausea or vomiting, headaches, paleness or flushing, drowsiness, fits or faints, loss of appetite, abdominal pain, jaundice and restlessness. Of the nicotinic acid group, 10/14 had flushing: two during the first week, another two during the second week, and a further two during the third week, three during the fourth week and one during the seventh week.

Five of the 14 patients in the placebo group also had flushing: two during the fourth week, two more during the eighth week and one during the ninth week.

There were also many other reports of symptoms, of which 50 reports were in the 15 patients with flushing and 28 in those without flushing, i.e. nearly a ratio of 2:1. These results suggested that the placebo patients 'caught' the flushing from the patients on nicotinic acid and that once a side effect is noticed more attention is focused on those patients or volunteers. The slow recognition of the flushing is also noticeable (Letemendia and Harris, 1959).

Another study in mental patients, mostly schizophrenics and all female, compared placebo and chlorpromazine. After a 2 week baseline period on their usual chlorpromazine dose, group A were changed to placebo but only the pharmacist knew of the change. Then,

2 weeks later group B was changed to placebo. After a further week, when group A had been on placebo for 1 month and group B for 1 week, the nurses were told to administer placebo previously believing that they had been on chlorpromazine. After a further week the placebo was withdrawn and the patients knew themselves to be without medication. The number of AE reports was as shown in Table 1.15.

Table 1.15 AE reports among psychiatric patients in chlorpromazine/placebo study; after Le Vay (1960)

Trial week	Group A reports		Group B reports	
1	Chlorpromazine	4	Chlorpromazine	8
2	Chlorpromazine	6	Chlorpromazine	6
3	Placebo	5	Chlorpromazine	9
4	Placebo	5	Chlorpromazine	5
5	Placebo	4	Placebo	4
6	Placebo	4	Placebo	9
7	Prescribed placebo	17	Prescribed placebo	23
8	No drugs	18	No drugs	27

It can be seen that substitution of placebo produced no deterioration, but on the nurses being told to administer placebo the reports trebled. Six patients were described as unmanageable. One ward sister who had predicted that withdrawal of chlorpromazine would have no effect had no rises in the number of reports of disturbances, whereas another sister, who had foretold of problems if chlorpromazine was withdrawn, found the number of disturbances per week rose from one to 17 and she threatened to resign (Le Vay, 1960). It would appear that the placebo by itself was as effective as chlorpromazine, but that its adverse effect on withdrawal was in the mind of the observer.

A three-way comparison of aspirin, sulfinpyrazone and placebo in patients with unstable angina took place at three different centres A, B and C, and they used a questionnaire to collect AE information. Minor GI symptoms were reported by 65 per cent in centre A, 66 per cent in centre B and 39 per cent centre C ($p < 0.001$). The only difference found between the three centres was that the consent form omitted mentioning GI symptoms in centre C (Myers *et al.*, 1987). Levine (1987) suggested that the way round the problem was to introduce some false side-effects into the consent form. This would only introduce more problems and cannot be recommended.

The possibility that a patient package insert (PPI) might encourage patients to report more side effects was excluded in a study in the USA of 249 mild hypertensives given thiazides (56 per cent black and 33 per cent Spanish Americans). Two-thirds were given a PPI and one-third were not. There was no difference in the number of AEs reported, but those given the PPI attributed more of them to the drug (Morris and Kanouse, 1982). Since physicians no longer prescribe placebos, complementary medicine has filled the void.

Herbal medicines

A UK survey showed that 13 per cent of the public used herbal remedies at least once a month, with 10 per cent using them at least weekly; but 17 per cent of all those who had used herbal remedies said that they would not tell their doctor that they were using them if prescribed a conventional medicine. In the USA the figure was 49 per cent for the year 1997, and for the same period the Canadian figure was 24 per cent (Brazier and Levine, 2003). Reports to the MCA relating to herbal medicines were less than 0.5 per cent of the total (NAO, 2003).

There has been a move towards making these require a licence (De Smet, 1995a); in the meanwhile their usage is increasing, and some are dangerous:

- Ephedra, also known as Ma Huang, but better known as ephedrine, causes deaths from cardiac arrhythmias, cerebral vascular accident (CVA), hypertension (Josefson, 1996).

- Respiratory distress (bronchospasm) with royal jelly (not herbal, but a bee product) (Peacock *et al.*, 1995).

- Hepatitis (Carlson, 1990) with horse chestnut leaf (*Aesculus hippocastanum*) and lactone, which is sometimes adulterated with other drugs (De Smet *et al.*, 1995b).

- Hepatotoxicity with chaparrel (*Larrea tridentata*).

- Chronic nutmeg (*Myristica fragrans*) psychosis (Brenner *et al.*, 1993).

- An outbreak of fibrosing interstitial nephritis in 70 Belgians was caused by a herbal slimming preparation.

- Cardiac arrhythmias (bi-directional tachycardia) and death with *Aconitum* species (Tai *et al.*, 1993a, b).

- Renal failure and carcinogenesis with *Aristolochic* species. Withdrawn from market.

- Neonatal hyperbilirubinemia with berberine (*Berberis vulgaris*) and Chuen-li.

- Hepatotoxicity and carcinogenicity with comfrey (*Symphytum officinale*).

- Pennyroyal (*Mentha pulegium*) has caused 22 cases of severe toxic effects: hepatotoxicity, renal damage, fatalities (Ernst, 2000).

- Germander (*Teucrium chamaedrys*) has been linked to 30 cases of acute liver failure (Ernst, 1998).

- Aplastic anaemia with pokeweed (*Pilocarpus pennatifolius*), contains pilocarpine.

- Carcinogenicity with sassafras (*Sassafras albidum*).

- Central nervous system depression and fatal hepatic veno-occlusive disease due to pyrrolizidine alkaloids (*Croalaria*, *Cynoglossum*, *Eupatorium*, *Heliotropium*, *Petasites*, *Senecio* and *Symphytum*) with herbal teas (Snodgrass, 2001).

- Kava (*Piper methysticum*) may be responsible for 30 cases of liver toxicity (Burros, 2002). Withdrawn from the market.

- Sparteine (*Cytisus scoparius*) can cause respiratory arrest, circulatory collapse and stimulates uterine motility. Withdrawn from the market.

- *Ginkgo biloba* increased bleeding time, anaphylaxis and arrhythmias. IV drug withdrawn from market in Germany.

- Echinacea (purple cornflower root) if used for more than 8 weeks can cause liver toxicity (Miller, 1998) and has been associated with allergic reactions.

- Ginseng can cause hypoglycaemia and inhibits platelet aggregation (Reactions 861, 2001).

Others are dangerous because they have been adulterated with metals (Pb, As, Hg, Cd, Ti) or pharmaceuticals, e.g. NSAIDs, paracetamol, corticosteroids or benzodiazepines (Karunanithy and Sumita, 1991; De Smet, 1995b; Ko, 1998). Five brands of Chinese anti-diabetics contained glyburide and phenformin. ADRs to herbal medicines are probably underreported, as 67 per cent of patients would not consult their doctor for a serious suspected ADR (Barnes *et al.*, 1998).

Herbal–drug interactions

Siberian ginseng, plantain and hawthorn can interact with digoxin. Licorice (*Glycyrrhiza glabra*) can interact with prednisone and spironolactone. Evening primrose oil and borage are contraindicated in patients taking anti-convulsants. Feverfew, garlic (*Allium sativum*), dong quai (*Angelica sinensis*), danshen (*Salvia militiorrhiza*), ginger, ginseng and *Ginkgo biloba* all affect bleeding time and, therefore, probably interact with Warfarin. St John's Wort (*Hypericum perforatum*) should not be taken with monoamine oxidase inhibitor (MAOI) or selective serotonin reuptake inhibitor (SSRIs). It induces cytochrome P450 (CYP2C9) and interacts with Warfarin, also may induce CYP3A4 probably interacting with oral contraceptives (Hartmann *et al.*, 2000).

Some final food for thought

It has been estimated that the average cost of developing a new drug is US$802 million (Tufts Center, 2001). The time from start of research until marketing is a minimum of 12 years, is usually 15 years and may be up to 30 years and of those that reach the market 80 per cent fail to cover their development costs (Gittens, 1996). Only five out of 5000 compounds ever make it to human testing (Sylvestri, 1996). Only 23 per cent of drugs that begin clinical testing receive marketing approval (DiMasi *et al.*, 1991). Since 1972, 3–4 per cent of new active substances licensed in the UK have been withdrawn for safety reasons (Rawlins, 1995). It should be clear from this chapter that separating the AEs due to a drug from the many other similar AEs due to normal physiological variation, disease, environmental chemicals, placebo, food allergies, food additives, drug excipients, drug withdrawal and rebound reaction is a difficult and complicated task. The drug disasters of the past and the number of drugs removed from the market because of ADRs indicate that, too often, their discovery is delayed until too many patients have suffered. The subsequent chapters attempt to describe the methods currently available for the early detection of the new ADRs.

References

Aberer W (1991). Homeopathic preparations – severe adverse effects, unproven benefits. *Dermatologica* **182**(4): 253.

Abraham J (1995). Opren/Oraflex – the making of a drug disaster. In *Science, Politics and the Pharmaceutical Industry*. UCL Press; 98–178.

Alexandra WJ (1991). Adverse events: a classification system for use in clinical trials. *Drug Inf J* **25**: 457–459.

Alvarez-Requejo A, Carvaajal A, Vega TL and Bégaud B (1994). Undereporting of adverse drug reactions in a Spanish regional centre of pharmacovigilance. *Drug Inf J* Abstr. 249 (Suppl. 1): S104.

Anon. (1880). *Leader. Br Med J*: 2984.

Anon (1981b). Pertussis vaccine. *Br Med J* **282**: 1563.

Anon. (1983). *Leader. Lancet* **ii**: 624.

Anon. (1985). MRC trial of treatment of mild hypertension: principal results. Medical Research Council Working Party [comment]. [Clinical Trial. Journal Article. Randomized Controlled Trial]. *Br Med J Clin Res Ed.* **291**(6488): 97–104.

Anon. (1994). Rules violated in Fialuridine trial. *Reactions*, 21st May, p. 3.

Arneborn P and Palmbled J (1982). Drug-induced neutropenia a survey for Stockholm 1973–1978. *Acta Med Scand* **212**: 289–292.

Aronson JK and White NJ (1996). *Principles of Clinical Pharmacology and Drug Therapy in Oxford Textbook of Medicine*. Third edition on compact disc. Oxford University Press.

Ashworth J (1997). *Science, Policy and Risk*. Royal Society of London.

Assenzo JR and Sho VS (1982). Use of statistics in the analysis of side-effect data from clinical trials of psychoactive agents. *Prog Neuro-psychopharmacol Biol Psychiatry* **6**: 543–550.

Atkin PA and Shenfield GM (1995). Medication related adverse reactions and the elderly: a literature review. *Adverse Drug React Toxicol Rev* **14**(3): 175–191.

Atkins MJ (1995). Who discovered inhalation anaesthesia? *Pharm Med* **9**: 33–34.

Audit Commission (2001). A spoonful of sugar. Medicines management in NHS hospitals.

Avery AA, Taylor RL, Partidge M, Neil K *et al.* (2001). Investigating preventable drug-related admissions to a medical admissions unit. *Pharmacoepidemiol Drug Saf* **10**(S103): 243.

Ayani I, Aguirre C, Gutierrez G, Madariaga A *et al.* (1999). A cost-analysis of suspected adverse drug reactions in a hospital emergency ward. *Pharmacoepidemiol Drug Saf* **8**: 529–534.

Bader J-P (1981). *Scrip*, No. 639, 1.

Bains N and Hunter D (1999). Adverse reporting on adverse reactions. *Can Med Assoc J* **160**(3): 350–351.

Bakke OM, Wardell WM and Lasagna L (1984). Drug discontinuations in the United Kingdom and the United States, 1964 to 1983: issues of safety. *Clin Pharmacol Ther* **35**(3): 559–567.

Bakke OM, Manocchia M, Abajo F, Kaitin KI *et al.* (1995). Drug safety discontinuations in the United Kingdom, the United States, and Spain from 1974 through 1993: a regulatory perspective. *Clin Pharmacol Ther* **58**(1): 108–117.

Barnes J, Mills SY, Abbot NC, Willoughby M *et al.* (1998). Different standards for reporting ADRs to herbal remedies and conventional OTC medicines: face-to-face interviews with 515 users of herbal remedies. *Br J Clin Pharmacol* **45**(5): 496–500.

Barros (1935). *Semana Med* **42**: 907.

Bass R (1987). Risk–benefit decisions in product licence applications. In *Medicines and Risk/Benefit Decisions*, Walker SR and Asscher AW (eds). MTP Press Ltd: 127–135.

Bateman DN, Lee A, Rawlins MD and Smith JM (1991). Geographical differences in adverse drug reaction reporting rates in the northern region. *Br J Clin Pharmacol*: 188–189.

Bates DW, Cullen DJ, Laird N, Petersoen LA *et al.* (1995). Incidence of adverse drug events and potential adverse drug events. *J Am Med Assoc* **274**: 29–34.

Bates DW, Spell N, Cullen DJ, Burdick E, *et al.* (1997). The cost of adverse drug events in hospitalised patients. *J Am Med Assoc* **277**: 307–311.

Baum C, Faich GA and Anello C (1987) Differences in manufacturers reporting of ADR to the FDA in 1984. *Drug Inf J* **21**: 257.

Baum C, Anello C, Faich GA, Dreis M, *et al.* (1988) National ADR surveillance. *Arch Intern Med* **148**: 785.

Beardon PHG, McGilchrist MM, McKendrick AD, McDevitt DG *et al.* (1993). Primary non-compliance with prescribed medication in primary care. *Br Med J* **307**: 846–848.

Beecher NH (1955). The powerful placebo. *J Am Med Assoc* **159**: 1602–1606.

Bégaud B (1993). Pharmacovigilance. In *Methodological Approaches in Pharmacoepidemiology*, Bégaud B, Péré J-C and Miremont G (eds). ARME-P/Elsevier, Bordeaux/Amsterdam.

Bégaud B, Péré J-C and Miremont G (eds) (1993). *Methodological Approaches in Pharmacoepidemiology*. ARME-P/Elsevier, Bordeaux/Amsterdam.

Bégaud B, Chaslerie A and Haramburu F (1994). [Organization and results of drug vigilance in France]. *Rev Epidemiol Med Soc Sante Publique* **42**(5): 416–423.

Bégaud B, Martin K, Haramburu F and Moore N (2002). Rates of spontaneous reporting of adverse drug reactions in France. *J Am Med Assoc* **288**(13): 1588.

Belton KJ and The European Pharmacovigilance Research Group (1997). Attitude survey of adverse drug-reaction reporting by health care professionals across the European Union. *Eur J Clin Pharmacol* **52**: 423–427.

Benichou C and Solal-Celigny P (1991). Standardisation of definitions and criteria for causality assessment of adverse drug reactions. Drug-induced blood cytopenias: report of an international consensus meeting. *Nouv Rev Hematol* **33**: 257–262.

Beral V (1977). Mortality among oral contraceptive users. Royal College of General Practitioners' Oral Contraception Study. *Lancet* **2**: 727–731.

Berry DC, Knapp P and Raynor DK (2002). Provision of information about drug side-effects to patients. *Lancet* **359**: 853–854.

Berry DC, Raynor DK, Knapp P and Bersellini E (2003). Patients' understanding of risk associated with medication use: impact of European Commission guidelines and other risk scales. *Drug Saf* **26**: 1–11.

Bhalla N, Duggan C and Dhillon S (2003) The incidence and nature of drug-related admission to hospital. *The Pharmaceutical Journal* **270**, 583–6.

Bhasin S, Reyburn H, Steen J and Waller P (1997). The effects of media publicity on spontaneous adverse reaction reporting with Mefloquine in the UK. *Pharmacoepidemiol Drug Saf* **6**: S32.

Bixler EO, Kales A, Manfredi RL, Vgontzas AN *et al.* (1991). Next-day memory impairment with triazolam use. *Lancet* **337**: 827–831.

Bjerre L and LeLorier J (1997). Beyond odds ratio: the number needed to harm one (NNTH). *Pharmacoepidemiol Drug Saf* **6**(Suppl 2): S51.

Bjene LM and Lelouir J (2000). Expressing the magnitude of adverse effects in case-control studies. "The number of patients needed to be treated to for one additional patient to be harmed." *British Medical Journal* **320**, 503–6.

Black J (1990). The puzzle of Pink disease. *J R Soc Med* **92**: 478–487.

Boardman H (2002). Fraud and misconduct in biomedical research. *Pharm. Physician* **12**(4): 18–22.

Bodenheimer T (2000). Clinical investigators and the pharmaceutical industry. *New Engl J Med* **342**(20): 1539–1543.

Bolton DPG and Cross KW (1974). Further observations on cost of preventing retrolental fibroplasia. *Lancet* **1**: 445–458.

Bongard V, Ménard-Taché S, Bagheri H, Kabiri K *et al*. (2002). Perception of the risk of adverse reactions: differences between health professionals and non-health professionals. *Br J Clin Pharmacol* **54**: 433–436.

Bordet R, Gautier S, Le Louet H, Dupuis B *et al*. (2001). Analysis of the direct cost of adverse drug reactions in hospitalized patients. *Eur J Clin Pharmacol* **56**: 935–941.

Borghi C and Canti D (1986). Il concetto storico di farmaco e di terapia. In *Tollerabilita di un Farmaco, Valutazione Clinica*. (Organizzazione Editoriale) Medico Farmaceutica, Srl, Milan; 3–23.

Bottiger LE and Westerholm B (1973). Drug-induced blood dyscrasias in Sweden. *Br Med J* **3**: 339–343.

Bottiger M, Romanus V, de Verdier C and Boman G (1982). Osteitis and other complications caused by generalised BCGitis. Experiences in Sweden. *Acta Paediatr Scand* **71**: 471–478.

Bowman L, Carlsedt BC, Hancock EF and Black CD (1996). Adverse drug reactions (ADR). Occurrence and evaluation in elderly patients. *Pharmacoepidemiol Drug Saf* **5**: 9–18.

Bradley CP (1992). Factors which influence the decision whether or not to prescribe: the dilemma facing general practitioners. *Br J Gen Pract* **42**: 454–458.

Brazier NC and Levine MAH (2003). Understanding drug–herb interactions. Pharmacoepidemiol Drug Saf **12**: 427–430.

Brennan TA, Hebert LE, Laird NM, Lawthers A *et al*. (1991). Hospital characteristics associated with adverse events and substandard care. *J Am Med Assoc* **265**(24): 3265–3269.

Brenner N, Frank OS and Knight E (1993). Chronic nutmeg psychosis. *J R Soc Med* **86**: 179–180.

Brodie KK (1986). Drugs and breast feeding. *Practitioner* **230**(1415): 483–485.

Brodovicz K, Sharrar R and Hostelley L (2001). The Weber effect – is it real? *Pharmacoepidemiol Drug Saf* **10**: S138.

Brown K, Sykes RS and Phillips G (2001). Is that adverse experience really expected? Guidelines for interpreting and formatting adverse experience information in the United States. *Drug Inf J* **35**: 269–284.

Brown MS, Wastila LJ, Berash CI and Lasagna L (1983). Patient perception of drugs risk and benefits. Drug Information OPE, study 67, Patient receipt of prescription drug information USA, F and DA. Available at www.fplc.edu/risk/vol1/summer/brown.htm [27 June 2003].

Brown P and Faloon L (2001). The incidence and reporting of adverse drug reactions in the division of psychiatry. *Pharm World Sci* **23**(5): 181–182.

Brown WJ, Buist NR, Gipson HT, Huston RK *et al*. (1982). Fatal benzyl alcohol poisoning in a neonatal intensive care unit. *Lancet* **1**: 1250.

Bryant GD and Norman GR (1980). Expressions of probability: words and numbers. *New Engl J Med* **302**: 411.

Buajordet I, Brørs O, Langslet A and Wesenberg F (1998) Adverse drug reactions in hospitalized children – intensive ADR monitoring in a paediatric unit at a Norwegian University hospital. *Pharmacoepidemiol Drug Saf* **7**(S98): 046.

Bucher HC, Weinbacher M and Gyr K (1994). Influence of method of reporting study results on decision of physicians to prescribe drugs to lower cholesterol concentration. *Br Med J* **309**: 761–764.

Bulpitt CJ (1974). A symptom questionnaire for hypertensive patients. *J Chronic Dis* **27**: 309–323.

Bulpitt CJ (1983). *Randomised Controlled Clinical Trials*. Martinus Nijhoff: The Hague.

Bulpitt CJ, Dollery CT and Carne S (1976). Change in symptoms of hypertensive patients after referral to hospital clinics. *Br Heart J* **38**: 121–128.

Burley DM (1988). The rise and fall of thalidomide. *Pharm Med* **3**: 231–237.

Burros M (2002). Herbal remedy tied to liver toxicity. *Bangkok Post*, 21 January, p. 8.

Calman K (1996). UK medical chief calls for risk debate. *Scrip* **5**: 2169.

Calman KC and Royston G (1997). Personal paper: risk language and dialects. *Br Med J* **315**: 939–942.

Calogero GF, Servello MM, Fava G, DiBernando N *et al.* (2001). Adverse drug events (ADEs) in emergency departments around the Strait of Messina. *Br J Clin Pharmacol* **51**: 363–391.

Carlsson C (1990). Herbs and hepatitis. *Lancet* **2**: 1068.

Chan TYK and Critchley AJH (1994). Drug-related problems as a cause of medical admissions in Hong Kong. *Pharmacoepidemiol Drug Saf* **3**(Suppl. 1, S41): 103.

Chrischilles EA, Segar ET and Wallace RB (1992). Self-reported adverse drug reactions and related resource use. *Ann Intern Med* **117**: 634–640.

Chyka PA (2000). How many deaths occur annually from drug reactions in the United States? *Am J Med* **109**(2): 122–130.

CIOMS Working Group III (1995). Guidelines for preparing core clinical safety information on drugs. CIOMS, Geneva.

CIOMS V (2001). Current challenges in pharmacovigilance: pragmatic approaches. *CIOMS*, Geneva.

Classen DC, Pestotnick SL, Evans RS and Burke JP (1991). Computerized surveillance of adverse drug events in hospital patients. *J Am Med Assoc* **266**: 2847–2851.

Classen DC, Pestotnik SL, Scott Evans R, Lloyd JF, *et al.* (1997). Adverse drug events in hospitalized patients. *J Am Med Assoc* **277**: 301–306.

Cluff LE, Thornton GF and Seidl LG (1964). Studies on the epidemiology of adverse drug reactions. *J Am Med Assoc* **188**(11): 976–983.

Cohen MR (1974). A compilation of abstracts and an index of articles published by the BCDSP. *Hosp Pharm* **9**: 437–448.

Committee of Principal Investigators (1978). A cooperative trial in the primary prevention of ischaemic heart disease using clofibrate. *Br Heart J* **40**(10): 1069–1118.

Committee of Principal Investigators (1980). WHO cooperative trial on primary prevention of ischaemic heart disease using clofibrate to lower serum cholesterol: mortality follow–up. *Lancet* **2**(8191): 379–385.

Conforti A, Leone R, Moretti L, Guglielomo L *et al.* (1995). Spontaneous reporting of adverse drug reactions in an Italian region: six years of analysis and observations. *Pharmacoepidemiol Drug Saf* **4**: 129–135.

Cook M and Ferner RE (1993). Adverse drug reactions: who is to know. *Br Med J* **307**: 480–481.

Cooper JW (1996). Adverse drug reactions and interactions in a geriatric nursing home population over 4 years. *J Am Geriatr Soc* **44**: 194–197.

Cosentino M, Leoni O, Oria C, Michielotto D *et al.* (1999). Hospital-based survey of doctors attitudes to adverse drug reactions and perception of drug-related risk for adverse reaction occurrence. *Pharmacoepidemiol Drug Saf* **8**: S27–S35.

Crooks J (1977). The detection of adverse drug reactions. *J R Coll Physicians London* **11**(3): 239–244.

Cross KW (1973). Cost of preventing retrolental fibroplasia. *Lancet* **2**: 954–956.

Cullen DJ, Sweitzer BJ, Bates DW, Burdick E *et al.* (1997). Preventable adverse drug events in hospitalized patients: a comparative study of intensive care and general care units. *Crit Care Med* **25**: 1289–1297.

Curien-Chevrier N, Louvat M, Clavey D and Demange C (1997). Adverse drug reactions: result of 4 months of prospective study at Remiremont hospital. *Pharm Hosp Fr* (Special issue): 19–21.

D'Arcy PF and Griffin JP (1994). Thalidomide revisited. *Adverse Drug React Toxicol Rev* **13**(2): 65–76. *Daily Telegraph* (1981). 3–25 June.

Dales L, Hammer SJ and Smith NJ (2001). Time trends in autism and in MMR immunisation coverage in California. *J Am Med Assoc* **285**: 1183–1185.

Dartnell JGA, Anderson RP, Chohan V, Galbraith KJ *et al.* (1996). Hospitalisation for adverse events related to drug therapy: incidence, avoidability and costs. *Med J Aust* **164**: 659–662.

Dawalibi S (2002). Quinze millards d'euros pour les médicaments. *Le Figaro Économie*, No 18076, Cahier No. 2, 20 September.

De Craen AJM, Kaptchuk TJ, Tijssen JGP and Kleijen J (1999). Placebos and placebo effects in medicine: historical overview. *J R Soc Med* **92**: 511–515.

De Deyn PP (2000). The ethical and scientific challenges of placebo control arms in clinical research. *Int J Pharm Med* **14**(3): 149–159.

Dekker E and Groen J (1956). Reproducible psychogenic attacks of asthma. *J Psychosom Res* **1**: 58–67.

Delamothe T (1992). Reporting adverse drug reactions. *Br Med J* **304**: 465.

Delay J and Pichot P (1973). *Medizinsche Psychologie*. Thieme: Stuttgart.

De Smet PAGM (1995a). Should herbal medicine-like products be licensed as medicines? *Br Med J* **310**: 1023–1024.

De Smet PAGM (1995b). Health risks of herbal remedies. *Drug Saf* **13**(2): 81–93

Dessertenne F (1966). La tachycardia ventriculaire á deux foyers opposées variable. *Arch Mal Cœur Vaiss* **59**: 263–272.

Detournay B, Fagnani F, Pouyanne P, Haramburu F *et al*. (2000). Cost of hospitalizations for adverse drug effects. *Thérapie* **55**(1): 137–139.

DeWitt JE and Sorofman BA (1999). A model for understanding patient attribution of adverse drug reaction symptoms. *Drug Inf J* **33**: 907–920.

Dharnidharka VR, Kandoth PN and Anad RK (1993). Adverse drug reactions in pediatrics with a study of in-hospital intensive surveillance. *Indian Pediatr* **30**(6): 745–751.

Di Masi JA, Hansen RW, Grabowski HG and Lasagna L (1991). Cost of innovation in the pharmaceutical industry. *J Health Econ* **10**: 107–142.

Dinman BD (1980a). Occupational health and the reality of risk – an eternal dilemma of tragic choice. *J Occup Med* **22**(3): 153–157.

Dinman BD (1980b). The reality and acceptance of risk. *J Am Med Assoc* **244**(11): 1226–1228.

Distillers Company (Biochemicals Ltd) (1961). Distival. *Lancet* **2**: 1262.

Domecq C, Naranjo CA, Ruiz I and Busto U (1980). Sex-related variations in the frequency and characteristics of adverse drug reactions. *Int J Clin Pharmacol Ther Toxicol* **18**: 362–366.

Dormann H, Muth-Sebach U, Krebs S, Criegge-Rieck M *et al*. (2000). Incidence and costs of adverse drug reactions during hospitalisation: computerised monitoring versus stimulated spontaneous reporting. *Drug Saf* **22**(2): 161–168.

Doucet J, Jego A, Noel D, Geffory CE *et al*. (2002). Preventable and non-preventable risk factors for adverse drug events related to hospital admission in the elderly. *Clin Drug Invest* **22**(6): 385–392.

Drici M-D, Raybaud F, De Lunardo C, Iacono P *et al*. (1995). Influence of the behaviour pattern on the nocebo response of healthy volunteers. *Br J Clin Pharmacol* **39**: 204–206.

Dukes MNG and Lunde I (1979). Common sense and communities. *Pharm Weekblad* **144**: 1283–1284.

Dyer C (2002). Government sued for 11 week delay in warning about aspirin. *Br Med J* **324**: 134.

Eaton L (2002). Adverse reactions to drugs increase. *Br Med J* **324**: 8.

Ebbesen J, Buajordet I, Erikssen J, Brørs O *et al*. (2001). Drug related deaths in a department of internal medicine. *Arch Intern Med* **161**: 2317–2323.

Edwards A, Elwyn G and Mulley A (2002). Explaining risks: turning numerical data into meaningful pictures. *Br Med J* **324**: 827–830.

Edwards IR, Wiholm B-E and Martinez C (1996). Concepts in risk–benefit assessment. A simple merit analysis of a medicine. *Drug Saf* **15**: 1–7.

Edwards R (2002). The International Society of Pharmacovigilance. *Pharmacoepidemiol Drug Saf* **11**: 253–254.

Eland IA, Grootheest AC, Belton KJ, Rawlins MD *et al*. (1998). Attitudinal survey of adverse drug reaction reporting by medical practitioners in the Netherlands. *Pharmacoepidemiol Drug Saf* **7**: S152.

Eland IA, Belton KJ, Van Grootheest AC, Meiners AP *et al*. (1999). Attitudinal survey of voluntary reporting of adverse drug reactions. *Br J Clin Pharmacol* **48**: 623–627.

Ellis H (1997). Penicillin: the early days. *Int J Pharm Med* **11**: 275–279.

Elting LS, Martin CG, Cantor SB and Rubenstein EB (1999). Influence of data display formats on physician investigators' decisions to stop clinical trials: prospective trial; with repeated measures. *Br Med J* **318**: 1527–1531.

Ernst E (1998). Harmless herbs? A review of the recent literature. *Am J Med* **104**: 170–178.

Ernst E (2000). Risks associated with complimentary therapies. In *Meyler's Side Effects of Drugs*, 14th edition, Dukes MNG and Aronson JK. Elsevier: chapter 48.

Ernst E and Resch KL (1995). Concept of true and perceived placebo effects. *Br Med J* **311**: 551–553.

Ernst E and Resch KL (1996). Risk–benefit ratio or risk–benefit nonsense. *J Clin Epidemiol* **49**(10): 1203–1204.

Evans RS, Pestotnik SL, Classen DC, Horn SD *et al* (1994). Preventing adverse drug events in hospitalised patients. *Ann Pharmacother* **28**(4): 523–527.

Farrington CP, Miller E and Taylor B (2001). MMR and autism: further evidence against a causal association. *Vaccine* **19**: 3632–3635.

Farrington P, Pugh S, Colville A, Flower A *et al*. (1995). A new method for active surveillance of adverse events from diphtheria/tetanus/pertussis and measles/mumps/rubella vaccines. *Lancet* **345**: 567–569.

Fattinger K, Roos M, Vergères P, Kind B *et al*. (1998) Comprehensive hospital drug monitoring (CHDM): 'event monitoring' of adverse drug reactions (ADRs) in inpatients. *Pharmacoepidemiol Drug Saf* **7**(S105): 061.

FDA Task Force (1993). Fialuridine: hepatic and pancreatic toxicity. Food and Drug Administration, 12 November.

Ferry M and Piette F (1993). Survey of the incidence of undesirable events in geriatric services. *Thérapie* **48**(1): 55–57.

Fields HL and Levine JD (1981). Biology of placebo analgesia. *Am J Med* **70**(4): 745–746.

Finn R (1992). Food allergy – fact or fiction: a review. *J R Soc Med* **85**: 560–564.

Finney DJ (1963). An international drug safety program. *J New Drugs* **3**: 262.

Fleming DM, Knox JDE and Crombie DL (1981). Debendox in early pregnancy and foetal malformation. *Br Med J* **283**: 99–101.

Fremont-Smith K (1998). Adverse drug reactions in hospitalized patients. *J Am Med Assoc* **280**: 20.

Fugh-Berman A (2000). Herb–drug interactions. *Lancet* **355**: 134–138.

Fung M, Thornton A, Mybeck K, Wu JH *et al*. (2001). Evaluation of the characteristics of safety withdrawal of prescription drugs from worldwide pharmaceutical markets – 1960 to 1999. *Drug Inf J* **35**: 293–317.

Garijo B, de Abajo FJ, Castro MAS, Lopo CR *et al*. (1991). Hospitalizaciones motivadas por fármacos: un estudio prospective. *Rev Clín Esp* **188**: 7–12.

Geiling EMK and Cannon PR (1938). Pathological effects of elixir of sulphanilamide (diethylene glycol) poisoning. *J Am Med Assoc* **111**: 919–926.

Gershanik J, Boecler B, Ensley H, McCloskey S *et al*. (1982). The gasping syndrome and benzyl alcohol poisoning. *New Engl J Med* **307**: 1384–1388.

Gill AM, Leach HJ, Hughes J, Barker C *et al*. (1995). Adverse drug reactions in a paediatric intensive care unit. *Acta Paediatr* **84**: 438–441.

Gittens J (1996). Quantitative methods in the planning of pharmaceutical research. *Drug Inf J* **30**: 479–487.

Gonzalez-Martin G, Caroca CM and Paris E (1998). Adverse drug reactions in hospitalized pediatric patients. A prospective study. *Int J Clin Pharmacol Ther* **36**(10): 530–533.

Gordon AJ (1985). Numerators, denominators, and other holy grails: management and interpretation of worldwide drug safety data. *Drug Inf J* **19**: 319–328.

Göttler M (1998). A literature-based meta-analysis on cost and preventability of adverse drug reactions leading to hospital admission. *Pharmacoepidemiol Drug Saf* **7**: S192, 268.

Göttler M (2000). ADRs in the elderly. In *Opinion & Evidence, Drug Safety*, 2nd edition, Edwards R (ed.). Adis International; IV-11.

Göttler M, Schneeweiss S and Hasford J (1997). Adverse drug reaction monitoring – cost and benefit considerations part II: cost and preventability of adverse drug reactions leading to hospital admission. *Pharmacoepidemiol Drug Saf* **3**: S79–S90.

Göttler M, Garcia-Gomez I and Hasford J (1998). Physicians' attitudes towards adverse drug reaction reporting in Germany. *Pharmacoepidemiol Drug Saf* **7**(S193).

Gottlieb S (2001). Drug effects blamed for fifth of hospital deaths among elderly. *Br Med J* **323**: 1025.

Grandjean P, Sandoe SH and Kimbrough RD (1991). Non-specificity of clinical signs and symptoms caused by environmental chemicals. *Hum Exp Toxicol* **10**: 167–173.

Grange JC (1990). Adverse or toxic effects of drugs in medical practice: a one-year follow-up. *Thérapie* **45**(4): 331–334.

Grawitz (1935). *Semana Med* **42**: 525.

Green DM (1964). Pre-existing conditions, placebo reactions and 'side effects'. *Ann Intern Med* **60**(2): 255–265.

Grenade LL, Graham DJ and Nourjah P (2001). Underreporting of haemorrhagic stroke associated with phenylpropanolamine. *J Am Med Assoc* **286**(24): December 26.

Griffin JP and Weber JCP (1986). Voluntary systems of adverse reaction reporting, Part II. *Adverse Drug React Acute Poisons Rev* **1**: 23–55.

Grohmann R, Rütter E, Sassim N and Schmidt LG (1989). Adverse effects of Clozapine. *Psychopharmacologia* **99**: s101–s104.

Gruner JE (1958). [Damage to the central nervous system after ingestion of an ethyl tin compound (Stalinon)]. *Rev Neurol* **98**: 109–116 (in French).

Grymonpre RE, Mitenko PA, Sitar DS, Aoki FY et al. (1988). Drug-associated hospital admissions in older medical patients. *J Am Geriatr Soc* **36**: 1092–1098.

Guruprasad P, Rawlins MD and Day CP (1999). Accuracy of hepatic adverse drug reaction reporting in one English health region. *Br Med J* **319**: 1541.

Hafner Jr JW (2002). Adverse drug events in emergency department patients. *Ann Emerg Med* **39**: 258–267.

Hallas J, Gram LF, Grodum E, Damsbo N et al. (1992). Drug related admissions to medical wards: a population based survey. *Br J Clin Pharmacol* **33**(1): 61–68.

Hamif M, Mobarek MR, Ronan A, Rahman D et al. (1995). Fatal renal failure caused by diethylene glycol in paracetamol elixir: the Bangladesh epidemic. *Br Med J* **311**: 88–91.

Haramburu F, Bégaud B and Moride Y (1997). Temporal trends in spontaneous reporting of unlabelled adverse drug reaction. *Br J Clin Pharmacol* **44**: 299–301.

Hartmann K, Bon S and Kuhn M (2000). Drug interactions with St John's Wort – case series from a spontaneous reporting scheme. *Pharmacoepidemiol Drug Saf* **9**: S23.

Hasford J, Goettler M, Munter K-H and Müller-Oerlinghausen B (2002). Physicians' knowledge and attitudes regarding the spontaneous reporting system for adverse drug reactions. *J Clin Epidemiol* **55**: 945–950.

Hayashi K and Walker AM (1996). Japanese and American reports of randomised trials: differences in the reporting of adverse effects. *Control Clin Trials* **17**: 99–110.

Headland FW (1859). *An essay on the action of medicines in the system or 'on the mode in which therapeutic agents introduced into the stomach produce their peculiar effects on the animal economy'*, 3rd edition. John Churchill; 391.

Hecht A (1987). Diet, drug dangers – déjà vu. *FDA Consumer*, 22 February, 22–27.

Heeley E, Riley J, Wilton LV and Shakir SAW (2001). Prescription event monitoring and reporting of adverse drug reactions. *Lancet* **356**: 1872–1873.

Heilman K (1988). The perception of drug-related risk. In *Therapeutic Risk: Perception, Measurement, Management*, Burley D and Inman WHW (eds). John Wiley: 1–11.

Heinrich J (2001). Drug safety: most drugs withdrawn in recent years had greater risks for women. United States General Accounting Office, 19 January.

Hemminki E (1980). Study of information submitted by drug companies to licensing authorities. *Br Med J* (22 March): 833–836.

Herbst AL, Ulfelder H and Poskanzer DC (1971). Association of maternal stilboestrol therapy and tumour appearance in young women. *New Engl J Med* **284**: 878.

Hiller JL, Benda GI, Rahatzad M, Allen JR *et al*. (1986). Benzyl alcohol toxicity: impact on mortality and intraventricular haemorrhage among very low weight infants. *Pediatrics* **77**: 500–506.

Hippius M, Filz H, Sicker T and Hoffmann A (1999). Adverse drug reactions – related hospital admissions. Length of stay and cost of hospitalisation. In *Annual Congress of Clinical Pharmacology*, Berlin, 10–12 June.

Hirokawa K (1996). Clinical pharmacologists and drug regulations – future perspectives in Japan. *Br J Clin Pharmacol* **42**: 63–71.

Hoek R, Stricker BHCh, Ottervanger JP and Van Der Velden K (1995). Reporting of suspected adverse reactions to drugs in primary care. *Pharmacoepidemiol Drug Saf* **4**: S23.

Hoigné RV (1997). Should 'Idiosyncrasy' be defined as equivalent to 'Type B' adverse drug reactions? *Pharmacoepidemiol Drug Saf* **6**: 213.

Hoigné R, D'Andrea Jaeger M, Wymann R, Egli A *et al*. (1990). Time pattern of allergic reactions to drugs. In *Agents and Actions, Risk Factors for ADR*, vol. 29. Birkhauser: Basel; 39–57.

Holden WL, Juhalri J and Dai W (2003). Benefit-risk analysis: a proposal using quantitative methods. *Pharmacoepidemiol Drug Saf.* **12**, 611–616.

Horton R (1994). The context of consent. *Lancet* **344**: 211–212.

Hróbjartsson A, Gótsche PC and Glund C (1998). The controlled clinical trial turns 100 years: Fibger's trial of serum treatment of diphtheria. *Br Med J* **317**: 1243–1245.

Hunter D and Bains N (1999). Rates of adverse events among hospital admissions and day surgeries in Ontario from 1992 to 1997. *Can Med Assoc J* **160**(11): 1585.

Hurwitz N and Wade OC (1969). Intensive hospital monitoring of adverse reactions to drugs. *Br Med J* **1**: 531–536.

Hutchinson TA (1986). Standardised assessment methods for adverse drug reactions: a review of previous approaches and their problems. *Drug Inf J* **20**: 439–444.

Hurwitz N and Wade (1969). Admissions to hospital due to drugs. *Br Med J* **1**: 539–540.

Imbs JL, Pouyanne P, Haramburu F, Welsch M *et al*. (1999). Iatrogenic medication: estimation of its prevalence in French public hospitals. Regional Centre of Pharmacovigilance. *Thérapie* **54**(1): 21–27.

Impicciatore P, Choonara I, Clarkson A, Provarsi D *et al*. (2001). Incidence of adverse drug reactions in paediatric in/out-patients: a systematic review and meta-analysis of prospective studies. *Br J Clin Pharmacol* **52**: 77–83.

Inman WHW (1972). Monitoring by voluntary reporting at national level. In *Adverse Drug Reactions*, Richards DJ and Rondel RK (eds). Churchill Livingstone.

Inman WHW (1977). Study of fatal bone marrow depression with special reference to phenylbutazone and oxyphenbutazone. *Br Med J* **1**: 1500–1505.

Inman WHW (1981). Postmarketing surveillance of adverse drug reactions in general practice. 1: Search for new methods. *Br Med J* **282**: 1131–1132.

Inman WHW (1986). The United Kingdom. In *Monitoring for Drug Safety*. MTP Press, Lancaster.

Inman WHW and Adelstein AM (1969). Rise and fall of asthma mortality in England and Wales in relation to pressurised aerosols. *Lancet* **2**: 279.

Inman WHW, Vessey MP, Westerholm B and Engelind A (1970). Thrombo-embolic disease and the steroid content of oral contraceptives. *Br Med J* **2**: 203.

Jamaa M, Laine-Cessac P, Victor J, Tadel A *et al*. (1993) Evaluation of drug side-effects over a year in a cardiology service. *Thérapie* **48**(3): 259–262.

James BC (1997). Every defect a treasure: learning from adverse events in hospitals. *Med J Aust* **166**: 484–487.

Jaramillo-Arango J (1953). In *The British Contribution to Medicine.* E & S Livingstone Ltd.

Jasanoff S (1993). Innovation and integrity, in biomedical research. *Acad Med* **68**(Suppl. 9): S91–S95.

Jewett DL, Fein G and Greenberg MH (1990). A double blind study of symptom provocation to determine food sensitivity. *New Engl J Med* **323**(7): 429–433.

Jha AK, Kuperman GJ, Rittenberg E, Teich JM *et al.* (2001). Identifying hospital admissions due to adverse drug events using a computer-based monitor. *Pharmacoepidemiol Drug Saf* **10**: 113–119.

Jick H (1984). Boston Collaborative Drug Surveillance Program. In *Monitoring for ADR*, Walker SR and Goldberg A (eds). MTP Press, Lancaster.

Joelson S, Joelson IB and Wallander MA (1997) Geographical variation in adverse event reporting rates in clinical trials. *Pharmacoepidemiol Drug Saf* **6**(Suppl. 3): S31–S35.

Johnson JA and Bootman JL (1995). Drug-related morbidity and mortality: a cost-of-illness model. *Ann Intern Med.* **155**: 1949–1956.

Jonville-Béra AP, Giraudeau B, Blanc P, Beau-Salinas F *et al.* (2002). Frequency of adverse drug reactions in children: a prospective study. *Br J Clin Pharmacol* **53**: 207–210.

Josefson D (1996). Herbal stimulant causes US deaths. *Br Med J* **312**: 1378–1379.

Joubert PH, Van Rijssen FWJ and Venter JP (1977) Drug side effects assessed in a 'naturalistic' setting. *S Afr Med J* **52**: 34–36.

Joyce CRB (1982). Placebos and other comparative treatments. *Br J Clin Pharmacol* **13**: 313–318.

Joyce CRB and Joyce J (1983). Pyramidal publication. *Eur J Clin Pharmacol* **25**: 1–2.

Juntti-Patinen L and Neuvonen PJ (2002). Drug-related deaths in an University Central hospital. *Eur J Clin Pharmacol* **58**: 479–482.

Karunanithy R and Sumita KP (1991). Undeclared drugs in traditional Chinese antirheumatoid medicine. *Int J Pharm Pract* **1**: 117–119.

Kaufman DW and Shapiro S (2000). Epidemiological assessment of drug-induced disease. *Lancet* **356**: 1339–1343.

Kaye JA, del Mar Melero-Montes M and Jick H (2001). Mumps, measles, and rubella vaccine and the incidence of autism recorded by general practitioners: a time trend analysis. *Br Med J* **322**: 460–463.

Kee F (1996). Patients' prerogatives and perceptions of benefit. *Br Med J* **312**: 958–960.

Kelly N (2001). Can the frequency and risks of fatal adverse drug events be determined? *Pharmacotherapy* **21**(5): 521–527.

Kennedy WP (1961). The nocebo reaction. *Med World* **91**: 203–205.

Kevany J (1996). Extreme poverty: an obligation ignored. *Br Med J* **313**: 65–66.

Key C, Layton D and Shakir SAW (2002). Results of a postal survey of the reasons for non-response by doctors in a prescription event monitoring study of drug safety. *Pharmacoepidemiol Drug Saf* **11**: 143–148.

Khosla PP, Bajaj VK, Sharma G and Mishra KC (1992). Background noise in healthy volunteers – a consideration in adverse drug reaction studies. *Indian J Physiol Pharmacol* **36**(4): 259–262.

Kimmel SE, Goldberg L, Sekeres M, Berlin J *et al.* (1995). Incidence and predictors of under reporting of serious adverse events following protamine administration. *Pharmacoepidemiol Drug Saf* **4**(Suppl. 1): S35, abstract 080.

Kitchener S, Malekottodjary N and McClelland GR (1996). Adverse effects from placebo-treated healthy volunteers. *Br J Clin Pharmacol* **41**: 473p.

Klebanoff MA, Read JS, Mills JL and Shiono PH (1993). The risk of childhood cancer after neonatal exposure to vitamin K. *New Engl J Med* **329**(13): 905–908.

Klein LE, German PS, Levine DM, Feroli Jr ER *et al.* (1984). Medication problems among outpatients. A study with emphasis on the elderly. *Arch Intern Med* **144**(6): 1185–1188.

Knowles JB and Lucas CJ (1960). Experimental studies of the placebo response. *J Ment Sci* **106**: 231–240.

Knox EG (1975). Negligible risks to health. *Commun Health* **6**: 244–251.

Ko RJ (1998). Adulterants in Asian patent medicines. *New Engl J Med* **339**: 847.

Kong A, Barnett GO, Mosteller F and Youtz C (1986). How medical professionals evaluate expressions of probability. *New Engl J Med* **315**: 740–744.

Kono R (1980). Trends and lessons of SMON research. In *Drug-induced Suffering. Medical, Pharmaceutical and Legal Aspects*, Soda T (ed.). Excerpta Medica, Princeton; 11.

Kravitz GR (1998). Adverse drug reactions in hospitalized patients. *J Am Med Assoc* **280**: 20.

Kurz X, Van Ermen A, Roisin T and Belton KJ (1996). Knowledge and practices of adverse drug reaction reporting by Belgian physicians. *Pharmacoepidemiol Drug Saf* **5**: S19.

Kvasz M, Allen IE, Gordon MJ, Ro EY *et al.* (2000). Adverse drug reactions in hospitalized patients: a critique of a meta-analysis. *Medgenmed: Medscape General Medicine*, 27 April.

Lacoste-Rousillon C, Pouyanne P, Haramburu F, Miremont G *et al.* (2001). Incidence of serious adverse drug reactions in general practice: a prospective study. *Clin Pharmacol Ther* **69**: 458–462.

Lagnaoui R, Moore N, Fach J, Longy-Boursier M *et al.* (2000). Adverse drug reactions in a department of systemic diseases-oriented internal medicine: prevalence, incidence, direct costs and avoidability. *Eur J Clin Pharmacol* **55**: 181–186.

La Grenade L, Graham DJ and Nourjah P (2001). Under-reporting of haemorrhagic stroke associated with phenylpropanolamine. *J Am Med Assoc* **286**(24).

Lane DA, Kramer MS, Hutchinson TA, Jones JK *et al.* (1987). The causality assessment of adverse drug reactions using a Bayesian approach. *Pharm Med* **2**: 265–283.

Lapeyre-Mestre M, Gary J, Machelard-Roumagnac M, Bonhomme C *et al.* (1997) Incidence and cost of adverse drug reactions in a French cancer institute. *Eur J Clin Pharmacol* **53**(1): 19–22.

Lasagna L (1980). The Halcion story, trial by media. *Lancet* **1**: 815.

Lasagna L, Laties VG and Dohan JL (1958). Further studies on the 'pharmacology' of placebo administration. *J Clin Invest* **37**: 533–537.

Lasagna L, Mosteller F, Von Felsinger JM and Beecher HK (1954). A study of placebo response. *Am J Med* **16**: 770–779.

Lazarou J, Pomeranz BH and Corey PN (1998). Incidence of adverse drug reactions in hospitalized patients: a meta-analysis of prospective studies. *J Am Med Assoc* **279**: 1200–1205.

Leape LL, Brennan TA, Laird N, Lawthers AG *et al.* (1991). The nature of adverse events in hospitalised patients: results of the Harvard Medical Practice Study II. *New Engl J Med* **324**: 377–384.

Lee TR (1987) Risks in society. In *Medicines and Risk/Benefit Decisions*, Walker SR and Asscher AW (eds). MTP Press; 5–13.

Lenz W (1962). Thalidomide neuropathy. *Lancet* **1**: 45.

Lenz W (1980). Thalidomide: facts and inferences. In *Drug-induced Suffering. Medical, Pharmaceutical and Legal Aspects*, Soda T (ed.). Excerpta Medica, Princeton; 103–109.

Lenz WM (1966). Malformations caused by drugs in pregnancy. *Am J Dis Child* **112**(2): 99–103.

Lenz W and Knapp K (1962). Die Thalidomid-Embryopathie. *Dtsch Med Wochenschr* **87**: 1232.

Lessof MH (1992). Reactions to food additives. *J R Soc Med* **85**: 513–515.

Letemendia FJJ and Harris AD (1959). The influence of side effects on the reporting of symptoms. *Psychopharmacologia* **1**: 39–47.

Le Vay MK (1960). Placebo effect in mental nursing. *Lancet*: 1403.

Levine RJ (1987). The apparent incompatibility between informed consent and placebo-controlled clinical trials. *Clin Pharm Ther* **42**: 247–249.

Levine JD, Gordon NC and Fields HL (1978). The mechanism of placebo analgesia. *Lancet* **23**: 654–657.

Levy M, Livshits T and Sadan B (1998). Computerised surveillance of adverse drug reactions in hospital. *Pharmacoepidemiol Drug Saf* **7**(Suppl. 2): S157, 187.

Lewis JA (1981). Post-marketing surveillance: how many patients? *Trends Pharmacol Sci* **2**(4): 93–94.

Lewis MA, Kühl-Habich D, Llauger-Boix M and Van Rosen J (1998). Adverse event monitoring in a population of German children. *Pharmacoepidemiol Drug Saf* **7**(Suppl. 2): S191, 265.

Lichenstein S (1978). Judged frequency of lethal events. *J Exp Psychol Hum Learn Mem* **4**: 551.

Lind JA (1753). *A Treatise on the Scurvy. Containing an inquiry into the nature, causes and cure of that disease, together with a critical and chronological view of what has been published on the subject.* A. Millar, London.

Longo DR, Brownson RC, Johnson JC, Hewett JE, *et al.* (1996). Hospital smoking bans and employee smoking behaviour. *J Am Med Assoc* **275**: 1252–1257.

Lumley CE, Walker SR, Staunton N and Grob PR (1986). The under-reporting of adverse drug reactions seen in general practice. *Pharma Med* **1**: 205–212.

Luparello T, Lyons HA, Blecker ER, McFadden Jr ER. (1968). Influences of suggestion on airway reactivity in asthmatic subjects. *Psychosom Med* **30**: 819–825.

Mackintosh DR and Zepp VJ (1996). Detection of negligence, fraud and other bad faith efforts during field auditing of clinical trial sites. *Drug Inf J* **30**: 645–653.

Madsen KM, Hviid A, Vestrgaard M, Schendel D *et al.* (2002). A population-based study of measles, mumps and rubella vaccination and autism. *New Engl J Med* **347**: 1477–1482.

Maistrello I, Morgutti M, Maltempi M and Dantes M (1995). Adverse drug reactions in hospitalized patients: an operational procedure to improve reporting and investigate under reporting. *Pharmacoepidemiol Drug Saf* **4**: 101–106.

Mäkelä A, Nuorti JP and Peloila H (2002). Neurologic disorders after measles–mumps–rubella vaccination. *Pediatrics* **110**: 957–963.

Malhota S, Karan RS, Pandhi P and Jain S (2001). Drug related medical emergencies in the elderly: role of adverse drug reactions and non-compliance. *Postgrad Med J* **77**(913): 703–707.

Mann R (1988). From Mythridatium to modern medicine: the management of drug safety. *J R Soc Med* **81**: 725–728.

Mann RD and Andrews EB (2002). Preface. In *Pharmacovigilance.* John Wiley; xvii.

Mannesse CK, Derks FHM, De Ridder MAJ, Man in't Veld AJ *et al.* (1997). Adverse drug reactions in elderly patients as contributing factor for hospital admission: cross sectional study. *Br Med J* **315**: 1057–1058.

Manning FJ and Swartz M (1995). *Review of the Fialuridine (FIAU) Clinical Trials.* National Academic Press.

Marion MN and Simon P (1984). Signification des adverbes utilisés pour indiquer la frequence des effets secondaires d'un médicament. *Thérapie* **39**: 47–63.

Martin R, Kapoor K, Wilton L and Mann R (1998). Underreporting of suspected adverse drug reactions to newly marketed, black triangle drugs in general practice. *Pharmacoepidemiol Drug Saf* **7**: S126.

Martinez-Mir I, Garcia-Lopez M, Palop V, Ferrer JM *et al.* (1996). A prospective study of adverse drug reactions as a cause of admission to a paediatric hospital. *Br J Clin Pharmacol* **42**(3): 319–324.

Martinez-Mir I, Garcia-Lopez M, Palop V, Ferrer JM *et al.* (1999). A prospective study of adverse drug reactions in hospitalised children. *Br J Clin Pharmacol* **47**(6): 681–688.

Martone WJ, Williams WW, Mortenson ML, Gayner RP *et al.* (1986). Illness with fatalities in premature infants associated with intravenous vitamin E preparation, E-Ferol. *Pediatrics* **78**: 591–600.

Martys CR (1979). Adverse reactions to drugs in general practice. *Br Med J* **2**: 1194–1197.

Mathieu MP (1999). *Pararexel's Pharmaceutical R & D Statistical Sourcebook 1998.* Parexel International Corporation, Waltham, MA.

Mayo E (1933). In *The Human Problems of an Industrial Civilization.* McMillans, New York; chapter 3.

McBride WG (1961). Thalidomide and congenital abnormalities. *Lancet* **2**: 1358.

McDonald CJ, Mazzuca SA and McCabe Jr GP (1983). How much of the placebo 'effect' is statistical regression? *Stat Med* **2**: 417–427.

McDonald CJ, Mazzuca SA and McCabe Jr GP (1989). How much of the placebo 'effect' is really statistical regression? (Authors' Reply) *Stat Med* **8**: 1301–1302.

McDonnell PJ and Jacobs MR (2002). Hospital admissions resulting from preventable adverse drug reactions. *Ann Pharmacother* **36**: 1331–1336.

McEwan J (1999). Adverse reactions – a personal view of their history. *Int J Pharm Med* **13**: 269–277.

McGettigan P and Feely J (1995). Adverse drug reaction reporting: opinions and attitudes of medical practitioners in Ireland. *Pharmacoepidemiol Drug Saf* **4**: 355–358.

McGettigan P, Golden J, Arthur N and Feely J (1996). Adverse drug reaction reporting by hospital doctors: knowledge, use of the system and response to intervention. *Br J Clin Pharmacol* **41**: 437–475.

McKenzie R, Fried MW, Sallie R, Conjeevaram H *et al.* (1995). Hepatic failure and lactic acidosis due to Fialuridine (FIAU), an investigational nucleoside analogue for chronic hepatitis B. *New Engl J Med* **333**: 1099–1105.

McNeil BJ, Pauker SG, Sox HC and Tversky A (1982). On the elicitation of preferences for alternative therapies. *New Engl J Med* **306**: 1259–1267.

McPherson K (1996). Third generation oral contraception and venous thrombo-embolism. *Br Med J* **312**: 68–69.

Meade TW (1981). Pertussis vaccine. *Br Med J* **281**: 59.

Mellin GW and Katzenstein M (1962). The saga of thalidomide. *New Engl J Med* **267**: 1184–1193.

Melmon KL and Nierenberg DW (1981). Drug interactions and the prepared observer. *New Engl J Med* **304**(12): 723–725.

Menniti-Ippolito F, Raschetti R, Da Cas R, Giaquinto C *et al.* (2000). Active monitoring of adverse drug reactions in children. *Lancet* **355**: 1613–1614.

Meyer FP, Tröger U and Röhl F-W (1996). Adverse non-drug reactions: an update. *Clin Pharmacol Ther* **60**: 347–352.

Millar S (2001). Consultations owing to adverse drug reactions in a single practice. *Br J Gen Prac* **51**: 130–131.

Miller DL, Ross EM, Alderslade R, Bellman MN *et al.* (1981). Pertussis immunization and serious acute neurological illness in children. *Br Med J* **282**(6276): 1565.

Miller LG (1998). Herbal medicinals. *Arch Intern Med* **158**: 220–211.

Mills A and Edwards IR (1999). Venous thrombo-embolism and the pill. The combined oral contraceptive pill – are poor communication systems responsible for loss of confidence in this contraceptive method? *Hum Reprod* **14**(1): 7–10.

Milstein JB, Faich GA, Hsu JP, Knapp DC *et al.* (1986). Factors affecting physician reporting of ADR. *Drug Inf J* **20**: 157–164.

Mitchell AA, Lacouture PG, Sheehan JE, Kauffman RE *et al.* (1988). Adverse drug reactions in children leading to hospital admission. *Pediatrics* **82**(1): 24–29.

Mjörndal T, Boman MD, Hägg S, Bäckström M *et al.* (2002). Adverse drug reactions as a cause for admissions to a department of internal medicine. *Pharmacoepidemiol Drug Saf* **11**: 65–72.

Montastruc P, Damase-Michel C, Lapeyre-Mestre M, Puget C *et al.* (1995). A prospective intensive study of adverse drug reactions in urban general practice. *Clin Drug Invest* **10**(2): 117–122.

Moore N, Briffaut C, Noblet C, Normand CA *et al.* (1995a). Indirect drug-related costs. *Lancet* **345**: 588–589.

Moore N, Lecointre D, Noblet C and Mabille M (1995b). Serious adverse drug reactions in a department of internal medicine: incidence and cost analysis. *Pharmacoepidemiol Drug Saf* **4**(Suppl. 1): S74, abstract 160.

Moore N, Mammeri M, Carrara O, Deschalliers J-P *et al.* (1995c). Incidence and cost of adverse drug reactions in a department of a general hospital management system. *Pharmacoepidemiol Drug Saf* **4**(Suppl. 1): S72, abstract 158.

Moore N, Lecointre D, Noblet C and Mabille M (1998). Frequency and cost of serious adverse drug reactions in a department of general medicine. *Br J Clin Pharmacol* **45**: 301–308.

Moride Y, Haramburu F and Bégaud B (1994). Assessment of under reporting of adverse events in pharmacovigilance. *Pharmacoepidemiol Drug Saf* **3**(Suppl 1): S73, abstract 179.

Moride Y, Haramburu F, Requejo AA and Bégaud B (1997). Under-reporting of adverse drug reactions in general practice. *Br J Clin Pharmacol* **43**: 177–181.

Morris LA and Kanouse DE (1982). Informing patients about drug side effects. *J Behav Med* **5**(3): 363–373.

Muehlberger N, Schneeweiss S and Hasford J (1997). Adverse drug reaction monitoring – cost and benefit considerations part I: frequency of adverse drug reactions causing hospital admissions. *Pharmacoepidemiol Drug Saf* **6**(Suppl. 3): S71–S77.

Mulroy R (1973). Iatrogenic disease in general practice: its incidence and effects. *Br Med J* **2**: 407–410.

Munoz MJ, Ayani I, Rodriguez-Sasiain JM, Gutierrez G *et al.* (1998). Adverse drug reaction surveillance in pediatric and adult patients in an emergency room. *Med Clin* **111**(3): 92–98.

Myers MG, Cairns JA and Singer J (1987). The consent form as a possible cause of side-effects. *Clin Pharm Ther* **42**: 250–253.

Nanda C, Fanale JE and Kronholm P (1990). The role of medication non-compliance and adverse drug reactions in hospitalisations of the elderly. *Arch Intern Med* **150**: 841–846.

NAO (2003). *Safety, Quality, Efficacy: Regulating Medicines in the UK*. National Audit Office. Stationary Office.

Napke E and Stevens DGH (1984). Excipients and additives: hidden hazards in drug products and in product substitution. *Can Med Assoc J* **131**: 1449–1452.

Nevin NC (1998). Gene therapy: supervision, obstacles and the future. *Int J Pharm Med* **12**: 19–23.

Newman TB (1995). If almost nothing goes wrong, is almost everything all right? Interpreting small numerators. *J Am Med Assoc* **274**: 1013.

Nicholls A, Elliman D and Ross E (1998). MMR vaccination and autism 1998. *Br Med J* **316**: 716–717.

Nicholls JJ (1977). The practolol syndrome: a retrospective analysis. In *Post-marketing Surveillance of Adverse Drug Reactions to New Medicine*. Medico-Pharmaceutical Forum, Publication No. 7.

Nickas J (1997). Clinical trial safety surveillance in the new regulatory and harmonization environment: lessons learned from the 'Fialuridine crisis'. *Drug Inf J* **31**: 63–70.

Norwegian Multicenter Study Group (1981). Timolol-induced reduction in mortality and reinfarction in patients surviving acute myocardial infarction. *New Engl J Med* **304**(14): 801–807.

O'Brien B (1986). *What Are My Chances Doctor? – A Review of Clinical Risk*. Office of Health Economics, London.

O'Brien KL, Selanikos JD, Hecdirert C, Placide MF *et al.* (1998). Evidence of pediatric deaths from acute renal failure caused by diethylene glycol poisoning. *J Am Med Assoc* **279**(15): 1175–1180.

Olivier P, Boubles O, Tubery M, Carles P *et al.* (2001). Preventability of adverse events in a medical emergency service. *Thérapie* **56**(3): 275–278.

Orme ML'E (1985). The Debendox saga. *Br Med J* **291**: 918–919.

Oswald I (1989). Triazolam syndrome 10 years on. *Lancet* **i**: 451–452.

Ottervanger JP, Van Witsen TB, Valkenburg HA, Grobbee DE *et al.* (1995). Differences in reporting of ADR: a specific drug between general practitioners and consumers. *Pharmacoepidemiol Drug Saf* **4**: S25.

Peacock S, Murray V and Turton C (1995). Respiratory distress and royal jelly. *Br Med J* **311**: 1473.

Pearce N, Beasley R, Crane J, Burgess C *et al.* (1995). End of the New Zealand asthma mortality epidemic. *Lancet* **345**: 41–44.

Péré J-C, Bégaud B, Haramburu F and Albin H (1984). Notions de fréquence et de gravité des effets indésirables. *Thérapie* **39**: 447–452.

Petrovic P, Kalso E, Petersson KM and Ingvar M (2002). Placebo and opioid analgesia – imaging shared neuronal network. *Science* **295**: 1737–1740.

Pochin FE (1975). The acceptance of risk. *Br Med Bull* **31**(3): 184.

Pogge RC (1963). The toxic placebo. *Med Times* **91**(8): 773–776.

Porter J and Jick H (1977). Drug-related deaths among medical in-patients. *J Am Med Assoc* **237**: 879.

Posner J and Burke CA (1985). The effects of Naloxone on opiate and placebo analgesia in healthy volunteers. *Psychopharmacology* **87**: 468–472.

Pouyanne P, Harmburu F, Imbs L and Bégaud B (2000). Admissions to hospital caused by adverse drug reactions: cross sectional incidence study. *Br Med J* **320**: 1036.

Pullar R, Wright V and Feely H (1990). What do patients and rheumatologists regard as an 'acceptable' risk in the management of rheumatoid disease. *Br Med J* **29**: 215–218.

Putnam RK (1990). Analysis of drug prescribing changes by physicians. Report to the Pharmaceutical Manufacturers Association of Canada, Ottawa.

Raschetti R, Menniti-Ippolito F, Morgutti M, Belisari A *et al.* (1997). Adverse drug events in hospitalized patients. *J Am Med Assoc* **277**: 1351–1352.

Rawlins MD (1986). Regulatory decisions and consumers. *Med Toxicol* **1**(Suppl. 1): 128–129.

Rawlins MD (1988a). Spontaneous reporting of adverse drug reactions I: the data. *Br J Clin Pharmacol* **26**: 1–5.

Rawlins MD (1988b). Spontaneous reporting of adverse reactions II: uses. *Br J Clin Pharmacol* **26**: 7–11.

Rawlins MD (1989). Trading risk for benefit. In *Risk and Consent to Risk in Medicine*, Mann RD (ed.). Parthenon Publishing Group, Carnforth; 193–202.

Rawlins MD (1995). The challenge to pharmacoepidemiology. *Pharmacoepidemiol Drug Saf* **4**: 5–10.

Rawlins MD and Jefferys DB (1993). United Kingdom product licence applications involving new active substances, 1987–1989: their fate after appeals. *Br J Clin Pharmacol* **35**: 599–602.

Rawlins MD and Thompson JW (1977). Pathogenesis of adverse drug reactions. In *Textbook of Adverse Reactions* (Davies DM (ed.)). Oxford University Press: P44.

Rawlins MD and Payne S (1997). Pharmacovigilance under the Commission. *Scrip* (February): 54–56.

Rawlins MD, Fracchia GN and Rodriguez-Farré E (1992). EURO-ADR: pharmacovigilance and research. A European perspective. *Pharmacoepidemiol Drug Saf* **1**: 261–268.

Reidenberg MM and Lowenthal DT (1968). Adverse non-drug reactions. *New Engl J Med* **279**(13): 678–679.

Rheingold PD (1968). The MER 29 story – an instance of successful mass disaster litigation. *Calif Law Reform* **56**(116): 19–68.

Richman V (1996). Early warnings about drugs. *Lancet* **347**: 1699.

Riethling A-K, Gordalla P, Haase G, Göttler M *et al.* (2000). Adverse drug reactions (ADR) leading to hospital admissions – systematic screening in Germany. *Eur J Clin Pharmacol* P56, AB, Abstr No. 41.

Roberts DE and Gupta G (1987). Evaluating expression of probability by medical professionals. *New Engl J Med* **316**: 550.

Roberts R (1996). Studies in pediatrics: special issues. In *DIA Conference, 15–16 April 1996, Assessing Safety of Investigational Drugs*.

Robson J (1997). Information needed to decide about cardiovascular treatment in primary care. *Br Med J* **314**: 277–280.

Rogers S (1976). Reflections on issues posed by recombinant DNA molecular technology II. *Ann N Y Acad Sci* **265**: 65–70.

Rose G (1982). Bias. *Br J Clin Pharmacol* **13**: 157–162.

Rosenzweig P, Brohier S and Zipfel A (1995). The placebo effect in healthy volunteers: influence of experimental conditions on physiological parameters during phase 1 studies. *Br J Clin Pharmacol* **39**(6): 657–664.

Ross C (1994). New drug approvals process under scrutiny. *Lancet* **344**: 1075.

Royal BW (1973). Monitoring adverse reactions to drugs. *WHO Chron* **27**: 469–475.

Royer RJ (1990). Pharmacovigilance. The French system. *Drug Saf* **5**(Suppl. 1): 137–140.

Royer RJ (1997). Mechanism of action of adverse drug reactions: an overview. *Pharmacoepidemiol Drug Saf* **6**: S43–S50.

Sachs RM and Bortnichak EA (1986). An evaluation of spontaneous ADR monitoring systems. *Am J Med* **81**(Suppl. 5B): 49–55.

Sampson HA (1996). Managing peanut allergy. *Br Med J* **312**: 1050–1051.

Schindel L (1972). Placebo-induced side effects. In *Drug Induced Diseases*, Meyer L. and Peck HM (eds). Excerpta Medica, Amsterdam; 323–330.

Schlienger RG, Oh PI, Knowles SR and Shear NH (1998). Quantifying the costs of serious adverse drug reactions to antiepileptic drugs. *Epilepsia* **39**(Suppl. 7): S27–S32.

Schneeweiss SG, Göttler M and Hasford J (1997). Adverse drug events in hospitalized patients. *J Am Med Assoc* **277**: 1352.

Schneeweiss SG, Hasford J, Göttler M, Hoffman A-K *et al.* (2001a). Hospital admissions caused by adverse drug events: a longitudinal population-based study. *Pharmacoepidemiol Drug Saf* **10**: S84.

Schneeweiss SG, Göttler M, Hasford J, Swoboda W *et al.* (2001b). First results from an intensified monitoring system to estimate drug related hospital admissions. *Br J Clin Pharmacol* **52**(2): 196–200.

Schneeweiss S, Hasford J, Göttler M, Hoffman A *et al.* (2002). Admissions caused by adverse drug events to internal medicine and emergency departments in hospitals: a longitudinal population-based study. *Eur J Clin Pharmacol* **58**: 285–291.

Schneider PJ, Gift MG, Lee Y-P, Rothermich EA *et al.* (1995). Cost of medication related problems at a university hospital. *Am J Health Syst Pharm* **52**: 2415–2418.

Schoenemann JH, Müller-Oerlinghausen B, Munter KH and Enayati-Kashani S (1998). Adverse drug reactions causing hospital admissions. *Pharmacoepidemiol Drug Saf* **7**: S1–S3.

Schonhofer P (1981). *Scrip* (638): 2.

Schwartzberg J (2001). http://www.npsf.org/download/FocusSummer.

Schweiger A, Parducci A (1981). Nocebo: the psychologic induction of pain. *Pavlov J Biol Sci* **16**: 140–143.

Scott HD, Thacher-Renshaw A, Rosenbaum SE, Waters WJ *et al.* (1990). Physician reporting of adverse drug reactions. Results of the Rhode Island Adverse Drug Reaction Reporting Project. *J Am Med Assoc* **263**: 1785–1788.

Senard J-M, Montastruc P and Herxheimer A (1996). Early warnings about drugs from the stock market. *Lancet* **347**: 987–988.

Shah RR (2001). Thalidomide, drug safety and early drug registration in UK. *Adverse Drug React Toxicol Rev* **20**(4): 199–285.

Shakir SAW and Layton D (2002). Causal association in pharmacovigilance and pharmacoepidemiology. *Drug Saf* **25**(6): 467–471.

Shapiro AK (1961). Factors contributing to the placebo effect. Their implications for psychotherapy. *Am J Psychother* **18**: 73–88.

Shapiro S (1977). Post-marketing assessment of drugs. In *Post-marketing Surveillance of Adverse Reactions to New Medicines*, Medico-Pharmaceutical Forum Publication No. 7.

Shapiro S, Slone D, Lewis GP and Jick H (1971). Fatal drug reactions amongst medical inpatients. *J Am Med Assoc* **216**: 467–472.

Silverstein M, Trinh D and Petterson T (1994). Adverse drug reactions resulting in hospitalisations in the elderly: a population-based study. *Pharmacoepidemiol Drug Saf* **3**(Suppl. 1): S31, 083.

Skolbekken J-A (1998). Communicating the risk reduction achieved by cholesterol reducing drugs. *Br Med J* **516**: 1956–1958.

Smalley W (2001). Drug safety: can simple interventions be effective in a complex world? *Pharmacoepidemiol Drug Saf* **10**: 209–210.

Smith CC, Bennett PM, Pearce HM, Harrison PI *et al.* (1996). Adverse drug reactions in a hospital general medical unit meriting notification to the Committee on Safety of Medicines. *Br J Clin Pharmacol* **42**: 423–429.

Smyth RL, Ashby D, O'Hea U, Burrows E *et al*. (1995). Fibrosing colonopathy in cystic fibrosis: results of a case-control study. *Lancet* **346**: 1247–1251.

Sneader W (2000). The discovery of aspirin: a reappraisal. *Br Med J* **321**: 1591–1594.

Snodgrass WR (2001). Herbal products: risks and benefits of use in children. *Curr Ther Res* **62**(10): 729.

Spriet-Pourra C and Auriche M (1988). Drug withdrawals from sale: an analysis of the phenomenon and its implications. In *Scrip Report* PGB Publications Ltd.

Spriet-Pourra C and Auriche M (1994). Drug withdrawal from sale. In *Scrip Report,* 2nd Edition. PGB Publications Ltd.

Spriet-Pourra C, Spriet A, Soubrie C and Simon P (1982). Les méthodes d'étude des effets indésirables des médicaments, II. *Thérapie* **37**: 13–22.

St George DAB (1996). Data from several sources are needed to show numbers taking drugs. *Br Med J* **312**: 1419.

Strom BL (1994). Study designs available for pharmacoepidemiologic studies. In *Pharmacoepidemiology*, Strom BL (ed.). John Wiley.

Strom BL (2000). Study designs available for pharmacoepidemiologic studies. In *Pharmacoepidemiology* 3rd edition, Strom BL (ed.). John Wiley.

Suh D-C, Woodall BS, Shin S-K and Santis EH-D (2000). Clinical and economic impact of adverse drug reactions in hospitalised patients. *Ann Pharmacother* **34**: 1373–1379.

Sundström A, Fahlgren B and Wiholm B-E (1998). Individual experiences of adverse drug reactions in a randomly selected control population. *Pharmacoepidemiol Drug Saf* **7**: S143, 155.

Sundström A, Jansson K and Wiholm B-E (2000a). The CCNet control-pool: a database of 2000 randomly selected community controls in Sweden. Poster at *8th Annual Meeting of ESOP*, Verona, 21–29 September.

Sundström A, Persson U, Jansson K and Wiholm B-E (2000b). Experiences of adverse drug reactions in a randomly selected control population: more common and more severe than expected? Poster at *8th Annual Meeting of ESOP*, Verona, 21–29 September.

Sylvestri A (1996). Water under the bridge: postmarketing concerns as related to pediatric populations. *Drug Inf J* **30**: 1163–1171.

Tai Y-T, Lau C-P, Put-Hay But P, Fong PC *et al*. (1993a). Bidirectional tachycardia induced by herbal aconite poisoning. *Pacing Electrophysiol* **15**: 831–839.

Tai Y-T, Put-Hay But P, Young K, Lau C-P (1993b). Cardiotoxicity after accidental herb-induced aconite poisoning. *Lancet* **340**: 1254–1256.

Tangrea JA, Adrianza ME and McAdams M (1991). A method for the detection and management of adverse events in clinical trials. *Drug Inf J* **25**: 63–80.

Thomas EJ and Brennan TA (2000). Incidence and types of preventable adverse events in elderly patients: population based review of medical records. *Br Med J* **320**: 741–744.

Thompson MS (1986). Willingness to pay and accept risk to cure chronic disease. *Am J Public Health* **76**: 392–396.

Thompson R (1982). Side-effects and placebo amplification. *Br J Psychiatry* **140**: 64–68.

Thuermann PA, Windecker R, Steffen J, Scaefer M *et al*. (2002). Detection of adverse drug reactions in a neurological department. *Drug Saf* **25**(10): 713–724.

Tierney S (1977). The testing of new drugs and the responsibility for their unforeseen effects. *J R Coll Physicians London* **11**(3): 237.

Toogood JH (1980). What do we mean by 'usually'? *Lancet* **i**: 1094.

Tramèr MR, Reynolds DJM, Moore RA and McQuay HJ (1997). Impact of covert duplicate publication on meta-analysis: a case study. *Br Med J* **315**: 635–639.

Tsubaki T, Homma Y and Hoshi M (1971). Epidemiological study related to clioquinol as etiology of SMON. *J Med J* **2448**: 29–34.

Tubert-Bitter P, Haramburu F, Bégaud B, Chaslerie A *et al.* (1998). Spontaneous reporting of adverse drug reactions: who reports and what? *Pharmacoepidemiol Drug Saf* 7: 323–329.

Tucker WB (1954). Effects of placebo administration and occurrence of toxic reactions. *J Am Med Assoc* **155**: 339.

Tufts Center for the Study of Drug Development (2001). News release, 30 November. Available at http://csdd.tufts.edu/newsEvents/RecentNews.asp?newsid=6.

Turk JL (1994). Sir James Simpson: leprosy and syphilis. *J R Soc Med* **87**: 549–551.

Urquhart J and Heilmann K (1983). Risk Watch. The Odds of Life. Publishers Facts on File Publications, New York and Bicester, UK. In the original German *Keine Angst vor der Angst* published in 1983 by Kindler Verlag, Munich.

Van den Bremt PMLA, Egberts ACG, Lenderink AW, Verzijl JM *et al.* (1998). Reporting of adverse drug reactions in hospital: a comparison of doctors, nurses and patients as sources of reports. *Pharmacoepidemiol Drug Saf* 7(Suppl. 2): S165, 208.

Van der Kroef C (1979). Reactions to triazolam. *Lancet* **2**: 526.

Vargas E, Garcia-Arenillas M, Portoles MM (1996). Adverse drug reactions in a cardiology department: cause of admission or appearance during hospitalisation. *Clin Drug Invest* **12**: 46–52.

Veatch RM (1993). Benefit/risk assessment: what patients can know that scientists cannot. *Drug Inf J* **27**: 1021–1029.

Vega P, Lapeyre-Mestre M, Damase-Michel C and Montastruc J-L (1996). Factors influencing spontaneous reporting of adverse drug reactions in hospital and private medicine in the southwest of France. *Pharmacoepidemiol Drug Saf* **5**: S8.

Venulet J (1974). From experimental to social pharmacology – natural history of pharmacology. *Int J Clin Pharmacol* **10**: 203–205.

Venulet J (1978). Aspects of social pharmacology. In *Progress in Drug Research* vol. 22, Jucker E (ed.). Birkhäuser Verlag, Basel und Stuttgart.

Venulet J (1993). The WHO drug monitoring programme: the formative years (1968–1975). In *Drug Surveillance International Cooperation Past, Present and Future*, Bankowski Z and Dunne JF (eds). CIOMS, Geneva; 13–22.

Venulet J (1999). Epidemiological pharmacology. *Pharmacoepidemiol Drug Saf* **8**: 57–60.

Vinar O (1969). Dependence on a placebo: a case report. *Br J Psychiatry* **115**: 1189–1190.

Vincent C, Neale G and Woloshynowy DM (2001). Adverse Events in British hospitals: preliminary retrospective record review. *Br Med J* **322**(7285): 517–519

Von Kries R (1998). Neonatal vitamin K prophylaxis: the Gordian knot still awaits untying. *Br Med J* **316**: 161–162.

Von Kries R, Göbel U, Hachmeister A, Kaletsch U *et al.* (1996). Vitamin K and childhood cancer: a population based case-control study in Lower Saxony, Germany. *Br Med J* **313**: 199–203.

Wakefield AJ, Murch SH, Linnell AAJ, Casson DM *et al.* (1998). Ileal-lymphoid-nodular hyperplasia, non-specific colitis and pervasive developmental disorder in children. *Lancet* **351**: 637–641.

Waller PC, Coulson RA and Wood SM (1996). Pharmacovigilance in the United Kingdom: current principles and practice. *Pharmacoepidemiol Drug Saf* **5**: 363–375.

Wasserfallen J-B, Buclin T, Tillet T, Yersin B *et al.* (2001). Rate, type and cost of adverse drug reactions in emergency department admissions. *Eur J Intern Med* **12**(5): 442–447.

Wax DM (1995). Elixirs, diluents and the passage of the 1938 Federal Food, Drug and Cosmetic Administration. *Ann Intern Med* **15**: 456–461.

Weber JCP (1984). Epidemiology of adverse reactions to non-steroidal antiinflammatory drugs. In *Advances in Inflammatory Research*, vol. 6, Rainsford KD and Velo GP (eds). Raven Press; 1–7.

Weber JCP and Griffin JP (1986). Prescriptions, adverse reactions and the elderly. *Lancet* i: 1220.

WHO (1991). Letter M10/372/2(A).

WHO (2001). Diethylene glycol contamination linked to child fatalities in India. *WHO Bulletin* 7 February.

Wiholm B-E (1991). Weighing risk/benefit assessment: views of a Swedish 'regulator'. In *Improving Drug Safety – a Joint Responsibility*, 131–135. Van Eimerson W (ed.). Springer-Verlag.

Williamson J and Chopin JM (1980). Adverse reactions to prescribed drugs in the elderly: a multicentre investigation. *Age Ageing* **9**: 73–80.

Wolf S (1950). Effects of suggestions and conditioning on the action of chemical agents in human subjects: the pharmacology of placebos. *J Clin Invest* **29**: 100.

Wolf S (1959a). Placebos. *Assoc Res Nerv Dis Proc* **37**: 147–161.

Wolf S (1959b). The pharmacology of placebos. *Pharmacol Rev* **II**: 689.

Wolf S and Pinsky RH (1954). Effects of placebo administration and occurrence of toxic reactions. *J Am Med Assoc* **155**(4): 339–341.

Wood S (1992). Handling of drug safety alerts in the European Community. *Pharmacoepidemiol Med* **1**: 139–142.

Wright PE (1974). Skin reaction to practolol. *Br Med J* **2**: 560.

Wright PE (1974). Skin reaction to practolol. *Br Med J* **1**: 595–598.

Yamagishi K (1997). When a 12.86 per cent mortality is more dangerous than 24.14 per cent: implications for risk communication. *Appl Cogn Psychol* **11**: 495–506.

Zeckhauser RJ and Viscusi WK (1990). Risk within reason. *Science* **248**: 559–564.

Ziegler DK, Mosier MC, Buenaver M and Okuyemi K (2001). How much information about adverse effects of medication do patients want from physicians? *Arch Intern Med* **161**: 706–713.

Zipursky A (1996). Vitamin K at birth. *Br Med J* **313**: 179–180.

Further reading

McEwan J. (1999). Adverse reactions – a personal view of their history, *Int J Pharm Med* **13**: 269–277.

Hardysides S (1999). All the history that you can remember. *Communicable Dis Public Health* **2**(4): 230–232.

Sebastian A (2000). *Dates in Medicine*. Parthenon Publishing Group.

Mann Rd (1988). From mithridatium to modern medicine: the management of drug safety. *J R Soc Med* **81**: 725–728.

Haramburu F, Pouyanne P, Imbs JL, Blayac JP and Bégaud B (2000). Incidence and prevalence of adverse drug reactions. *Presse Med* **29**(2): 11–14.

Martin U and George C (2002). Drugs and the elderly. In *Pharmacovigilance*, Mann R and Andrews E (eds). John Wiley; **88**.

Wilson R and Crouch EAC (2001). *Risk–Benefit Analysis*, 2nd edition. Harvard University Press.

Benefit–risk balance for marketed drugs: evaluating safety signals. *Report of CIOMS Working Group IV*, Geneva, 1998.

'Benefit/risk assessment; What patients can know that scientists cannot' (Veatch, 1993).

Reactions: No. 835, 3; 838, 3; 839, 3; 841, 5; 843, 3; 851, 3; 854, 3; 857, 2; 862, 3; 868, 2; 872, 5; *Br Med J* **322**: 183–4; **322**: 460–463; **322**: 1083; **323**: 163–164; **323**: 838–840.

Barsky J, Saintfort R, Rogers MP and Borus JF (2002). Nonspecific medication side effects and the nocebo phenomenon. *J Am Med Assoc* **287**(5): 622–627.

Guess HA, Kleinman A, Kusek JW and Engel LW. BMJ Books. *The Science of the Placebo: Towards an Interdisciplinary Research Agenda*.

Vogt EM (2002). Effective communication of drug safety information to patients and the public. *Drug Saf* **25**(5): 313–321.

Living with Risk, The British Medical Association guide published by Wiley Medical Publications in 1987 as a paperback, which is also suitable for patients.

Mann R (ed.). (1989). *Risk and Consent to Risk in Medicine*. The Parthenon Publishing Group.

Risk Watch. The Odds of Life. Urquhart J and Heilmann K. Publishers Facts on File Publications, New

York and Bicester, UK. Or, in the original German: *Keine Angst vor der Angst* published in 1983 by Kindler Verlag, Munich (out of print).

Ernst E (2000). Risks associated with complementary therapies. In *Meyler's Side Effects of Drugs*, 14th edition, Dukes MNG and Aronson JK (eds). Elsevier; chapter 48.

Adverse Effects of Herbal Drugs (see Bibliography).

Huxtable RJ (1990). The harmful potential of herbal and other plant products. *Drug Saf* **5**(Suppl. 1): 126–136.

De Smet PAGM (1997). Adverse effects of herbal remedies, *Adverse Drug Reaction Bulletin* 183. 1997.

Ernst E. Harmless herbs? A review of the recent literature. *Am J Med* vol. **104**: 170–178, 1998.

Herb-Drug Interactions by A Fugh-Berman. *Lancet* **355**: 134–138, 2000.

Communicating risks: illusion or truth The BMJ, 7417, 27th September 2003 is devoted to this subject.

2

Adverse Drug Reactions and Interactions: Mechanisms, Risk Factors, Detection, Management and Prevention

P. A. Routledge

Introduction

Adverse drug reactions (ADRs), of which adverse interactions are a special case, are a major cause of morbidity in the community. They are also reported to account for up to 5 per cent of all medical admissions to hospital (Grahame-Smith and Aronson, 1992; Aronson and White, 1996) and they are occasionally fatal. In the USA, it has been suggested that they are between the fourth and sixth commonest cause of death in hospitalized patients (after heart disease, cancer and stroke and around the same frequency as pulmonary disease and road-traffic accidents) (Lazarou *et al.*, 1998).

ADRs are often difficult to differentiate from non-drug-related disease. Many factors, such as concomitant treatment and disease, can cloud their identification, and there are few specific laboratory or clinical methods to confirm them. In clinical practice it is thus often difficult to separate adverse events from adverse reactions, particularly in the case of previously unrecognized reactions. Most doctors often rely on their own experience or the experience of others of similar problems before accepting that a drug might have caused the event. For these reasons, ADRs remain an important clinical and public health problem, although many ADRs are predictable and, therefore, potentially avoidable from the known pharmacology of the drug and the characteristics of the patient.

Classification of adverse drug reactions

ADRs can occur in two forms: commonly they are 'type A' or 'dose-related' adverse reactions, which are an 'accentuation' of normal drug effect (Rawlins and Thompson, 1977). Thus, digoxin slows the heart rate in a dose-dependent fashion, but this may become an adverse effect if the heart rate becomes too slow. Type A reactions make up perhaps 75

Stephens' Detection of New Adverse Drug Reactions Fifth Edition edited by John Talbot and Patrick Waller
© 2004 John Wiley & Sons, Ltd   ISBN: 0 470 84552 X

per cent of all adverse reactions, but they are proportionately less likely to have fatal consequences than type B reactions (Table 2.1). Nevertheless, because their onset is often gradual, they may remain unrecognized for some time and produce considerable morbidity to the patient.

Table 2.1   A classification of adverse reactions, revised from Rawlins and Thompson (1977)

	Type A (accentuated)	Type B (bizarre)
Dose relationship	Yes	No
Frequency	Common	Rarer
Mortality	Low	Higher
Morbidity	High	Lower
Treatment	Stop drug or reduce dose	Stop drug

Type B reactions are unpredictable and often 'bizarre' reactions to a drug, which may be present at an extremely low concentration. These reactions tend to be sudden and often dramatic in onset and are usually quickly recognized, although some, particularly those involving anaphylaxis, may be fatal.

Grahame-Smith and Aronson (1992) have extended the original Rawlins and Thompson classification described above to include type C ADRs and type D reactions. Type C (chronic) reactions are long-term drug effects including adaptive changes (e.g. drug tolerance) and withdrawal (rebound) effects. Type D (delayed) reactions involve carcinogenesis and effects associated with reproduction. Although this classification highlights ADRs that may have been given inadequate consideration in the past, it relies on both temporal and mechanistic features. In this chapter, these issues will be addressed within the context of the original classification.

Risk factors for type A adverse reactions

Type A reactions, being an extension of the normal pharmacological effect of the drug, occur when the concentration of the drug at the site(s) of action is increased above the normal therapeutic level (Table 2.2). This may occur when the dose administered is excessive for that individual either because:

- elimination mechanisms are compromised (pharmacokinetic causes), or

Table 2.2   Risk factors for type A ADRs

Pharmacokinetic	Pharmacodynamic
Renal disease	Renal disease
Liver disease	Liver disease
Cardiac failure	Cardiac failure
Extremes of age	Extremes of age
Pharmacogenetic	

- the target organ is excessively sensitive to a given drug concentration (pharma-codynamic causes)

Both of these mechanisms tend to go hand in hand and are seen at the extremes of life, as well as in patients with renal or liver disease. Other individuals may be at increased risk because of genetically inherited factors, and these will also be described.

Pharmacological and pharmaceutical factors

Certain drugs are associated with an increased risk of adverse reactions or interactions. These tend to be agents with a low therapeutic ratio (i.e. the difference between a therapeutic and toxic dose is low) and include oral anticoagulants, oral hypoglycaemic agents, some antihypertensives, many cytotoxic agents, corticosteroids, nonsteroidal anti-inflammatory drugs (NSAIDs) and digoxin. In addition to these pharmacological factors, the pharmaceutical formulation may predispose to ADRs. Changes in formulation have, in the past, been associated with increased bioavailabiity of certain drugs with a low therapeutic ratio (e.g. phenytoin and digoxin) and subsequent type A toxicity. The likelihood of this problem is now low because of the strict bioequivalence criteria insisted upon by national licensing bodies. Nevertheless, the formulation may cause local toxicity, e.g. the intestinal perforation seen in association with a certain form of indomethacin in the early 1980s (Day, 1983) or the colonic strictures reported in association with high-dose pancreatic enzyme supplements (Fitzsimmons et al., 1997). It is also rare now for the fillers, binders, surfactants, dyes or other excipients, which constitute around 90 per cent of the mass of many formulations, to cause type A toxicity. However, serious problems have occurred, such as fatal renal failure in Bangladeshi children caused by diethylene glycol in paracetamol elixir (Hanif et al., 1995).

Pharmacokinetic risk factors

These include several situations when elimination mechanisms are impaired. These include reduction in renal excretion of drugs, as well as impaired drug metabolism, largely due to liver disease (Routledge, 2002).

Renal disease

Most drugs are lipid soluble and, therefore, are first metabolized to more polar (water-soluble) compounds before the metabolites can be excreted in the urine. Several clinically important compounds (e.g. digoxin, aminoglycoside antibiotics, lithium, captopril and potassium-sparing diuretics) are already relatively water soluble and are not markedly bound to plasma proteins and so undergo glomerular filtration. In other cases, the active metabolite of an inactive drug (prodrug) may be excreted largely unchanged by the kidney – examples include oxypurinol, the active metabolite of allopurinol, and enalaprilat, which is the active metabolite of enalapril. In renal failure, glomerular filtration rate (GFR) declines progressively and is a useful marker of renal dysfunction. Normally, the GFR in an adult is around 120 ml/mm and the clearance of drugs exclusively by this process cannot exceed this value. Mild renal failure is defined by a GFR of 20–50 ml/min, moderate renal failure by a GFR of 10–20 ml/min and severe renal impairment by a GFR of less than 10 ml/mm. Drugs for which glomerular filtration is an important pathway may accumulate in renal failure unless the dose is reduced accordingly.

Active tubular secretion is the other important excretory process in the kidney. Weak electrolytes (acids and bases) are secreted into the proximal tubular fluid and digoxin may be secreted by the distal tubule. This is an energy-dependent process and drugs can be effectively cleared, with a tubular secretion of ampicillin of around 400 ml/min in subjects with normal renal function. Tubular secretion is relatively spared in renal impairment, so dose reduction of those drugs for which this process contributes significantly to total clearance may not be necessary unless renal impairment is severe.

Liver disease

The liver is the largest metabolic organ and quantitatively the most important, although the skin, gut, lungs, kidney and white cells have some limited metabolic capacity. Many drugs are lipid soluble, and even if a substantial proportion was not protein bound in the blood and, therefore, could undergo glomerular filtration, they would be passively reabsorbed through the renal tubular cell down a concentration gradient. Several metabolic pathways are present to convert these agents to more water-soluble metabolites, which are generally less active than the parent compound, although there are several important exceptions.

Phase 1 metabolism involves the mono-oxygenase system in the smooth endoplasmic reticulum of the hepatocyte. Here, a variety of subtypes of cytochrome P450 enzymes (CYP450) catalyse oxidation, reduction, hydrolysis and dealkylation reactions. These enzymes are not specific, and drugs may compete with each other for metabolism via one particular pathway and a given drug may be metabolized via several routes mediated by several subtypes of CYP450. Some of the most clinically relevant subtypes and substances for which they are quantitatively important metabolic pathways are shown in Table 2.3.

Phase 2 metabolism involves the conjugation of parent drug or metabolite with a water-soluble molecule such as glucuronic acid (glucuronidation), sulphate, amino acid (such as glutathione or glycine) or acetyl coenzyme A (acetylation). As with phase 1 reactions, the metabolites are generally less active and, therefore, of low toxicity. However, there are important exceptions.

Finally, drugs with a high molecular weight (e.g. rifampicin) may be excreted in the bile, particularly as conjugates. The drug or its conjugate may be reabsorbed, either directly or after deconjugation by intestinal microflora, resulting in an enterohepatic recycling, which offsets the effects of biliary excretion. In obstructive jaundice the enterohepatic circulation is impaired, leading to an accumulation of drugs excreted in the bile (e.g. rifampicin and fusidic acid).

In liver disease, phase 1 metabolism is often relatively more affected than phase 2 metabolic reactions. The effect of liver disease is most marked for those drugs that are normally efficiently removed by hepatic metabolism (high-clearance compounds). These agents normally have high presystemic (first pass) metabolism, resulting in low bio-availability after oral administration despite complete absorption. Important examples include morphine, nifedipine and propranolol. Not only is the metabolic activity of the liver affected in liver disease, but also the intra- and extra-hepatic shunting results in a smaller proportion of the drug being metabolized on its first passage through the liver.

There is no ideal marker of the likely reduction in drug metabolic processes in chronic liver disease. The simplest clinical marker is the serum albumin, although strictly speaking

Table 2.3 Some clinically important subtypes of cytochrome P450 and some important substrates and inhibitors of metabolism

Cytochrome P450 subtype	Some important substrates	Some important inhibitors
CYP1A2	Clozapine R-Warfarin Tacrine Theophylline	Cimetidine Ciprofloxacin Erythromycin
CYP2C9	Amitriptyline Phenytoin S-Warfarin	Amiodarone Cimetidine Fluconazole Metronidazole Sulphapyridine
CYP2C19	Diazepam Mephenytoin Omeprazole	Fluoxetine Fluvoxamine
CYP2D6	Codeine Haloperidol Imipramine Paroxetine Risperidone Thioridazine Venlafaxine	Amiodarone Fluoxetine Fluvoxamine Quinidine
CYP2E1	Ethanol Isoniazid Paracetamol	Disulfiram
CYP3A4	Astemizole Carbamazepine Corticosteroids Ciclosporin Erythromycin Lidocaine Nifedipine Quinidine Terfenadine Verapamil	Cimetidine Clarithromycin Erythromycin Grapefruit juice Ketoconazole

this is a marker of biosynthetic rather than metabolic function. Although the serum albumin gives a measure of the likely degree of liver damage and also of the patient's prognosis, it is relatively crude. However, serum bilirubin, transaminase enzymes and alkaline phosphatase may be normal, even in the presence of severe chronic liver dysfunction, and may therefore be unhelpful. In acute liver damage, the albumin concentration may be normal at first because of the long half-life of the protein (20 days) and the reduction in vitamin K-dependent clotting factors, particularly factor XII, which has a half-life of 4 h, is a more useful guide. The International Normalized Ratio (INR), a derivative of the one-stage prothrombin time that is particularly sensitive to changes in factor VII, is normally used for this purpose.

In cardiac failure, cardiac output (normally around 6 l/min) is reduced. This results in a disproportionate reduction in hepatic blood flow (normally around 1.5 l/min) and a reduction in the systemic clearance of compounds that are normally efficiently cleared (e.g. lidocaine) for which hepatic blood flow is a major determinant of clearance. In addition, the liver can be affected by the increased venous back-pressure caused by failure of the right side of the heart consequent to left ventricular failure (biventricular or congestive heart failure). This results in increased size and congestion of the liver and derangement of liver function, which can progress in severe cases to jaundice.

Drug metabolism can decrease so that clearance even of drugs that are normally poorly cleared (e.g. theophylline) may be further decreased. In addition, the increased venous pressure may result in intestinal mucosal oedema and reduced absorption of relatively inefficiently absorbed drugs (e.g. furosemide).

Extremes of age

Neonates   The neonatal period covers the first 30 days of life. Prematurity amplifies many of the problems encountered in the drug treatment of this group, but even the healthy full-term neonate is prone to ADRs because of the immaturity of pharmacokinetic processes (Routledge, 1994). Absorption of drugs may be more complete in the neonate as transit delays are compensated for by increased mucosal contact times. If a rapid drug response is needed, then routes other than the oral route should be used. Reduced gastric acidity may result in increased absorption of drugs, such as with amoxycillin. Reduced body fat and increased body water result in changes in the volume of distribution for lipid- and water-soluble drugs.

Other influences include reduced plasma albumin and alpha-1-acid glycoprotein (AAG) concentrations, resulting in reduced plasma protein binding affinity and increased competition for binding from free fatty acids and bilirubin. These effects tend to prolong the half-life of the drug. Despite increased hepatic size relative to body size, phase 1 (and most phase 2) metabolic enzyme systems are immature, so hepatic metabolism of drugs may be reduced. Chloramphenicol produces the 'grey baby' syndrome via inefficient glucuronidation for example. Renal function is globally reduced in neonates, with the GFR being about 40 per cent of the normal adult value. This results in delayed excretion of drugs such as digoxin and gentamicin. In general, smaller weight-related doses of all drugs are required in the neonatal period (Rylance and Armstrong, 1997).

The elderly   The increased risk of ADRs in the elderly is well described, and around 10 per cent of all admissions to geriatric units are directly due to an ADR, generally a type A reaction (Williamson and Chopin, 1980).

Pharmacokinetic factors are important contributors to the increased risk of type A ADRs in the elderly. The GFR tends to decline with increasing age from 30 years onwards (Lindeman, 1992) so that the average GFR of an 80-year-old is 30 per cent less, even in the absence of overt renal disease. This decline does not occur in all elderly subjects and may be partly related to underlying pathophysiological changes rather than the inevitable consequence of age. Nevertheless, the decline in renal function is important in relation to renally excreted drugs with a low therapeutic index, as mentioned above. The relationship between age and drug metabolism is less clear-cut. There does tend to be a slow decline in the metabolism of some drugs with increasing age, but wide variability at any age indicates that factors other than chronological age are more important determinants of the rate of metabolism. Perhaps the most important of these is the presence of physical frailty (Owens *et al.*, 1994). Biological (rather than chronological) age more accurately reflects nutritional state and protein energy malnutrition. This is particularly seen in the housebound or nursing home resident and is associated with a reduction in the activity of several important pathways of drug metabolism (O'Mahony and Woodhouse, 1994).

Pharmacogenetic factors

Genetic factors play a major role in determining drug response and handling, as well as in susceptibility to ADRs. Although receptors, transport processes and metabolic pathways may all be affected, most is known about the metabolic processes, many of which are responsible for handling foreign substances (xenobiotics), of which drugs are an important group. Allelic variations affecting drug handling (pharmacokinetics) with a frequency of at least 1 per cent are often termed polymorphisms (e.g. acetylation), whereas less common variants are often classified as rare inborn errors of metabolism (e.g. porphyria), but the distinction is relatively arbitrary.

The extent to which an individual metabolizes a drug is often, if only partly, genetically determined. Twins derived from the same ovum (monozygotic) metabolize many drugs at a similar rate, whereas dizygotic twins differ more in clearance values. For most drugs the variability in metabolism is unimodally distributed. A bimodal or trimodal distribution may suggest the existence of separate populations capable of metabolizing those drugs at markedly different rates. Some pathways of drug metabolism showing such polymorphism are acetylation, oxidation, succinylcholine hydrolysis (de-esterification) and thiopurine *S*-methylation. These issues are discussed in detail in recent reviews by Ingelman-Sundberg *et al.* (1999), Meyer (2000) and Weinshilboum (2003). Polymorphisms affecting drug target genes, and gene products other than drug metabolizing enzymes (e.g. receptors) or disease-modifying or treatment-modifying genes that can influence drug response, are reviewed by Evans and McLeod (2003). However, the clinical significance of these polymorphisms to the risk of ADRs is generally less well studied than polymorphisms affecting drug metabolism.

Acetylation

This metabolic pathway with its polymorphic distribution was discovered over 40 years ago. The enzyme *N*-acetyltransferase mediates acetylation of some drugs. At least two populations exist with different rates of acetylation. The gene controlling the *N*-acetyltransferase in the liver (NAT2) is on chromosome 8 and the slow phenotype is inherited as an autosomal recessive trait. For reasons that are not clear, the proportion of slow acetylators varies markedly between different races, being 55 per cent in European Caucasians, 10 per cent in Japanese and 5 per cent in the Inuit of northern Canada and in Egyptians. Drugs that undergo genetically determined acetylation are dapsone, isoniazid, hydralazine, phenelzine, procainamide and some sulphonamides, such as the sulphapyridine, which forms part of the sulphasalazine molecule used for the treatment of ulcerative colitis. Slow acetylators require lower doses of hydralazine than fast acetylators in the treatment of hypertension and are more likely to have dose-related toxicity with high doses of sulphasalazine. They are also more likely to develop the lupus erythematosus-like syndrome caused by isoniazid or hydralazine, and the pyridoxine-deficient peripheral neuropathy caused by isoniazid. Phenytoin toxicity due to inhibition of its metabolism by isoniazid occurs more frequently in slow acetylators receiving isoniazid for treatment or prophylaxis of tuberculosis. Drug-related lupus (DRL) is very rarely seen in fast acetylators of hydralazine, but not all slow acetylators develop the complication. It is clear, therefore, that the mechanism is multifactorial, and several studies have examined other causes of susceptibility. Studies of human leucocyte antigen (HLA) associations with DRL have given conflicting results, but immunogenetic differences are associated with systemic lupus erythematosus and it is likely that they will also pertain to the drug-induced form of this condition. The acetylator status of an individual may be easily assessed by giving isoniazid (200 mg orally) and measuring the ratio of the concentration of acetylisoniazid and isoniazid in a plasma or saliva sample 3 h later (Hutchings and Routledge, 1986). Genotyping only requires a sample of blood without administering a drug and may be available for clinical use in the future.

Oxidation

Certain metabolic pathways involving oxidation are polymorphically inherited, with poor and extensive metabolizer phenotypes.

CYP2D6   One of the most important examples is the autosomal recessive defect of cytochrome P450, CYP2D6. The gene is located on chromosome 22 and the poor metabolizer phenotype is inherited in an autosomal recessive fashion. This phenotype occurs in about 7 per cent of Caucasians and up to 20 per cent of Ethiopians, but has a lower prevalence in other racial types (e.g. 1 per cent in Oriental populations). It affects the metabolism of codeine, debrisoquine, haloperidol, imipramine, paroxetine and several other antidepressants, phenformin, propafenone and several other antiarrhythmic agents, sparteine, metoprolol and several other beta adrenoceptor blocking drugs, and up to 100 other drugs. The dose-related adverse effects of some of these drugs (e.g. peripheral neuropathy with perhexiline and central nervous system (CNS) toxicity with some tricyclic antidepressants) are more likely in poor hydroxylators. Quinidine inhibits this pathway, and its concurrent administration may result in a genotypically extensive metabolizer behaving as a poor metabolizer.

The lactic acidosis that has been described in approximately 10 per cent of subjects receiving phenformin was first reported in 1959, 10 years before the drug was marketed in the UK (Walker and Linton, 1959). The drug was not withdrawn until around 1980, after approximately 50 fatal case of lactic acidosis associated with its use had been reported. Despite this, phenformin is still used in some countries outside the USA and Europe and lactic acidosis is still reported.

Prolongation of the QT interval of the electrocardiogram (and increased risk of torsades de pointes and other serious ventricular arrhythmias) may be commoner in poor metabolizers of certain neuroleptic drugs (e.g. thioridazine and droperidol) by this pathway. This has resulted in licence variations (or voluntary drug withdrawal) in some countries. It is discussed later in this chapter. Ultrarapid metabolism may also rarely occur via this pathway due to gene amplification in some subjects, and failure of antidepressant therapy has been associated with this abnormality (Bertilsson *et al.*, 1993).

CYP2C9   The metabolism of the most potent enantiomer of warfarin, S-warfarin is predominantly via hydroxylation, mediated by CYP2C9. Individuals requiring low doses of warfarin to provide adequate anticoagulation are more likely to be poor metabolizers, because they possess a variant allele CYP2C9*2 or CYP2C9*3 rather than the wild-type allele CYP2C9*1. It has been suggested that such individuals may be at increased risk of warfarin-induced bleeding (Aithal et al., 1999), although this has been disputed (Taube et al., 2000). They also have lower clearance values of the anticonvulsant diphenylhydantoin (phenytoin), which is also metabolized largely by this route (van der Weide et al., 2001).

CYP2C19   The metabolism of mephenytoin (an anticonvulsant drug similar to phenytoin) and the proton pump inhibitor omeprazole is mediated by cytochrome CYP2C19, whose activity is bimodally distributed. The normal (wild-type) gene is absent in 2–6 per cent of Caucasians and up to 20 per cent of Southeast Asians (Japanese, Koreans and Chinese) in an autosomal recessive inheritance, and these people are therefore poor metabolizers. These individuals are more likely to develop drowsiness during mephenytoin treatment, but they may have better eradication rates when omeprazole is used in combination with amoxycillin in the treatment of gastrointestinal *Helicobacter pylori* infection (Furuta et al., 1998).

Succinylcholine de-esterification

Succinylcholine is a depolarizing neuromuscular blocking agent used in induction of general anaesthesia. Normally, it is rapidly metabolized in the plasma by a non-specific esterase called pseudocholinesterase (butyrylcholinesterase) and has a short half-life and duration of action. Some individuals possess pseudocholinesterase of abnormal affinity or amount, and metabolize the succinylcholine much more slowly, resulting in a prolonged neuromuscular blockade. Prolonged apnoea was first recognized in 1953 (Forbat et al., 1953). It is now known that there are three types of abnormality of pseudocholinesterase, each inherited in autosomal recessive fashion: the dibucaine-resistant, fluoride-resistant and gene types (Kalow and Genest, 1957). The prevalence of the homozygous poor metabolism phenotype is only 1 in 3500 in Europeans, so it is not a common polymorphism like acetylation or CYP2D6 oxidation. The gene for the trait is located on chromosome 3.

In some individuals there is an increase of up to threefold in the concentration of plasma pseudocholinesterase with consequent resistance to the effects of succinylcholine (Cynthiana variant). The prevalence may be as high as 1 in 1000 (i.e. three times more frequent than the deficiency state).

Thiopurine S-methylation

Thiopurine methyltransferase (TPMT) is one of three major enzymes responsible for the metabolism of azathioprine, via its active metabolite 6-mercaptopurine to 6-methylmercaptopurine. TPMT activity is determined by an allelic polymorphism for either high (TPMT H) or low (TPMT L) enzyme activity. Homozygotes for the low activity allele (0.3 per cent of the population) are known to be at risk of profound myelosupression on recommended doses of azathioprine and heterozygotes (11 per cent) may also be at risk. In such individuals, more drug is metabolized via one of the other pathways (mediated by hypoxanthine guanine phosphoribosyl transferase) to toxic 6-thioguanine nucleotides. On the other hand, homozygotes for the high TPMT activity allele may be inadequately immunosuppressed with conventionally recommended doses of this drug. The gene is located on chromosome 6.

Pharmacodynamic risk factors

In general, many of the groups with pharmacodynamic reasons for susceptibility to ADRs are also those with pharmacokinetic differences. In addition, pharmacogenetically determined differences in pharmacodymamics may increase the risk of adverse reactions.

Renal disease

In renal failure, there is an accumulation of toxic waste products, resulting eventually in severe uraemia and encephalopathy with confusion, loss of memory and other neurological signs. It is thought that purine metabolites, amines, indoles, phenols and other substances may contribute to uraemia, and retained middle molecules (molecular weight 500–5000 Da) may also contribute to the problem. It is likely that subclinical accumulation may contribute to the increased sensitivity to psychoactive drugs, particularly opiates, although pharmacokinetic factors may also be important for several drugs.

Liver disease

Encephalopathy may occur in severe liver disease. Even before this, however, a subclinical phase may be detected by psychometric or electrophysiological testing. It is thought to be due to decreased hepatic extraction of substances that tend to inhibit neuronal function. The precise mechanism by which psychoactive drugs cause a further deterioration of cerebral function in these circumstances is not yet known; however, in the case of benzodiazepines it is thought to be related to an interaction at the GABA receptor complex. Liver disease (both acute and chronic) is associated with a reduced production of vitamin K-dependent clotting factors, even after parenteral vitamin K administration. This (together with other defects of haemostasis) contributes to an increased risk of bleeding *per se*; in addition, bleeding risk due to drug therapy (e.g. aspirin and other NSAIDs) is increased. The increased sensitivity to warfarin is caused by a combination of this effect and the reduced clearance of warfarin in liver disease, although the pharmacodynamic sensitivity is probably the more important factor.

Sex

Females appear to be more susceptible to ADRs than males (Hurwitz and Wade, 1969; Hoigné *et al.*, 1984; Jacubeit *et al.*, 1990; Bowman *et al.*, 1996), with a study by Domecq *et al.* (1980) giving figures of 37.9 per cent for women and 29.6 per cent for men. This remained the case even after due consideration of the duration of hospitalization, number of drugs, age, and the presence of liver and renal disease. The increases may be due to pharmacokinetic factors (women tend to have lower ratios of lean body mass to adipose tissue mass) and hormonal influences, e.g. tardive dyskinesia (Kando *et al.*, 1995). In seven phase-1 studies, females reported spontaneously 2.3 times more frequently than males, and side effects due to laboratory abnormalities were higher in women (26 per cent) than in men (15 per cent; Vomvouras and Piergies, 1995). There may also be differences in pharmacokinetics (e.g. serum propranolol levels are twice as high in women as in men; Walle *et al.*, 1994). Androgens and oestrogen affect the QT interval and women are more prone to torsades de pointe (Drici and Clement, 2000). Female patients are estimated to have a 1.5- to 1.7-fold greater risk of developing an ADR than are male patients (Heinrich, 2001). Eight out of ten prescription drugs withdrawn during the period 1997 to 2001 posed a greater risk for women than for men (White, 1999).

Extremes of age

Neonates   The blood–brain barrier regulates the entry of drugs to the brain. It is less efficient at birth, especially in preterm neonates, who are particularly sensitive to psychoactive agents such as opiates or lithium.

Elderly   Increasing age is associated with several pharmacodynamic changes that may increase the risk of drug toxicity. Lamy (1991) has classified these as:

- primary (physiological) ageing factors
- secondary (pathophysiological) ageing factors
- tertiary (psychological) ageing factors.

All these factors may affect response. Primary factors include the slower metabolic processes, the reduction in brain mass, neurone density, cerebral blood flow and capacity for autoregulation, and possible increased permeability of the blood–brain barrier, all of which occur with increasing age. Secondary factors include the many diseases to which the elderly are more prone. Tertiary factors include the effects that psychological stresses may have upon motivation, nutrition and other aspects of self-care. Physiological ageing of the CNS contributes to the increased risk of toxicity of drugs acting on the CNS. Reduced ability to respond to stress (reserve capacity) results in reduced ability to maintain homeostasis, so that drugs that affect balance (e.g. CNS sedatives), temperature regulation (e.g. phenothiazines), bowel and bladder function (e.g. anticholinergic agents) and blood pressure (e.g. vasodilators) may all cause adverse effects at normal adult doses.

Risk factors for type B reactions

Type B reactions are 'bizarre', in that they cannot be predicted from the drug's known pharmacology. They include allergic reactions to drugs, and because of their often dramatic onset may be associated with a proportionately higher mortality than type A reactions, although they are less common. Type B reactions may occur to the excipients, preservatives or vehicle in the formulation. This problem is discussed at length by Uchegbu and Florence (1996). In the case of L-tryptophan-associated eosinophilia-myalgia syndrome, an unidentified contaminant occurring during the production of one formulation may have been responsible (Kilbourne *et al.*, 1996). The mechanisms of type B reactions are often poorly understood, but many involve allergic or pseudoallergic mechanisms (Rieder, 1994).

Allergic reactions

Allergic reactions to drugs are often known as hypersensitivity reactions.

Type I hypersensitivity

The commonest form of hypersensitivity is the immediate hypersensitivity associated with hay fever and asthma. This was classified by Gell and Coombs as type I (or immediate) hypersensitivity, and certain drugs (e.g. penicillins and cephalosporins) can also cause this problem. Mast cells, which are common in the gut and lung, and basophils have a high affinity receptor for the Fc domain of the immunoglobulin (IgE). When two such IgE molecules bound together as a dimer on the cell wall are crosslinked by a previously circulating antigen molecule, mediators such as histamine, leukotrienes and prostaglandins are released. If these are released in large amounts, then systemic anaphylaxis may ensue, with bronchospasm and circulatory collapse, sometimes with fatal consequences.

Type II hypersensitivity

In type II, or antibody-mediated cytotoxic hypersensitivity, the antigen (rather than the antibody as in type I reactions) is bound to the surface of a cell membrane, often a red cell or platelet. Circulating immunoglobulin (IgG, IgM or IgA) reacts with the antigen to stimulate complement as well as cytotoxic cells, resulting in lysis of the target cell. This is the mechanism of certain drug-induced haemolytic anaemias (e.g. due to methyldopa) and thrombocytopenias (e.g. due to quinine).

Type III hypersensitivity

In type III hypersensitivity reactions, antigen–antibody complexes are deposited in areas of turbulent flow or filtration (e.g. the glomerulus of the kidney). This type of reaction, known as immune complex hypersensitivity, results in complement activation and the lysosomes released by polymorphonuclear cells cause vascular damage. In addition to glomerulone-phritis, this reaction may result in fever, lymphadenopathy, arthritis and rashes and may be induced by several drugs, including gold and penicillamine.

Type IV hypersensitivity

Type IV, or delayed-type (cell-mediated) immunity, occurs in the absence of detectable circulating antigen or antibody. Specific helper T lymphocytes may be stimulated by a drug that acts as a hapten and has complexed with a tissue macromolecule to form an antigen. This results in the release of cytokines and the accumulation of other cells (particularly monocytes) in the area, and resulting granulomata, oedema or widespread rash, normally several days after exposure to the drug. It appears that people with human immunodeficiency virus (HIV) infection may be more prone to such drug-induced allergic reactions, particularly in response to sulphonamides.

Pseudoallergic reactions

Pseudoallergic reactions are so called because they mimic allergic hypersensitivity, particularly of type I hypersensitivity. Such reactions, if severe, are often termed anaphylactoid and can occur on first exposure to a drug, particularly a neromuscular blocker or radiographic contrast dye. It is not known why certain individuals are predisposed to such reactions, but asthmatics, especially those with nasal polyps, are more likely than others to experience such reactions with aspirin, for example. There is cross-reactivity with other NSAIDs and with tartrazine, a dye that was once commonly used in drugs but which is now restricted in use.

Drug metabolism and type B adverse drug reactions

As well as its role in type A toxicity, drug metabolism may have an important role in determining type B ADRs. Although metabolism generally results in detoxification of a drug, it may sometimes produce chemically reactive metabolites in a process termed bioactivation (Pirmohamed *et al.*, 1996). If the body's defence mechanisms against this metabolite are overwhelmed, or repair processes are inadequate, then it can combine with tissue macromolecules (e.g. protein or DNA) to cause toxicity, either directly or via activation of immune processes. The risk of this occurring is determined by a variety of factors, including age, gender, HLA status and a variety of still unrecognized host-dependent factors. For this reason, type B toxicity caused by bioactivation is still unpredictable in most cases.

Pharmacogenetic factors

Glucose-6-phosphate dehydrogenase deficiency

Some individuals have erythrocytes that are genetically deficient in glucose-6-phosphate dehydrogenase (G6PD), which is at least partly responsible for preventing the oxidation of various red-cell proteins. Haemolysis occurs if the abnormal erythrocyte is exposed to oxidizing agents, probably because of unopposed oxidation of sulphydryl groups in the cell membrane. Common causative agents include aspirin, sulphonamides, some antimalarials, antileprotics and pharmacological doses of vitamins K or C. The gene is on the X chromosome, and inheritance of the deficiency state therefore occurs in a sex-linked (X) recessive mode. It is relatively common (up to 14 per cent) in African Americans and in Mediterranean races, but the severity of reactions appears to be greater in G6PD-deficient Caucasians.

Porphyria

People with hepatic porphyrias (acute intermittent porphyria or porphyria cutanea tarda) have abnormalities of haem biosynthesis and symptoms may be precipitated by many drugs, particularly alcohol, the oral contraceptive, barbiturates and sulphonamides. (For a fuller and up-to-date list, contact the Welsh Medicines Information Centre, University of Wales, Cardiff CF14 4XW, UK, tel.: +44 (0)2920 742979).

Malignant hyperthermia

This is a serious and occasionally fatal condition that may occur in association with general anaesthesia with halothane or methoxyflurane used in conjunction with succinylcholine. It occurs in about 1 in 20 000 anaesthetized patients and is inherited in an autosomal dominant fashion. Body temperature may rise to 41 °C with increased muscle tone, tachycardia, sweating, cyanosis and tachypnoea. Creatine kinase activity may rise due to muscle damage, and muscle death (rhabdomyolysis) may occur. The muscle relaxant, dantrolene, and diazepam, which acts as a general relaxant, are sometimes effective in preventing muscle damage. The gene is thought to lie on the long arm of chromosome 19.

Coumarin resistance

Coumarin resistance is a very rare defect that has been reported in only two human kindreds. In this condition, up to 20 times the usual dose of warfarin or other coumarin anticoagulant may be required to produce satisfactory anticoagulation. It has an autosomal dominant inheritance and the mechanism appears to be resistance of the enzyme vitamin K epoxide reductase in the vitamin K–K epoxide shuttle to the normal inhibitory effect of coumarins. The site of the gene is not known.

Aminoglycoside antibiotic-induced deafness

Susceptibility to the ototoxic effects of aminoglycoside antibiotics, such as gentamicin, may be genetically determined in some individuals. The prevalence is thought to be at least 1 in 10 000, and in Shanghai it is thought that 25 per cent of all deaf mutes may have become deaf after exposure to these widely used agents (Hu *et al.*, 1991).

Inheritance is solely through the maternal line, and both sexes are equally affected, supporting the evidence that transmission is dependent upon the mitochondrial genome, a rare mechanism for inheritance of disease. Recently, the 1555A $\rightarrow$ G mitochondrial mutation has been shown to be associated with a susceptibility to aminoglycoside antibiotics. It has been found in 3 per cent of outpatients with hearing problems, making it the most prevalent mitochondrial mutation found in the hearing-impaired population (Usami *et al.*, 2002).

Long QT syndrome

This condition is characterized by an increased delay between the QRS complex and T wave in the electrocardiogram associated with a susceptibility to life-threatening ventricular arrhythmias, such as *torsades de pointes* (Figure 2.1), which may progress to ventricular

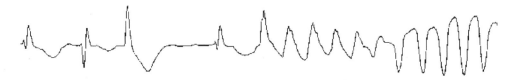

Figure 2.1   An electrocardiogram showing *torsades de pointes*

fibrillation in 20 per cent of cases. In addition, sudden death may be described more commonly in individuals with long QT syndrome. QT interval prolongation may occur spontaneously or during therapy with some drugs (e.g. some antihistamines, antiarrhythmic drugs, neuroleptics and tricyclic antidepressants). Congenital long QT syndromes are associated with mutations in the genes encoding potassium or sodium channels, which mediate the depolarization of cardiac conducting tissue. There seems to be several forms of the condition, with linkages between chromosomes 3, 7 and 11 in three of these. Clinical syndromes caused by theses phenotypes include the Romano–Ward and Jervell–Lange-Neilsen syndromes. The recently described Brugada syndrome is an important cause of sudden death in Southeast Asia and is caused by a mutation in a sodium channel (Roberts and Brugada, 2003). The QT interval duration and morphology are not always very sensitive, and specific diagnostic markers (and the penetrance of some of the mutations) may not be great, making the identification of affected individuals and carriers difficult.

The list of drugs that may prolong the QT interval continues to increase, and an up-to-date list is available at http://www.torsades.org/. It is not known how many cases of severe ventricular arrhythmias are related to an excessive concentration of the drug, since toxicity appears to be type A in nature. In addition, the presence of known risk factors, e.g. underlying bradycardia, hypokalaemia, hypomagnesemia, female gender (two- to four-fold increased risk), recent conversion from atrial fibrillation to sinus rhythm, or the presence of left ventricular hypertrophy, may markedly increase the risk. These factors are of particular concern in those with underlying congenital long QT syndromes caused by abnormalities in 'channelopathy genes', so that many cases are likely to be multifactorial in nature. Many of the drugs causing QT prolongation are CYP3A4 substrates, whose physicochemical characteristics mean that they may also affect the rapid inward potassium channel (I_{kr} or HERG) in cardiac conducting tissue. Others are CYP2D6 substrates, which may have homology in sometimes also affecting the inward sodium channel (I_{Na}).

Genetic predisposition to adverse drug reactions

Factors associated with an increased risk of ADRs include a history of allergic disorders, such as atopic disease or hereditary angioedema (Grahame-Smith and Aronson, 1992). HLA status may also be important:

- The risk of nephrotoxicity from penicillamine is increased in patients with the HLA types B8 and DR3, whereas patients with HLA-DR7 may be protected.

- The risk of skin reactions with penicillamine is associated with HLA-DRw6, and the risk of thrombocytopenia is associated with HLA-DR4; patients with HLA-DR4 also have a greater risk of the lupus-like syndrome (see above) associated with hydralazine.

- The risk of a hypersensitivity reaction to the HIV-1 reverse transcriptase inhibitor abacavir is associated with HLAB*5701, HLA-DR7 and HLA-DQ3 (Mallal et al., 2002).

Detection of adverse drug reactions

Vere (1976) described the tendency of ADRs to masquerade as natural illness over 25 years ago. He gave five main reasons why so many adverse reactions escape unnoticed:

- The reaction may be so odd or bizarre that an often used and apparently innocent drug escapes suspicion.

- The drug-induced disorder can closely mimic a common natural disease.

- There is a long delay in the appearance of the adverse effect.

- The drug evokes a relapse of natural disease or may evoke a disorder in a naturally susceptible subject.

- The clinical situation may be so complex that its drug-related components pass unnoticed.

Even today, iatrogenic disease may still go unrecognized. If the delay in onset of iatrogenic disease is very prolonged, then the effects are even more difficult to detect. Autoimmune haemolytic anaemia has been described 9 years after uneventful antihypertensive treatment with methyldopa for example (Terol *et al.*, 1991), so continued vigilance is required in all patients throughout the course of their treatment.

Another difficulty in identifying drug-induced disease is that there may be a significant prevalence of the non-drug-induced condition in the community. Vere (1976) pointed out that the risk of adenocarcinoma of the vagina in female children born to mothers who took high doses of the oestrogen stilboestrol in pregnancy was probably recognized largely because it was so unusual that there was no 'background noise'. The same argument applies to the unusual maldevelopment of limbs seen in phocomelia caused by thalidomide, which was therefore recognized reasonably quickly.

Drugs that aggravate already existing disease may escape suspicion for some time, particularly if the natural disease is common. Fialuridine is a nucleoside that was undergoing trials for the treatment of hepatitis B. Unfortunately, the major adverse effect of this drug was on the liver, and the worsening liver function in treated patients appeared to be explained by the monitoring physicians as worsening of the hepatitis rather than as direct drug toxicity. The incorporation of the nucleoside in patients into the cell nuclear protein ensured that the toxicity was quite persistent, even after withdrawal of the drug, and several patients died of the complications of lactic acidosis associated with the hepatitis (McKenzie *et al.*, 1995).

Finally, ADRs may be difficult to detect because of the confounding effects of other treatments being administered at the same time. Some agents (e.g. blood products or contrast media) may be administered for therapeutic or diagnostic purposes while the patient is undergoing treatment, and other drugs (e.g. corticosteroids or antihistamines) may affect the natural history of iatrogenic disease and prevent it from being recognized.

Biochemical and histological confirmation

There are relatively few specific investigations to confirm the presence of an ADR. Biochemical pictures associated with iatrogenic disease may mimic those from other idiopathic causes. Histological evidence, although often difficult to obtain, may sometimes be more helpful:

- The ductopenia associated with flucloxacillin-induced liver damage is relatively specific for this drug-induced hepatic damage.

- Although not specific for drug-induced glomerulonephritis, the granular deposition of immune complexes shown on immunocytochemical stains of renal biopsy material contrasts with the more linear deposition seen in other forms of immune complex glomerulonephritis, such as Goodpasture's syndrome.

Some *in vitro* investigations, such as the radioallergosorbent test (RAST), which detects antigen-specific antibodies in serum, or the histamine release test, may be valuable in determining anaphylactic or anaphylactoid reactions, particularly to anaesthetic induction agents. The histamine release test and basophil degranulation test may have an advantage over RASTs in that they will demonstrate anaphylactoid reactions (i.e. those that are non-IgE mediated) as well as those that are anaphylactic and mediated by IgE. Tryptase is the most important protein in mast cell granules and is released in anaphylactoid as well as in anaphylactic reactions. Plasma tryptase concentrations are maximal 1–6 h after the reaction, but may be detected in concentrations above normal for up to 12–14 h, making this test a useful but nonspecific confirmatory test in severe reactions, particularly those occurring in anaesthesia. Urine methylhistamine concentrations have also been used for this purpose, but they are more difficult to interpret (Association of Anaesthetists of Great Britain and Ireland and The British Society of Allergy and Clinical Immunology, 1995).

Tests using other cellular components of blood, such as the basophil degranulation test, passive haemagglutination, lymphocyte transformation and leukocyte/macrophage migration inhibition tests, may have some value in certain allergic type B reactions; however, the sensitivity of these tests is relatively poor, and negative tests do not always exclude the possibility of drug-induced disease (Pohl *et al.*, 1988). The major difficulty with many of the *in vitro* tests is that the challenge agent is normally the parent drug. Since the responsible compound may be a metabolite or breakdown product, and unless this specific agent is present or generated in the *in vitro* situation, the test may be falsely negative (Pohl *et al.*, 1988).

Skin testing and direct drug rechallenge

Skin tests are essentially a form of *in vivo* rechallenge at reduced drug dose. Such tests may be insensitive and nonspecific. In addition, they can be potentially dangerous, and deaths have been reported with intradermal testing to penicillin, for example, although this is rare with a careful technique and newer reagents. Scratch tests and intradermal tests may be particularly helpful in the investigation of immediate-type anaphylactic/anaphylactoid reactions to drugs used during anaesthesia. Skin patch testing may be helpful in the investigation of fixed drug eruptions, but should not be used in Stevens–Johnson syndrome or toxic epidermal necrolysis (Breathnach, 1995).

Systemic drug rechallenge is fraught with even more potential risk than skin testing. It is generally only considered when a suspected drug is the only agent known to be effective in a particular condition (e.g. allopurinol in long-term prophylaxis of gout). Rechallenge with the protease inhibitor abacavir has, for example, resulted in severe (and sometimes fatal) reactions and is absolutely contraindicated (Hetherington *et al.*, 2001).

Other evidence

Since direct evidence is often difficult to obtain, circumstantial evidence may be important in detecting ADRs. A useful criterion for determining whether a reaction is drug induced is the timing of the onset of the symptoms relative to the start of drug therapy:

- Type A reactions normally occur when the drug has accumulated; thus, it may take five half-lives of the drug for the ADR to reach maximum intensity.

- Type B reactions are often immunological in nature and so sometimes require a latent period of up to 5 days before being seen. Most occur within 12 weeks of initiation of drug therapy.

The time course for type B reactions may, however, be clouded by several factors. Drug-induced agranulocytosis, for example, may take two or more weeks to occur after initial drug exposure and may, therefore, present after the drug has been discontinued. The same is true of drug-induced jaundice, particularly when it occurs after the agent is used for short-course therapy (e.g. co-amoxiclav or flucloxacillin). Some type B reactions (e.g. halothane-induced jaundice) appear more rapidly on re-exposure after a previous reaction has occurred.

The time course to resolution after stopping the drug (dechallenge) may also be of help in assessing causality. Some ADRs take a considerable time to disappear after drug discontinuation, particularly if the drug has a long half-life of elimination (e.g. amiodarone), whereas others may be associated with irreversible effects (e.g. pulmonary fibrosis after busulphan or nitrofurantoin).

The absence of an alternative explanation is an important criterion in considering a drug-related cause, but the latter should still be considered and relevant information sought without waiting to rule out non-drug-related causes. Finally, it has been shown that doctors rely to a large extent on whether previous reports of ADRs have been published in association with the drug. It is important that clinicians are trained to have a much higher level of suspicion of the possibility of iatrogenic disease, since it is a situation in which prompt treatment (e.g. drug withdrawal) may result in a permanent cure.

Management of adverse drug reactions

Type A reactions will generally respond to a reduction in dose of the drug, although temporary drug discontinuation may be necessary if the reaction is significant. Unfortunately, some adverse effects are permanent (e.g. lung fibrosis with busulphan or liver fibrosis with methotrexate), although withdrawal of treatment as soon as the condition is recognized may reduce the eventual magnitude of toxicity.

For type B reactions the clinician should withdraw the suspected drug immediately and refer the patient for specialist investigations (e.g. skin testing if appropriate) on recovery. It is sometimes necessary to give supportive therapy, particularly for anaphylactic and anaphylactoid reactions, and corticosteroids may sometimes be used to suppress inflammatory or potentially fibrotic processes.

In rare circumstances, when no alternative agents are available for treatment of a particular condition, desensitization by administration of gradually increasing doses of the drug may eventually allow the patient to tolerate the agent at full dose. This approach has been used successfully in some patients with aspirin or allopurinol hypersensitivity, for example.

Part of the management of ADRs is to report them to the regulatory authorities. This allows the appropriate bodies to assess the risk–benefit of particular medications, which can contribute to safe drug use in susceptible subjects in the future. In the UK, the Committee on Safety of Medicines (CSM) (Medicines and Healthcare products Regulatory Agency, MHRA) asks health professionals to report all suspected serious reactions to established medicines and all suspected adverse reactions to newly introduced (the so-called black triangle '▼') drugs, whatever their severity.

Prevention of adverse drug reactions

The goal of therapeutics is to obtain optimum efficacy and minimum toxicity of drug therapy. This ideal is difficult to achieve because of the wide variability in drug response within patients. Bespoke prescribing aims to achieve this by tailoring initial doses to the individual patient and titrating drug dose subsequently to avoid toxicity. Bespoke prescribing has been used for the initiation of warfarin and heparin therapy (Routledge, 1986). The approach is primarily of value in avoiding type A adverse reactions, although the avoidance of excessive doses of certain drugs in high-risk individuals may also reduce the risk of type B reactions (e.g. there is a higher risk of severe allergic-type skin reactions with excessive doses of allopurinol in patients with renal disease).

In renal dysfunction, the creatinine clearance is closely related and similar in magnitude to the GFR. Thus, GFR can be calculated by measuring the patient's serum creatinine (which has little diurnal variation) and age, gender and body weight. The Cockroft–Gault equation uses the relationship:

$$\text{Creatinine clearance} = \frac{(140 - \text{age (y)}) \times \text{Body weight (kg)}}{0.82 \times \text{Plasma creatinine } (\mu\text{mol/l})}$$

For females, who have less muscle mass at any given weight, the result must be multiplied by 0.85. This equation is relevant only when the renal function is relatively constant and in the absence of concomitant liver disease. It is a useful guide to dose adjustment in renal disease and in the elderly when glomerular filtration is the major renal excretory mechanism. The proportional dose adjustment will also depend upon the proportion F of the drug excreted unchanged by the kidney (since some drug may be cleared by metabolic pathways) in the following formula:

$$\text{Dose (as proportion of normal)} = \frac{(1 - F) + F \times \text{GFR (patient)}}{\text{GFR (normal)}}$$

This relationship can be used to aid in the calculation of the dose of digoxin or gentamicin, for example. The situation is more difficult if renal tubular secretion is a major excretory mechanism, since no clinically applicable direct measurement of this pathway is available.

Dose adjustment is more difficult in liver disease, although the serum albumin concentration is of some help in deciding upon the starting dose. The initial induction dose of warfarin should be reduced by at least 50 per cent if the INR is greater than 1.3 (Fennerty *et al.*, 1988).

Therapeutic drug monitoring

Monitoring drug concentration in the plasma is also of value in avoiding some ADRs. The ideal way to monitor drug therapy is to have a simple measure of drug effect (e.g. oral anticoagulant therapy), but this is rarely available. In the absence of a pharmacodynamic measure, and particularly when the only endpoint is the absence of features of the illness (e.g. absence of seizures during anticonvulsant treatment or arrhythmias during antiarrhythmic treatment), the plasma drug concentration is a useful surrogate marker of efficacy and safety. To be applicable, the drug should have a concentration-related and reversible effect without the development of tolerance, and the metabolites should be relatively inactive unless active metabolite concentrations are also measured. Relatively few drugs fulfil these strict criteria, but therapeutic drug monitoring (TDM) is used to adjust the doses of ciclosporin, digoxin, gentamicin and other aminoglycoside antibiotics, lithium, phenytoin (diphenylhydantoin) and theophylline (Routledge and Hutchings, 2001).

Since drugs are normally given at fixed intervals, the plasma concentration varies between doses during the processes of absorption, distribution, metabolism and excretion. Samples taken some time after the dose are therefore more reflective of the average concentration between doses and should be taken at least 8 h after digoxin administration and 12 h after lithium. Peak levels are sometimes required (e.g. with gentamicin) and occur around 30—60 min after an intramuscular injection or immediately at the end of an intravenous infusion. Peak levels of orally administered drugs are achieved at 30–180 min after conventional formulations and later after modified-release preparations. For many drugs, a sample taken just before the next dose is due (trough concentration) will correlate best with the average (steady-state) concentration.

It takes approximately five half-lives before the plasma concentrations of a drug reach their maximum steady state level. Sampling before this time has elapsed is therefore most valuable if drug toxicity due to excessive accumulation is expected. Ideally, five half-lives should elapse before steady-state plasma concentrations are measured, but this may take some time in certain cases (e.g. 9 months in the case of amiodarone, which has a half-life of 45 days). Details of sampling time relative to dose, time of last dose change and present daily dose schedule should always be stated on the assay request form to aid interpretation of the plasma concentration.

In clinical practice, total rather than free (active) drug concentrations are measured by conventional assay methodologies. Although, in most circumstances, these will correlate with free drug concentrations, this is not always the case:

- In neonates, the frail elderly and in liver disease, plasma albumin may be reduced due to impaired production.

- In renal dysfunction, particularly nephrotic syndrome, plasma albumin may be reduced due to loss into the urine.

- In renal failure, accumulation of inhibitors of protein binding may further reduce binding, so the measurement of total concentration may underestimate free concentrations in all these conditions.

For some drugs (e.g. diphenylhydantoin and theophylline), saliva concentrations may reflect the free drug concentration more accurately and some laboratories can also measure free drug concentrations directly by ultrafiltration or equilibrium dialysis techniques.

AAG is an acute-phase protein that avidly binds many basic drugs (e.g. lidocaine, disopyramide, quinidine and verapamil). In situations where AAG may be raised, for instance after acute myocardial infarction, surgery, trauma or burns, or in rheumatoid arthritis and other inflammatory conditions, total drug concentrations may overestimate free drug concentrations. Conversely, AAG may be reduced in neonates, nephrotic syndrome and severe liver disease and the opposite holds true. Measurement of free drug concentration may thus be more helpful in such circumstances, although direct measurement of AAG concentration in plasma may allow the free concentration of some compounds to be calculated with reasonable accuracy (Routledge, 1986).

Surveillance and the prevention of adverse drug reactions

Many type B reactions occur in patients who are prescribed the same drug or a very similar agent to which they have had a previous adverse reaction. For this reason, the general practitioner and hospital medical records and the inpatient prescription sheets should all be clearly marked with a bright label so that the prescriber is aware of previous serious ADRs. Computerized systems have been developed to alert physicians to previous type B reactions to drugs and of appropriate drug administration rates, and their use has resulted in a reduced frequency of type B reactions (Classen *et al.*, 1991; Evans *et al.*, 1994). Unfortunately, these systems are not yet widely available, and the vigilance of healthcare professionals is still the most important factor in avoiding such episodes.

Drug interactions

Interactions between drugs have been observed for nearly 100 years and have been described under the classical headings of antagonism, synergism and potentiation. Many interactions have been, and still are, deliberately used with therapeutic benefit, but adverse interactions are becoming an increasingly important problem for several reasons:

- Newly introduced drugs are often much more potent than their predecessors and act on fundamental biochemical and enzymatic pathways or receptors.

- Progress in therapeutics, together with an increasingly aging population, has resulted in increased polypharmacy.

Drug interactions have been estimated to account for 6–30 per cent of all ADRs (Orme *et al.*, 1991). Since adverse reactions are relatively common and interactions involve many different types of drugs, it may appear at first sight an almost impossible task for any physician to retain a perspective on the subject. Fortunately, although more than 1000 drug interactions have been described, the number that are clinically important is much smaller and involves a relatively small number of pharmacological groups of drugs (Seymour and Routledge, 1998). It is also important to recognize that perhaps more than 50 per cent of drug interactions result in some loss of action of one or other of the drugs. These are more likely to be overlooked, since alternative explanations, such as poor compliance, may be considered as reasons for inefficacy of the treatment.

Mechanisms

Interactions may occur outside or inside the body:

- The former are referred to as pharmaceutical incompatibilities and they generally occur when two or more agents are mixed in infusions or in the same syringe, or when a drug reacts with the infusion fluid itself.

- Interactions occurring within the body result from either an alteration in the delivery of the drug to its site of action (pharmacokinetic interactions) or from a drug-induced alteration in receptor or organ response to another agent (pharmacodynamic interactions). Often, these characteristics are altered when other drugs are given.

Both pharmacokinetic and pharmacodynamic interactions are equally important. Pharmacokinetic interactions will be discussed first, because these must generally first be excluded before the possibility of a pharmacodynamic interaction is investigated.

Pharmacokinetic interactions

These may occur during any one or more of the pharmacokinetic processes whereby the drug reaches its site of action and is then eliminated (i.e. absorption, distribution, metabolism and excretion). Such interactions may result in either an increased or decreased drug concentration at the site of action. Although the former may result in drug toxicity, a decreased efficacy may put the patient at increased risk from the effects of the disease.

Absorption

For most drugs, absorption is a passive process that is dependent upon the properties of the drug and its particular formulation, the pH of the absorption medium and the length of time the drug remains at the site of absorption. Drugs may interact with each other during all these processes, as well as directly with each other by formation of poorly absorbed complexes. It is important to distinguish in this context between changes in the rate and extent of drug absorption:

- Alteration of the rate of absorption alone will change the shape of the concentration–time curve after oral administration, but it will not alter the average or steady-state drug concentration. Such changes may be important, however, in the case of drugs given in single doses and in which a threshold concentration for drug effect exists (e.g. analgesics). A delay in absorption under these circumstances, especially if the rate of elimination of the drug is high, may result in an inability to reach a drug concentration associated with drug efficacy.

- In contrast, a change in extent of absorption will result in a change in variation in delivery of drug to its site of action both after a single dose and repeated doses.

Drug-induced changes in the pH of the gastrointestinal media may increase or decrease the rate and extent of drug absorption. Alkalis may aid dissolution of poorly soluble acidic drugs (e.g. aspirin) and stimulate gastric emptying. Alterations in gut motility induced by one drug may alter the rate and/or extent of absorption of another. Sparingly soluble drugs (e.g. digoxin) may be unable to undergo complete disintegration and dissolution when gastric emptying and intestinal transit rates are increased by such drugs as metoclopramide and their extent of absorption may therefore be reduced. In contrast, since the greatest proportion of drug absorption occurs in the small intestine, the rate-limiting step for absorption of well-absorbed drugs is the rate of gastric emptying. Metoclopramide, therefore, increases the absorption rate of paracetamol by increasing the gastric emptying rate. The opposite effects are seen with anticholinergic and opiate drugs.

Certain agents may complex with drugs and reduce their absorption. Aluminium, calcium, or magnesium antacids may thus reduce the absorption of several drugs, including 4-quinolone antibiotics, tetracyclines and iron. Ion-exchange resins, such as cholestyramine and colestipol, have been shown to bind to, (and thereby to decrease the extent of absorption of) warfarin, thyroxine and triiodothyronine, and digitalis glycosides.

Drugs may also interfere with absorption of other drugs more indirectly by causing malabsorption syndromes. Colchicine, neomycin and *para*-amino salicylic acid (PAS) may impair the absorption of folate, iron and vitamin B_{12} by this means. The causes of drug absorption interactions are therefore numerous. Their importance may have been underestimated, since physicians are more likely to attribute inadequate response to other factors, such as poor compliance with prescribed therapy.

Drug distribution

Most drugs do not merely distribute throughout body fluids, they are bound or in some cases actively transported into blood and tissue elements. Drugs that are relatively inefficiently cleared by the organ of elimination (e.g. liver or kidney) have been termed 'restrictively eliminated' compounds, since their clearance, either by glomerular filtration or by liver metabolism, is limited by their degree of binding in the blood. Restrictive elimination occurs when the extraction ratio of the drug is less than the free fraction of that drug in blood. Displacement of such compounds from plasma protein binding sites will cause an immediate rise in free drug concentration. This increase will only be temporary, however, since the increase in free fraction will allow more of the drug to be eliminated until a new steady state is reached when the unbound (free) concentration returns to its original level. Permanent changes will be seen in the total plasma concentration, since total clearance of the drug has been increased. This will only be detected if total plasma concentration is measured (this is the moiety most often measured by laboratories), since the effect at steady state will be unchanged. The magnitude of the temporary increase of unbound drug will depend upon:

- the original volume of distribution of the displaced drug
- the original degree of binding in the blood
- the degree of binding to tissues.

Thus, it is likely plasma protein displacement interactions will cause (and then only temporarily) a significant increase in free drug concentration only when poorly cleared drugs have a high degree of binding in plasma and poor binding to tissues. Although warfarin fulfils these criteria, several drugs that have been shown to displace warfarin from plasma binding sites, such as phenylbutazone, also interact in more important ways with warfarin, e.g. competition for metabolism. Therefore, it is difficult to estimate what (if any) effect is produced by the transient increase in free-drug concentration.

Many drugs are effectively cleared by the body, so that the extraction ratio of the eliminating organ(s) is greater than (and therefore not limited by) the fraction of drug free in the blood. Displacement of these compounds from plasma binding sites will theoretically result in a permanent increase in free drug concentration, but only a temporary increase in total drug concentration in blood. The magnitude of the permanent increase in free drug concentration will also depend upon the relative degrees of initial binding in blood and tissues, being greatest for drugs with high binding in blood and poor tissue binding. To date, no clinically important interactions involving this mechanism alone have been described for highly cleared drugs.

Elimination

Drugs are either excreted directly in the urine or are first metabolized by other organs (e.g. the liver or gut) to more water-soluble products, which can be more easily excreted by the kidney. Interactions may occur during any of these processes and result in enhancement or diminution of drug effect.

Hepatic metabolism

The chemical reactions involved in drug metabolism are generally classified as either:

- phase 1 (oxidation, reduction or hydrolysis), or
- phase 2 (conjugation with glucuronic acid, sulphates or acetate).

Any drug may undergo one or more of these types of metabolism before being excreted by the kidney, but the most important of these are oxidation and glucuronic acid conjugation. Because of its size, enzyme content and plentiful blood supply, the liver is the major site of drug metabolism, although the intestine, lung and kidney have been shown to be other minor sites of metabolism.

The major group of drug-metabolizing enzymes, the cytochrome P450 system, is extremely versatile and is responsible for the biotransformation of many drugs and endogenous compounds. Because of the relative nonspecificity of these pathways, several interactions can take place between drugs using this route of metabolism. Cytochrome P450 is now known to be made up of several subtypes or isozymes, and enzyme inhibition interactions have been reported with at least six of these (see Table 2.3). Some drugs are metabolized by several of these isozymes, either concurrently or sequentially. In addition, some drugs metabolized by these pathways can act competitively to inhibit metabolism of each other via that route. Other drugs (e.g. cimetidine or erythromycin) can inhibit more than one isozyme non-competitively, and so act on more than one pathway.

Drug clearance is a measure of the efficiency of removal of the compound and, unlike the elimination half-life $T_{1/2}$, is unaffected by drug distribution. For those drugs in which intrinsic clearance, and therefore efficiency of removal (extraction ratio), is high, systemic (intravenous) clearance is rate limited by blood flow to the organ. In contrast, the systemic clearance of poorly extracted compounds is limited predominantly by the intrinsic clearance ability of the organ. The lower the initial efficiency of removal, the more a given change in enzyme activity will alter systemic clearance. After oral administration, however, changes in intrinsic clearance will equally affect the clearance of drugs that are both poorly and well extracted by the liver. This occurs despite the fact that the systemic clearance of the oral dose of a highly extracted drug will be much less affected by any change in intrinsic clearance analogous to post-intravenous administration. The reason for this phenomenon is that increasing intrinsic clearance will increase the hepatic extraction ratio so that a much smaller proportion F of the highly extracted drug will reach the systemic circulation, even for the first time. Thus, for all drugs that are completely absorbed from the gut and metabolized by the liver, the area under the plasma concentration–time curve (AUC) is independent of changes in blood flow.

Two important consequences emerge from these theoretical considerations:

- In contrast to poorly extracted drugs, changes in enzyme activity caused by other compounds will affect plasma levels of highly extracted drugs much more after oral administration than after the intravenous route. Poorly extracted drugs will be affected approximately equally, whatever the route of administration.

- Secondly, $T_{1/2}$ of orally administered highly extracted drugs will be much less affected by changes in intrinsic clearance than the half-life of poorly extracted compounds.

One example is the difference in lidocaine kinetics between patients with epilepsy receiving enzyme-inducing drugs and drug-free controls given oral and intravenous doses of lidocaine on separate occasions (Perrucca and Richens, 1979). The patients did not differ significantly from controls in $T_{1/2}$ after oral or intravenous administration or clearance after intravenous administration. Despite this, intrinsic (apparent oral) clearance (as measured by the AUC) was increased more than twofold in the subjects after oral administration. Thus, $T_{1/2}$ may be a poorer indicator of changes in hepatic drug metabolism than clearance or AUC, particularly for already highly efficiently cleared drugs (Routledge and Shand, 1981).

Enzyme induction   Induction of the metabolism of one drug by another is an important mechanism for interactions. Several agents (e.g. phenobarbitone, diphenylhydantoin, primidone, carbamazepine and rifampicin) can increase the activity of many isozymes of cytochrome P450. The delay between commencement of the inducing agent and the full effect (7–10 days) can make recognition of the interaction difficult. The offset of the interaction occurs over a similar period after the inducing agent is stopped, producing similar difficulties in identification.

Several agents have been implicated as inducers of hepatic drug metabolism. The more important ones are listed in Table 2.4. It is important to remember that not all patients receiving these agents will necessarily be affected since there is wide inter-individual variation.

Table 2.4   Some clinically important drugs that induce oxidative metabolism

Barbiturates
Carbamazepine
Oxcarbazepine
Phenytoin
Primidone
Rifampicin
Rifabutin
St John's Wort
Ethanol (CYP2E1)
Cigarette smoke (CYP1A2)

The herbal medicine used for treatment of depression, St John's Wort is derived from *Hypericum perforatum*, which is found widely across Europe. The extract contains many pharmacologically active constituents, some of which can induce microsomal oxidation down a variety of pathways, as well as the activity of the efflux pump, P-glycoprotein (Pgp), which will be discussed later. This results in increases in the clearance of several HIV protease inhibitors, HIV non-nucleoside reverse transcriptase inhibitors, ciclosporin, oral contraceptives (all metabolized via CYP3A4), some anticonvulsants, the *S*-enantiomer of warfarin (CYP2C9), and theophylline (CYP1A2).

Although interactions involving induction usually result in decreased drug action, toxicity may occur if toxic metabolite production is increased. Phenobarbitone increases the demethylation of pethidine to norpethidine, which may cause CNS depression and prolonged sedation in enzyme-induced subjects.

Enzyme inhibition   Inhibition of drug metabolism is also a well-established and potentially more serious phenomenon, since it may lead directly to toxic concentrations of some drugs. As inhibition is, in many cases, competitive, two simultaneously administered drugs may inhibit the metabolism of each other. Several of the compounds observed to cause clinically significant inhibition of metabolism are listed in Table 2.5. One important interaction illustrating both inhibition and induction of drug metabolism is that between phenylbutazone and warfarin. Warfarin (like many other drugs) consists of a racemic mixture of equal parts of the dextro (*R*) and laevo (*S*) enantiomers (stereoisomer).

Table 2.5 Some clinically important inhibitors of drug metabolism

---

Allopurinol[a]
Amiodarone
Cimetidine
Some macrolides
Monoamine oxidase inhibitors[a]
Some 4-quinolones
Some antifungals
Some HIV agents
Metronidazole
Some selective serotonin re-uptake inhibitors
Some sulphonamides

---

[a] Relatively selective inhibitors of certain metabolic pathways.

Phenylbutazone increases the clearance of *R*-warfarin and simultaneously decreases the clearance of *S*-warfarin. It does not, therefore, affect the clearance of warfarin when it is measured as the racemate. Since *S*-warfarin is approximately five times more potent as an anticoagulant than *R*-warfarin, however, the overall effect of the interaction is to increase the anticoagulation produced by the racemic drug.

Renal excretion

Drugs are excreted by the kidney both by glomerular filtration and tubular secretion. They may then be reabsorbed by active tubular reabsorption. Changes in any of these processes induced by one agent may result in altered excretion of another compound. Furosemide in low doses may reduce the renal clearance of cephaloridine and gentamicin, and this has been attributed to a furosemide-induced reduction in GFR. However, other work has indicated that furosemide may increase GFR; so, although furosemide may increase the nephrotoxicity of cephalosporins and the ototoxicity of gentamicin, the role of altered GFR in these interactions is unclear. Tubular secretion is an active process by which some acids and bases are transported into tubular fluid against a concentration gradient. Competition for this relatively nonspecific process between two acidic or two basic drugs may lead to diminished excretion of one or both agents. Clinically significant interactions will only occur, however, if this process is responsible for a major proportion of the total excretion of the drug(s). Probenecid and salicylates can reduce the elimination of methotrexate by this mechanism and may lead to severe toxicity if methotrexate dosage is not adjusted accordingly. Weak bases are less ionized when the urine is alkalinized by other agents. Acetazolamide and antacids, which render urine alkaline, have thus caused toxicity due to impaired excretion of the basic compound, amphetamine, and also reduce quinidine excretion by the kidney. Conversely, alkalinization of urine may increase the excretion of acidic drugs, such as salicylates and phenobarbitone, and this interaction has been put to clinical use in the treatment of poisoning by these agents with forced alkaline diuresis.

Drug transport

It is becoming increasingly clear that the penetration of some drugs into cells and tissues, and the bioavailabilty and excretion of certain compounds by the liver and kidneys, is affected by a group of energy-dependent membrane transporters found in a variety of cells throughout the body. The best known of these is the ATP-dependent multidrug efflux transporter Pgp. It is a surface phosphoglycoprotein found in the gut, heart, kidney, liver, brain, testes, placenta and adrenal glands, where it pumps drugs out of the cell. It is coded for by the multidrug resistance locus, MDR-1, and substrates include a variety of compounds, particularly those metabolized via CYP3A4, with which it appears to share some homology. Substrates for Pgp include digoxin, quinidine, ciclosporin, some HIV protease inhibitors, and many agents used in cancer chemotherapy and some antihistamines. Pgp, by acting as an absorption barrier and excreting drugs into the intestinal lumen, can cause reduced bioavailability of certain compounds. It can also prevent accumulation of drugs into cells in the vascular compartment as well as the interstitial space. Finally, it has a role in enhancing excretion of xenobiotics via the urine and bile. Teleologically, it appears to be a defence mechanism to prevent uptake of certain substances into organs such as the brain (Ambudkar *et al.*, 1999).

In addition, there are energy-dependent organic anion transporters (OATs), which mediate the hepatic uptake of organic anions, canalicular multispecific OATs which are probably involved in the gastrointestinal uptake of organic anions, OAT polypeptides (which mediate renal uptake of organic anions) and multidrug resistance proteins, responsible for the biliary excretion of organic anions (Kusuhara and Sugiyama, 2002). Some interactions (e.g. the inhibition of digoxin clearance by quinidine) may be caused in large part by competition for a transporter (Pgp in the case of quinidine and digoxin). Recently, a relational database with details of this rapidly changing field has become available (Yan and Sadee, 2000) at http://lab.digibench.net/transporter/.

Pharmacodynamic factors

Pharmacodynamic interactions occur when one drug alters the response of another by interaction at the receptor site or acts at a different site to enhance or diminish the first drug's effects. The interactions that were first recognized were those in which drugs act at the same receptor site:

* Drugs that combine with the receptor to initiate a response are termed agonists.

* Drugs that interact with the receptor to inhibit the action of an agonist, but do not initiate a response themselves, are termed antagonists.

Antagonism may be competitive, when increasing the agonist concentration restores its effects completely, or it may be non-competitive (irreversible). Partial agonists act on the same receptor as the agonist to initiate a minor response, but by occupying a significant fraction of the receptors they antagonize the action of more potent agonists. Thus, naloxone is a potent antagonist of the agonist action of morphine. Nalorphine, however, although possessing antagonist activity, is also a partial agonist and may add to respiratory depression produced by morphine.

Many of the interactions at the receptor site are used to advantage clinically, either to antagonize or augment the effect of endogenous mediators or to counteract toxicity due to overdose of administered agents. Unwanted interactions most commonly occur when one fails to realize that a drug acting at one receptor may also act at another receptor. Antihistamines, which block H_1 receptors, also have muscarinic anticholinergic activity, for example, as do some phenothiazines and tricyclic antidepressants; co-administration of two or more of these agents can lead to excessive anticholinergic activity.

Pharmacodynamic interactions may also occur when two drugs act at separate sites to cause potentiation, summation or antagonism of their normal actions. Such interactions are often used clinically in the treatment of:

- angina (e.g. beta blockers and vasodilators)

- hypertension (beta blockers and diuretics)

- malignant disease (combined cytotoxic chemotherapy).

However, these interactions may also occur inadvertently. Several drugs, including anabolic steroids, clofibrate, quinidine and salicylates, act on the synthesis of vitamin K-dependent clotting factors or the normal coagulation mechanism to potentiate the anticoagulant action of warfarin. Another long-recognized example is the ability of diuretic-induced hypokalaemia to potentiate digoxin toxicity. Even if the effects are only additive rather than synergistic, they may be sufficient to cause adverse effects in some cases.

Sometimes the effect may be more than additive. The estimated relative risk of peptic ulcer in elderly subjects receiving NSAIDs is around 4 (Griffin *et al.*, 1991). The relative risk in comparable subjects receiving corticosteroids is only 1.1 (Piper *et al.*, 1991). Patients taking both types of compound concomitantly have a risk for peptic ulcer disease 15 times greater than that of non-users of either drug (Piper *et al.*, 1991).

Pharmacodynamic interactions that occur when drugs act at different sites may also result in a loss of drug efficacy. For example, the use of NSAIDs in patients receiving antihypertensive therapy with beta blockers, thiazides and angiotensin-converting enzyme (ACE) inhibitors can result in a loss of antihypertensive action, probably because NSAIDs promote sodium retention.

Risk factors for drug–drug interactions

It is well known that the potential for drug–drug interaction increases both with age and with the number of medications prescribed. As increasing numbers of effective strategies for primary and secondary prevention of disease are discovered, the number of agents that patients receive is also increasing (e.g. in ischaemic heart disease), so this issue will increase in importance in the future. It is clear that the more dependent patients in institutionalized settings (e.g. nursing homes or long-stay medical wards) have an increased risk of ADRs, including interactions. This may be explained partly by the fact that patients cared for in these establishments are more frail and ill and, therefore, receive many drugs. Thus, residents of nursing homes are often prescribed an average of five to eight regular medications. Increased frailty is an important risk factor for ADRs, even in outpatients, and excessive psychotropic medication, which may be used in such individuals, is a particular concern because of the risk of adverse reactions and interactions. A recent study showed that the number of prescribing physicians was a determinant of the risk of potentially inappropriate drug combinations. The use of a single primary care physician, but particularly the use of a single dispensing pharmacy, lowered this risk significantly (Tamblyn *et al.*, 1996).

Detection and management

These issues are essentially the same as for ADRs in general. The physician should maintain a high level of surveillance, particularly when drugs with a low therapeutic ratio are prescribed to patients with a high risk for an adverse interaction. A recent study of patients attending a cardiology outpatient service revealed 545 discrepancies in 239 patients (76 per cent) between what doctors prescribed and what patients were taking. There was a correlation between the discrepancies and the patients' age and number of recorded medications. Over-the-counter or herbal therapies were involved in one-third of the discrepancies (Bedell *et al.*, 2000), so that a careful history of *all* agents taken should be elicited. Some adverse drug events, including ADRs, can be detected using computerized decision-support systems (Hunt, 1998; Wiffen *et al.*, 2002), and their use in the clinical situation should be encouraged.

Prevention

Guides to intravenous admixture incompatibility exist, but the possibility of their occurrence can be minimized by taking the following precautions:

- Never add a drug to an infusion fluid unless absolutely necessary.

- Never add more than one drug to the syringe or infusion fluid.

- Do not add drugs to whole blood or blood products, amino acid or lipid solutions, mannitol or sodium bicarbonate.

An inordinate proportion of serious adverse interactions occur with relatively few therapeutic agents. These are generally drugs in which the therapeutic ratio is small, such as oral anticoagulants, cytotoxic drugs, anticonvulsants, and hypotensive and hypoglycaemic agents. The decision to use these agents should be considered carefully and the patient monitored closely.

Drugs may be prescribed for many years without any assessment of their continuing therapeutic role. The list of drugs a patient receives should, therefore, be regularly reviewed. On some occasions it may be appropriate to withdraw one or more drugs and subsequently monitor the patient. For example, in the elderly it may be possible to consider stopping:

- NSAIDs in osteoarthritis

- digoxin in individuals in sinus rhythm

- diuretics for idiopathic oedema

- neuroleptics, such as prochlorperazine, prescribed for nausea or 'dizzy turns'.

Great care is recommended in those situations where patients have been on drugs that can produce dependence (e.g. long-term benzodiazepines or barbiturates), since sudden withdrawal can result in a severe withdrawal syndrome. Similarly, gradual withdrawal may be necessary for many agents (e.g. nitrates or beta blockers used in angina or anticonvulsants used in epilepsy) to avoid rebound, with worsening of the condition. Nevertheless, a shorter drug list is an important factor in reducing the risk of interactions.

Drug–drug interactions may not be immediately obvious when combinations are first prescribed, so patients should be encouraged to form a 'prescribing partnership', alerting doctors and other prescribers to symptoms that occur when new drugs are introduced. Nonspecific complaints, such as confusion, lethargy, weakness, dizzy turns, incontinence, depression and falling, should all prompt a closer look at the patient's drug list. The patient should be warned of the dangers of taking new medications (particularly over-the-counter remedies) without obtaining advice concerning potential interactions. The fewer people prescribing for the patient, the lower the risk that an interaction will occur iatrogenically (Tamblyn *et al.*, 1996).

On a broader front, more sensitive and reliable parameters of drug effect are needed. It is reassuring to note that when physicians have a reliable and simple measure of drug effect (e.g. for anticoagulants with the one-stage prothrombin time or INR) drug interactions are often quickly recognized and therapy can be adjusted appropriately.

Pharmacogenetics and the prevention of adverse drug reactions

As our understanding of pharmacogenetic (and environmental) influences on inter-individual differences in pharmacokinetics and pharmacodynamics increases, bespoke prescribing (choosing the right dose of the right drug for the right patient) will hopefully be increasingly possible. Indeed, *Pharmacogenomics* has been defined as 'The science of increasing the effectiveness of drugs and minimizing their side effects by matching drugs to people according to their genetic make up'.

Pharmacogenomics shows great promise in relation to drug safety (McLeod and Evans, 2001). However, phenotyping individuals for certain polymorphisms of drug metabolism or response can be time consuming and often requires administration of exogenous agents (Hutchings and Routledge, 1986). Even when specific phenotyping tests can be performed directly on blood samples, the uptake is variable (Holme *et al.*, 2002). Genotyping may also be time consuming and expensive, and not all relevant alleles may yet have been identified for some important polymorphisms. For these reasons, genotyping is not yet used routinely in clinical practice, and prescribers tend to avoid using drugs in which genetic polymorphism may result in potential toxicity for a small proportion of their patients. Increased availability of pharmacogenetic testing may help us to identify those at risk of toxicity to specific agents and avoid specific medicines in at-risk groups (Ozdemir *et al.*, 2001).

When testing is available for a range of polymorphisms, personal pharmacogenetic profiling may then become a possibility in the clinical setting. Pharmacogenetically based prescribing guidelines could then be developed, and the pharmaceutical industry can then concentrate its efforts on developing new drugs based on specific genotypes ('drug stratification'; Roses 2000, 2002a, b; Wolf *et al.*, 2000). For example, screening using probe drugs and inhibitory monoclonal antibodies to identify the major contributory CYP450s (including those showing genetic polymorphisms) responsible for the metabolism of potential new chemical entities is already being used in early drug discovery (Donato and Castell, 2003; Soars *et al.*, 2003).

Conclusions

Adverse drug reactions, of which drug–drug interactions are a special category, are a significant cause of morbidity and occasionally cause fatality. The risk of serious ADRs is highest for only a few drug groups (e.g. cytotoxics, hypotensives, NSAIDs, hypoglycaemics and oral anticoagulants) and in certain groups (e.g. the frail elderly and those with renal or liver disease or heart failure). Adverse drug reactions may be difficult to detect because they can mimic other diseases and may have very few specific features. In addition, there are often few specific or sensitive *in vitro* tests, and rechallenge to the agent may be precluded because of a possible severe response. The diagnosis of ADRs may, therefore, have to rely on circumstantial evidence, based on the time course of onset relative to the introduction of the drug or change in dose and the response to dose withdrawal or drug discontinuation.

Fortunately, many ADRs and adverse drug interactions can be avoided with a knowledge of basic pharmacological principles and judicious choice of drugs and doses. When an ADR is suspected, a report to the regulatory authority and company will help identify risks and inform decisions about risk–benefit, and thus help to protect others from similar problems in the future. Although the use of pharmacogenetic testing may help us to avoid toxicity in at-risk groups, as things stand at present, our limited understanding of type A and type B toxicity and the changing environmental influences determining risk of ADRs means that vigilance will continue to be a vital part of drug safety. Because medicines can only ever have a 'provisional licence' for drug safety, careful surveillance safety should continue during the drug development process and throughout the life span of the drug as a therapeutic agent (Rawlins, 1995). Complacency in this respect can end in disaster (Routledge, 1998).

References

Aithal GP, Day CP, Kesteven PJ and Daly AK (1999). Association of polymorphisms in the cytochrome P450 CYP2C9 with warfarin dose requirement and risk of bleeding complications. *Lancet* **353**: 717–719.

Ambudkar SV, Dey S, Hrycyna CA, Ramachandra M *et al.* (1999). Biochemical, cellular, and pharmacological aspects of the multidrug transporter. *Annu Rev Pharmacol Toxicol* **39**: 361–398.

Aronson JK and White NJ (1996). Principles of clinical pharmacology and drug therapy. In *Oxford Textbook of Medicine*, third Edition, Weatherall D, Ledingham JGJ and Warrel DA (eds). Oxford University Press: Oxford (CDROM).

Association of Anaesthetists of Great Britain and Ireland and The British Society of Allergy and Clinical Immunology (1995). Suspected anaphylactic reactions associated with anaesthesia. Revised edition 2. http://www.aagbi.org/pdf/Anaphyld.pdf.

Bedell SE, Jabbour S, Goldberg R, Glaser H *et al.* (2000). Discrepancies in the use of medications: their extent and predictors in an outpatient practice. *Arch Intern Med* **160**: 2129–2134.

Bertilsson L, Dahl ML, Sjoqvist F, Aberg-Wistedt A *et al.* (1993). Molecular basis for rational megaprescribing in ultrarapid hydroxylators of debrisoquine. *Lancet* **341**: 63.

Bowman L, Carlsted TBC, Hancock EF and Black CD (1996). Adverse drug reactions (ADR) occurrence and evaluation in elderly inpatients. *Pharmacoepidemiol Drug Saf* **5**: 9–18.

Breathnach SM (1995). Management of drug eruptions: part II. Diagnosis and treatment. *Australas J Dermatol*, **36**: 187–191.

Classen DC, Pestotnick SL, Evans RS and Burke JP (1991). Computerized surveillance of adverse drug events in hospital patients. *J Am Med Assoc* **266**: 2847–2851.

Day TK (1983). Intestinal perforation associated with slow release indomethacin capsules. *Br Med J* **287**: 1671–1672.

Domecq C, Naranjo CA, Ruiz I and Busto U (1980). Sex-related variations in the frequency and characteristics of adverse drug reactions. *Int J Clin Pharmacol Ther Toxicol* **18**: 362–366.

Donato MT and Castell JV (2003). Strategies and molecular probes to investigate the role of cytochrome p450 in drug metabolism: focus on *in vitro* studies. *Clin Pharmacokinet* **42**: 153–178.

Drici M-D and Clément N (2001) Is gender a risk factor for Adverse Drug Reactions? The example of drug-induced long QT syndrome. *Drug Safety* **24**(8), 575–585.

Drici M-D, Raybaud F, De Lunardo C, Iacono P, *et al.* (1995). Influence of the behaviour pattern on the nocebo response of healthy volunteers. *Br J Clin Pharmacol* **39**: 204–206.

Evans RS, Pestotnick SL, Classen DC, Horn SD *et al.* (1994) Preventing adverse drug reactions in hospitalised patients. *Ann Pharmacother* **28**: 523–527.

Evans WE and McLeod HL (2003). Pharmacogenomics – drug disposition, drug targets and side effects. *N Engl J Med* **348**: 538–549.

Fennerty A, Campbell I and Routledge PA (1988). Anticoagulants in venous thrombo-embolism. Guidelines for optimum treatment. *Br Med J* **197**: 1285–1288.

FitzSimmons SC, Burkhart GA, Borowitz D, Grand RJ *et al.* (1997). High-dose pancreatic-enzyme supplements and fibrosing colonopathy in children with cystic fibrosis. *N Engl J Med* **336**: 1283–1289.

Forbat A, Lond MB, Lehmann H and Silk E (1953). Prolonged apnoea following injection of succinylcholine. *Lancet* **2**: 1067–1068.

Furuta T, Ohashi K, Kamata T, Takashima M *et al.* (1998). Effect of genetic differences in omeprazole metabolism on cure rates for *Helicobacter pylori* infection and peptic ulcer. *Ann Intern Med* **129**: 1027–1030.

Grahame-Smith DG and Aronson JK (1992). *Oxford Textbook of Clinical Pharmacology and Drug Therapy*. Oxford University Press: Oxford.

Griffin MR, Piper JM, Daugherty JR, Snowden M *et al.* (1991). Nonsteroidal anti-inflammatory drug use and increased risk for peptic ulcer disease in elderly persons. *Ann Intern Med* **114**: 257–263.

Hanif M, Mobarek MR, Ronan A, Rahman D *et al.* (1995). Fatal renal failure caused by diethylene glycol in paracetamol elixir: the Bangladesh epidemic. *Br Med J* **311**: 88–91.

Heinrich J (2001). Most drugs withdrawn in recent years had greater health risks for women. General Accounting Office-01-286R.

Hetherington S, McGuirk S, Powell G, Cutrell A *et al.* (2001). Hypersensitivity reactions during therapy with the nucleoside reverse transcriptase inhibitor abacavir. *Clin Ther* **23**: 1603–1614.

Hoigné R, Sollberger J, Zopp M, Müller U, *et al.* (1984). Die bedeutung von alter, geschelch Nierenfunktion, Atopie und Anzahl verabreichter Medikamente für das Auftreten von Nebenwirkungen, untersucht mit methoden der multivariatenStatistik. Ergebnisse aus dem komprehensiven Spital-Drug-Monitoring Bern (C.H.D.M.B.). *Schweiz Med Wochenschr* **114**: 1854–1857.

Holme SA, Duley JA, Sanderson J, Routledge PA *et al.* (2002). Erythrocyte thiopurine methyl transferase assessment prior to azathioprine use in the UK. *Q J Med* **95**: 439–444.

Hu DN, Qin WQ, Wu BT, Fang LZ *et al.* (1991). Genetic aspects of antibiotic-induced deafness: mitochondrial inheritance. *J Med Genet* **28**: 79–83.

Hunt DL, Haynes RB, Hanna SE and Smith K (1998). Effects of computer-based clinical decision support systems on physician performance and patient outcomes. A systematic review. *J Am Med Assoc* **280**: 1339–1346.

Hurwitz N and Wade OC (1969). Intensive hospital monitoring of adverse reactions to drugs. *Br Med J* **1**: 531–536.

Hutchings AD and Routledge PA (1986). A simple method for determining acetylator phenotype using isoniazid. *Br J Clin Pharmacol* **22**: 343–345.

Ingelman-Sundberg M, Oscarson M and McLellan RA (1999). Polymorphic human cytochrome P450 enzymes: an opportunity for individualised drug treatment. *Trends Pharmacol Sci* **20**: 342–349.

Jacubeit T, Drisch D and Weber U (1990). Risk factors as reflected by an intensive drug monitoring system. In Weber E, Lawson DH and Hoigné R (eds). *Risk Factors for ADR – Epidemiological Approaches. Agents and Actions. Supplements*, vol. 29. Birkhauser: 117–125.

Kalow W and Genest K (1957). A method for the detection of atypical forms of serum cholinesterase. Determination of dibucaine numbers. *Can J Biochem* **35**: 339–346.

Kando JC, Yonkers KA and Cole JO (1995). Gender as a risk factor for adverse events to medications. *Drugs* **50**(1): 1–6.

Kilbourne EM, Philen RM, Kamb ML and Falk H (1996). Tryptophan produced by Showa Denko and epidemic eosinophilia-myalgia syndrome. *J Rheumatol Suppl* **46**: 81–88.

Kusuhara H and Sugiyama Y (2002). Role of transporters in the tissue-selective distribution and elimination of drugs: transporters in the liver, small intestine, brain and kidney. *J Control Release* **78**: 43–54.

Lamy PP (1991). Physiological changes due to age: pharmacodynamic changes of drug action and implications for therapy. *Drugs Aging* **1**: 385–404.

Lazarou J, Pomeranz BH and Corey PN (1998). Incidence of adverse drug reactions in hospitalized patients: a meta-analysis of prospective studies. *J Am Med Assoc* **279**: 1200–1205.

Lindeman RD (1992). Changes in renal function with aging; implications for treatment. *Drugs Aging* **2**: 423–431.

Mallal S, Nolan D, Witt C, Masel G et al. (2002). Association between presence of HLA-B*5701, HLA-DR7, and HLA-DQ3 and hypersensitivity to HIV-1 reverse-transcriptase inhibitor abacavir. *Lancet* **359**: 727–732.

McKenzie R, Fried MW, Sallie R, Conjeevaram H et al. (1995). Hepatic failure and lactic acidosis due to fialuridine (FIAU), an investigational nucleoside analogue for chronic hepatitis B. *N Engl J Med* **333**: 1099–1105.

McLeod HL and Evans WE (2001). Pharmacogenomics: unlocking the human genome for better drug therapy. *Annu Rev Pharmacol Toxicol* **41**: 101–121.

Meyer U (2000). Pharmacogenetics and adverse drug reactions. *Lancet* **356**: 1667–1671.

O'Mahony MS and Woodhouse KW (1994). Age, environmental factors and drug metabolism. *Pharmacol Ther* **61**: 279–287.

Orme M L'E (1991) Drug interactions of clinical importance. In: Davis DM (ed) *Textbook of Adverse Drug Reactions*, Oxford University Press, 788–810.

Owens NJ, Fretwell MD, Willey C and Murphy SS (1994). Distinguishing between the fit and frail elderly, and optimising pharmacotherapy. *Drugs Aging* **4**: 47–55.

Ozdemir V, Shear NH and Kalow W (2001). What will be the role of pharmacogenetics in evaluating drug safety and minimising adverse effects? *Drug Saf* **24**: 75–85.

Piper JM, Ray WA, Daugherty JR and Griffin MR (1991). Corticosteroid use and peptic ulcer disease: role of nonsteroidal anti-inflammatory drugs. *Ann Intern Med* **114**: 735–740.

Pirmohamed M, Madden S and Park BK (1996). Idiosyncratic drug reactions: metabolic activation as a pathogenic mechanism. *Clin Pharmacokinet* **31**: 215–230.

Pohl LR, Satoh H, Christ DD and Kenna JG (1988). The immunological and metabolic basis of drug hypersensitivities. *Annu Rev Pharmacol* **28**: 367–387.

Rawlins MD (1995). Pharmacovigilance: paradise lost, regained or postponed? *J R Coll Physicians London* **29**: 41–49.

Rawlins MD and Thompson JW (1977). Pathogenesis of adverse drug reactions. In *Textbook of Adverse Reactions*, Davies DM (ed.). 44.

Rieder MJ (1994). Mechanisms of unpredictable adverse drug reactions. *Drug Saf* **11**: 196–212.

Roberts R and Brugada R (2003). Genetics and arrhythmias. *Annu Rev Med* **54**: 257–267.

Roses AD (2000). Pharmacogenetics and the practice of medicine. *Nature* **405**: 857–865.

Roses AD (2002a). Genome-based pharmacogenetics and the pharmaceutical industry. *Nat Rev Drug Discov* **1**: 541–549.

Roses AD (2002b). Pharmacogenetics place in modern medical science and practice. *Life Sci* **70**: 1471–1480.

Routledge P (1998). 150 years of pharmacovigilance. *Lancet* **35**: 1200–1201.

Routledge PA and Shand DG (1981). Drug interactions. In *Recent Advances in Medicine 18*, Dawson AM, Compston N and Besser GM (eds). Churchill-Livingstone: London; 39–54.

Routledge PA (1986). The plasma protein binding of basic drugs. *Br J Clin Pharmacol* **22**: 499–506.

Routledge PA (1994). Pharmacokinetics in children. *J Antimicrob Chemother* **94**(Suppl A): 19–24.

Routledge PA (2002). Therapeutics and toxicology. In *Textbook of Medicine*, (4th edition, Souhami RL and Moxham J (eds). Churchill Livingstone: Edinburgh.

Routledge PA and Hutchings AD (2001). Therapeutic drug monitoring (TDM). In *The Immunoassay Handbook*, 2nd edition, Wild D (ed.). Nature Publishing Group: London.

Rylance G and Armstrong D (1997). Adverse drug events in children. *Adverse Drug React Bull* **184**: 699–702.

Seymour RM and Routledge PA (1998). Important drug–drug interactions in the elderly. *Drugs Aging* **12**: 485–494.

Soars MG, Gelboin HV, Krausz KW and Riley RJ (2003). A comparison of relative abundance, activity factor and inhibitory monoclonal antibody approaches in the characterization of human CYP enzymology. *Br J Clin Pharmacol* **55**: 175–181.

Tamblyn RM, McLeod PJ, Abrahamowicz M and Laprise R (1996). Do too many cooks spoil the broth? Multiple physician involvement in medical management of elderly patients and potentially inappropriate drug combinations. *Can Med Assoc J* **154**: 1174–1184.

Taube J, Halsall D and Baglin T (2000). Influence of cytochrome P-450 CYP2C9 polymorphisms on warfarin sensitivity and risk of over-anticoagulation in patients on long-term treatment. *Blood* **96**: 1816–1819.

Terol MJ, Cervantes F, Pereira A and Rozman C (1991). Autoimmune hemolytic anaemia after 9 years of treatment with alphamethyldopa. *Med Clin Barc* **10**: 598.

Uchegbu IF and Florence AT (1996). Adverse drug events related to dosage forms and delivery systems. *Drug Saf* **14**: 39–67.

Usami S, Koda E, Tsukamoto K, Otsuka A *et al.* (2002). Molecular diagnosis of deafness: impact of gene identification. *Audiol Neurootol* **7**: 185–190.

Van der Weide J, Steijns LS, van Weelden MJ and de Haan K (2001). The effect of genetic polymorphism of cytochrome P450 CYP2C9 on phenytoin dose requirement. *Pharmacogenetics* **11**: 287–291.

Vere DW (1976). Drug adverse reactions as masqueraders. *Adverse Drug React Bull*, **60**: 208–211.

Vomvouras S and Piergies AA (1995). Gender differences in study events during phase 1 trials. *Clin Pharmacol Ther* **136**: PI-3.

Walker RS and Linton AL (1959). Phenethyldiguanide: a dangerous side-effect. *Br Med J* **2**: 1005–1006.

Walle JK, Fagan TC, Topmiller MJ, Conrad EC, *et al.* (1994). The influence of gender and sex steroid hormones on the plasma binding of propanolol enantiomers. *Br J Clin Pharmacol* **37**: 21–25.

Weinshilboum R (2003). Inheritance and drug response. *New Eng J Med* **348**: 529–537.

White C (1999). Gender effects on pharmacotherapy. At *Conference on Biologic and Molecular Mechanisms for Sex Differences in Pharmacokinetics, Pharmacodynamics and Pharmacogenetics*, 5 May.

Wiffen P, Gill M, Edwards J and Moore A (2002). Adverse drug reactions in hospital patients. *Bandolier Extra* 1–15, www.bandolier.com.

Williamson J and Chopin JM (1980). Adverse reaction to prescribed drugs in the elderly: a multicentre investigation. *Age Ageing* **9**: 73–80.

Wolf CR, Smith G and Smith RL (2000). Science, medicine, and the future: pharmacogenetics. *Br Med J* **320**: 987–990.

Yan Q and Sadee W (2000). Human membrane transporter database: a Web-accessible relational database for drug transport studies and pharmacogenomics. *AAPS PharmSci* **2**: E20.

3

Toxicology and Adverse Drug Reactions

D. J. Snodin

Introduction

Toxicology has two main goals in relation to adverse drug reactions (ADRs). The first is to identify and characterize the potential for harmful effects that can be produced in biological systems, particularly laboratory animals, by a drug,[1] and to suggest therapeutic circumstances in which toxic responses may occur and/or are unlikely to occur. The second is necessary when unexpected adverse clinical reactions are detected, i.e. those not predicted by conventional animal and clinical studies, and to investigate the mechanism in additional toxicological studies, often of nonstandard design, in order to understand these reactions and possibly how to avoid or ameliorate them.

Toxicity testing

Pharmacotoxicological tests

The term 'pharmacotoxicology' is often used to describe the experimental study of pharmacodynamic and toxicological effects of the ingredients of medicinal products.[1] Toxicological testing of pharmaceuticals employs basic concepts, laboratory animal species, study types and designs that are similar to those used in other industrial sectors, such as chemicals and food ingredients, but there are several special features.

The intended biological activity of test materials has a number of consequences, such as:

* Selection of an appropriate species that is pharmacologically responsive, but in which responses reducing the effectiveness of a particular model (such as the production of

---

[1] Most tests are undertaken on active ingredients rather than the formulated medicinal product. Exceptions include vaccines (may contain adjuvants and preservatives), topical products and modified-release formulations, where excipients may alter the pharmacotoxicological responses.

Stephens' Detection of New Adverse Drug Reactions Fifth Edition edited by John Talbot and Patrick Waller
© 2004 John Wiley & Sons, Ltd   ISBN: 0 470 84552 X

neutralizing antibodies following administration of human-specific proteins) are minimized.

- Occurrence of both pharmacological effects and toxicological effects; the detection of toxicological effects can often be confounded by exaggerated pharmacodynamic responses.

Human data from clinical trials, not normally available for non-pharmaceuticals, for the most part supersede the results of animal studies, except in the case of those endpoints (such as genotoxicity, carcinogenicity and reproductive toxicity) where it is impractical and/or unethical to undertake human studies. An important role of toxicological studies during drug development is to provide sufficient safety data to evaluate the risk to patients participating in a particular clinical trial. Thus, the timing of studies is closely related to the key clinical elements (e.g. phase 1, 2 and 3 trials) of the clinical development programme. Toxicokinetic measurements are performed to enable comparison of systemic exposure in animals with that in patients who are exposed to the drug. This may not always be practicable, e.g. with topically applied drugs where systemic exposure is often negligible.

The nature and purposes of the principal non-clinical studies normally required for a new conventional (chemical) pharmaceutical active ingredient (new chemical entity; NCE) are described in Tables 3.1 and 3.2.

Good laboratory practice

All safety studies must be performed in compliance with GLP – a guiding set of principles with the aim of ensuring that laboratories design, perform and report all safety studies on pharmaceuticals (and other materials, such as industrial chemicals) carefully and document all activities in such a way that studies can be reconstructed at any time afterwards (Könemann, 1990; Hawkins, 1993; Department of Health, 2000; CFR, 2003). Many aspects of laboratory activities can influence the results produced and their subsequent interpretation, and so competent authorities in the major industrial countries (as well as organizations such as OECD: www.sourceoecd.org/content/templates/co/co_main_oecdguid.htm?comm= oecdguid) have promulgated GLP regulatory guidance documents. The role of GLP regulations (in the UK these are 'The Good Laboratory Practice Regulations, 1999') is to codify the components of GLP, the principal ones being:

- test facility organisation and personnel

- quality assurance programme

- facilities

- apparatus, materials and reagents

- test systems

- test and reference items

- standard operating procedures

- performance of the regulatory study

- reporting of regulatory study results

- storage and retention of records and materials

- inspections

- study audits.

Animal welfare

Strict controls exist over the use and welfare of experimental animals. The principal UK legislation is 'The Animals (Scientific Procedures) Act 1986'. This controls experimental and other scientific work carried out on living animals that may cause pain, suffering or other distress to the animals. Both project and personal (i.e. the experimenter) licences, as well as a certificate of designation relating to the place where the work is undertaken, are required under the act and a variety of codes of practice regarding housing and care and humane killing, etc. have been published (Home Office, 2002). Similar provisions for the maintenance of animal welfare apply in other countries (European Biomedical Research Association www.ebra.org/; FRAME www.frame.org.uk/). GLP requirements also impact on animal welfare in respect of 'support facilities and conditions for their (test animals) care, housing and containment which are adequate to prevent stress and other problems which could affect the test system and hence the quality of the data' (Department of Health, 2000).

Determination of toxic potential

The overall aim of the non-clinical tests is to determine the potential for toxic reactions by examining a variety of endpoints that may be affected:

- *Functional or dynamic.* For example, a potentially adverse change in blood pressure or cardiac function (typically evaluated in safety pharmacology studies).

- *Biochemical.* For instance, a change in the concentration of a serum enzyme such as aspartyl amininotransferase (AST) indicating liver damage. On the other hand, direct (and possibly intended) enzyme inhibition (e.g. acetyl cholinesterase inhibition) may also occur.

- *Haematological.* For example, a treatment-related reduction in haematocrit indicating anaemia, or changes in lymphocytes suggesting immunological effects or a response to inflammation or infection.

- *Structural.* For example, pathological changes in organ weight and/or structure, such as liver hypertrophy and/or necrosis.

- *Behavioural.* Drug-related behavioural dysfunction, in most cases not obviously correlated with specific deficits in nervous structure or function.

- *Developmental.* For example, reduced body weight gain not accompanied by reduced food consumption often indicates a toxic response; impaired foetal development may be associated with foetal abnormalities.

Table 3.1 Non-clinical safety studies: good laboratory practice (GLP) required

Test type	Test system	Results/evaluation
Safety pharmacology	Standard pharmacological procedures on organ system(s) such as cardiovascular, respiratory, renal, urinary and central nervous system (CNS)	Evaluation of any functional effect at a range of single doses
Acute toxicity	Limit test using single high dose (or a range of doses) by therapeutic route (plus parenteral route for orally administered drugs) in rodent and non-rodent; observation period normally 14 days	Clinical responses to treatment (e.g. lethargy, prostration), mortality and necropsy (on decedants and survivors), providing an early gross indication of organ systems likely to be affected by toxicity
Repeated-dose toxicity (sub-acute to chronic)	Administration of drug at three dose levels (plus control group) using intended therapeutic route usually over 2–26 weeks in rat and 2–39 weeks in appropriate non-rodent species (normally the dog)	Variety of clinical observations, body weight, food consumption, haematology, clinical chemistry, macro- and micro-pathology. ECG monitoring sometimes included in non-rodent. Data evaluated to assess target organ(s) for toxicity, dose-exposure-response relationships and reversibility
Genetic toxicity	Standard three-test battery for gene mutation in bacteria (Ames test), chromosome aberrations or mutations in mammalian cells *in vitro* and *in vivo* cytogenetic test (normally rodent bone-marrow micronucleus assay). *In vitro* assays performed in the absence and presence of induced rat liver S9 microsomal fraction as exogenous metabolizing system	Evaluation of DNA damage producing effects at the level of the gene or chromosome (clastogenicity)

Carcinogenicity	Control group plus three dose levels of drug using intended therapeutic route in rat for 24 months. Second study in mouse, either conventional 24-month bioassay or study in an acceptable alternative model (e.g. 6-month study in p53+/− mouse). Blood samples taken for measurement of drug plasma concentration	Adequate survival and demonstration that >25-fold human exposure or maximum tolerated dose (MTD) was achieved to ensure a valid test. Incidence, dose–response and statistical analysis of organ-specific tumours assessed, distinguishing different tumour types and metastases. Distinction between genotoxic and nongenotoxic carcinogens (tumour profile, threshold, mechanistic studies, etc.)
Toxicity to reproduction	Segment I study for fertility and general reproductive performance in the rat. Segment II studies in rat and rabbit for embryotoxicity/ teratogenicity and Segment III study in the rat for peri-/post-natal toxicity. Tests can be combined (e.g. I/II) if appropriate.* Three dose levels and control group in each test. Blood samples taken from pregnant or non-pregnant animals for measurement of drug plasma concentration	Determination of mating, reproductive parameters, fetal development, pup skeletal and soft-tissue abnormalities, nursing behaviour, postnatal development and pup survival. Evaluation of dose-response relationships and maternal and foetal no-effect levels
Local tolerance	Particularly for drugs administered parenterally (e.g. i.v., s.c.) or topically, tests (e.g. in rabbit ear model) to assess reactions of adjacent tissues	Determination of nature, severity, dose–response of any local tolerance effects
Special studies	Sensitization/immunogenicity, phototoxicity	Depends on specific test

*In ICH S5A, Reproductive Toxicology: Detection of Toxicity to Reproduction for Medicinal Products, the sequence of events from premating and conception in one generation to conception in the next generation is divided into six stages, A–F inclusive, rather than three segments.

Table 3.2   Other nonclinical tests (not necessarily to GLP)

Test type	Test system	Results/evaluation
Pharmacology	*In vitro* and *in vivo* tests for primary and secondary pharmacological activity; e.g. mode of action and receptor binding	Demonstration of pharmacological rationale, and specificity of action on target entity (e.g. enzyme, cofactor, chemokine). Extent of unwanted pharmacodynamic activity
Drug interactions	Co-administration, in appropriate *in vitro* or animal models, of other drugs likely to be prescribed in the intended patient group	Evaluation of both kinetic and pharmacodynamic interactions
Pharmacokinetics	Studies (single- and repeated-dose) in various laboratory animal species (particularly those used for toxicity testing) on absorption, distribution, metabolism and excretion (ADME). A: kinetic parameters such as T_{max}, C_{max} and area under plasma concentration–time curve (AUC) at various doses. D: tissue distribution studies using radiolabelled drug; plasma protein binding. M: detection and identification of metabolites in plasma (urine and faeces). E: proportions of drug (and metabolites) excreted by major routes (e.g. urine, faeces, bile). Other studies: melanin binding; enzyme induction. *In vitro* studies using hepatocytes/microsomes from various species to identify metabolites and major P450 isoforms	Cross-species comparisons of kinetic parameters and metabolic profile – often useful in understanding any interspecies differences in pharmacological and toxicological responses. Information also useful in evaluating potential for human kinetic drug interactions

Any effects or abnormalities noted in standard *in vivo* tests are considered in relation to the drug dose administered, usually expressed in mg/kg/day or mg/m^2/day, as well as to the systemic exposure (conventional metrics being C_{max} and/or AUC). There is a reasonable expectation that toxic responses, other than those at the site of application, are likely to be dose related. If this is not the case then it is possible that the findings may be of doubtful significance for man (or there may be an effect only at the high dose). Toxicokinetic monitoring is now established as an essential component of repeated-dose toxicity studies and can help identify a variety of factors that can affect dose–response relationships and data interpretation (Dahlem *et al.*, 1995; Schwartz, 2001). These include: first-pass metabolism and possible saturation thereof, enzyme induction, saturation of metabolic clearance and plasma accumulation of the drug and/or its metabolites.

It is often important to assess the reversibility of toxicological findings, and so a recovery phase is frequently included in repeated-dose toxicity studies. For example, in a 3-month toxicity study a 4-week post-treatment reversibility phase would be typical and would normally involve the inclusion of additional animals, at least in the control and high-dose groups.

Testing in special types of animal (e.g. ovariectomized animals for osteoporosis products or juvenile animals for paediatric products) is sometimes advocated to assess pharmacodynamic and/or toxic responses. Although the former is quite well established (e.g. Vahle *et al.*, 2002), use of juvenile animals is still being evaluated in the EU (CPMP Safety Working Party, 2001).

Toxicity testing guidelines

National guidelines on non-clinical testing requirements for pharmaceuticals have been available for the last 20–30 years. Such documents are intended to serve a number of purposes in terms of providing guidance to companies involved in drug development, such as:

- selection of an appropriate study package

- suitable study designs

- interpretation of results.

International Conference on Harmonization

Guidance in EU countries has been subject to two types of harmonization. Firstly, EU Notes for Guidance (NfGs) replaced all national guidelines (occurring mainly in the 1980s), and more recently a global harmonization procedure has been undertaken under the auspices of the International Conference on Harmonization (ICH; www.ich.org/). The ICH process (International Harmonization of Technical Requirements of Pharmaceuticals for Human Use) was initiated in October 1989 and was hosted by the International Federation of Pharmaceutical Manufacturers Associations (IFPMA; www.ifpma.org/). The principal objectives of the initial and subsequent conferences have been:

- To identify and eliminate the differing requirements in the three participating states/ regions (USA, Japan and EU).

- To avoid repetition of all types of tests.

- To accelerate development of medicinal products, thus giving patients quicker access to new medicinal products without negatively affecting quality, safety and efficacy.

The technical discussions and drafting of guidelines is undertaken by expert working groups in quality, safety and efficacy supervised by the ICH Steering Committee. (Multidisciplinary working groups are also involved in some topics.) The working groups consist of representatives of each participating authority (Japan's Ministry of Health and Welfare, the United States' Food and Drug Administration (FDA) and the European Commission) and the pharmaceutical trade association from each region (Japan Pharmaceutical Manufacturers Association, Pharmaceutical Research and Manufacturers of America and European Federation of Pharmaceutical Industries' Associations). Two observers (WHO and Canada) are part of the ICH global cooperation group.

Five steps, ranging from initiation to implementation, are involved in the ICH guideline process:

- Step 1. Preparation of concept paper and draft guideline by an expert working group.

- Step 2. A draft consensus guideline is signed by all six parties (authorities and associations) and released for 6 months' consultation. A unanimous decision is required at this stage in order for the particular draft guideline to progress to the consultation stage. For example, a proposal for a guideline on immunotoxicity testing failed to secure unanimous agreement at the 2002 steering committee meeting in Brussels.

- Step 3. Comments received during the consultation period are evaluated by the competent authorities in the three regions and incorporated, as appropriate, into the existing draft. This draft is signed by the authorities and submitted to the steering committee for approval.

- Step 4. The final draft is approved by the steering committee and confirmed by the signatures of the regulatory authorities.

- Step 5. The process is concluded by implementation of the guideline in the three regions in compliance with legal and regulatory procedures.

Guideline maintenance has now become an issue after over 10 years of the ICH process, and some guidelines have been subjected to revision (denoted by R in parentheses) in recognition of scientific progress and/or the need for clarification. Some others have been updated using a maintenance procedure (M). ICH guidelines relevant to nonclinical testing are listed in Table 3.3.

EU- and US-specific guidelines

Although the ICH process has led to guideline harmonization for the major areas of nonclinical investigation, there remains scope (and probably this will always be the case) for national guidelines covering more specialized topics. In the EU, the CPMP, via its expert preclinical group, the Safety Working Party, has released guidance on a variety of topics either in the form of NfGs, Points to Consider (PTC) or Position Paper (PP) documents (Table 3.4).

US-specific guidelines may be located under 'Guidance for Industry' on the website of the FDA (www.fda.com).

Biotechnology-derived and biological drugs

During the last 10–15 years there has been a dramatic rise in the development and therapeutic use of biotechnological and biological products, sometimes called new biological entities (NBEs) or 'biologics'. These drugs comprise a wide range of product types, including

Table 3.3 ICH guidelines relating to nonclinical testing

Field	ICH topic	Guideline title	Status
Safety	S1A	Guideline on the need for carcinogenicity studies of pharmaceuticals	Step 5
	S1B	Carcinogenicity: testing for carcinogenicity of pharmaceuticals	Step 5
	S1C	Carcinogenicity: dose selection for carcinogenicity studies of pharmaceuticals	Step 5
	S1C(R)	Addendum: addition of a limited dose and related notes	Step 5
	S2A	Genotoxicity: specific aspects of regulatory genotoxicity tests for pharmaceuticals	Step 5
	S2B	Genotoxicity: a standard battery for genotoxicity testing of pharmaceuticals	Step 5
	S3A	Toxicokinetics: the assessment of systemic exposure in toxicity studies	Step 5
	S3B	Pharmacokinetics: guidance for repeated-dose tissue distribution studies	Step 5
	S4A	Duration of chronic toxicity testing in animals (rodent and non-rodent)	Step 5
	S5A	Reproductive toxicology: detection of toxicity to reproduction for medicinal products	Step 5
	S5B(M)	Reproductive toxicology: toxicity to male fertility	Step 5
	S6	Preclinical safety evaluation of biotechnology-derived pharmaceuticals	Step 5
	S7A	Safety pharmacology studies for human pharmaceuticals	Step 5
	S7B	Safety pharmacology studies for assessing the potential for delayed ventricular repolarization (QT interval prolongation) by human pharmaceuticals	Step 3
Quality*	Q3A(R)	Impurities testing: impurities in new active substances	Step 3
	Q3B(R)	Impurities in new medicinal products	Step 3
Multidisciplinary	M3(M)	Nonclinical safety studies for the conduct of human clinical trials for pharmaceuticals	Step 5

*ICH Q3C(M), Note for guidance on impurities: residual solvents, is not included since, although the permitted residues of specified solvents are derived on the basis of toxicological data, there is no obvious opportunity for applicants to make independent safety-based assessments that will be acceptable to all regulatory authorities.

vaccines, blood cells, rDNA versions of endogenous hormones, deliberately modified versions of natural hormones, cofactors and a variety of antibody-related entities (e.g. antibody fragments – mainly for diagnostic applications, humanized monoclonal antibodies). Non-clinical testing strategies for NBEs are highly case-specific, depending on product type, clinical indication and availability of suitable animal models (especially for human proteins in nonhomologous animal species) for both pharmacological and safety evaluation, leading to the frequent use of nonhuman primate species (Terrell and Green, 1994; Dayan, 1995; Griffiths and Lumley, 1998; Pilling, 1999; Serabian and Pilaro, 1999; Black *et al.*, 2000; Dempster, 2000; Green and Black, 2000; Galluppi *et al.*, 2001; Descotes *et al.*, 2002; Verdier, 2002). Toxicity tests on the murine version of a recombinant product may provide useful

Table 3.4 EU-specific guidance on nonclinical testing

Reference	Title	Status
CPMP/SWP/465/95	Preclinical pharmacological and toxicological testing of vaccines	Adopted NfG
CPMP/SWP/728/95	Replacement of animal studies by in vitro models	Adopted NfG
CPMP/SWP/997/96	Pre-clinical evaluation of anticancer medicinal products	Adopted NfG
CPMP/SWP/1042/99	Repeated dose toxicity	Adopted NfG
CPMP/SWP/2145/00	Non-clinical local tolerance testing of medicinal products	Adopted NfG
CPMP/SWP/112/98	Safety studies for gene therapy products	Draft NfG
CPMP/SWP/2877/00	Carcinogenic potential	Adopted NfG
CPMP/SWP/4446/00	Specification limits for residues of metal catalysts	Draft NfG
CPMP/SWP/398/01	Photosafety testing	Draft NfG
3CC29a	Investigation of chiral active substances	Adopted NfG
CPMP/986/96	Assessment of the potential for QT interval prolongation by non-cardiovascular medicinal products	PTC
CPMP/SWP/372/01	Non-clinical assessment of the carcinogenic potential of insulin analogues	PTC
CPMP/SWP/2600/01	Need for the assessment of reproductive toxicity of human insulin analogues	PTC
CPMP/SWP/2592/02	CPMP SWP conclusions and recommendations with regard to the use of genetically modified animal models for carcinogenicity assessment	Recommendations

information, as reported for recombinant interferon gamma (Terrell and Green, 1993). Nevertheless, whenever possible, NBEs should be tested using the same range of study types as for NCEs with appropriate modifications in respect of dose levels, species and endpoints (e.g. determination of serum neutralizing antibodies). Where an evaluation of carcinogenic potential is feasible and appropriate (e.g. for a chronic indication such as diabetes or osteoporosis), use of only one rodent species (normally the rat) is acceptable (ICH S6 Guideline). Most biological products are of a proteinaceous nature and so would not be expected to exhibit genotoxic properties, unless, for example, residues of linker molecules were unexpectedly present. But nongenotoxic proteins, especially those with higher potency trophic activity in rodents compared with man, can still produce a neoplastic response, as has been reported for recombinant human parathyroid hormone (1–34) when evaluated in a conventional rat bioassay (Vahle *et al.*, 2002). The latter finding seems unlikely to represent a hazard for patients when factors such as relative potency and duration and extent of exposure are considered, but data from additional studies will be required to confirm this.

Dossier compilation and Common Technical Document

For reasons of consistency and ease of assessment, regulatory authorities have established detailed requirements for dossier content and order of presentation. As well as copies of actual study reports, different types of summary, overview and critical assessment have been specified by authorities as part of the application dossiers for new drugs, called new drug applications (NDAs) in the USA and marketing authorization applications (MAAs) in the EU. An initiative by ICH (www.ich.org/) has produced the Common Technical Document (CTD) – a global guideline on dossier format (Table 3.5). The nonclinical modules are 2.4, 2.6 and 4. This format, accompanied by an optional electronic version (eCTD), is expected to become mandatory in the next 1–2 years on a worldwide basis; its introduction should lead to considerable time and cost savings in dossier preparation. It seems unlikely, however, that the ultimate goal of the global dossier (i.e. one identical dossier acceptable to all regulatory authorities worldwide) will be achieved in the foreseeable future owing to inter-regional differences in legal systems, medical practice and testing guidelines.

Table 3.5 Outline of Common Technical Document (CTD)

Module	Description
1	Administrative information and prescribing information
2	Common Technical Document summaries
	2.1 CTD table of contents
	2.2 CTD introduction
	2.3 Quality overall summary
	2.4 Nonclinical overview
	2.5 Clinical overview
	2.6 Nonclinical written and tabulated summaries
	Pharmacology
	Pharmacokinetics
	Toxicology
	2.7 Clinical summary
3	Quality
4	Nonclinical study reports
	4.1 Module 4 table of contents
	4.2 Study reports
	4.3 Literature references
5	Clinical study reports

Drug development

Introduction

Drug development is an exceedingly complex, high-risk and costly process involving scientists from many disciplines. At the time of writing (late 2002), the development programme from discovery to authorization for a typical NCE would be expected to take at least 6 years and cost not less than £500M (House of Lords, 2002). A recent UK report indicates that the UK drug failure rate is still high; of 320 compounds reported to be in development in 1998, only 47 are now available as approved medicines; about 150 of these were discontinued and the remainder are still in development (Anonymous, 2002). This pattern is being replicated worldwide. It is claimed that of half a million chemical structures/compounds initially considered, computational and other (*in vitro*) preclinical lead optimization screening reduces the number tested in animals to ten, and the results of animal studies cause seven to be rejected; three compounds go into clinical trials and just one is eventually authorized for human use (House of Lords, 2002). Higher success rates have been reported (e.g. 0.01–0.02 per cent; Dorato and Vodicnik, 2001), but such estimates may go back some years, when more targets amenable to simple rational approaches remained available for commercial exploitation, and may predate the advent of high-throughput screening techniques.

Increasing attention in the pharmaceutical industry is being focused on the declining numbers of new molecular entities (NMEs; includes NCEs and biologics) going into clinical development and achieving regulatory approval in spite of an *increase* in NMEs entering preclinical development (Jones, 2002). Reasons suggested to explain this include the increasing complexity of the clinical workup and the rarity of unmet therapeutic need in 'easy' disorders (with clear clinical endpoints and well-understood pathophysiology). Even modest clinical gains in diseases that tend to be chronic and the result of aging, and which are not readily treatable using current drug therapies, can be quite difficult to achieve (Cohen, 2002).

Toxicological requirements for conventional clinical trial programmes

Clinical trials in drug development are normally divided into three phases: phase 1, phase 2 and phase 3. Table 3.6 summarizes the essential elements of such trials, including toxicological data requirements for a typical NCE. Some authors add one or two further phases: phase 0 (nonclinical discovery phase) and phase 4 (post-marketing studies for further evaluation of safety in normal clinical use and/or assessment of comparative risk–benefit). The division of phase 2 into two parts (e.g. 2A and 2B), and sometimes similarly with phase 1, can provide a more stepwise and cautious approach (Lesko *et al.*, 2000).

Table 3.6 Conventional clinical trial programme for a typical NCE

Phase	Description	Number of patients	Normal toxicological requirements
1	Initial studies normally in (male) volunteers, but sometimes in patients, to determine tolerance, safe dosage range and basic kinetics and metabolism	30–50	2–4 weeks in rodent and non-rodent[a] basic genotoxicity and pharmacokinetics
2	Early controlled trials in a limited number of patients under closely monitored conditions to determine preliminary efficacy and short-term safety at a range of doses	250–500	3–6 months in rodent and non-rodent extensive genotoxicity and pharmacokinetics rat and rabbit teratology
3	Extended large-scale controlled trials to obtain definitive evidence of efficacy and safety, and to characterize the adverse-event profile. Studies on drug interactions and in special patient groups (e.g. elderly, hepatic/renal impairment)	300–3000	6 months in rodent and 9 months in non-rodent segments I and III reproductive toxicity carcinogenicity

[a] See text comments on single-dose toxicity studies.

Drug discovery phase

'Conventional' drug discovery involving 'rational' design of small organic molecules based on structure–activity considerations relating to drug target (e.g. inhibition or augmentation of a particular enzyme, cytokine or neurotransmitter) is still undertaken. A range of techniques, such as chemoinformatics (e.g. to assemble virtual compound libraries), combinatorial chemistry, genomics, proteomics and high-throughput screening are now employed to complement the traditional approaches (Atterwill and Wing, 2000; Johnson *et al.*, 2001; Schmid *et al.*, 2001; Alaoui-Ismaili *et al.*, 2002; Augen, 2002; Törnell and Snaith, 2002; Valler, 2002; van Dongen *et al.*, 2002).

Following candidate selection and the application of various screening procedures (for potential pharmacotoxicological activity), the more promising compounds would be further evaluated using *in vitro* and *in vivo* pharmacological models (Caldwell, 2001). Surviving candidates would then be eligible for an initial toxicity evaluation, usually involving *in vitro* assays for genotoxicity and single- and/or repeated-dose toxicity studies in one or two animal species. A preliminary ADME assessment *in vitro* and in animals would also be undertaken in normal circumstances. Although a drug may show activity *in vitro* and also possibly in some *in vivo* (rodent) models, kinetic and metabolic factors may alter the nature and magnitude of this response in man and in animal species that provide better models for man. Therefore, it is important at this early stage, and throughout the development programme, to integrate the available pharmacodynamic and pharmacokinetic information. Incorporating initial evaluations of toxicity and pharmacokinetics within the drug discovery phase may provide sufficient information to enable, where appropriate, some 're-engineering' of the chemical structure of a promising candidate in order, for example, to improve bioavailability or minimize toxicity. A major objective of the initial toxicological assessment is to provide sufficient reassuring safety information to proceed with a first-dose-in-man (sometimes called first-into-man, FIM) study, subject of course to ethics committee review (Johnson and Wolfgang, 2001).

Parallel programmes of chemical (or biotechnological) and pharmaceutical development, carefully coordinated with the non-clinical and clinical programmes, need to be undertaken, and are crucial to the eventual authorization and commercialization of any new drug. The specification of the test material used in non-clinical studies is likely to change as its synthesis progresses from a bench- to pilot-plant- and eventually to commercial-scale process. Detailed analytical information should be available on batches of test material used in non-clinical (and clinical) studies to evaluate the consistency of the impurity profile and whether the material toxicologically tested is representative in terms of chemical composition of the proposed commercial active ingredient. Owing to difficulties in achieving adequate physicochemical characterization of biotechnology and biological products, extremely close attention to process control is required in order to manufacture a consistent active ingredient.

FIM studies to assess tolerability and kinetics are usually undertaken in healthy (male) volunteers (Meulenbelt *et al.*, 1998). Such a study (studies) would be the first in the phase 1 programme. Other studies in patients in order to obtain an indication of pharmacodynamic effects, potential efficacy and dose–response relationships, possibly using a surrogate marker, would follow as soon as possible in clinical development. Increasingly, companies are attempting to accelerate evaluation in humans, one approach being to employ low-dose proof-of-concept (POC) studies in phase 1 rather than phase 2 (Lesko *et al.*, 2000).

Toxicological requirements for FIM and most other phase 1 studies in the EU include two 14-day repeated-dose studies in a rodent and non-rodent species (normally the rat and dog – ICH M3 guideline). However, in the USA, the FDA can authorize a single-dose clinical trial on the basis of data from extended single-dose toxicity studies in the rodent and non-rodent. A recent draft position paper issued by the EU Committee on Proprietary Medicinal Products (CPMP) proposes a somewhat similar but more restrictive approach of using an extended single-dose toxicity study in one species to support single low-dose exploratory screening trials in humans, e.g. in order to characterize pharmacokinetic properties or receptor selectivity using positron emission tomography (PET) imaging or other sensitive analytical techniques (Table 3.4).

A high proportion of early development projects, especially in small companies, involve anticancer drugs, since there remain significant unmet therapeutic needs and development times tend to be somewhat shorter than those in most other therapeutic areas. For anticancer drugs in general, and cytotoxics in particular, initial development has a number of special features (DeGeorge et al., 1998; Den Otter et al., 2002):

- All studies have to be undertaken in patients, for ethical reasons.

- As all cytotoxics exhibit relatively similar toxicity profiles (targeting cell populations with a rapid turnover), toxicological evaluation tends to be focused on revealing any important deviations from the expected toxicity profile, establishing a no-observed-adverse-effect level (NOAEL) and providing basic information on pharmacokinetics. In the past, virtually all of this work was successfully undertaken in one species, usually the rat, but use of additional species such as the dog is being increasingly recommended (Clark et al., 1999).

- A safe starting dose for entry into patients can be derived from the toxicological data; one-third of the rodent LD_{10} or one-third of the dog toxic high dose, both in mg/m^2, is suggested by Clark et al. (1999) for platinum-based anticancers. Pharmacokinetically guided approaches can also be applied (Reigner and Blesch, 2002).

Drug development phase

Strategic considerations

The selection of which candidate drug(s) to take from discovery into development is frequently rated as the most important decision in the drug-development process (Parkinson et al., 1996). All toxicological information available at this early stage plays a major role at this go/no-go decision point, and further toxicological studies play an enabling role in providing key safety data to support phase 2 and phase 3 trials. The timing of toxicological studies in relation to important milestones in the clinical programme is an important strategic issue that has to be decided by individual companies on a case-by-case basis. Some companies may adopt a cautious, cost-effective approach and undertake just enough studies to support the next clinical trial, whereas others may be less risk averse and decide to commission carcinogenicity studies on the basis of early results from phase 2A trials, essentially taking a calculated risk on a positive outcome to the phase 2 programme and associated toxicological studies.

Statistical aspects

Of necessity, owing to a range of considerations including animal usage, consumption of test material, cost and time, many compromises are involved in the design of toxicity studies, particularly in respect of the number of dose groups and the number animals per group. In repeated-dose toxicity studies, group sizes of 10–20 rodents and four to six non-rodents/sex are normally employed. In conventional carcinogenicity studies, the usual group size is 50 animals/sex. Thus, toxicity studies tend to have less statistical power than most phase 3 studies, typically involving hundreds of patients. For example, consider a case where the desired α-level (type I error) is set at 0.05 (single-sided test) and the β-level (type II error) is set at 0.1 (i.e. 90% chance of detecting a unidirectional effect at the 95 per cent confidence level. For two groups of animals (control and test), if the historical control response is 50 units with a standard deviation of 20 units and one wishes to detect a difference in response of 10 units (i.e. $\delta = 10/20 = 0.5$), then group sizes of 36 animals would be required. For a two-sided test with $\alpha = 0.05$, 44 animals per group would be required (Lee, 1993). However, one is able to administer multiples of the (anticipated) therapeutic dose in animals which may partially compensate for the low number of animals. Dosage selection in toxicological studies has traditionally been based on a high degree of empiricism, but the use of toxicokinetic data from dose-ranging studies can provide a more rational approach (Bus and Reitz, 1992; Spurling and Carey, 1992; Morgan *et al.*, 1994; Swenberg, 1995).

Species selection

Species selection in drug development is usually based on pilot toxicity and general pharmacology studies in rodent and non-rodent species together with supporting kinetic and metabolic information. In practical terms, choices are limited to species that are available from laboratory animal suppliers, which are of a suitable size and for which there is an adequate database for parameters such as survival, haematology and clinical chemistry on control animals and in which appropriate investigations and measurements are feasible. Within the limited range of options, selection of the most appropriate species can be crucial, particularly in respect of toxicity studies in non-rodents and embryotoxicity studies (Morton, 1998; Dixit, 2000; Smith *et al.*, 2001).

Effectiveness of standard nonclinical studies

Toxicological studies are considered by those involved in drug development to be indispensable in respect of highlighting the principal target organs that are at risk of exhibiting toxic responses; development of a significant number of drug candidates is curtailed based on the results of nonclinical studies (Broadhead *et al.*, 2000). Unfortunately, little information on this valuable function of identifying drug candidates that are toxic and/or appear to have an inferior benefit–risk profile are in the public domain, presumably because commercial pressures force pharmaceutical companies to concentrate on developing leading candidates without diverting resources to compile and publish data on those that have been discarded. On the other hand, standard toxicological studies have, at the margin, inherent limitations associated mainly with statistical considerations (see above) and the less-than-perfect nature of animal models. Consequently, it must be accepted that not all human adverse events will be predicted, particularly those that occur with low frequency (the latter generally not being well predicted in clinical trials).

Zbinden (1991) highlights a number of examples of human drug tragedies (such as those associated with chloramphenicol, hexachloraphene, gossypol and methoxyflurane) that, with hindsight, could have been prevented by undertaking appropriate animal studies combined with taking suitable precautionary measures. Although such examples of drug toxicity that would have been detected with current testing strategies are of largely historical interest, they illustrate the continuing improvements in pharmaceutical toxicology and the potential dangers of moving prematurely to alternative (non-animal) methods (House of Lords, 2002).

As a drug development programme proceeds, pre-clinical data are, to a large extent, progressively superseded by clinical safety data gathered in clinical trials, provided that the safety monitoring is of sufficient breadth and depth to evaluate appropriate target organs and toxic responses found in animals. Some non-clinical toxicity endpoints, such as reproductive toxicity, genotoxicity and carcinogenicity, are not amenable to clinical experimentation owing to a variety of practical and ethical factors. For newly authorized drugs there is almost total reliance on animal and *in vitro* data for safety assessments in these three areas.

At the clinical trial stage, and immediately following authorization, companies and regulatory agencies generally take a cautious approach regarding the use of a new drug in pregnant women. Even when a drug causes no adverse effects in the standard battery of reproductive toxicity tests (Table 3.1), pregnant women would normally be advised to avoid the drug unless its use is absolutely essential (European Commission, 1999). The availability of reassuring information on accidental or deliberate foetal exposure during clinical trials may lead to less restrictive labelling. These would be unusual circumstances, however, since pregnant women are normally excluded from clinical trials. Some relaxation in pregnancy labelling is possible if evidence can be presented to regulatory authorities demonstrating that there is no association with adverse reproductive effects after several years of clinical use.

Nonstandard studies

Nonstandard and/or special investigative studies are often commissioned during drug development in an attempt to answer specific questions. For example, non-clinical studies may predict a particular toxic response that is, in fact, not observed in clinical trials. It is more convincing to be able to explain *why* a toxic effect occurred in animals but not in clinical-trial patients rather than just relying on the absence of clinical adverse events. Special studies could be undertaken *in vitro* and/or in animals in order to understand the causative factors of the effect and whether the mechanism involved excludes the likelihood of a human response. Some examples are:

- Animal toxicity attributable to species-specific kinetic, metabolic or pharmacodynamic effects (Warrington *et al.*, 2002; Tabacova and Kimmel, 2001; Soars *et al.*, 2001; Van Gelder *et al.*, 2000; Molderings *et al.*, 2000; Honma *et al.*, 2001).

- Validation and use of the rhesus monkey as a suitable model for testing the effects of finasteride, a type 2 5-α-reductase inhibitor, on external genital differentiation of the male foetus (Prahalada *et al.*, 1997).

- Various studies on tamoxifen demonstrating that the formation of liver tumours in the rat is not relevant to the use of the drug in women (De Matteis *et al.*, 1998; White *et al.*, 2001).

Validity and relevance of non-clinical testing programme

Through a process of continual improvement and capture of best practice in regulatory guidelines, non-clinical testing programmes in drug development tend to be similar across a broad range of therapeutic categories. But there still remains a degree of flexibility that enables individual programmes to be improved, for instance by 'backtracking' and undertaking more detailed investigations in problem areas and/or using special studies. In this way it is possible to produce a robust non-clinical database of optimum relevance to human safety assessment. Some of the more important factors that need to be considered in this optimization process are summarized in Table 3.7.

Table 3.7 Principal scientific factors affecting the validity and relevance of a drug toxicity testing programme

Factor	Main considerations
Scope	• All appropriate endpoints incorporated, e.g. potential carcinogenic effects of growth factors
Species suitability	• Pharmacodynamically responsive to drug • Similar metabolic profile to that in man
Receptor profiles	• Adequate separation in targeting of desired and undesired receptors in terms of pharmacodynamic responses in animal models and humans Applicability of highly specific receptor targeting in animal models to clinical situation
Kinetics	• Linear or non-linear kinetics? • Reasons for non-linearity (e.g. saturation of excretion mechanisms, liver enzyme induction) • Plasma accumulation on repeated dosing?
Metabolism	• Safety evaluation of any significant human metabolites not detected in animal models
Study design and implementation	• Adequate number of dose groups and numbers of animals • Use of one animal gender or two as appropriate • Suitable and validated endpoints and test methods • Duration of dosing relevant to indication • Use of recovery groups • GLP considerations
Dose levels and exposure	• Dose levels justified by range-finding studies • Adequate toxicokinetic monitoring incorporated into toxicity studies
Genotoxicity	• Confirmation that metabolic activating system employed in *in vitro* assays is capable of simulating *in vivo* metabolism • If not confirmed, separate studies on the principal metabolites may be necessary • Relationship between concentration of test material used in *in vitro* assays and human plasma C_{max} • Dose- or concentration-related changes in metabolism
Mechanistic studies	• Direct or indirect consequence of exaggerated pharmacology? • Species specificity and reasons for this • Disruption of homeostatic mechanisms, e.g. by modification of endocrine system

Data interpretation and risk assessment

Interpretation of nonclinical toxicity data

Routine toxicity tests deliberately incorporate a plethora of different endpoints (Table 3.1) selected on the basis of experience to be effective at detecting toxic responses. It is common for statistically significant differences to be observed between parameters for test and concurrent control animals, but such differences may occur by chance or through normal biological variation, not reflecting a genuine treatment-related effect. The greater the number of different endpoints, the higher will be the probability that some differences will occur by chance. Careful scrutiny of the data from individual studies is required in order to assess whether the effects observed fit a logical pattern indicative of a toxic response. Subsequently, data from several studies should be evaluated to ascertain consistency of response. Any major inter-study inconsistencies should be thoroughly investigated in an attempt to establish the reasons for the variable response.

The processes involved in non-clinical data interpretation include:

- Establishment of pattern of toxic response

  - endpoints affected

  - route/dose/exposure/time relationships

  - reversibility

  - inter-species variation

- Determination of target organ(s)

  - confirmed by multiple endpoints

  - inter-species differences explained (e.g. by kinetic, metabolic and/or known species sensitivities)

  - pharmacodynamic and/or toxicological effects

- Assessment of no-adverse-effect and lowest-effect doses and the systemic exposures corresponding to these doses.

- Proposed toxicological mechanism(s)

  - use of established precedents and information on class effects

  - special studies commissioned as appropriate.

A toxic effect in a particular organ will normally be associated with changes in a variety of parameters. For example, a toxic response in the liver would be expected to be associated with a change in bodyweight-related organ weight, increases in serum enzymes associated with hepatotoxicity (e.g. alanine aminotransferase and aspartate aminotransferase) and histopathological changes. Although slight alterations in one parameter (e.g. in serum enzymes) may be suggestive of liver damage, without confirmatory evidence from other sources, hepatotoxicity would not in this case normally be considered as a major concern.

Thus, a variety of separate effects may often be consequences of the same toxicological process. Gaining an understanding of the pattern of toxicity may suggest a causal mechanism that is often a critical prerequisite for effective extrapolation of non-clinical toxicological findings to man.

Risk assessment: extrapolation of toxicological data to man

Introduction

Risk assessment is the process of determining the types and likelihoods of adverse reactions in humans that may result from exposure to chemical, biological or physical hazards (Brecher, 1997). In the context of drug development, particularly at the early stages, the essence of risk assessment is the extrapolation of the non-clinical data to man. Most of the information is derived from *in vivo* experiments in animals using high doses of the drug substance. The relevance of responses in animals to patients using the intended therapeutic dose will be assessed by a number of interested parties (company, regulatory agency/ethics committee for clinical trials, regulatory agency at the MAA stage) at various time points during development.

Allometry

In the early days of drug toxicology there was a search, ultimately futile, to find a test species that metabolized drugs in the same way as humans. Eventually, it became apparent that drug metabolism in animals hardly ever proceeds at the same rate as in humans. Several investigators noted that drug clearance per unit of body weight was nearly always considerably higher in small animals compared with larger animals such as man. Determination of biological half-life and clearance of drugs in several species suggested that these and other pharmacokinetic parameters were proportional to some power of the body mass. In other words, several fundamental pharmacokinetic parameters appeared to obey allometric principles (i.e. the study of size and its consequences).

The general allometric equation linking morphological and biological functions Y and body weight W is

$$Y = aW^b \tag{3.1}$$

where a is the allometric coefficient and b is the allometric exponent.

A corollary of this equation is that the traditional bases for extrapolation of data, i.e. $W^{1.0}$ (mg/kg body weight) and $W^{0.67}$ (mg/m^2 body surface area) have no unique justification; they are just two examples of the general case and provide quantitatively different scaling factors.

Logarithmic transformation of equation (3.1) yields:

$$\log Y = \log a + b \log W \tag{3.2}$$

Equation (3.2) is of the form $y = mx + c$, and so it is possible to plot $\log Y$ versus $\log W$ for different animal species and from the linear relationship to predict values of Y for man. Alternatively, the data can be analysed by linear regression using a statistical software package.

Unfortunately, the application of allometric interspecies scaling to animal toxicity and pharmacokinetic data has led to somewhat disappointing results (Vocci and Farber, 1988; Bachmann, 1989; Chappell and Mordenti, 1991; Mordenti *et al.*, 1992; Ritschel *et al.*, 1992; Lin, 1998; Mahmood, 1998, 1999a,b, 2000a, 2001a, 2002; Lave *et al.*, 1999; Mahmood and Balian, 1999; Mahmood and Sahajwalla, 2002).

Scaling of toxicity data has been reasonably successful (e.g. up to 80% of compounds) for single-dose studies. Acute toxicity data (e.g. LD_{10}, MTD) for chemotherapeutic drugs have been extensively evaluated with exponents ranging from 0.6 to 0.9 (Chappell and Mordenti, 1991); an exponent of 0.75 appears to be more effective than use of surface-area relation-ships ($b = 0.67$) (Travis and White, 1988; Mahmood, 2001b). Travis (1991) also recom-mends in the more general case the use of 0.75 as exponent in preference to the conventional parameters (0.67 or 1.0). In a survey of 26 NCEs evaluated by the Medicines Evaluation Board in the Netherlands in the early 1990s, extrapolation on the basis of 'metabolism equivalents' using 0.75 as exponent was found to produce the closest fit to extrapolations based on pharmacokinetic data (Peters-Volleberg *et al.*, 1994).

There are many examples of successful pharmacokinetic interspecies scaling, particularly for drugs that are completely or largely renally excreted (Chappell and Mordenti, 1991; Lin, 1998). Determination of the most important pharmacokinetic parameters (e.g. distribution volumes, half-life, clearance, AUC) from experiments using young adults of four animal species followed by linear regression is recommended (Chappell and Mordenti, 1991). Drugs cleared by hepatic extraction are more difficult to evaluate by interspecies scaling, though some success has been achieved by correlating half-life with liver blood flow rather than body weight (Aviles *et al.*, 2001). The need to use brain weight as well as body weight in these situations brings a multivariate aspect to the problem (Lin, 1998).

Extrapolation to humans is often not straightforward, owing to the many intrinsic minor biochemical and physiological differences between animals and humans. Various minor modifications can be made to the basic allometric pharmacokinetic model, such as employ-ing free-fraction drug concentration [rather than the total (free + bound) concentration] and lifespan potential (physiological time). However, the value of using free-fraction concentra-tions has been disputed (Mahmood and Balian, 1999; Mahmood, 2000b).

A more sophisticated approach, physiologically based pharmacokinetics (PB-PK), in-volves mass balance models in which it is generally assumed that organs and tissues with similar behaviour can be combined into compartments and connected by the fluid motion through the compartments. This is a reductionist paradigm in contrast to the predominantly empirical approach in allometric scaling (Chappell and Mordenti, 1991). Setting up PB-PK models is time consuming, data intensive and costly (Campbell, 1996), and has not achieved a significant uptake in pharmaceutical toxicology.

NOAEL safety factor (or margin of exposure) approach combined with conventional dosimetry

This classical approach to risk assessment relies on applying a safety factor to the NOAEL obtained in the 'most sensitive species'. The conventional safety factor is 100 (10 each for intra- and inter-species variation), as is still employed in the assessment of food additives and other materials (Gaylor, 1983; Feron *et al.*, 1990; Newman *et al.*, 1993; Walker, 1998). For drug substances, where the (intended) maximum human dose (MHD) is known, individual safety factors (sometimes called margin of exposure, MoE, when used in this context) can be calculated for each toxicological effect by dividing the NOAEL by the MHD (both in mg/kg/day).

Many deficiencies in this approach have been identified (Garattini, 1985; Berry, 1988). These include:

- Absence of mechanistic/pharmacokinetic considerations, particularly in respect of why one species is more sensitive than another, and the relevance of this to man.

- Reliance on the applied dose, leading for example to exaggeration of safety factors, particularly those based on rodent data.

- Frequent nonlinearity of dose–exposure relationships, especially in animals at higher doses.

Body-surface-area-based doses are employed in interspecies scaling for some drug classes (e.g. anticancers and antivirals), and this metric has been described as a more accurate and conservative method (compared with using mg/kg doses) for general use in regulatory toxicology (Voisin et al., 1990). However, scaling on the basis of mg/m^2 doses is probably better described as over-conservative since animal:human safety margins tend to be under-estimated compared with those based on kinetic data (Table 3.8; Peters-Volleberg et al., 1994). This is further illustrated in the phenolphthalein example (Table 3.9).

Table 3.8 Body weights and scaling factors based on exponents of 0.67 and 0.75[a]

Parameter	Man	Beagle dog	Monkey (cynomolgus)	Rabbit	Rat	Mouse
Body weight (kg)	70	8	6	2	0.20	0.025
Exponent 0.67	1	2.0	2.2	3.2	6.9	14
Exponent 0.75	1	1.7	1.8	2.4	4.3	7.3

[a] Example: to scale on the basis of exponent 0.75, a dose of 4.3 mg/kg/day in the rat corresponds to 1 mg/kg/day in man.
Scaling factors are calculated from $(W_a/W_h)^{b-1}$, where W_a is the body weight of animal, W_h is the human body weight, b is an exponent. For derivation see Rodricks et al., (2001).

Given the above criticisms, the NOAEL safety factor approach is generally avoided in pharmaceutical toxicology, although its use has been recommended in risk assessment of reproductive toxicity data (Newman et al., 1993). The technique may be employed with reluctance in situations where no comparative kinetic data are available. The risk assessment of impurities, such as solvents based on sub-acute (rodent) NOAELs, is an important example (see ICH Q3C). Special considerations apply in respect of the comparative dosimetry of inhaled drugs (Dahl et al., 1991; Bide et al., 2000; Mahmood, 2001c).

In spite of its many deficiencies, the NOAEL safety factor approach has been used since the 1950s by the FAO/WHO Joint Expert Committee on Food Additives (JECFA), and appears to have been successful in terms of preventing adverse effects in consumers. This probably reflects the intrinsic conservatism of the JECFA procedure, which generally employs high safety factors (≥ 100).

Table 3.9 Phenolphthalein: animal: man exposure multiples (EMs) based on three different metrics in rat and mouse dietary carcinogenicity studies[a]

Species	Dose in mg/kg/day (EM)		Dose in mg/m²/day (EM)		Animal AUC$_{24}$ (h.µmol/l)	EM based on AUC$_{24}$
Rat, F344 (male)	24.9	(12.5)	129	(1.74)	1090	4.84
	58.8	(24.4)	306	(4.14)	1550	6.84
	176	(88)	915	(12.4)	4290	19.0
	606	(303)	3150	(42.6)	9620	42.6
	2780	(1390)	14 500	(196)	9100	40.2
Mouse, B6C3F1 (male)	38.2	(19.1)	115	(1.55)	983	4.35
	65.9	(33.0)	198	(2.68)	2350	10.4
	143	(72)	429	(5.80)	3970	17.5
	551	(276)	1650	(22.3)	9110	40.3
	2140	(1070)	6410	(86.6)	15 200	67.2

[a] Human data from study in male volunteers: dose 2.0 mg/kg, 74 mg/m²; AUC$_{24}$ 226 h.µmol/l; data based on measurement of total (free plus glucuronide conjugate) plasma phenolphthalein. Data are taken from Collins *et al.*, (2000). Note: (a) subproportional dose-related increase in animal AUC (due to saturation of absorption, possibly plus some enzyme induction in the rat); (b) over- and under-estimation of exposure margins by mg/kg and mg/m² metrics respectively (except for mg/m² at highest doses in the rat, where absorption is saturated).

Use of NOAEL and relative systemic exposure

In this commonly used technique, safety factors are based on systemic exposure of the drug in animals at the NOAEL relative to that in man at the maximum human dose (MHD):

$$\text{Safety Factor} = \frac{\text{Animal AUC at NOAEL}}{\text{Human AUC at MHD}}$$

Exposure margins in carcinogenicity studies can also be calculated in a similar fashion using the animal AUC at the high dose (or other dose) for the numerator.

AUC tends to be the default, but C_{max} or other appropriate metrics related to systemic exposure may also be employed. The measure of systemic exposure can be based on parent drug substance alone and/or important (active) metabolites. Stereochemical preferences in the disposition of racemic drugs often differ among species, e.g. in relation to the nature and extent of chiral inversion. Consequently, exposure extrapolations for chiral drugs from one species to another should be made with caution (Ruelius, 1987).

Scaling on the basis of relative systemic exposure avoids a variety of problems associated with other approaches (Voisin *et al.*, 1990):

- Drugs that are extensively metabolized cannot be compared across species using models that rely on body weight.

- Although numerous mammalian physiological parameters are related to body surface area ($W^{0.67}$) rather than body weight, the specific metabolic profile of many drugs does not correlate with overall metabolic rate, and thus with surface area.

- Quantitative interspecies differences in ADME profiles are highly drug specific and often confound body-weight-related interspecies relationships.

As well as being drug specific, using relative systemic exposure for scaling purposes enables data obtained by different routes of administration to be compared. For example, oral long-term bioassays may be employed to evaluate the carcinogenic potential of drugs that are intended for parenteral or inhalation administration in patients.

The NOAEL has been criticized in relation to its inferior statistical properties, e.g. for its sensitivity to sample size and its high sampling variability from experiment to experiment (Leisenring and Ryan, 1992; Brand *et al.*, 1999). Although alternative approaches have often been advocated, the NOAEL is still used quite extensively.

Pre-authorization risk assessment: species susceptibility and mechanistic studies

When a drug substance produces adverse effects in an animal model that are considered unlikely to be relevant to human safety, existing information on species sensitivity (e.g. exaggerated gastrointestinal toxicity in rodents to NSAIDs, gastric carcinoids produced by chronic administration of proton pump inhibitors, formation of liver tumours in mice) and/ or new data from drug-specific mechanistic studies are often extremely helpful in terms of risk assessment (Williams, 1997).

A number of mechanisms have been proposed to account for carcinogenic responses to nongenotoxic drugs, the strength of the evidence being quite variable from one case to another (Alden, 2000; Silva Lima and van der Laan, 2000). Chronic prolactin stimulation has been identified as a promoter of carcinogenicity (Yokoro *et al.*, 1977; Johnson *et al.*, 1995; Cook *et al.*, 1999; Suwa *et al.*, 2001) but confirmatory evidence such as serum prolactin data is important in regulatory decision making in individual cases. Interspecies differences in metabolism are known to account for differences in cancer susceptibility and toxicity (Hengstler *et al.*, 1999).

Unexpected adverse events detected in clinical trials may sometimes be amenable to investigation in animal models. HER-2 (human epidermal growth factor receptor 2 protein) is a member of the c-erbB family of receptor tyrosine kinases and is overexpressed by 20–30 per cent of human breast cancers. HER-2 overexpression is an independent adverse prognostic factor. Trastuzumab, a humanized monoclonal antibody that binds with high affinity to the extracellular domain of HER-2, is effective when used in combination with cytotoxics in the second-line treatment of advanced metastatic breast cancer (Harries and Smith, 2002; Ligibel and Winer, 2002). However, in combination with anthracyclines, in patients there is a marked increase in cardiotoxicity: 24.5 per cent heart failure versus 7.4 per cent with anthracyclines alone (Garattini and Bertele, 2002; Keefe, 2002; Page *et al.*, 2002; Tham *et al.*, 2002). Attempts were made to develop an animal model for this interaction in order to investigate the mechanism with the aim of eliminating or minimizing the cardiotoxic response. But, at the time of marketing authorization in the EU, all such attempts had been unsuccessful (European Medicines Evaluation Agency (EMEA: www. eudra.org/humandocs/humans/epar.htm; European Public Assessment Report (EPAR) for Herceptin).

In summary, species susceptibility and mechanisms of toxicity play critical (generally qualitative) roles in risk assessment. Many useful drugs would have failed to gain registration without this type of evidence.

Predictivity of nonclinical studies

The effectiveness of non-clinical studies, particularly animal studies, at predicting human toxic responses to pharmaceuticals is difficult to assess because, as already noted, virtually all of the relevant data are owned by pharmaceutical companies and there are distinct commercial barriers to the release of this information. Even though it is possible in theory to make an assessment of data available in the public domain, or available to regulatory authorities, both of these would be highly biased datasets since they would fail to include data on the significant number of drugs whose development was terminated based solely on internal company decisions.

The problems inherent in the above situation have been addressed by the Health and Environmental Safety Institute/International Life Sciences Institute who compiled relevant data via a multinational survey of pharmaceutical companies (Olson *et al.*, 2000). The survey included data from 12 companies on 150 compounds with 221 different human toxicities (HTs) being reported. Multiple HTs were reported in 47 cases. The results showed the true positive HT concordance rate of 71 per cent for rodent and non-rodent species, with non-rodents alone being predictive for 63 per cent of HTs and rodents alone for 43 per cent. The highest incidence of overall concordance was seen in haematological, gastrointestinal and cardiovascular HTs, and the least was seen in cutaneous HT. Where animal models, in one or more species, identified concordant HT, 94 per cent were first observed in studies of 1 month or less in duration. Of the 29 per cent of effects not detected in animal tests, the majority were of a type that animal tests were not designed to detect, or were intrinsically undetectable in this type of test, e.g. headache, dizziness and certain skin reactions.

Although the concept of undertaking repeated-dose toxicity studies in both rodents and non-rodents considerably predates the concordance survey described above, it is noteworthy that inclusion of the non-rodent markedly improves predictivity. In addition, techniques such as receptor and ADME profiling can help assess the degree of relevance to man of a particular species, and thus improve predictivity (Zbinden, 1993).

Adverse drug reactions detected after authorization

Adverse reactions and drug withdrawals

With long-term monitoring all drugs can be expected to exhibit side effects (i.e. unwanted effects of no therapeutic value) in some patients. Collection of safety data during clinical trials (especially phase 3 trials) enables detailed adverse event profiles to be compiled for a closely defined patient population. Such information is essential to the assessment of the benefit–risk of a particular drug. Rare adverse reactions, unlikely to be apparent in clinical trials, are detected only after the drug has been marketed and used by large numbers of patients, possibly including some more sick or less sick than those in the clinical trial population. Although a more comprehensive risk profile may begin to emerge only after widespread use, possibly leading to drug withdrawal, various confounding 'lifestyle' and other factors can often make determination of causation a tricky and complex process (Corrigan, 2002).

Since few relevant data are in the public domain, it is generally not possible to assess whether any inadequacies in non-clinical safety evaluation have contributed to the withdrawal of drugs on grounds of safety (see Chapter 1 and Appendix 1). However, quite a few drugs developed during the era of extensive pre-authorization toxicological evaluation have been withdrawn, suggesting that the observed human toxic responses were not clearly predicted by animal studies (or by clinical trials). Retrospective analysis might, in some cases, have shown weak signals. Newly introduced toxicological tests (for QT prolongation, ICH S7B) might have been helpful in the case of fluoroquinolone antibiotics, e.g. grepafloxacin (Owens and Ambrose, 2002).

Types of adverse drug reactions and their toxicological investigation

Type A adverse reactions are dose dependent and predictable based on the pharmacology (and kinetics) of the drug; about 80 per cent of all reported ADRs are type A. On the other hand, according to Knowles *et al.* (2000), idiosyncratic drug reactions (type B) cannot be explained on the basis of the conventional pharmacology of the drug, and although they may be dose dependent in susceptible individuals, they do not occur at any dose in most patients. Type B adverse reactions can affect any organ system; they include IgE-mediated anaphylaxis and allergy. In addition, there can be reactive metabolite effects, such as:

- Hypersensitivity-syndrome reactions. These are usually defined by the triad of fever, skin eruption and internal organ involvement; such reactions have been associated with anticonvulsants (phenytoin, phenobarbital, carbamazepine and lamotrigine), sulphonamide antibiotics, dapsone, minocycline and allopurinol.

- Serum-sickness-like reactions. These are distinct from serum sickness and defined by fever, rash, usually urticaria, and arthralgias occurring 1–3 weeks after drug exposure, immune complexes, hypocomplementaemia, vasculitis and renal lesions being absent; drugs implicated in such reactions are antibiotics such as cefaclor, cefprozil and minocycline.

- Drug-induced lupus. This is characterized by frequent musculoskeletal complaints, fever and weight loss, pleuropulmonary involvement in more than half of the patients, with no cutaneous findings of lupus erythematosus, symptoms and serological changes generally occurring more than a year after starting therapy. Drugs implicated in the causation of drug-induced lupus include procainamide, isoniazid, hydralazine, chlorpromazine, methyldopa and penicillamine.

Type B ADRs are generally unpredictable and often result in the post-marketing failure of otherwise useful therapies. Examples of recent cases include zileuton, trovafloxacin, troglitazone and felbamate. Zileuton, a 5-lipoxygenase inhibitor authorized in the USA (but not in the EU) to prevent and relieve the symptoms of chronic asthma, has been shown to cause liver toxicity in some patients (Sorkness, 1997). It is not widely used, owing to the need for four times daily dosing and the requirement for liver function monitoring during the first few months of therapy. US post-marketing surveillance data on trovafloxacin, a fluoroquinolone antibiotic, indicated the possibility of serious hepatic reactions and pancreatitis, leading to significant restrictions in its use (Ball, 2000; Bertino and Fish, 2000). Troglitazone and felbamate are discussed below.

Deciding whether a particular ADR is likely to be type A or B may not be possible until data on symptomatology and patient characteristics (e.g. race, gender, genetic polymorphisms, concurrent disease status and medications) have been analysed on a cohort of affected patients. Key factors in clinical assessment are the temporal relationship between drug intake and the appearance of symptoms, skin tests and provocation tests (Ring and Brockow, 2002).

Toxicological investigation of type A adverse drug reactions

Toxicological evaluation of predictable type A ADRs would normally be targeted on pharmacodynamic–pharmacokinetic mechanisms. Causative factors could include one or more of:

- Excess systemic exposure leading to an exaggerated pharmacodynamic response
    - impaired elimination of active drug due to interactions (e.g. P450 inhibition)
    - slow active drug clearance due to genetic polymorphism.
- Formation of toxic metabolite specific to humans.
- Other biological human-specific mechanisms, such as different receptor specificity or sensitivity.

The starting point for toxicological evaluation would be the establishment of appropriate *in vitro* and/or *in vivo* models based on pharmacodynamic and kinetic considerations. Studies would then be focused on a case-by-case basis on appropriate endpoints, such as enzyme induction/inhibition, interactions and genetic variability.

Variations in genes coding for drug-metabolizing enzymes, drug receptors and drug transporters have been associated with individual variability in the efficacy and toxicity of drugs. It is difficult to disentangle the contribution of environmental and genetic factors in an individual patient. Genotyping can predict the extremes of phenotypes, but less definable factors (such as other variant genes) and environmental factors (such as smoking and diet) contribute to the patient's phenotype.

Possibly the most actively researched area in genetic polymorphism relates to the contribution of genetically determined variability in drug metabolizing enzymes to inter-patient differences in response to drugs (Lu, 1998; Meyer, 2000). The most important clinically relevant drug-metabolizing enzyme polymorphisms relate to:

- CYP2C9, e.g. warfarin, tolbutamide, phenytoin, glipizide, losartan;
- CYP2D6, e.g. antiarrhythmics, antidepressants, antipsychotics, opioids;
- CYP2C19, e.g. omeprazole, diazepam;
- N-acetyltransferase, e.g. sulphonamides, procainamide, hydralazine, isoniazid;
- UDP-glucuronosyltransferase (UGT), e.g. irinotecan.

Toxicological studies in extensive- and poor-metabolizer animals (particularly non-rodents) may be helpful in assessing the possible safety impact of some human genetic polymorphisms.

Toxicological investigation of type B adverse drug reactions

Little is known with certainty about the mechanisms involved in the majority of idiopathic ADRs. Circumstantial, rather than direct, evidence suggests that drug reactive metabolites (DRMs) are responsible for most type B ADRs. The current hypothesis (Knowles *et al.*, 2000) linking reactive metabolites to ADRs suggests that there are basically three possibilities for further reaction of a newly formed DRM:

- Deactivation by nucleophiles and radical scavengers, e.g. glutathione, epoxide hydrolases.

- Reaction with macromolecules leading to cytotoxicity.

- Hapten formation – covalent binding to proteins and altered protein triggers an immune response.

A more recent 'multiple determinant hypothesis' states that the low frequency ($<1/5000$) of idiosyncratic drug toxicity is due to the requirements for occurrence of multiple critical and discrete events. The principal determinants of these events are proposed to be: chemical properties (including potential for DRM production), patient exposure, environmental and genetic factors (Li, 2002).

The generation and fate of reactive metabolites are determined by activating, inactivating and precursor-sequestering enzymes. In turn, these enzymes are controlled by long-term induction and repression, as well as the short-term control of post-translational modification and low-molecular-weight activators and inhibitors. The effectiveness of such enzyme systems in preventing DRM-mediated toxicity relates principally to their subcellular compartmentalization and isoenzyme multiplicity. Susceptibility differences to DRM-related toxic challenges between species and individuals are frequently thought to be causally linked to differences in these control factors (Oesch *et al.*, 1990).

The formation of an epoxide DRM has been postulated for some anticonvulsants (carbamezepine, phenobarbital and phenytoin), and enhanced individual susceptibility was thought to be related to a deficiency of epoxide hydrolaze. More recent studies have thrown some doubt on this hypothesis and alternative DRMs have been postulated such as free radicals and an orthoquinone for phenytoin and an iminoquinone for carbamezepine (Knowles *et al.*, 2000).

The potential of a drug to stimulate idiosyncratic reactions probably relates more to its chemical structure than its pharmacological mechanism. If biotransformation can yield products containing structural elements such as quinones, phenols, acyl halides, aromatic or hydroxyl amines, then the potential for type B ADRs is increased (Petersen, 2002). Examples supporting this hypothesis are tacrine (Figure 3.1; primary aromatic amine, hepatotoxic cholinesterase inhibitor for treatment of Alzheimer's disease superseded by drugs such as donepezil and rivastigmine (Figure 3.1) with less potential to produce DRMs) and troglitazone (can be transformed into a quinone, a property not shared by its successors such as rosiglitazone and pioglitazone; see Figure 3.1). However, an alternative to this suggestion by Peterson to explain the hepatotoxicity of troglitazone is advanced by Haskins *et al.*, (2001); see Figure 3.2.

Some researchers believe that it is currently impossible to predict which chemical species will cause idiosyncratic ADRs and advocate the need for a more thorough understanding of basic drug metabolism before attempting to relate chemical species formation to biological function (Williams and Naisbitt, 2002). Many drugs that are associated with idiosyncratic toxicity contain nitrogen which is relatively easy to oxidize and many nitrogen-containing compounds undergo redox cycling, which can generate active oxygen species. Moreover, several nitrogen-containing substances, including aromatic amines, nitro compounds, hydrazines and compounds that can be oxidized to iminoquinones and related substances, have been associated with adverse reactions. However, in addition to the presence of such structural elements, various other factors, such as dose, electron density and patient susceptibility, may play a role (Uetrecht, 2002).

Modern biochemical, molecular and immunochemical techniques have enabled identification of specific target proteins of xenobiotic covalent binding, and it is apparent that binding is not random but rather selective in its targeting. Selective protein binding may correlate better with target organ toxicity, and evidence on several compounds (e.g. paracetamol, halothane and 2,5-hexanedione) tends to support this proposal (Cohen et al., 1997).

Many idiosyncratic reactions appear to have an immunological aetiology; hapten formation followed by uptake, antigen processing and T-cell proliferation appear to be the critical parts of the mechanism (Naisbitt et al., 2000, 2001; Park et al., 2000, 2001; Ju and Uetrecht, 2002). Drugs associated with a high incidence of hypersensitivity appear to be capable of ready formation of DRMs, but this appears not to apply to all drugs that can form DRMs. One possible explanation is that orally administered drugs may lead to oral tolerance in most individuals through mechanisms similar to those found with orally administered antigens (i.e. interaction with gut-associated lymphoid tissue of the small intestine). Following oral administration of the NSAID diclofenac (Figure 3.1) to rats, a series of diclofenac protein adducts (55 to 142 kDa) were detected in small intestine homogenates. Two of the adducts were identified as aminopeptidase N (CD13) and sucrase-isomaltase and were localized primarily in the mid-villus and villus-tip enterocytes and also in the dome overlying Peyer's patches. Similar adducts were detected in villus-tip enterocytes of rats treated with halothane or paracetamol. It is possible that such intestinal protein adducts of drugs formed in gut-associated lymphoid tissue may lead to down-regulation of drug-associated allergic reactions in many individuals (Ware et al., 1998).

The liver is the principal site of drug metabolism and it is a common target for idiosyncratic drug reactions (Jaeschke et al., 2002). In the case of immune reactions directly involving leukocytes, the enzyme system most likely to be responsible for the formation of reactive metabolites is the NADPH oxidase/myeloperoxidase system found in neutrophils and monocytes. In addition to the proposed hapten/T-lymphocyte pathway, other mechanisms may exist, such as molecular mimicry (caused by a common alteration in the processing and presentation of antigens due to non-drug stimuli such as viruses) and direct alteration of the class II major histocompatibility (MHC) molecule by a DRM leading to a graft versus host reaction (Uetrecht, 1997). Hepatitis of the type triggered by drugs such as halothane, tienilic acid and dihydralazine appears to have a range of immunological features, including dose independence, immune system manifestations such as fever and eosinophilia, delay between drug treatment and disease onset, shortened delay on rechallenge and occasional presence of serum autoantibodies (Beaune and Lecoeur, 1997; Dansette et al., 1998; Castell, 1998). Genetic imbalance between bioactivation and detoxification pathways, as well as reduced cellular defences against DRMs due to disease or concomitant drug therapy, may act as risk factors to the onset and severity of ADRs (Hess and Rieder, 1997).

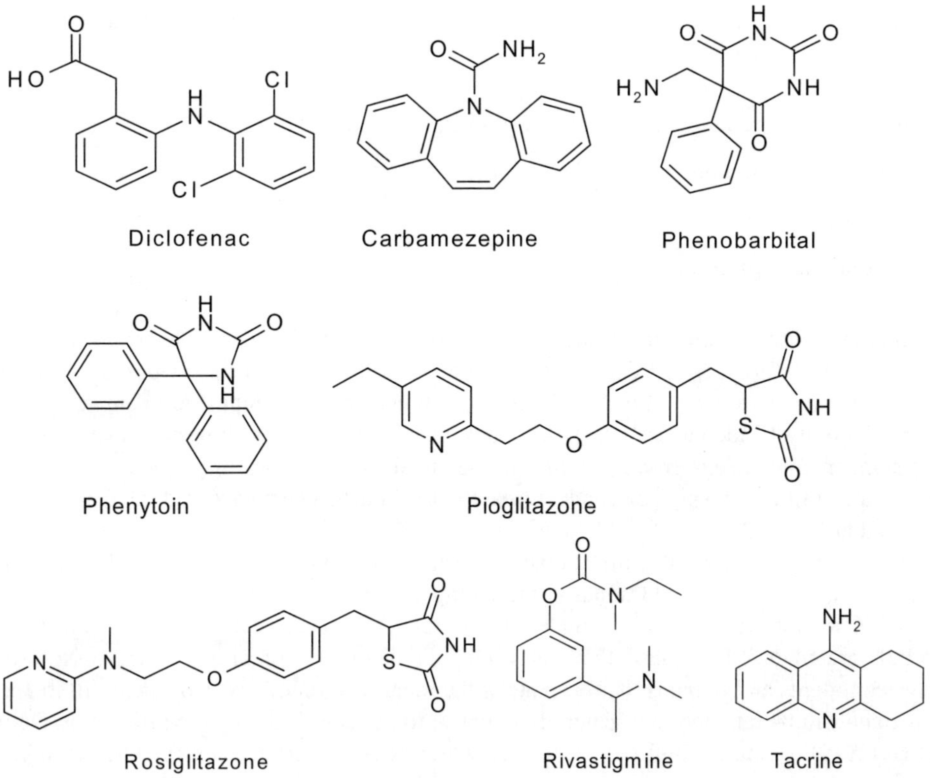

Figure 3.1 Chemical structures of some drugs discussed in the text

Tolcapone, a catechol-O-methyltransferase inhibitor used for treatment of motor fluctuations in Parkinsons's disease, had been associated with numerous cases of hepatotoxicity, including three cases of fatal fulminant hepatic failure. The structurally similar drug entacapone appears not to stimulate this type of toxic response. *In vitro* studies suggest that CYP P450-catalysed oxidation of amine and acetylamine human tolcapone metabolites leads to formation of reactive intermediates that may form covalent adducts to hepatic proteins, resulting in damage to liver tissues (Smith *et al.*, 2003). Use of the broad-spectrum antiepileptic drug felbamate has been limited due to reports of treatment-related hepatotoxicity and aplastic anaemia. It has been proposed that bioactivation leads to formation of a highly reactive electrophilic metabolite, atropaldehyde (ATPAL), an α,β-unsaturated aldehyde, that is capable of forming covalent protein adducts *in vivo*. *In vitro* studies on ATPAL support this hypothesis and suggest that both direct covalent binding with critical macromolecules and indirect interference with cellular detoxication mechanisms may be involved (Dieckhaus *et al.*, 2002; Kapetanovic *et al.*, 2002).

Cutaneous reactions are the most frequently occurring adverse reactions to drugs, with the incidence amongst hospitalized patient normally ranging from 1 to 3 per cent, although the frequency of cutaneous reactions to specific drugs may exceed 10 per cent. Anti-infectives and anticonvulsants are most commonly associated with adverse skin reactions. The varied nature of cutaneous reactions, even with specific drugs, indicates a multiplicity of mechanisms. Dividing cutaneous reactions into four mechanistically based categories has been proposed (Svensson *et al.*, 2001):

- immediate-type immune-mediated reactions;

- delayed-type immune-mediated reactions;

- photosensitivity reactions;

- autoimmune syndromes.

Important predisposing factors are viral infection and female gender. To account for the latter, gender differences in T-cell activation and proliferation have been proposed, as well as the increased prevalence of skin diseases, such as systemic lupus erythematosus and photosensitivity (Rademaker, 2001). Although it has been well established for many years that sulphonamide drugs produce delayed-type cutaneous reactions that severely limit their therapeutic utility, in spite of much research, the mechanisms involved remain unclear (Reilly and Ju, 2002).

Gender differences in the metabolism of xenobiotics in both humans and laboratory animals may provide an additional confounding factor in the toxicological evaluation of ADRs. Xenobiotic metabolism by male rats can reflect human metabolism when CYP1A or CYP2E are involved, because there is strong regulatory conservation of these isoforms between rodents and humans. Unfortunately, the identification of sex-dependent differences in metabolism by rats does not generally translate to humans. The major confounding factor is that CYP2C, a major subfamily in the rat, which is expressed in a sex-specific manner, is not found in humans. In addition, sex-specific isoforms of cytochrome P450 appear to be absent in humans, indicating that the commonly used male rat is unlikely to be an accurate model for the prediction of sex-related differences in metabolism in humans (Mugford and Kedderis, 1998).

Rare, but serious, ADRs associated with some carboxylic-acid-containing drugs have been investigated in a variety of toxicological studies. Drugs containing a carboxylic acid moiety can be bioactivated by two distinct pathways: by UGT-catalysed conjugation with glucuronic acid, resulting in the formation of acyl glucuronides, or by acyl-CoA synthetase-catalysed formation of acyl-CoA thioesters. Both metabolites are electrophilic species that, if they escape inactivation by glutathione, can acylate target proteins. Although there is accumulating evidence that acyl glucuronides can alter cellular function by a variety of mechanisms, including haptenation of peptides, glycation or acylation of specific proteins, and direct stimulation of neutrophils and macrophages, the roles of acyl-CoA are less clear (Boelsterli, 2002).

In summary, the underlying immunological and other mechanisms of idiosyncratic drug toxicity are poorly understood, which greatly hampers the development of suitable animal models. Each type of immunopathology is thought to result from a specific cluster of immunologic and biochemical phenomena, and other factors such as genetic predisposition, metabolic variability and concomitant diseases. It may thus be difficult to find common mechanisms that lead to nonclinical models able to predict specific types of systemic hypersensitivity reaction. However, there are already adequate models for detecting drugs that induce contact sensitization, and it may be possible to develop screening tests for signs indicative of a general hazard for immune-based reactions (Hastings, 2001). New technologies, such as toxicogenomics, proteomics and metabonomics, offer the potential to identify human toxicants during drug development (Steiner and Anderson, 2000; Castle *et al.*, 2002; Wilkins, 2002). Use of transgenic models, including mouse models that have been 'humanized' in various ways, e.g. by changing receptors that regulate cytochrome P450 enzymes, may be helpful in understanding mechanisms of toxicity involved in the causation of idiosyncratic ADRs (Wolf and Henderson, 1998; Rudmann and Durham, 1999; Xie and Evans, 2002). One approach may be to classify compounds in various ways, e.g. relating to reactivity/adduct formation, and to identify predictive markers for screening purposes (Uetrecht, 2000, 2001; Nelson, 2001). In respect of candidate drugs in the discovery phase, key questions (Baillie and Kassahun, 2001) might include:

- What level of covalent binding to proteins in liver (or other relevant target tissue) might be acceptable?

- Which protein targets are critical to the viability of the cell, and which are likely to be adducted by a specific reactive intermediate?

- Is there a dose threshold for toxicity, and what factors influence this?

- Is it possible to predict the human immunogenicity of potential drug–protein conjugates?

Sites of metabolic activation within a new drug candidate series have been rapidly identified by trapping the reactive intermediates formed on incubation with rat and human liver microsomes as their glutathione conjugates and mass-spectral characterization of these thiol adducts. A strategy of iterative structural modification of the chemical series in order to block bioactivation sites led to a significant reduction in the propensity to undergo metabolic activation, as evidenced by decreases in the irreversible binding of radioactivity to liver microsomal material on incubation of tritium-labelled compounds *in vitro* (Samuel *et al.*, 2003).

Proteomics might also be employed as a diagnostic tool for recognizing a drug signature in a tissue exhibiting an adverse response (Hellmond *et al.*, 2002). The development of these technologies in repsect of predicting or diagnosing ADRs is still at an early stage, and major breakthroughs seem unlikely in the short term.

Examples of toxicological investigation of adverse drug reactions

Many drugs that produce ADRs have been investigated using nonclinical models; each drug will have a particular aetiology and the nonclinical investigations are likely to be tailored to this. Two cases are described below in order to provide examples of typical approaches.

Hepatotoxicity of thiazolidinediones

Thiazolidinediones (TZDs), particularly troglitazone (Figure 3.2), when used in the treatment of type 2 diabetics, are associated with sporadic clinical hepatotoxicity not predicted by conventional animal studies. In isolated rat and human hepatocytes, multiprobe fluores-

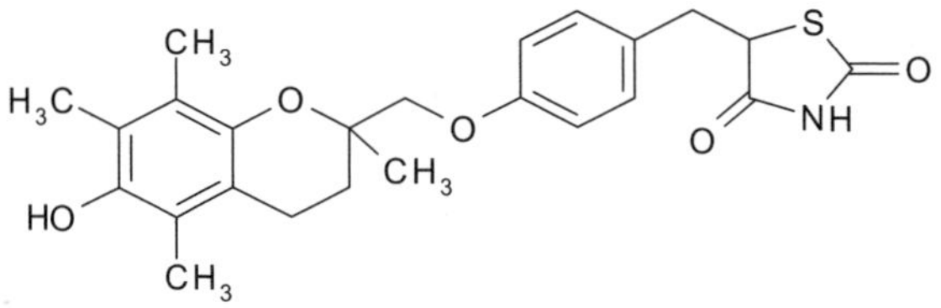

Figure 3.2 Structure of troglitazone

cence analysis showed disruption of mitochondrial activity as an initiating event followed by increased membrane permeability, calcium influx and nuclear condensation. Other effects included treatment-related hepatic enzyme leakage, decreased reductive metabolism and cytoplasmic ATP depletion. The relative potency of TZDs for causing these effects was: troglitazone > pioglitazone > rosiglitazone. The authors conclude that hepatic alterations *in vitro* are characteristic of TZDs, with only quantitative differences in subcellular organelle dysfunction (Haskins *et al.*, 2001).

Indinavir-induced hyperbilirubinemia

Up to 25 per cent of patients receiving indinavir (Figure 3.3) for the treatment of HIV infection develop unconjugated hyperbilirubinemia, prompting discontinuation of treatment in some patients.

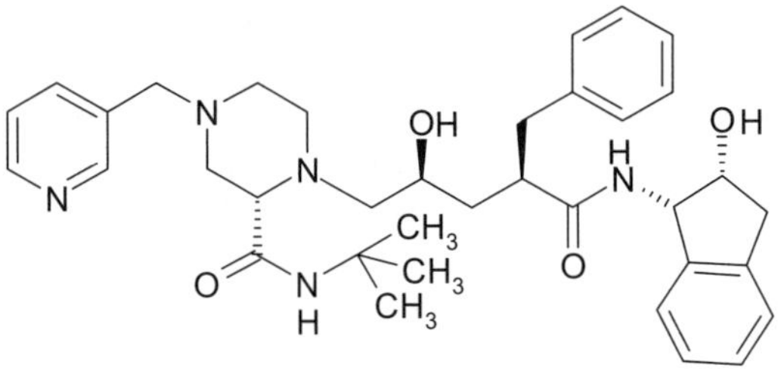

Figure 3.3 Structure of indinavir

The hypothesis that the side effect occurred by indinavir-mediated inhibition of bilirubin UGT was tested in two ways: (a) evaluation of patients with Gilbert's polymorphism (reduced hepatic UGT activity); (b) studies in the Gunn rat model of UGT deficiency. Serum bilirubin increased by a mean of 0.34 mg/dl in indinavir-treated patients lacking Gilbert's polymorphism versus 1.45 mg/dl in those who were heterozygous or homozygous for the mutant allele.

Indinavir competitively inhibits UGT activity ($K_i = 183\ \mu\text{M}$) and concomitantly induces hepatic bilirubin UGT mRNA and protein expression. Although saquinavir also competitively inhibits UGT activity, there is no association with hyperbilirubinemia, probably because of the higher K_i (360 μM) and the lower therapeutic plasma levels compared with indinavir.

Oral indinavir increased plasma bilirubin in wild-type and heterozygous Gunn rats, the mean rise being markedly greater in the latter group.

The findings of the various studies are considered to indicate that clinical hyperbilirubine-mia results from indinavir-mediated inhibition of bilirubin conjugation (Zucker *et al*., 2001).

Conclusions

Pharmacotoxicology has developed out of all recognition since the thalidomide tragedy (Dally, 1998); mandatory prelicensing nonclinical tests of largely standardized design perform a critical function in drug discovery and development. With careful study design, species selection, study performance and data interpretation, taking particular account of kinetic and metabolic differences between the animal models and man, the tests are generally highly predictive for most toxic responses encountered in clinical trials. A recent industry survey found that human gastrointestinal, cardiovascular and haematological toxicities were best predicted, whereas cutaneous effects were most difficult to detect in animal models.

Low-frequency ADRs of the type likely to be identified at the post-marketing stage after large numbers of patients have been exposed to a particular drug are, unsurprisingly, not well predicted by standard animal studies. The majority of these ADRs have been found to result from unanticipated pharmacodynamic and kinetic factors, and the mechanisms involved are often amenable to nonclinical investigation using *in vitro* and/or *in vivo* systems. On the other hand, a minority of ADRs are idiosyncratic and the processes leading to their causation are poorly understood. The formation of DRMs is thought to be involved; although this hypothesis is consistent with some of the evidence, a major anomaly is why *more* patients do not suffer such adverse reactions, since DRMs are thought to be produced by many drugs.

There is good evidence that most idiosyncratic ADRs have an immunological basis; the need for suitable animal models for mechanistic studies has been stressed by many investigators, but this may be difficult to achieve given the clinical variability in suscept-ibility, thought to be due to the genetic, metabolic and concomitant disease status of the individual patient. Use of genetically modified animals could lead to suitable models, and toxicogenomics and proteomics may also provide useful contributions. The process of screening new drug candidates for metabolic activation potential and introducing structural modifications in order to block bioactivation sites seems to show great potential for minimizing idiosyncratic ADRs. However, even with the benefit of these new technologies, developing reliable models for the prediction and evaluation of idiosyncratic ADRs possibly represents the greatest current challenge in pharmacotoxicology.

Acknowledgements

The valuable contribution of Dr C. J. Powell in terms of developing the outline for this chapter and reviewing an early draft is acknowledged. Thanks are also due to Professor A. D. Dayan for his most helpful comments.

References

Alaoui-Ismaili MH, Lomedico PT and Jindal S (2002). Chemical genomics: discovery of disease genes and drugs. *Drug Discov Today* 7: 292–294.

Alden CL (2000). Safety assessment for non-genotoxic rodent carcinogens: curves, low-dose extra-polations, and mechanisms in carcinogenesis. *Hum Exp Toxicol* **19**: 557–560.

Anonymous (2002). UK drug failure rate still high. *Scrip* no. 2751, 31 May, 4.

Atterwill C and Wing M (2000). *In vitro* preclinical lead optimization technologies (PLOTs) in pharmaceutical development. *Altern Lab Anim* **28**: 857–867.

Augen J (2002). The evolving role of information technology in the drug discovery process. *Drug Discov Today* **7**: 315–323.

Aviles P, Pateman A, Roman RS, Guillen MJ *et al.* (2001). Animal pharmacokinetics and interspecies scaling of sordarin derivatives following intravenous administration. *Antimicrob Agents Chemother* **45**: 2787–2792.

Bachmann K (1989). Predicting toxicokinetic parameters in humans from toxicokinetic data acquired from three small mammalian species. *J Appl Toxicol* **9**: 331–338.

Baillie TA and Kassahun K (2001). Biological reactive intermediates in drug discovery and develop-ment: a perspective from the pharmaceutical industry. *Adv Exp Med Biol* **500**: 45–51.

Ball P (2000). Safety of the new fluoroquinolones compared with ciprofloxacin. *J Chemother* **12** (Suppl 1): 8–11.

Beaune PH and Lecoeur S (1997). Immunotoxicology of the liver: adverse reaction to drugs. *J Hepatol* **26**(Suppl 2): 37–42.

Berry CL (1988). The no-effect level and optimal use of toxicity data. *Regul Toxicol Pharmacol* **8**: 385–388.

Bertino Jr J and Fish D (2000). The safety profile of the fluoroquinolones. *Clin Ther* **22**: 798–817.

Bide RW, Armour SJ and Yee E (2000). Allometric respiration/body mass data for animals to be used for estimates of inhalation toxicity to young adult humans. *J Appl Toxicol* **20**: 273–290.

Black LE, Green JD, Rener J, Dayan A *et al.* (2000). Safety evaluation of immunomodulatory biopharmaceuticals: can we improve the predictive value of preclinical studies? *Hum Exp Toxicol* **19**: 205–207.

Boelsterli UA (2002). Xenobiotic acyl glucuronides and acyl CoA thioesters as protein-reactive metabolites with the potential to cause idiosyncratic drug reactions. *Curr Drug Metab* **3**: 439–450.

Brand KP, Rhomberg L and Evans JS (1999). Estimating noncancer uncertainty factors: are ratios of NOAELs informative? *Risk Anal* **19**: 295–308.

Brecher RW (1997). Risk assessment. *Toxicol Pathol* **25**: 23–26.

Broadhead CL, Betton G, Combes R, Damment S *et al.* (2000). Prospects for reducing and refining the use of dogs in the regulatory toxicity testing of pharmaceuticals. *Hum Exp Toxicol* **19**: 440–447.

Bus JS and Reitz RH (1992). Dose-dependent metabolism and dose setting in chronic studies, *Toxicol Lett* **64–65**: 669–676.

Caldwell GW, Ritchie DM, Masucci JA, Hageman W *et al.* (2001). The new pre-preclinical paradigm: compound optimization in early and late phase drug discovery. *Curr Top Med Chem* **1**: 353–366.

Campbell DB (1996). Extrapolation from animals to man. The integration of pharmacokinetics and pharmacodynamics. *Ann N Y Acad Sci.* **801**: 116–135.

Castell JV (1998). Allergic hepatitis: a drug-mediated organ-specific immune reaction. *Clin Exp Allergy* **28**(Suppl 4): 13–19.

Castle AL, Carver MP and Mendrick DL (2002). Toxicogenomics: a new revolution in drug safety. *Drug Discov Today* **7**: 728–736.

Chappell WR and Mordenti J (1991). Extrapolation of toxicological and pharmacological data from animals to humans. *Advances in Drug Research* vol. 20, Testa B (ed.) Academic Press: 1–116.

CFR (2003). Code of Federal Regulations (USA), Part 58, Good Laboratory Practice for Nonclinical Laboratory Studies. http://www.access.gpo.gov/nara/cfr/waisidx_03/21cfr58_03.html [1 July 2003].

Clark DL, Andrews PA, Smith DD, DeGeorge JJ *et al.* (1999). Predictive value of preclinical toxicology studies for platinum anticancer drugs. *Clin Cancer Res* **5**: 1161–1167.

Cohen A (2002). New safe medicines faster . . . why does it still take so long and why isn't the pipeline bursting. *Eur J Pharm Sci.* **17S**: S23.

Cohen SD, Pumford NR, Khairallah EA, Boekelheide K *et al.* (1997). Selective covalent binding and target organ toxicity. *Toxicol Appl Pharmacol* **143**: 1–12.

Cook JC, Klinefelter GR, Hardisty JF, Sharpe RM *et al.* (1999). Rodent Leydig cell tumorigenesis: a review of the physiology, mechanisms, and relevance to humans. *Crit Rev Toxicol* **29**: 169–261.

Collins BJ, Grizzle TB and Dunnick JK (2000). Toxicokinetics of phenolphthalein in male and female rats and mice. *Toxicol Sci* **56**: 271–281.

Corrigan OP (2002). A risky business: the detection of adverse drug reactions in clinical trials and post-marketing exercises. *Soc Sci Med* **55**: 497–507.

CPMP Safety Working Party (2001). Concept paper on the development of a Committee for Proprietary Medicinal Products (CPMP) note for guidance on the need for preclinical testing of human pharmaceuticals in juvenile animals. www.emea.eu.int [1 July 2003].

Dahl AR, Schlesinger RB, Heck HD, Medinsky MA *et al.* (1991). Comparative dosimetry of inhaled materials: differences among animal species and extrapolation to man. *Fundam Appl Toxicol* **16**: 1–13.

Dahlem AM, Allerheiligen SR and Vodicnik MJ (1995). Concomitant toxicokinetics: techniques for and interpretation of exposure data obtained during the conduct of toxicology studies. *Toxicol Pathol* **23**: 170–178.

Dally A (1998). Thalidomide: was the tragedy preventable? *Lancet* **351**: 1197–1199.

Dansette PM, Bonierbale E, Minoletti C, Beaune PH *et al.* (1998). Drug-induced immunotoxicity. *Eur J Drug Metab Pharmacokinet* **23**: 443–451.

Dayan AD (1995). Safety evaluation of biological and biotechnology-derived medicines. *Toxicology* **105**: 59–68.

DeGeorge JJ, Ahn CH, Andrews PA, Brower ME *et al.* (1998), Regulatory considerations for preclinical development of anticancer drugs. *Cancer Chemother Pharmacol* **41**: 173–185.

De Matteis F, White IN and Smith LL (1998). Species differences in the metabolic activation of tamolifen into genotoxic derivatives: risk assessment in women. *Eur J Drug Metab Pharmacokinet* **23**: 425–428.

Dempster AM (2000). Nonclinical safety evaluation of biotechnologically derived pharmaceuticals. *Biotechnol Annu Rev* **5**: 221–258.

Den Otter W, Steerenberg PA and Van der Laan JW (2002). Testing therapeutic potency of anticancer drugs in animal studies: a commentary. *Regul Toxicol Pharmacol* **35**: 266–272.

Department of Health (2000). *The GLP Pocket-Book: The Good Laboratory Practice Regulations 1999 and Guide to UK GLP Regulations*. MCA Publications.

Descotes J, Ravel G and Ruat C (2002). Vaccines: predicting the risk of allergy and autoimmunity. *Toxicology* **174**: 45–51.

Dieckhaus CM, Thompson CD, Roller SG and Macdonald TL (2002). Mechanisms of idiosyncratic drug reactions: the case of felbamate. *Chem Biol Interact* **142**: 99–117.

Dixit R (2000). Applications and limitations of developmental toxicokinetic studies: mechanistic vs. risk assessment. *Teratology* **61**: 468–475.

Dorato MA and Vodicnik MJ (2001). The toxicological assessment of pharmaceutical and biotechnology products. In *Principles and Methods of Toxicology*, fourth edition, edited by Wallace Hayes A. Taylor and Francis: Philadelphia.

European Commission (1999). A Guideline on Summary of Product Characteristics. http://dg3.eudra.org/f2/eudralex/vol-2/C/SPCGuidRev0-Dec99.pdf [1 July 2003].

Feron VJ, van Bladeren PJ and Hermus RJ (1990). A viewpoint on the extrapolation of toxicological data from animals to man. *Food Chem Toxicol* **28**: 783–788.

Galluppi GR, Rogge MC, Roskos LK, Lesko LJ (2001). Integration of pharmacokinetic and pharmacodynamic studies in the discovery, development, and review of protein therapeutic agents. *Clin Pharmacol Ther* **69**: 387–399.

Garattini S (1985). Toxic effects of chemicals: difficulties in extrapolating data from animals to man. *Crit Rev Toxicol* **16**: 1–29.

Garattini S and Bertele V (2002). Efficacy, safety and cost of new anticancer drugs. *Br Med J* **325**: 269–271.

Gaylor DW (1983). The use of safety factors for controlling risk. *J Toxicol Environ Health* **11**: 329–336.

Green JD and Black LE (2000). Overview status of preclinical safety assessment for immunomodulatory pharmaceuticals. *Hum Exp Toxicol* **19**: 208–212.

Griffiths SA and Lumley CE (1998). Non-clinical safety studies for biotechnology-derived pharmaceuticals: conclusions from an international workshop. *Hum Exp Toxicol* **17**: 63–83.

Harries M and Smith I (2002). The development and use of trastuzumab (Herceptin). *Endocr Relat Cancer* **9**: 75–85.

Haskins JR, Rowse P, Rahbari R and de la Iglesia FA (2001). Thiazolidinedione toxicity to isolated hepatocytes revealed by coherent multiprobe fluorescence microscopy and correlated with multiparameter flow cytometry of peripheral leukocytes. *Arch Toxicol* **75**: 425–438.

Hastings KL (2001). Pre-clinical methods for detecting the hypersensitivity potential of pharmaceuticals: regulatory considerations. *Toxicology* **158**: 85–89.

Hawkins R (1993). Good laboratory practice. In *Experimental Toxicology – The Basic Issues*, Anderson D and Conning DM (eds). Royal Society of Chemistry.

Hellmold H, Nilsson CB, Schuppe-Koistinen I, Kenne K *et al.* (2002). Identification of end-points relevant to detection of potentially adverse drug reactions. *Toxicol Lett* **127**: 239–243.

Hengstler JG, van der Burg B, Steinburg P and Oesch F (1999). Interspecies differences in cancer susceptibility and toxicity. *Drug Metab Rev* **31**: 917–970.

Hess DA and Rieder MJ (1997). The role of reactive drug metabolites in immune-mediated adverse drug reactions. *Ann Phamacother* **31**: 1378–1387.

Home Office (2001). Animals (Scientific Procedures) Inspectorate. www.homeoffice.gov.uk/ [1 July 2003].

Honma W, Kamiyama Y, Yoshinari K, Sasano H *et al.* (2001). Enzymatic characterization and interspecies differences of phenol sulfotransferases, ST1A forms. *Drug Metab Dispos* **29**: 274–281.

House of Lords (2002). Report by the Select Committee on Animals in Scientific Procedures. www.parliament.the-stationery-office.co.uk/pa/ld/ldanimal.htm [1 July 2003].

Jaeschke H, Gores GJ, Cederbaum AI, Hinson JA *et al.* (2002). Mechanisms of hepatotoxicity. *Toxicol Sci* **65**: 166–176.

Johnson DE and Wolfgang GH (2001). Assessing the potential toxicity of new pharmaceuticals. *Curr Top Med Chem* **1**: 233–245.

Johnson DE, Ochieng J and Evans SL (1995). The growth inhibitory properties of a dopamine agonist (SKF 38393) on MCF-7 cells. *Anticancer Drugs* **6**: 471–474.

Johnson DE, Blower Jr PE, Myatt GJ and Wolfgang GH (2001). Chem-tox informatics: data mining using a medicinal chemistry building block approach. *Curr Opin Drug Discov Devel* **4**: 92–101.

Jones R (2002). Early candidate selection – have we progressed? *Eur J Pharm Sci* **17S**: S22–23.

Ju C and Uetrecht JP (2002). Mechanism of idiosyncratic drug reactions: reactive metabolite formation, protein binding and the regulation of the immune system. *Curr Drug Metab* **3**: 367–377.

Kapetanovic IM, Torchin CD, Strong JM, Yonekawa WD *et al.* (2002). Reactivity of atropaldehyde, a felbamate metabolite in human liver tissue *in vitro*. *Chem Biol Interact* **142**: 119–134.

Keefe DL (2002). Trastuzumab-associated cardiotoxicity. *Cancer* **95**: 1592–1600.

Knowles SR, Uetrecht J and Shear NH (2000). Idiosyncratic drug reactions: the reactive metabolite syndromes. *Lancet* **356**: 1587–1591.

Könemann WH (1990). Foreword. In *Good Laboratory and Clinical Practices*, Carson PA and Dent NJ (eds). Heinemann Newnes.

Lave T, Coassolo P and Reigner B (1999). Prediction of hepatic metabolic clearance based on interspecies allometric scaling techniques and *in vitro–in vivo* correlations. *Clin Pharmacokinet* **36**: 211–231.

Lee PN (1993). Statistics. In *Experimental Toxicology – The Basic Issues*, Anderson D and Conning DM (eds). Royal Society of Chemistry.

Leisenring W and Ryan L (1992). Statistical properties of the NOAEL. *Regul Toxicol Pharmacol* **15**: 161–171.

Lesko LJ, Rowland M, Peck CC and Blaschke TF (2000). Optimizing the science of drug development: opportunities for better candidate selection and accelerated evaluation in humans. *J Clin Pharmacol* **40**: 803–814.

Li AP (2002). A review of the common properties of drugs with idiosyncratic hepatotoxicity and the 'multiple determinant hypothesis' for the manifestation of idiosyncratic drug toxicity. *Chem Biol Interact* **26**: 7–23.

Ligibel JA and Winer EP (2002). Trastuzumab/chemotherapy combinations in metastatic breast cancer. *Semin Oncol* **29**: 38–43.

Lin JH (1998). Applications and limitations of interspecies scaling and *in vitro* extrapolation in pharmacokinetics. *Drug Metab Dispos* **26**: 1202–1212.

Lu AY (1998). Drug-metabolism research challenges in the new millennium: individual variability in drug therapy and drug safety. *Drug Metab Dispos* **26**: 1217–1222.

Mahmood I (1998). Interspecies scaling of renally secreted drugs. *Life Sci* **63**: 2365–2371.

Mahmood I (1999a). Prediction, clearance, volume of distribution and half-life by allometric scaling and by use of plasma concentrations predicted from pharmacokinetic constants: a comparative study. *J Pharm Pharmacol* **51**: 905–910.

Mahmood I (1999b). Allometric issues in drug development. *J Pharm Sci* **88**: 1101–1106.

Mahmood I (2000a). Can absolute oral bioavailability in humans be predicted from animals? A comparison of allometry and different indirect methods. *Drug Metabol Drug Interact* **16**: 143–155.

Mahmood I (2000b). Interspecies scaling: role of protein binding in the prediction of clearance from animals to humans. *J Clin Pharmacol* **40**: 1439–1446.

Mahmood I (2001a). Interspecies scaling: is a priori knowledge of cytochrome P450 isozymes involved in drug metabolism helpful in prediction of clearance in humans from animal data? *Drug Metabol Drug Interact* **18**: 135–147.

Mahmood I (2001b). Interspecies scaling of maximum tolerated dose of anticancer drugs: relevance to starting dose for phase 1 clinical trials. *Am J Ther* **8**: 109–116.

Mahmood I (2001c). Interspecies scaling of inhalational anesthetic potency minimum alveolar concentration (MAC): application of a correction factor for the prediction of MAC in humans. *Am J Ther* **8**: 237–241.

Mahmood I (2002). Interspecies scaling: predicting oral clearance in humans. *Am J Ther* **9**: 35–42.

Mahmood I and Balian JD (1999). The pharmacokinetic principles behind scaling from preclinical results to phase 1 protocols. *Clin Pharmacokinet* **36**: 1–11.

Mahmood I and Sahajwalla C (2002). Interspecies scaling of biliary excreted drugs. *J Pharm Sci* **91**: 1908–1914.

Meulenbelt J, Mensinga TT, Kortboyer JM, Speijers GJ et al. (1998). Healthy volunteer studies in toxicology. *Toxicol Lett* **102–103**: 35–39.

Meyer UA (2000). Pharmacogenetics and adverse drug reactions. *Lancet* **356**: 1667–1671.

Molderings GJ, Bonisch H, Bruss M, Likungu J et al. (2000). Species-specific pharmacological properties of human alpha(2A)-adrenoceptors. *Hypertension* **36**: 405–410.

Mordenti J, Chen SA, Moore JA, Ferraiolo BL et al. (1992). Interspecies scaling of clearance and volume of distribution for five therapeutic proteins. *Pharm Res* **8**: 1351–1359.

Morgan DG, Kelvin AS, Kinter LB, Fish CJ et al. (1994). The application of toxicokinetic data to dosage selection in toxicology studies. *Toxicol Path* **22**: 112–123.

Morton DM (1998). Importance of species selection in drug toxicity testing. *Toxicol Lett* **102–103**: 545–550.

Mugford CA and Kedderis, GL (1998). Sex-dependent metabolism of xenobiotics. *Drug Metab Rev* **30**: 441–498.

Naisbitt DJ, Gordon SF, Pirmohamed M and Park BK (2000). Immunological principles of adverse drug reactions: the initiation and propagation of immune responses elicited by drug treatment. *Drug Saf* **23**: 483–507.

Naisbitt DJ, Williams DP, Pirmohamed M, Kitteringham NR *et al.* (2001). Reactive metabolites and their role in drug reactions. *Curr Opin Allergy Clin Immunol* **1**: 317–325.

Nelson SD (2001). Structure toxicity relationships – how useful are they in predicting toxicities of new drugs? *Adv Exp Med Biol* **500**: 33–43.

Newman LM, Johnson EM and Staples RE (1993). Assessment of the effectiveness of animal developmental toxicity testing for human safety. *Reprod Toxicol* **7**: 359–390.

Oesch F, Doehmer J, Friedberg T, Glatt HR *et al.* (1990). Toxicological implications of enzymatic control of reactive metabolites. *Hum Exp Toxicol* **9**: 171–177.

Olejniczak K, Gunzel P and Bass R (2001). Preclinical testing strategies. *Drug Inf J* **35**: 321–336.

Olson H, Betton G, Robinson D, Thomas K, *et al.* (2000). Concordance of the toxicity of pharmaceuticals in humans and animals. *Regul Toxicol Pharmacol* **32**: 55–67.

Owens RC and Ambrose PG (2002). Torsades de pointes associated with fluoroquinolones. *Pharmacotherapy* **22**: 6663–6668.

Page E, Assouline D, Brun O, Coeffic D *et al.* (2002). Cardiac dysfunction in clinical trials of trastuzumab. *J Clin Oncol* **20**: 4119–4120.

Park BK, Kitteringham NR, Powell H and Pirmohamed M (2000). Advances in molecular toxicology – towards understanding idiosyncratic drug toxicity. *Toxicology*: **153**: 39–60.

Park BK, Naisbitt DJ, Gordon SF, Kitteringham NR *et al.* (2001). Metabolic activation in drug allergies (2001). *Toxicology* **158**: 11–23.

Parkinson C, Thomas KE and Lumley CE (1996). The timing of preclinical toxicological studies: pharmaceutical company approaches to toxicity testing in support of initial clinical investigations. *Regul Toxicol Pharmacol* **23**: 162–172.

Petersen KU (2002). From toxic precursors to safe drugs. Mechanisms and relevance of idiosyncratic drug reactions. *Arzneimittelforschung* **52**: 423–429.

Peters-Volleberg GWM, De Waal EJ and van der Laan JW (1994). Interspecies extrapolation in safety evaluation of human medicines in the Netherlands (1990–1992): practical considerations. *Regul Toxicol Pharmacol* **20**: 148–258.

Pilling AM (1999). The role of the toxicologic pathologist in the preclinical safety evaluation of biotechnology-derived pharmaceuticals. *Toxicol Pathol* **27**: 678–688.

Prahalada S, Tarantal AF, Harris GS, Ellsworth KP, Clarke AP, Skiles GL, MacKenzie KI, Kruk LF, Ablin DS, Cukierski MA, Peter CP, vanZwieten MJ, Hendrickx AG (1997), 'Effects of finasteride, a type 2 5-alpha reductase inhibitor, on fetal development in the rhesus monkey' (*Macaca mulatta*), *Teratology* **55**, 119–131.

Rademaker M (2001). Do women have more adverse drug reactions? *Am J Clin Dermatol* **2**: 340–351.

Reigner BG and Blesch KS (2002). Estimating the starting dose for entry into humans: principles and practice. *Eur J Clin Pharmacol* **57**: 835–845.

Reilly TP and Ju C (2002). Mechanistic perspectives on sulfonamide-induced cutaneous drug reactions. *Curr Opin Allerg Clin Immunol* **2**: 307–315.

Ring J and Brockow K (2002). Adverse drug reactions: mechanisms and assessment. *Eur Surg Res* **34**: 170–175.

Ritschel WA, Vachharajani NN, Johnson RD and Hussain AS (1992). The allometric approach for interspecies scaling of pharmacokinetic parameters. *Comp Biochem Physiol C Pharmacol Toxicol Endocrinol* **103**: 249–253.

Rodricks JV, Gaylor DW and Turnbull D (2001). Quantitative extrapolations in toxicology. In *Principles and Methods of Toxicology* fourth edition, Wallace Hayes A, (ed). Taylor and Francis: Philadelphia.

Rudmann DG and Durham SK (1999). Utilization of genetically altered animals in the pharmaceutical industry. *Toxicol Pathol* **27**: 111–114.

Ruelius HW (1987). Extrapolations from animals to man: predictions, pitfalls and perspectives. *Xenobiotica* **17**: 255–265.

Samuel K, Yin W, Stearns RA, Tang YS *et al.* (2003). Addressing the metabolic activation potential of new leads in drug discovery: a case study using ion trap mass spectrometry and tritium labeling techniques. *J Mass Spectrom* **38**: 211–221.

Schmid EF, James K and Smith DA (2001). The impact of technological advances on drug discovery today. *Drug Inf J* **35**: 41–45.

Schwartz S (2001). Providing toxicokinetic support for reproductive toxicology studies in pharmaceutical development. *Arch Toxicol* **75**: 381–387.

Serabian MA and Pilaro AM (1999). Safety assessment of biotechnology-derived pharmaceuticals: ICH and beyond. *Toxicol Pathol* **27**: 27–31.

Silva Lima B and van der Laan JW (2000). Mechanisms of nongenotoxic carcinogenesis and assessment of the human hazard. *Regul Toxicol Pharmacol* **32**: 135–143.

Smith D, Trennery P, Farningham D and Klapwijk J (2001). The selection of marmoset monkeys (*Callithrix jacchus*) in pharmaceutical toxicology. *Lab Anim* **35**: 117–130.

Smith KS, Smith PL, Heady TN, Trugman JM *et al.* (2003). *In vitro* metabolism of tolcapone to reactive intermediates: relevance to tolcapone liver toxicity. *Chem Res Toxicol* **16**: 123–128.

Soars MG, Riley RJ, Findlay KA, Coffey MJ *et al.* 2001). Evidence for significant differences in microsomal drug glucuronidation by canine and human liver and kidney. *Drug Metab Dispos* **29**: 121–126.

Sorkness CA (1997). The use of 5-lipoxygenase inhibitors and leukotriene receptor antagonists in the treatment of chronic asthma. *Pharmacotherapy* **17**: 50S–54S.

Spurling NW and Carey PF (1992). Dose selection for toxicity studies: a protocol for determining the maximum repeatable dose. *Hum Exp Toxicol* **11**: 449–457.

Steiner S and Anderson NL (2000). Pharmaceutical proteomics. *Ann N Y Acad Sci* **919**: 48–51.

Suwa T, Nysaka A, Peckham JC, Hailey JR, *et al.* (2001). A retrospective analysis of background lesions and tissue accountability for male accessory sex organs in Fischer-344 rats. *Toxicol Pathol* **29**: 467–478.

Svensson CK, Cowen EW and Gaspari AA (2001). Cutaneous drug reactions. *Pharmacol Rev* **53**: 357–379.

Swenberg JA (1995). Bioassay design and MTD setting: old methods and new approaches. *Regul Toxicol Pharmacol* **21**: 44–51.

Tabacova SA and Kimmel CA (2001). Enalapril: pharmacokinetic/dynamic inferences for comparative developmental toxicity. A review. *Reprod Toxicol* **15**: 467–478.

Terrell TG and Green JD (1993). Comparative pathology of recombinant murine interferon-gamma in mice and recombinant human interferon-gamma in cynomolgus monkeys. *Int Rev Exp Pathol B* **34**: 73–101.

Terrell TG and Green JD (1994). Issues with biotechnology products in toxicologic pathology. *Toxicol Path* **22**: 187–193.

Tham YL, Verani MS and Chang J (2002). Reversible and irreversible cardiac dysfunction associated with trastuzumab in breast cancer. *Breast Cancer Res Treat* **74**: 131–134.

Törnell J and Snaith M (2002). Transgenic systems in drug discovery: from target identification to humanized mice. *Drug Discov Today* **7**: 461–470.

Travis CC (1991). Interspecies extrapolation in risk analysis. *Ann 1ˢᵗ Super Sanita* **27**: 581–593.

Travis CC and White RK (1988). Interspecies scaling of toxicity data. *Risk Anal* **8**: 119–125.

Uetrecht JP (1997). Current trends in drug-induced autoimmunity. *Toxicology* **119**: 37–43.

Uetrecht JP (2000). Is it possible to more accurately predict which drug candidates will cause idiosyncratic drug reactions? *Curr Drug Metab* **1**: 133–141.

Uetrecht JP (2001). Prediction of a new drug's potential to cause idiosyncratic reactions. *Curr Opin Drug Discov Dev* **4**: 55–59.

Uetrecht JP (2002). N-oxidation of drugs associated with idiosyncratic drug reactions. *Drug Metab Rev* **34**: 651–665.

Vahle JL, Sato M, Long GG, Young JK *et al.* (2002). Skeletal changes in rats given daily subcutaneous injections of recombinant human parathyroid hormone (1–34) for 2 years and relevance to human safety. *Toxicol Pathol* **30**: 312–321

Valler MJ (2002). HTS and uHTS: strategies for success. *Eur Pharm Rev* (1): 23–30.

Van Dongen M, Weigelt J, Uppenberg J, Schultz J *et al.* (2002). Structure-based screening and design in drug discovery. *Drug Discov Today* **7**: 471–478.

Van Gelder J, Shafiee M, De Clercq E, Penninckx F *et al.* (2000). Species-dependent and site-specific intestinal metabolism of ester prodrugs. *Int J Pharm* **205**: 93–100.

Verdier F (2002). Non-clinical vaccine safety assessment. *Toxicology* **174**: 37–43.

Vocci F and Farber T (1988). Extrapolation of animal toxicity data to man. *Regul Toxicol Pharmacol* **8**: 389–398.

Voisin EM, Ruthsatz M, Collins JM and Hoyle PC (1990). Extrapolation of animal toxicity data to humans: interspecies comparisons in drug development. *Regul Toxicol Pharmacol* **12**: 107–116.

Walker R (1998). Toxicity testing and derivation of the ADI. *Food Addit Contam* **15** (Suppl): 11–16.

Ware JA, Graf ML, Martin BM, Lustberg LR *et al.* (1998). Immunochemical detection and identification of protein adducts of diclofenac in the small intestine of rats: possible role in allergic reactions. *Chem Res Toxicol* **11**: 164–171.

Warrington JS, Von Moltke LL, Shader RI and Greenblatt DJ (2002). *In vitro* biotransformation of sildenafil (Viagra) in the male rat: the role of CYP2C11. *Drug Metab Dispos* **30**: 655–657.

White IN, Carthew P, Davies R, Styles J *et al.* (2001). Short-term dosing of alpha-hydroxytamoxifen results in DNA damage but does not lead to liver tumours in female Wistar/Han rats. *Carcinogenesis* **22**: 553–557.

Wilkins MR (2002). What do we want from proteomics in the detection and avoidance of adverse drug reactions? *Toxicol Lett* **127**: 245–249.

Williams DP and Naisbitt DJ (2002). Toxicophores: groups and metabolic routes associated with increased safety risk. *Curr Opin Drug Discov Dev* **5**: 104–115.

Williams GM (1997). Safety assessment of pharmaceuticals: examples of inadequate assessments and a mechanistic approach to assuring adequate assessment. *Toxicol Path* **25**: 32–38.

Wolf CR and Henderson CJ (1998). Use of transgenic animals in understanding molecular mechanisms of toxicity. *J Pharm Pharmacol* **50**: 567–574.

Xie W and Evans RM (2002). Pharmaceutical use of mouse models humanized for the xenobiotic receptor. *Drug Discov Today* **7**: 509–515.

Yokoro K, Nakamo M, Ito A, Nagao K *et al.* (1977). Role of prolactin in rat mammary carcingenesis: detection of carcinogenicity of low-dose carcinogens and of persisting dormant cancer cells. *J Natl Cancer Inst* **58**: 1777–1783.

Zbinden G (1991). Predictive value of animal studies in toxicology. *Regul Toxicol Pharmacol* **14**: 167–177.

Zbinden G (1993). The concept of multispecies testing in industrial toxicology. *Regul Toxicol Pharmacol* **17**: 85–94.

Zucker SD, Qin X, Rouster SD, Yu F *et al.* (2001). Mechanism of indinavir-induced hyperbilirubinemia. *Proc Nat Acad Sci USA* **98**: 12 671–12 676.

4

Clinical Trials: – Collection of Safety Data and Establishing the Adverse Drug Reaction Profile

J. Talbot and M. D. B. Stephens

Introduction

All clinical trials should have a safety component as a primary or secondary objective. In early Phase I and Phase II trials, safety and tolerability are often a primary objective and the main reason for conducting the study. In later Phase II and Phase III trials the primary objective is usually efficacy, but safety and tolerability must also be included as a secondary objective.

Safety data from clinical trials can be broadly divided into the following three types, although these can overlap:

- adverse events (AEs)

- laboratory safety data

- vital signs and physical findings.

Safety monitoring in clinical trials can be considered as non-specific, i.e. general safety monitoring, or specific, i.e. looking for particular safety issues based on animal data, pharmacology or experience with other similar drugs or from earlier trials; see below.

Clinical trials have some general safety goals:

- To detect and characterize common adverse drug reactions (ADRs), usually type A.

- To determine tolerability in volunteers or patients, i.e. how is the ADR tolerated, does it resolve or improve on repeated dosing, is it so unpleasant that the subject has to stop treatment or can they put up with it?

- To identify any predisposing or risk factors for particular ADRs.

Stephens' Detection of New Adverse Drug Reactions Fifth Edition edited by John Talbot and Patrick Waller
© 2004 John Wiley & Sons, Ltd   ISBN: 0 470 84552 X

In studies where a range of doses is used and in studies with a pharmacokinetic component, an additional safety goal will also be to determine the relationship between ADRs and dose or plasma concentrations of the drug.

The nature and frequency of the safety monitoring used in a trial will depend on experience with the drug and the type of study being conducted. In early Phase I safety and tolerability studies in volunteers, there will be extensive and frequent monitoring (electro-cardiogram (ECG), blood pressure, etc.), blood sampling and questioning of the subjects. In large Phase III trials, standard questions and routine laboratory screens at appropriate time intervals are typically used. In some Phase IV studies, only certain clinical outcomes, e.g. death, hospitalization or a clinical event such as stroke, may be collected. This chapter will focus mainly on AEs. Laboratory safety data are dealt with in Chapter 5.

Adverse Events

The term AE was defined by Finney (1965) as 'a particular untoward happening experienced by a patient, undesirable either generally or in the context of his disease'. AEs are not necessarily recognized drug reactions and a causal relationship to treatment is not implied, as in the term ADR. Thus, all ADRs are AEs but only some AEs are ADRs.

The concept of collecting AEs rather than ADRs was adopted after the failure of clinical trials to detect severe skin and eye problems with practolol. Skegg and Doll (1977) proposed that the value of clinical trials in detecting unwanted effects of new medicines would be enhanced if doctors recorded all AEs experienced by subjects, not just those regarded as adverse reactions to drugs. All events should be reported to the centre coordinating the trial and analysed in treated subjects and controls. This is the basis for how AE monitoring in clinical studies is conducted today. Events should be treatment-emergent. This can be defined as an event that was not present before the start of treatment and became apparent after treatment began, or an event that was present before the start of treatment but worsened after treatment began. In controlled studies, the profile of AEs in the different treatment groups can be compared; see Figure 4.1.

This simple example, taken from either a single parallel group, placebo controlled trial or pooled data from a number of such trials, shows only ten different AEs. In reality, there will be many more different AEs, maybe hundreds, which then need to be grouped by system organ class and preferred terms; see Chapter 12. Figure 4.1 shows that patients on both drug and placebo experience AEs, with the placebo group giving the background nature and frequency of AEs in the patient population. Some AEs are more frequent on drug; in this example, rash and diarrhoea are significantly more frequent. This serves to flag these AEs for closer scrutiny as possible ADRs, and common clinical characteristics, similar time to onset, etc. would strengthen their association. However, with such multiple comparisons, some AEs will be significantly more frequent by chance, e.g. if the frequencies for 100 different AEs were compared, five would be significantly different at $p = 0.05$ by chance; see below and also Chapter 6.

Furthermore, if an AE is not more frequent in the group receiving drug, then this does not exclude individual cases of the AE being drug induced. It could simply be an ADR of low frequency; this is often seen with serious events such as hepatitis or agranulocytosis, where the numbers in a trial are likely to be very small and not statistically significant.

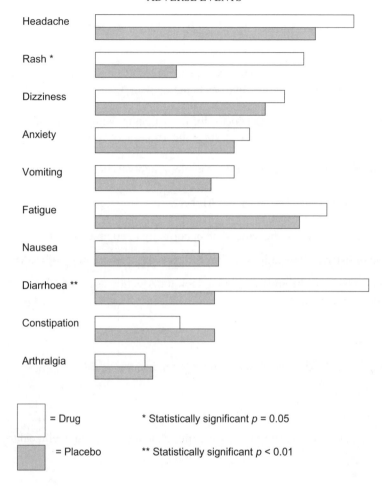

Figure 4.1   An example of an AE profile – drug versus placebo

Factors affecting collection of adverse events

In order to collect AEs efficiently it is necessary to know which factors might hinder their collection so that they can be circumvented. Between the occurrence of an AE and its final assessment the AE must be communicated. Factors preventing this communication include failure of the patient to recognize the AE or to communicate it to the clinical investigator and failure of the investigator to recognize or report it. The patient may fail to recognize the AE because:

- There are no symptoms (i.e. biochemical change, hypertension, etc.).
- There is a change in mood, *which* is only recognized by relatives or friends.
- There is a lack of intelligence or mental illness.

The patient may fail to communicate the AE to the investigator because:

- The patient does not associate the AE with the drug and, therefore, does not consider it to be relevant.

- The patient recognizes the event as a possible ADR (e.g. from the patient consent information), but presumes that one has to put up with it.

- The patient does not inform the doctor for fear of being thought neurotic or because the doctor inhibits the patient by tone of voice, interruptions or poor bedside manner.

- The patient has a poor memory or there are long intervals between patient visits.

The investigator may fail to recognize the AE because:

- The doctor does not give the patient the opportunity to communicate the AE.

- The doctor listens to the patient, but fails to consider the possibility of an AE.

- The doctor fails to take positive steps to look for AEs (i.e. does not ask questions and/or examine patient adequately).

The investigator recognizes the AE but does not report it because of:

- Complacency, thinking that it is too minor to report.

- Fear of litigation.

- Guilt at causing the patient to suffer.

- Ignorance of the mechanism of reporting (this should not happen in clinical trials).

- Lethargy – too busy.

Filtration of adverse events using protocols and case report forms

Bearing in mind the factors that can prevent the reporting of an AE to the pharmaceutical company or trial coordinator, steps can be taken to overcome them by using the study protocol and case report forms (CRFs) for collecting data in addition to the explanation by the study monitor. The wording of the protocol and the form design need to be appropriate to the indication and the stage in the drug's development.

Collection of adverse events

A specific illness does not preclude patients from experiencing many of the same AEs as a healthy person, in addition to those due to their illness. Should details of all AEs be collected? This will depend upon several factors:

- The indication for the drug. If the drug is given for a minor illness, then even very mild AEs may be relevant. If the drug is given for a disease that leads to death, such as secondary cancer or AIDS, then minor discomforts are less relevant.

- The stage or phase of the clinical trial programme. Details of minor symptoms are relevant for Phase I studies, but once an ADR has been characterized then counting the numbers of AEs may suffice.

- The type of potential ADR. Standardized enquiry is often needed for psychiatric studies, and laboratory tests are necessary for some drug-induced diseases.

- It is important that the clinical investigator makes a diagnosis wherever possible, rather than just listing signs and symptoms. When the diagnosis is in the form of a syndrome, such as an organ failure, the cause should be recorded by the investigator whenever possible (e.g. left-sided cardiac failure due to hypertension (Nickas, 1995)).

- A signal of a possible ADR halfway through a clinical trial programme may require changes to the methods of collecting data.

- AE collection during a clinical trial programme does not need to be standardized throughout the programme, but it must be consistent. The addition of a questionnaire to one study should not interfere with the analysis as long as the other standard methods of collection are included. Different questionnaires for a single drug programme should only be used if the drug programme is for two separate indications.

During treatment

The basic principle is to collect AEs that have appeared whilst the patient is on treatment and in the immediate period after stopping treatment, as well as any AE that was present at baseline but has since become worse on treatment. These are sometimes called 'treatment-emergent signs and symptoms' (TESS). A recent history of any AE immediately before the study may influence the assessment if it (or a related event) then occurs on treatment.

It is usual practice for companies to collect AEs with specifically designed company forms, and Astra was one of the pioneers in this area (Wallander and Palmer, 1986); however, they discovered that a substantial number of AEs were recorded not on the special form, but elsewhere in the CRF (73.7 per cent were on the correct form, 26.3 per cent were found elsewhere). In older studies, the percentage found elsewhere was 33–36 per cent, whereas for studies starting in 1986 the figure was only 13 per cent. Moreover, in the older studies, those found elsewhere were often serious events: 42 per cent compared with 26 per cent on the correct form. This ratio subsequently reversed, so that by 1989 no serious AEs and only 14 per cent of non-serious AEs were not on the correct form. Drug safety staff should hence ensure that the whole of the CRF is checked for AEs and that there is a good CRF design, instructions and investigator training (Wallander et al., 1992).

If a checklist or questionnaire is going to be used then it needs to cover the same time interval on each occasion, and since minor events are soon forgotten then the interval should generally not be longer than 2 weeks. Wallander et al. (1991) found that a questionnaire revealed events primarily from the preceding week, despite asking about the previous month. This means that there should be a baseline question, questionnaire or checklist that covers the previous 1 or 2 weeks followed by the same question, questionnaire or checklist 1 or 2 weeks later. This allows easy recognition of increased frequency of headaches for example. The subsequent intervals between visits should preferably be the same; but this is not always practical or essential, since it is possible to compare the events occurring with the trial drug and comparator over the same period. If the study is for longer than 4 weeks then it is preferable to have at least two visits while on the drug (one in the middle of treatment and another on the last day of treatment) and a post-treatment visit. In a long study, weekly questionnaires may overburden the patient and their enthusiasm to complete them might diminish. The only way to circumvent this problem might be to use the questionnaire to highlight crucial points (e.g. the week before adding the study medication and the week after, so as to pick up the most common type A ADRs).

The post-treatment visit

Spilker (1984) considers that the main purpose of the post-treatment visit is to check for any withdrawal effects and to ensure the patient's safety, but says that they may also be used to study residual effects of treatment. He lists five factors that should govern whether or not a post-treatment period is needed:

- previous experience with the drug in similar patient populations;
- whether the drug dosage is being tapered slowly or stopped abruptly;
- the clinical status of the patient;
- whether patients are in a secure and/or controlled environment;
- the pharmacokinetic characteristics of the drug.

Friedman *et al.* (1985) described two types of post-study follow-up. The first was a short-term follow-up, which should be considered when 'intervention' is stopped at the previous visit in order to find out how soon the laboratory values or symptomatology return to baseline. The second type was a long-term follow-up, monitoring possible toxicity or benefit.

The guidelines of the Fogarty Conference (Davidson *et al.*, 1979) for the detection of hepatotoxicity recommend that, in early clinical trials of new drugs (Phase II), laboratory tests should be performed at 24 h, 5–7 days and 4–6 weeks after the last dose. In short-term studies (less than 6 months) the follow-up should be for 2 months and that following long-term studies (6 months or more) should be for 2 years, and 20 years in a small subset of patients. These recommendations are obviously intended to detect adverse reactions with a very delayed onset, such as fibrosis, cirrhosis, vascular lesions or neoplasms.

A routine post-treatment visit that includes examination and a routine laboratory screen is essential for all pre-marketing studies for the reasons outlined below:

- *To review the laboratory data from the samples taken at the last visit whilst on treatment.* The results of a laboratory test will take time to reach the investigator. If of clinical significance then it needs to be followed up until it is normal or a cause is found, since it may represent an ADR, a new disease, or a complication of an underlying disease. If it is abnormal, but of no clinical significance, then it may be an early sign of an ADR, a new disease or complication of an old disease, or a chance variation from normal. A repeated individual test value is unlikely to be abnormal by chance. Clinical enquiry and, if necessary, examination and further tests may resolve whether or not the abnormality is due to the drug or disease.

- *To detect any delayed ADR*. A rare type B ADR may not appear until after a drug has been stopped, e.g. jaundice or aplastic anaemia. The fialuridine disaster, in which 5 of 15 patients with chronic hepatitis B died from drug-induced hepatotoxicity, developed 9–13 weeks after treatment (McKenzie *et al.*, 1995).

- *To detect any signs or symptoms due to drug withdrawal or a rebound phenomenon*. It is important to show that drugs used in psychiatric disease are not followed by drug withdrawal symptoms similar to those with benzodiazepines (Busto *et al.*, 1986). Any rebound phenomena usually occur during the first week after stopping treatment, e.g. beta blocker rebound.

- *To ascertain the response of AEs to dechallenge*. The response to dechallenge is an important factor in the assessment of an AE occurring whilst on treatment.

Disadvantages of a post-treatment visit   The visit is an additional inconvenience for both the patient and the investigator and an additional cost to the patient and the pharmaceutical company. These are counterbalanced by the assurance that no lasting harm has been caused to the patient. However, if a chronic disease requires replacement of the trial drug by another treatment, then this latter treatment may cause an ADR by itself and it may be difficult to distinguish between a delayed ADR due to the trial drug and that caused by the replacement treatment. This problem could be overcome by replacement with a well-established drug with known side effects.

A more frequent problem occurs when the AE itself is treated, thereby confounding the response to dechallenge; this should only occur rarely, since most ADRs reverse rapidly when treatment is stopped. Any complications or sequelae of the underlying disease may be difficult to differentiate from a delayed ADR. These can be countered, as there should be an equal incidence in the control group.

The reasons for the post-treatment visit dictate the duration of the follow up period.

The results of the laboratory tests must be available at the time of the visit and sufficient time must be given for AEs to reverse and for any withdrawal symptoms and any rebound phenomena to manifest themselves. These events should have occurred within 1 week; a delayed ADR may take longer, and a 2 week interval is probably reasonable. However, cholestatic hepatitis may appear up to 5 weeks later, as in the case of co-amoxiclav. A visit at 1 month may be more reasonable.

When the study has a crossover design, the intermediary washout period should act as a post-treatment period following the first drug and be equal in duration to the post-treatment observation periods following the second drug (Stephens, 1988).

It is also reasonable to recommend a routine post-treatment visit following post-marketing clinical trials for subgroups of patients who may be prone to ADRs, such as the young, the elderly and those with organ failure. There may also be hypotheses arising from animal work or from clinical experience with similar drugs that will require long-term follow up for specific purposes. Long-term follow up to ensure that no serious ADRs, such as aplastic anaemia or a fialuridine-type problem, have occurred (i.e. at about 9 months) might be done by regular telephone interviews with the patient and/or GP.

Conclusion   The increased protection for the patient, the additional information obtained for assessment of any AEs and better knowledge of the safety of a drug that should result from routine post-treatment visits make them essential. They may need to be repeated under certain circumstances.

Post-study serious adverse events

AEs occurring after the final visit (usually the post-treatment visit) should not be actively sought or collected unless long-term follow up is indicated; see below. However, on occasions, investigators report deaths and other serious AEs that have occurred weeks or months after the study. It is important to establish why they have been reported, particularly serious AEs not due to underlying disease. Is there a possibility of a delayed drug effect or did the investigator misunderstand their responsibilities for reporting? When received, such post-study serious AEs will usually be entered onto the drug safety database but probably not onto the clinical study database. They are not usually included in the statistical analysis of the study but may be added as an addendum to the clinical study report (CSR) and, if appropriate, discussed in the safety section of the CSR.

Long-term follow up

For some drugs it may be appropriate to undertake long-term safety monitoring and follow-up of outcomes after patients have completed treatment. This has been done with some immuno-modulatory drugs such as tumour necrosis factor (TNF) antagonists, where there are concerns regarding infections, particularly tuberculosis, cancers, etc. (Klareskog *et al.*, 2001). Such a long-term follow up will either require a special protocol or an extension to the existing protocol and informed consent. Contact with the patient can be made by post, telephone or Internet and validated by the original investigator or the patient's GP. A control group is essential, preferably patients who have been randomly assigned to a comparator or placebo in the original study.

Separation of adverse drug reactions from placebo reactions

Since adverse symptoms not caused by drugs are common (Reidenberg and Lowenthal, 1968) and are not easily separated from drug-induced symptoms, both must be collected for analysis if a profile of ADRs is to be made. However, this technique can only be used in controlled studies, ideally with placebo. In principle, the frequency of ADRs may be estimated by subtraction of the number of patients affected by a particular AE in the placebo group from the number affected in the active drug group as follows (Lasagna, 1984):

$$\text{Drug group} - \text{Placebo group} = \text{Number of ADRs}$$

However, this is an oversimplification because:

- The difference may have arisen by chance.

- Having established that there is a significant difference between the two treatment groups for the number of events and the number of patients afflicted, the severity of the ADRs in the two groups should then be compared.

- The difference may be due to bias (see below), e.g. because of inadequate blinding.

A further problem is classification. Some terms may include more than one type of abnormality. For example, the incidence of 'blurred vision' may be equal in both groups; but there may be several cases of tunnel vision with the trial drug, but because there is no code for tunnel vision it is coded under a more general term. Another problem is that the symptoms forming a syndrome are often reported and coded separately; individually, there may be no difference between two treatments, but when the cases are examined there may be a combination of symptoms with one drug that warrant being called a syndrome. It is essential, therefore, essential to know the individual original description of the AEs before making a judgement. This area has been explored more fully by Bernheim (1994), and he has added bias to the equation:

$$\text{Attributable AEs} = \text{Drug group AEs} - \text{Placebo group AEs} \pm \text{Bias}$$

Bias is equal to the B (baseline frequency) and severity of the AE, multiplied by pharmacological clinical activity of the drug A_D, minus the pharmacological clinical activity of the placebo A_P:

$$\text{Bias} = B(A_D - A_P)$$

ADRs that are similar to common non-drug AEs are rarely described or investigated sufficiently for a causal relationship for each individual event to be established. If they cannot be distinguished qualitatively, then the correct quantitative procedure is to compare them using non-parametric statistics, giving the confidence limits for the incidences of ADRs. Small studies ($n < 30$) have little chance of separating ADRs from placebo or non-drug events unless they are very common and specific to the drug (Simpson et al., 1980). The situation can be worsened in volunteers receiving placebo who have a tendency to 'catch' AEs from the active drug group, therefore changing a relatively specific ADR to a non-specific event.

Methods for collecting symptomatic adverse events

Collection of all AEs or symptoms should only be done if:

- it is possible to compare the AEs of one group with those of another, since the 'background noise' of the non-drug symptoms can overwhelm the drug-induced symptoms in uncontrolled studies;

- they can be collected at the beginning and end of the study as a minimum.

Methods for collecting adverse events

- diary card,
- questionnaire,
- checklist,
- standard question.

The patient can be prompted to report all adverse symptoms if the investigator uses a diary card, a patient questionnaire or a checklist with a standard question. Since the majority of ADRs occur within the first week of drug treatment, the first visit should be within a week or so of starting treatment if all the minor events are to be collected. There is a steep fall-off in recollection of minor events, even in young intelligent volunteers, and this is likely to be greater with elderly sick patients.

Differences in reporting rates with different instruments

Studies with temafloxacin showed the following reporting rates (Norrby and Pernet, 1991):

- spontaneous reporting, 1.5–5.1 per cent

- standard question, 29–49 per cent

- studies using diary cards, 41.5 per cent

- studies not using diary cards, 23.5 per cent.

Patient diary cards

In trials where a patient diary card is used for recording patient information (e.g. daily peak flow rates in asthma trials) it can also be used for recording AEs. It is, in fact, the equivalent of answering a daily standard question or checklist. If sufficient space is allotted to the daily recording of any AEs in sufficient detail then the diary card is likely to be large. The large amount of unstructured data that is likely to be collected over any period longer than a few days would be difficult to manage. Daily recording of objective data with weekly recording of AEs makes the data easier to handle without the loss of important events.

In cancer studies, the known side effects due to chemotherapy vary from day to day and diary cards have been used very successfully. The Medical Research Council (MRC) Tuberculosis and Chest Diseases Unit, the Clinic of Oncology and the Radiotherapeutic Unit Daily Diary Card has three pages, one for each week (Fayers and Jones, 1983; Jones *et al.*, 1987); see also www.atsqol.org/ddc-mrc.asp.

The five standard questions asked each day relate to:

- sickness (vomiting)

- activity

- mood

- anxiety

- overall condition.

Each of these questions is given a range of five answers:

- Sickness – (i) none; (ii) poor appetite; (iii) felt sick but wasn't; (iv) sick once; (v) sick more than once.

- Activity – (i) normal work/housework; (ii) normal work, but with effort; (iii) reduced activity, but not confined to home; (iv) confined to home or hospital; (v) confined to bed.

- Mood – (i) very happy; (ii) happy; (iii) average; (iv) miserable; (v) very miserable.

- Anxiety – (i) very calm; (ii) calm; (iii) average; (iv) anxious; (v) very anxious.

- Overall condition – (i) very well; (ii) well; (iii) fair; (iv) poor; (v) very ill.

Many of the problems of a patient diary have been eliminated with the electronic patient diary (Donovan *et al.*, 1996), and it has been successfully used for rheumatology, urology, Parkinson's, psychiatry and pulmonary disease. It works like a daily questionnaire rather than a diary, since it does not need to allow free text entries. It can have a built-in alarm to remind the patient to fill it in. It has multiple-choice questions and a visual analogue scale (VAS) can be added. Electronic patient diaries have been found to be cost effective and do not present problems for elderly patients (Lundström, 1993). Symfo S. A., from Belgium, market hand-held electronic patient diaries for clinical trials and surveys Phases I to IV; see www.symfo.com.

Questionnaire or checklist?

Whereas diary cards generally collect the AEs experienced by the patient in an unstructured fashion on a daily basis, the questionnaire or checklist collects the AEs in a structured fashion so that valid statistical comparisons can be made between an active drug group and a control group. When the patient diary is limited to answering set questions it acts as a daily questionnaire. In many earlier papers the terms 'questionnaire' and 'checklist' have been used loosely to mean any question, whether delivered directly to the patient (self-answering questionnaire) or via a third person (i.e. doctor, nurse, social worker). The advantages and disadvantages of these two approaches are outlined in Tables 4.1 and 4.2.

There are advantages and disadvantages to using any form of multiple-question question-naire compared with the use of a single standard open question, such as 'Have you had any medical problems since your last visit?' The multiple-question questionnaire will collect symptoms present in normal healthy subjects in addition to those due to disease or drugs. A comparison between an open question and a 38-item checklist showed that 15 per cent of healthy persons had symptoms in the previous 3 days when the open question was used compared with 82 per cent when the checklist was used (Reidenberg and Lowenthal, 1968). The parallel figures for patients who had been ill or taken medication in the previous 3 days were 69 per cent for the open question and 87 per cent for the checklist. An open question tends to collect only the more severe symptoms, whereas the incidence of irrelevant complaints is higher with the multiple-question questionnaire.

The multiple-question questionnaire is likely to lead to the conclusion that the incidence of AEs with a given drug is higher than that resulting from placebo (Downing *et al.*, 1970); this is especially true for neurotic patients (Rickels and Downing, 1970; Lapierre, 1975) and with depressed patients, where 5–10 times more side effects will be listed with the multiple questionnaire than with the open question. Relevant side effects are more likely to be detected if a checklist is not used (Huskisson and Wojtulewski, 1974; Fisher *et al.*, 1987). Known side effects were recorded more frequently using active questioning, whereas unknown side effects were more likely to be described by spontaneous reports (Hagman *et al.*, 1977).

Table 4.1   Self-administered questionnaire

Advantages	Disadvantages
They can be given directly to the patient and returned to the organizer bypassing the investigator	Needs more organization and the costs to print, distribute, collect and analyse are greater
Questions involving sexual behaviour can be answered more frankly than by any other method	If the questionnaire bypasses the investigator then the patient may forget to report important AEs, forgetting that the investigator does not see the answers to the questionnaire
The involvement of the investigator can be minimal	Great care is needed in the wording of questions, since there is no interpretation by the investigator
Answers to very precise questions can be given and there is almost no limit to the number of questions posed	Tends to overestimate the real incidence of adverse events (Fisher *et al.*, 1987)
Confidentiality can be guaranteed by the use of the patient trial number	May suggest symptoms to patients
It is more likely to lead to the conclusion that the incidence of side effects resulting from a given drug is higher than that resulting from placebo	

Table 4.2   Checklist (questionnaire administered by a third party)

Advantages	Disadvantages
The actual words used to the patient can be tailored according to the patient's intelligence and background	Unless the person administering the checklist reads out the question to the patient then there will be individual variations in terminology, etc.; therefore, the resulting answers may not be comparable
	The number of questions is more limited, since it involves the administrator's time
	Questions involving sex may cause more embarrassment than with the self-administered questionnaire

These comments are not as contradictory as they may first appear if one relates the use of the open question and the multiple-question questionnaire to the phase of drug development. During Phases I and II, before the nature of the ADR profile is known, the open question is probably more appropriate. In large-scale Phase III and IV studies, however, where the relative incidence of common ADRs of the new drug can be compared with those of its main competitor, the multiple-question questionnaire is more likely to differentiate between the two.

Questionnaires

There are two types of questionnaire:

- A generic questionnaire that has been developed for use over a wide field, e.g. quality of life (QoL) questionnaires. Its disadvantage is that it needs to be very extensive if it is to cover the range of possible AEs. If it has a restricted number of questions then it must have an open question: 'Were there any other AEs?'

- A questionnaire designed specifically for a trial with particular drugs. Use of such a questionnaire is only advised for early randomized clinical trials when the new drug is similar to a standard drug, since a questionnaire designed to pick up the known ADRs of the standard drug may be inadequate for identifying the as yet unknown ADRs of the new drug. This may well bias the study in favour of the new drug, since the established ADRs of the standard treatment will be well represented in the questionnaire.

Designing a questionnaire   The 10 stages in this process are (Stone, 1993):

- decide what data you need
- select items for inclusion
- design individual questions
- compose wording
- design layout
- think about coding
- prepare first draft and pre-test
- pilot and evaluate
- perform survey.

Read (Stone, 1993) and (Charlton, 2000) before starting.

Quantification of symptoms

The two main methods for quantifying a symptom are:

- descriptive scales
- Visual Analogue Scales (VAS).

Descriptive scales (fixed interval scales or Likert scales)   Denis Likert first described a five-point scale in 1932. It uses graded descriptive terms:

- Absent or present (score 0 or 1). This is the method used by most questionnaires, but it may lack sensitivity when comparing two similar drugs in a relatively small trial.

- If present, is it mild, moderate or severe? (Score 2, 3, 4 respectively). Patients' understanding of the words mild, moderate and severe is likely to differ, so they should be defined.

- A five-point scale (e.g. very drowsy, slightly drowsy, normal, more alert, very alert) (Yuen *et al.*, 1985). The WHO handbook for reporting the results of cancer treatment has a five-grade scheme (0–4) for both clinical and laboratory AEs (WHO, 1979). Available at http://whqlibdoc.who.int/publications/.

- A seven-point scale (Jaeschke *et al.*, 1990):

  (i)   extremely short of breath

  (ii)   very short of breath

  (iii) quite a bit short of breath

  (iv)   moderately short of breath

  (v)   some shortness of breath

  (vi)   a little shortness of breath

  (vii) not at all short of breath.

- Another seven-point scale can be used for the frequency of the event (Guyatt *et al.*, 1987):

  (i)   all of the time

  (ii)   most of the time

  (iii) a good bit of the time

  (iv)   some of the time

  (v)   a little of the time

  (vi)   hardly any of the time

  (vii) none of the time.

- A further seven-point scale has been used with the SAFETEE general inquiry questionnaire. Patients were asked to rank each of the 76 possible symptoms on a scale of 1 to 7. The rankings were based upon the patients' willingness to exchange their current disease state for a situation where they would now be afflicted with that symptom. A rank of 1 would indicate a complete willingness to exchange and a rank of 7 would be an absolute refusal. Using weighted values for the SAFETEE symptoms obtained from the ranking procedure, an index was created to measure the impact of non-life-threatening AEs associated with drug therapy. This adverse drug effect index has been validated (Levine *et al.*, 1990).

- A 10-point scale (Lewis *et al.*, 1985a): the patient is asked to allocate a score between 1 and 10 for different symptoms.

Visual analogue scale   A VAS is shown in Figure 4.2. It is a 10 cm scale; it may be vertical or horizontal, with some practical advantage with the horizontal scale. There should not be any intermediate points (Aitken, 1969; Scot and Huskisson, 1976) that might cause clustering. However, there is always a tendency towards clustering at the extremes of the scale, at the midpoint and at 6.18 cm (Benjafield and Adams-Webber, 1976). It has been suggested that patients should see their previous scores when making serial assessments, but others disagree (Joyce *et al.*, 1975; Scott and Huskisson, 1979; Carlsson, 1983). Some 7 per cent of patients find the VAS difficult to understand despite instruction (Lewis, 1987; Jaeschke *et al.*, 1990) and it has been suggested that patients who score inaccurately for all symptoms should be screened out (Lewis *et al.*, 1985c).

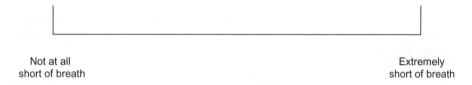

| Not at all | Extremely |
| short of breath | short of breath |

Figure 4.2   A visual analogue scale (VAS)

Grant *et al.* (1999) compared the reproducibility and sensitivity of a VAS, Borg scale (12 points) and a Likert scale (five points) in normal subjects. The VAS performed best in terms of reproducibility for breathlessness and general fatigue and in terms of sensitivity for breathlessness.

Drug effects were significantly more marked for volunteers who were not depressed compared with those who were depressed (Peat *et al.*, 1981). A VAS has been found to be more sensitive than a 10-point scoring system when used for testing beta adrenoceptor blockers (Lewis *et al.*, 1985c), a five-point scale or a standard question when used to measure sedation (Yuen *et al.*, 1985), a sleep and mood scale (Lundberg, 1980), and a four-point pain scale (Joyce *et al.*, 1975).

Errors can occur using a VAS, and Maxwell (1978) has suggested that it should be combined with either a four-point scale or a simple global assessment. In a VAS assessment of angina using 'No pain at all' and 'Pain as bad as I could ever bear', afterwards the patients were asked which of the following did they use: number of attacks, duration of attacks, severity of an individual attack or a combination of these; it was found that the patients' VAS scores correlated best with the severity of pain, which was considered ;the least clinically important variable. It is important, therefore, to take care in phrasing the question (Vandenburg, 1987). In multi-national studies it is also necessary to be aware of cultural differences, for instance in perception of pain, between countries. An alternative to using a scale is the use of a VAS meter, which gives an immediate reading without the need for subsequent measurement and produces a similar assessment to the conventional VAS (Hounslow *et al.*, 1987).

VASs have been used for:

• Pain (Huskisson, 1974; Joyce *et al.*, 1975; Scott and Huskisson, 1976; Carlsson, 1983; Vandenberg, 1987; McCormack *et al.*, 1988).

- Quality of sleep (Parrott and Hindmarsh, 1978).

- Dyspnoea (Jaeschke *et al.*, 1990).

- Subjective sensation of resistance to breathing (Aitken, 1969).

- Depression (Zealley and Aitken, 1969; McCormack *et al.*, 1988).

- Anxiety (McCormack *et al.*, 1988).

- Beta blocker side effects (Lewis *et al.*, 1984; Lewis *et al.*, 1985a,b; Lewis, 1987; Dimenäs *et al.*,1989).

- Quality of life (Jaeschke *et al.*, 1990).

Bulpitt and Fletcher (1990) did not use a VAS because of the difficulty in explaining the concept to many patients, the lack of data on validity and repeatability, and the difficulty in interpreting the results.

Conclusions   A VAS is best used as an efficacy assessment when the symptom is due to the underlying disease and the drug is likely to improve the symptom (i.e. a change in severity). In a large-scale placebo-controlled clinical trial using a questionnaire for AEs, there are disadvantages in having just absent or present (i.e. a tick in a box if present). It is only where the trial compares a new drug and the standard therapy under similar circumstances and where it is important to detect a difference that it is worth using a four-point scale. If a large-scale study is not possible and a limited questionnaire is used yet it is vital to discover whether the two treatments differ, then it is worth using a VAS, but probably only in a single-centre study with an enthusiastic investigator.

Questionnaire/checklist

A questionnaire can qualify a symptom by asking further questions about the type of sensation, location, duration, quality, etc., but if it aims to cover all body sensations then it will be prohibitively long. Questionnaires devised for one clinical trial may not be suitable in a different context and, therefore, the investigator needs to check whether:

- the questionnaire is acceptable to the study population;

- it is easily completed;

- it will produce responses consistent with those obtained in normal doctor–patient interviews;

- it is reproducible when administered on two separate occasions;

- it will be of value or use when completed (Lewis *et al.*, 1984).

Questionnaires are likely to identify milder symptoms than those volunteered spontaneously or in answer to a general question and will include body sensations experienced by normal subjects. This increases the background noise and may entail the use of larger groups if ADRs are to be distinguished (Borghi *et al.*, 1984).

Types of questionnaire   Questionnaires used in clinical trials can be divided into:

- Specific questionnaires designed for a specific trial(s) or for a specific drug where possible side effects are elicited by individual specific questions.

- Generic questionnaires, which can be divided into ADR questionnaires and QoL questionnaires.

The ADR questionnaires are designed to cover all reasonable ADRs. Rare ADRs are too specific and can occur in too many areas to be covered in a questionnaire of limited size. QoL questionnaires cover the physical state, emotional wellbeing, sexual and social functioning, and cognitive acuity of patients (Croog *et al.*, 1986). In general, an ADR questionnaire is used for identifying the AEs suffered by the patient, whereas the QoL assessment indicates how the adverse and beneficial events have affected the patient's general wellbeing.

Examples of such questionnaires are described in Chapter 5 of the fourth edition of this book. More recent examples include:

- a new instrument to assess drug safety (Sacristan *et al.*, 2001);

- standardizing assessment of adverse effects in rheumatology trials (Woodworth *et al.*, 2001);

- patient-based method of assessing AEs in rheumatology clinical trials (Welch *et al.*, 2001).

An early evaluation of side effects should take place at baseline and within 1–2 weeks of the start of a trial, since most ADRs are evident within that period. Possible long-term ADRs can be assessed using QoL 3 to 6 months later, when adaptation has occurred and placebo effects have worn off. The period covered by the questionnaire should be identical throughout the study. Where and how the questionnaire is completed is important; answering a questionnaire in the home setting may not have the same results as within the hospital environment. It is rarely possible to organize a prospective randomized study of an ADR, due to ethical problems, but it has been done with angiotensin converting enzyme (ACE) inhibitors and cough (Ramsay and Yeo, 1995; Tanser *et al.*, 2000).

Drawbacks of adverse drug reaction questionnaires   In all structured systems for the collection of AEs there is a tendency to lose information. A patient's graphic description of an event may help to separate the drug-induced event from naturally occurring events, but information can be lost on coding. In early studies the quality of the patient's description must be retained. Although in a structured system there should be space for additional description, there will inevitably be loss of descriptive information. There is a continuum from the individualized approach with a single event reported spontaneously to the counting of events in epidemiological surveys. There is a need to characterize the AEs in detail early in clinical development of a new drug until an accurate description is developed; thereafter they can be counted.

Standard/open question

This should be the standard method for all clinical trials and some of its characteristics have already been mentioned. An alternative approach is to record only 'spontaneously volunteered side effects'. When the list of factors that can prevent reporting of AEs is studied in relationship to this method, it can be seen that it has the following disadvantages compared with a standard question:

- The doctor may not give the patient the opportunity to mention an AE.

- If the doctor assessing the spontaneously volunteered AE judges that it was not due to the drug, then it may not be recorded.

The standard question should be unambiguous and worded in such a way that it is not mistaken for a social courtesy. Examples of standard questions from clinical studies include:

- 'Have you noticed any change in body function or had any physical complaints in the past week?' (Avery *et al.*, 1967). This was used in a study in America in hospitalized depressed patients. It very pointedly does not ask for any mental changes. The wording might not be so easily understood by other English-speaking patients.

- 'How are you feeling?', followed by 'How else are you feeling?', and finally by 'How does the drug make you feel?'. This was used in a study of neurotic outpatients in America (Downing *et al.*, 1970).

- 'Have you noticed any new symptoms which might be related to the treatment?' (Huskisson and Wojtulewski, 1974).

- 'Did you experience any unpleasant effects from the medicine you took?' (Lasagna, 1981).

- 'Any problems?' (New Zealand Hypertension Study Group, 1979).

- 'Has the treatment upset you in any way?' (Aitken, 1969).

- 'Have you noticed any symptoms since your last examination?' (Jackson, 1990a,b).

- 'Have you had any health problems since we last met?' (Wallander *et al.*, 1991).

Some of these imply that patients make decisions as to causality and will, therefore, vary in their interpretation of AEs. These examples should be avoided. Two alternative standard questions are:

- 'Have you had any medical problems since your last visit?' (Lapierre, 1975), or 'Have you had any problems since your last visit?', or 'Have you had any problems during the last week?'

- 'Have you felt different in any way since your last visit?'

The standard question is a suitable method for all clinical trials, being usable in addition to patient questionnaires or checklists, as well as independently. If the question is worded correctly then it should collect all drug-associated events, but not stimulate the production of too many non-drug-associated events. If the standard question is worded to collect all events defined by Finney (1965), then it includes non-medical events (i.e. social). The problem of dealing with large amounts of social data in clinical studies has not yet been solved in the drug trial context. Until methodology of collecting, recording and analysing social events has advanced and the pattern established, first for the healthy population and second for disease groups, then the definition of AEs should be restricted to medical events.

Sequence for collecting subjective adverse events

If all four methods of collecting subjective AEs (spontaneous, standard question, checklist and questionnaire) are to be used, then instinctively they should be used in this order. After a social greeting, the patient needs to be given the opportunity to mention any medical problem bothering them. Then the standard question should be asked and then, lastly, a checklist used. A questionnaire can be handed to the patient on leaving, so that it can be filled in either in the waiting room or at home. The alternative, which is usually used with QoL questionnaires, is to have the questionnaire filled in prior to the consultation on the grounds that the doctor/nurse cannot then influence its completion. This approach has the theoretical disadvantage that having mentioned their symptoms on the questionnaire they might think it unnecessary to repeat them to the investigator and, therefore, they will not be recorded on the CRF. However, the influence of a patient-completed symptom checklist on the subsequent reporting of AEs in a clinical trial interview was examined in a study of 128 patients receiving anti-epileptic medication. The patients were randomized to receive a 16-symptom checklist either before the clinician assessed the AEs or afterwards. The difference was small and not significant; the authors suggested that giving the checklist first does not affect subsequent reporting (Wagner *et al.*, 1994).

Investigator assessments

Having decided how collection of the AEs occurring in a clinical trial is to be done, a decision must be made as to whether one needs to collect the investigator's opinion about whether the AE was due to the drug. Where a questionnaire or a checklist has been used, a statistical assessment of the numbers of each type of AE with the trial drug and the comparator drug/placebo will be made and the investigator's opinion is not necessary. However, does one require an opinion on all spontaneous reports and those elicited by a standard question? The number of these AEs is likely to be relatively few and will probably be more severe than those elicited by questionnaire or checklist. The investigator knows more about the patients and their diseases, both past and present, and is frequently an expert in the latter. Although the investigator may be an expert in the disease under treatment, they may well not be expert in the area of the AE. Most general physicians have a good knowledge of common ADRs of drugs in general use, but physicians specialized in a branch of medicine frequently have knowledge on only a narrow range of drugs and diseases; however, their opinion may be invaluable if the AE comes within their speciality. One possibility is to collect the investigator's opinion in all studies except where data have been collected by a questionnaire or checklist. The investigator's opinion on all serious AEs is essential.

Choice of alternatives

Two categories include:

- Drug related or not drug related.

- P (possible or probable) or N (not assessable or unlikely) – used by the Swedish regulatory authority.

- Is there a reasonable possibility that the event may have been caused by the trial therapy? Yes or no?

Three categories include:

- Possible, probable or certain.

- Probably not, possible, probable.

- Improbable, possible, probable.

Four categories include:

- Unlikely, possible, probable, definite (Kramer and Hutchinson, 1984; Weber, 1984).

- General list – implies unlikely, possible, probable, certain (Mashford, 1984).

- Doubtful, possible, probable, definite (Naranjo *et al.*, 1980).

- Unlikely, possible, probable, almost certain (Stephens, 1984).

- Remote, possible, probable, highly probable (Turner, 1984; Ruskin, 1985).

Five categories include:

- Unrelated, doubtful possible, probable, almost definite, definite (Emanueli, 1984).

- Unrelated, unlikely, possible, probable, definite.

- Doubtful, coincidental, possible, probable, certain.

- Appears to be excluded, doubtful, possible, probable, very probable (French regulatory authority).

- Unrelated, conditional, possible, probable, almost definite, definite (Karch and Lasagna, 1977).

- Negative, coincidental, possible, probable, causative.

- Not related, remote, possible, probable, definite.

How many alternatives and which terms?

There are certain principles, as follows:

- The terms themselves should not require explanation or definition. Their lack of definition is an advantage.

- The investigator should not be forced into an either/or situation because of a lack of alternatives. In the clinical world there are all shades of opinion and the choices should cover the whole range.

- The more alternatives there are the narrower the use of each term becomes.

- Absolute terms, such as 'unrelated' and 'definitely not', can only be used in exceptional circumstances because they are almost impossible to prove and, therefore, should be avoided.

- No term has an absolute meaning and terms mean different things to different people. The very indistinct limits are suitable for an area where differences of opinion are extremely common and the data are very rarely reliable.

Decisions regarding collection of adverse events

Consider:

- Animal toxicology and pharmacology and potential type A effects or class effects.

- ADRs of other treatments for the same indication and possible control groups.

- The drug development plan – Phases I–IV. Consider which methods of collection would be suitable, whether translation into different languages will be necessary, and whether the results can be pooled if more than one method is being used.

- All studies should include the opportunity for spontaneous reporting and a standard question. If a diary card, checklist or questionnaire is added to these two standard methods, then have the implications been considered?

- Check with data management personnel for design of forms, coding, etc. Will the data be collected by more than one company, e.g. a clinical research organization (CRO)? If so, then problems of standardization and coordination increase.

- Does the method of collecting AEs suit the aim of the study?

- Can the method be simplified?

- Is the method consistent with methods used in the rest of the trial programme?

- Have all the essential staff involved in the study been approached?

Pre-marketing studies

The pre-marketing programme for the detection of new ADRs can be divided into:

- The general non-specific search for ADRs. This aims to detect all ADRs, not just those previously foreseen.

- The specific search for ADRs that may be foreseen for historical, toxicological, pharmacological or clinical reasons.

Non-specific monitoring

This is the search for ADRs that is undertaken for all drugs and excludes the specific search for particular ADRs that might be foreseen from previous information. An ADR may manifest itself either by subjective symptoms or objective findings, or a combination of both.

Subjective symptoms   The Phase I and early Phase II studies should aim to identify the minor AEs, which may be fairly common. If a particular AE is shown to be more common in the drug group than in the placebo group, then later studies can be planned with this in mind.

Most minor AEs are described inadequately by clinicians (e.g. 'headache'). However, if they are recognized early in the clinical trial programme, then a specific questionnaire or form can be designed to obtain a full description. If the minor AE has some special characteristics, then its relationship to the drug may be recognized and possibly the drug will not need to be stopped unnecessarily. The questionnaire or form must, therefore, try to identify the particular clinical characteristics of the event.

The background characteristics of the patients suffering the AE must be identified to see whether a susceptible subgroup can be identified as being more at risk (e.g. the elderly, those with renal failure). Further investigation of these patients may also indicate the mechanism of action.

Treating the AE often confounds the effect of stopping the drug, so that stopping should precede treatment whenever possible. Minor events are usually completely reversible on stopping the drug, but it is helpful if the speed of reversibility can be ascertained.

Objective findings   These are usually covered by standard laboratory investigations and the standard clinical investigations, but then are of special importance when considering the effect of the drug on the course of any chronic diseases that may be present in addition to the primary disease. In these circumstances, it is important to measure the effect of the drug on chronic disease and the parameters usually used for its diagnosis and prognosis.

Specific monitoring

Some ADRs may be predicted because of the known pharmacology of the drug, experience with drugs of the same class, animal toxicology, or previous use in humans. Their discovery will be a function of the number of patients studied and the investigations undertaken.

Phase I studies

The purpose of Phase I studies is to obtain information on:

- initial safety
- tolerability
- bioavailability
- pharmacokinetics
- drug metabolism
- drug interactions
- proof of principle.

Certain physiological parameters that measure the function of an organ with limited power of repair and regeneration are ideally evaluated in Phase I. These include the special senses and the central and peripheral nervous system (i.e. ophthalmological screen, audiometry, etc. (Goldberg *et al.*, 1975).

Volunteer studies uncover the following types of ADR:

- ADRs masked or modified in patients by disease or concomitant medication.

- ADRs likely to be induced by higher doses of study drug (i.e. in dose escalating studies).

- ADRs that are extensions of the pharmacological action of the drug.

- ADRs related to interaction between drug and common events in normal life, e.g. alcohol (Idänpään-Heikkilä, 1983).

Rarity of serious adverse drug reactions in volunteers

Serious ADRs are extremely rare in volunteers. In a survey in the USA there was only one drug-related sequel in one of 29 162 volunteers used over 12 years and only one clinically significant medical event occurring in every 26.3 years of an individual volunteer's participation (Zarafonetis *et al.*, 1978). However, in 1985 there were two deaths. The first occurred in Dublin, when, unbeknown to those in charge of the study, a volunteer had received a depot injection of flupenthixol the day before receiving an injection of trial drug. The volunteer had not revealed that he was under a psychiatric clinic (Darragh *et al.*, 1985). The second death occurred in Cardiff and was due to aplastic anaemia 9 months after taking part in the study of a new benzodiazepine. It was not possible to say whether the disease was due to the investigational drug (Anon., 1985). These two deaths resulted in a re-examination of the problems of research in healthy human volunteers.

More recently, a 24-year-old female research volunteer at Johns Hopkins University died of adult respiratory distress syndrome in 2001, following inhalation of hexamethonium used to block bronchial nerve ganglia in an asthma study. The Food and Drug Administration

(FDA) said that Johns Hopkins had not sought FDA approval to use an unlicenced drug and that they had failed to report a previous unanticipated ADR (persistent cough) in an earlier volunteer (Altman, 2001). The report of the internal investigation into this death has been published: www.hopkinsmedicine.org (report of internal investigation).

The Association of the British Pharmaceutical Industry (ABPI) published the results of a 1984 survey of its member companies on their experience in this area, including both in-house and external studies (Royle and Snell, 1986). The number of serious suspected reactions in in-house studies was five (0.27/1000 subjects exposed) and in external studies it was eight (0.91/1000). A reappraisal in 1986 from the USA cited a further death in a volunteer who had anorexia nervosa unbeknown to the investigator. The author of that paper, therefore, suggests that investigators ask themselves a series of questions prior to the study:

- Do some studies pay subjects so much that they are willing to give inaccurate histories?

- Are you so busy that you do not actually participate in screening subjects or in conducting the study?

- Is the study conducted in an environment and with appropriate medical supervision to respond to a medical emergency?

- Is the research question asked either trivial or predictable in outcome?

- Should the research question be asked in the population for which the drug is intended?

- Have you made adequate provision to cover medical expenses of the subject and liability expenses for yourself? (Powell, 1986).

A survey among members of the British Pharmacological Society in 1987 showed that 69 per cent of volunteers ($n = 8163$) had AEs. They were moderately severe in 0.55 per cent and these, in order of frequency, were postural hypotension, abdominal pain, nausea and vomiting, palpitations, bronchoconstriction, drowsiness and headache. There were three severe life-threatening effects; viz. anaphylaxis, perforated duodenal ulcer and a skin reaction, but all made a complete recovery. Orme *et al.* (1989) suggested that GPs should be given exclusions for studies and thereby prevent those who match an exclusion criterion from entering the study.

Another study from France in 430 volunteers had an overall incidence rate of 13.5 per cent, covering 69 different types of AE. Severe AEs accounted for only 0.36 per cent of AEs. A total of nine deaths and life-threatening AEs had been reported in clinical research up to 1992 (Sibille *et al.*, 1992). The same group have updated this study with 1015 volunteers. The incidence rate for AEs with active drugs was 13.7 per cent and for placebo it was 7.9 per cent (Sibille *et al.*, 1998).

The ABPI, in 1998, issued a booklet that summarizes the situation, *Medical Experiments in Non-patient Human Volunteers*. The Royal College of Physicians' report on research in healthy volunteers was published in 1986 (RCP, 1986).

Problems with including women in Phase I studies

It is not generally expected that reproductive toxicology studies will be completed before Phase II studies. Therefore, it is essential that adequate reproductive precautions are taken after counselling. Current reproductive toxicology information must be given to the participant. This should cover the risk of study participation, the importance of adequate contraception, lists of contraceptive choices with risk–benefit drug interactions, information on teratology and the need to avoid pregnancy during drug exposure (Johnson-Pratt and Bush, 1996).

The new drug must be shown not to be an enzyme-inducing agent, lest the volunteer/patient on oral contraceptives should become pregnant whilst on the new drug. If this is not possible, then the contraceptive pill cannot be relied on. Normal contraceptive failure rates are high; therefore, females of childbearing potential should have a pregnancy test and a test for recent occurrence of ovulation before and at appropriate intervals during and at the end of the study (Larson et al., 1982).

A survey of 28 clinical pharmacology units showed that whereas 79 per cent conducted clinical trials in women of childbearing potential only 86 per cent did pregnancy tests routinely at screening and immediately before the first dose and only 18 per cent did so at the post-study visit. Although 91 per cent specified that volunteers should be using a reliable form of contraceptive, only 9 per cent on the oral contraceptive were asked if they had missed any pills, and of those using other methods only 36 per cent were asked if they had used adequate contraception while in the study. The following recommendations were made:

- All female volunteers should have their menstrual history taken at screening.

- All post-menopausal females should have their hormone levels checked at screening.

- All women of childbearing potential should be tested for pregnancy at screening and this should be repeated at the beginning of each study session and again at the post-study visit (Higginbotham and Rolan, 1997).

Women in Phase I studies have 2.3 times the frequency of AEs as men, with a higher percentage due to laboratory abnormalities (males:females, 15 per cent: 26 per cent) (Vomvouras and Piergies, 1995). In addition, the presence of women suffering from premenstrual tension could increase the background noise in the control and trial drug groups, and if distributed unevenly between the two groups in controlled studies this could produce misleading ADR data. This can be dealt with by stratifying the randomization by sex.

Difference between adverse events in volunteers and patients

AEs occurring in healthy volunteers need to be considered separately from those occurring in patients for the following reasons:

- Due to absence of disease. The volunteer does not have the disease that the drug can correct. Therefore, there may be an exaggerated pharmacological reaction in volunteers that would not occur in patients or would occur to a lesser extent, thus producing either objective or subjective effects, e.g. hypertension.

- Some of the AEs in volunteers are due to the environment in which the studies are conducted, e.g. no caffeine, confinement.

- Due to incorrect dosage. The dosage used may be outside the subsequent recommended therapeutic range.

- Due to different age, intelligence and psychological make-up. Excluding the absence of disease, volunteers are likely to differ from patients who subsequently take the drug.

- Due to a different relationship with the investigator. The relationship between the volunteer and the person responsible may be that of a junior (the volunteer) to a senior investigator, and this could affect the reporting of AEs.

Because of these differences between patients and volunteers, it has been advocated that volunteer patients should be used more often (Oates, 1972; Weissman, 1981).

Screening

The screening of new volunteers before they participate in clinical studies is essential and will cover medical history of the volunteer, history of allergy, family medical history, smoking and drinking. Inclusion criteria will cover age, weight, fluency of literacy in relevant language, absence of significant physical abnormality, laboratory examination for hepatitis and for drugs of abuse plus the usual pre-study laboratory screen (clinical chemistry, haematology and urinalysis) (Jackson, 1990a,b), ECG, ophthalmological examination and chest X-ray. These are followed by exclusion criteria relating to abnormalities in the medical history, alcohol and current treatment, if any.

Drug abuse

Screening for drug abuse is essential. In the USA 7.7 per cent of volunteers used illicit drugs, 5.8 per cent cannabinoids, 3.6 per cent amphetamines, 1.2 per cent barbiturates, 1.1 per cent cocaine, 1.0 per cent opiates and 0.3 per cent benzodiazepines (De Vries et al., 1991). Screening for drugs of abuse would normally be carried out at least at the pre-study medical and randomly thereafter. They should cover morphine, amphetamines, cocaine, cannabis, benzodiazepines and barbiturates.

Electrocardiography

Normal values for ECGs in healthy volunteers have been published (Adamson et al., 1998). The value of 24 hour continuous ECG monitoring was shown in a paper from Simbec Research Ltd, where the use of a 24 hour Holter monitoring in 57 healthy male volunteers aged 18–46 revealed:

- sinus bradycardia in 53

- sinus tachycardia in 54

- sinus arrhythmia in 30

- ventricular ectopics in 25

- atrial premature beats in 43

- first-degree block in seven

- pause of more than 2 seconds in three

- second block in five

- atrial bigeminy in one

- two consecutive unifocal ventricular ectopics in two

- three consecutive unifocal ventricular ectopics in one

The authors recommend 24 hour ambulatory monitoring before drug treatment with new chemical entities (Barrington *et al.*, 1990).

Screening of 156 volunteers found that only 20 (13 per cent) had normal sinus rhythm throughout, 83 per cent had supraventricular ectopics, 11 per cent had ventricular ectopics, 2 per cent had unsustained ventricular tachycardia and 6.5 per cent had sinus pauses. One volunteer was in atrial fibrillation throughout. The authors also gave some guidelines for the management of ambulatory cardiac monitoring in volunteers (Stinson *et al.*, 1995).

QTc interval prolongation

Extension of the QTc interval on the ECG has been an issue of much debate in recent years following withdrawal of several non-cardiac drugs, e.g. terfenadine, astemizole, droperidol and cisapride, which caused QTc prolongation to such a degree that potentially life-threatening or fatal ventricular arrhythmias, e.g. torsades de pointes, may occur. These were either with the drugs alone or as a result of drug–drug interactions (De Ponti *et al.*, 2000). See also Chapter 2.

Phase I studies should be directed at the early identification of a change in repolarization, usually QT or QTc (corrected) prolongation. Important questions include (Haverkamp *et al.*, 2000):

- What electrocardiographic repolarization signal should be measured?

- What threshold QTc signal is of concern and what are the clinical implications of a small, yet statistically significant, QTc prolongation?

- Since QTc quantifies a complex relationship between the duration of ventricular repolarization and heart rate, what are the heart rate correction issues for drugs that slow or accelerate heart rate?

- Which heart rate correction is preferred, e.g. Bazett, Fredericia?

The European Committee for Proprietary Medicinal Products (CPMP) have published guidelines on monitoring of the QTc interval during early clinical studies (CPMP, 1997) as have the International Society for Holter and Non-invasive Electrocardiology (ISHNE),

October 2001 (http://www.ishne.org) and more recently the FDA (2002) have published a preliminary concept paper for discussion.

Malik and Camm (2001) have written an extensive review on this subject and its implications for drug approval and labelling.

Screening for viral infectivity

Taking a good medical and social history and clinical chemistry will detect potential volunteers in high risk groups, and many centres would routinely exclude such subjects from participating in clinical studies (Harry et al., 1995).

Serological tests for hepatitis B surface antigen (HBsAg) are required to exclude those with a positive test who may risk infecting others. Three volunteers had acute hepatitis B and another had positive serology following a trial where this screening was not done. One of the volunteers was a carrier who infected the others, probably via contamination of the gloves worn by the staff (Mehlman et al., 1994).

Screening for previous hepatitis C infection is also required prior to participation in Phase I clinical studies.

Although screening for hepatitis B and C is usual, there has been much more debate about screening routinely for HIV because of the perceived consequences for potential volunteers of a positive test (Thompson et al., 1993). It has been recommended that all volunteers should be tested (Sanchez et al., 1994; Vickers et al., 1994), but this policy has not been widely adopted. An academic unit reported that all of its 500 subjects tested negative for HIV1 and HIV2 antibodies, despite drawing 41.8 per cent of volunteers from South Africa (Jagathesan et al., 1995).

Because of the low rate of genuine positive results in the 'healthy volunteer' population the problem of false positive results is relatively greater than for patients.

Monitoring during the study

Phase I studies can be separated into two different categories:

- Studies that occur between first dose in man and the first patient studies.

- Studies that are carried out later in the programme in parallel with Phases II and III.

Studies that occur in parallel with Phases II and III contribute to the general AE profile but are usually carried out to address specific questions, such as the effect of renal impairment on pharmacokinetic profile. These studies are not considered further.

Phase I studies that occur prior to initiation of patient studies (hereafter described as 'early Phase I studies') have as their primary aim the establishment of the maximum tolerated single and multiple doses, and hence the likely therapeutic margin. The therapeutic margin is generated based on the maximum tolerated dose compared with the efficacious plasma concentrations or pharmacodynamic end-points. This will be vital information in determining whether a drug progresses beyond initial patient studies.

Safety end-points in early Phase I studies

Adverse event recording   In many ways, AE recording during early Phase I studies is the same as recording AEs at other stages of drug development. The same issue of the weakness of data in open studies applies, and early studies should be carried out as double-blind placebo-controlled studies. During dose escalation the AE profile and other safety parameters should be reviewed between each dose level and provision made for unblinding of the data if safety concerns arise.

A specific feature of the early Phase I studies is the lack of prior human experience with the drug. In contrast to the later studies, the only data on which to predict the AE profile are data from animals, which has limited predictivity; see Chapter 3. The main burden of data comes from toxicology studies, but an understanding of the pharmacology is also important. Furthermore, there needs to be an appreciation that certain AEs, e.g. nausea or dizziness, may be hard to detect in animals and may occur at lower doses than associated findings in animals, e.g. where only vomiting and gross unsteadiness are observable.

Vital signs and electrocardiogram recordings   These are a standard component of early Phase I studies. It is usual to make frequent recordings of vital signs, i.e. pulse and blood pressure, during early Phase I studies; the timing of such recordings is determined from an understanding of the predicted pharmacokinetic profile and a knowledge of the safety pharmacology studies, which will have documented the occurrence of changes in vital signs in animals at low multiples of the therapeutic dose. Often, the standing, as well as lying, blood pressure is recorded to look for postural changes. Vital signs may be expanded to include respiratory rate and/or temperature, depending on the observation in safety pharmacology studies and the known pharmacology of the compound being tested.

Likewise, ECG recording will often be frequent, depending on preclinical findings, and follow regulatory guidance (CPMP, 1997). Holter monitoring for 24 hours is recommended.

Safety bloods   It is usual for safety bloods to be taken during the screening process and to include full blood count, clinical chemistry and urinalysis before dosing and then at 24 and 48 or 72 hours after dosing.

Pharmacodynamic end-points   It may be appropriate to include safety assessments that evaluate predictable pharmacodynamic end-points, such as cognitive function testing after dosing a central nervous system (CNS) active compound. Increasingly, genomics, proteomics and metabonomics are being used to assess pharmacodynamic effects in early studies and these may, through advanced technology, be able to evaluate patterns of change across a range of assessed parameters.

Possible improvements in adverse event collection from volunteers   It is important that maximum use is made of the opportunity to collect AEs efficiently. This may be improved by:

- A list of specific symptoms, depending upon the pharmacology and toxicology – a VAS could be used (Jackson, 1990a,b). The use of a questionnaire so early in the clinical trial programme means that only predictable ADRs can be covered, unless a very exhaustive questionnaire is used. There is always the concern that new minor AEs may not be mentioned when a questionnaire is used. The relationship in a Phase I unit between staff and volunteers is usually such that minor AEs are mentioned with the use of a single standard question (Jackson, 1990a,b).

- Use of an anonymous questionnaire in controlled studies on possible sexual effects. The completed questionnaire, identified only by a number, can be placed in an envelope to be given to a person outside the unit, who also has the randomization code.

- The use of a follow-up question 24 hours after a single-dose study.

- The use of a standard question in all studies, i.e. 'Have you noticed any physical or mental changes during the study?'

- Rechallenge – the consideration of rechallenge using placebo and active drug in volunteers with non-serious type A symptoms only.

- An initial single-blind placebo period, which might reduce the number of placebo reactions whilst in the controlled part of the study. In a small study using an 'All Body Organs and Functions' (ABOF) questionnaire there were 13 AEs in the initial placebo period and nine during the controlled part of the study (Nony et al., 1994)

The Institute of Medicine in the USA has published a comprehensive report recommending better protection for participants in clinical research. The report, Responsible research: a systems approach to protecting research participants, is available at http://national-academies.org.

Phase II studies

The purpose of Phase II studies is to test whether the new drug is effective for one or more clinical indications and to determine doses for further study. These studies should only include patients with the target disease, and preferably those with no other concomitant disease. The number of patients involved is relatively small. These studies should detect the most frequent ADRs and may predict target organ systems for other ADRs to be found later in Phase III studies. They are seldom able to define any precise or comparative incidence of ADRs or discover ADRs that typically appear in a subgroup of patients (Idänpään-Heikkilä, 1983).

The monitoring of patients in Phase II studies is similar, whenever possible, to that used in Phase I studies. Where possible, there should be two laboratory examinations before starting treatment. The first should be 1–2 weeks before the study, so that the results are available before treatment is started and patients can be excluded if necessary. The second is immediately before treatment is taken on day one. Problems met in early clinical trials have been described in the CIOMS (1983) review of safety issues in early clinical trials of drugs:

- Collaboration between sponsor and investigator may be less interactive than is desirable.

- Potentially serious ADRs may be poorly documented and the relevant forms not completed properly.

- Patients who do not fulfil the selection criteria may be admitted to trials, making interpretation of potential AEs difficult.

- Pretreatment assessment is inadequate and incomplete and, therefore, it is difficult to interpret AEs occurring during treatment.

- Appropriate actions that are needed to evaluate a potential ADR properly are often not instituted.

- Treatment may be instituted before appropriate safety assessments have been taken or before the results have been received.

- Rechallenge after an AE may be undertaken without appropriate monitoring.

- Parochial attitudes may be adopted and the sponsoring organization and experts in the evaluation of ADRs may not be involved until very late.

- Occasionally, ADRs are published without adequate investigation and may lead to problems in determining the true situation.

- Often, there seems to be a lack of appreciation of the regulatory and legal implications of handling ADRs sensibly.

These can be overcome by the protocol and CRF clearly describing the exact procedures to be undertaken if there is an AE including a rigorous follow up procedure for withdrawals. This emphasizes the need for good and thorough protocol and CRF design and development.

A single serious AE in an early Phase II study may abort an entire new drug programme if sufficient information is not collected and a proper assessment is not made. Spilker (1984) covers the various safety parameters that can be measured in clinical studies covering laboratory tests, ophthalmological testing, psychological and performance tests in his guide to clinical studies and developing protocols.

The death of a clinical trial patient during the pre-marketing phase may be due to many reasons, but if due to the drug then it may be disproportionately catastrophic for the future of that compound. The steps to take in these circumstances are dealt with by Cato and Cached (1988).

Some ECG monitoring will continue in Phase II studies and maybe into Phase III to confirm safety in the target population with co-morbidities and concomitant medications. The nature and extent of this will be based on the type of drug and the ECG findings, including QTc prolongation, from Phase I; see above. ECGs should be statistically analysed and reported according to predefined standards; Steare and Morganroth (2002) advocate centralized ECG collection and analysis.

For chronic treatments there is a requirement to have treated at least 100 patients for 1 year before a marketing application. A survey of 27 drugs showed that only 4 per cent (25 serious AEs) of first occurrences appeared in the second 6 month period. Of these 25 ADRs there were 13 type A reactions; the ADRs in this context were AEs possibly, probably or definitely due to the drug (Brown *et al.*, 1996). It is sensible, therefore, to try to recruit patients from Phase II studies into long-term extension studies.

Phase III studies

The FDA comments concerning the pre-marketing programme and the resultant New Drug Application (NDA) (Temple, 1991a) were:

- Sponsors exclude patient populations deemed 'too sick' even when the drug is clearly going to be used in such populations.

- Some safety databases are not adequate enough to support the planned dose or the planned duration of use.

- Existing databases are not examined because doing so would require more time.

- Sometimes there is complete indifference to finding the right dose of the drug.

- There is a tendency to focus on the good effect of the drug and to forget that it may also have other less desirable effects that need study.

A subsequent review in 1995 of the 1993 cohort of new molecular entities approved by the FDA said that the FDA did not receive data analysed in the way it would like to have it. With 'nuisance' AEs there were seldom any subgroup summaries, by age, gender, race, or ethnicity, and analyses seldom accounted for the length of exposure or dose. If the AE limits the dose or causes discontinuation, then, although reported, it was seldom analysed statistically. There was also little assessment of the range of discomfort or the timing relative to the start of treatment or relative to the disease state.

With serious AEs there was usually no attempt to analyse them statistically and they were not discussed in relation to the patient's condition, demographics or pharmacokinetics. The time course of therapy and the AE were usually not examined systematically. As far as laboratory data were concerned, movements within the normal range were generally ignored (Fairweather, 1996).

In March 2003, the FDA published for comment a Concept Paper on pre-marketing risk assessment that focused on clinical development, particularly Phase III studies. The design of the trials programme is critical to ensure that sufficient safety data are generated to allow for product appproval, proper risk management and to inform post-marketing safety assessment. The size of the safety database supporting a new product depends on its novelty, the intended patient population, proposed indication and intended duration of use.

Ideally, programmes should include long-term controlled safety studies to allow for comparisons of event rates and for accurate attribution of AEs, particularly for detecting changes in rates of frequent events in the population and especially when the AE could be part of the disease being treated. The safety database in Phase III should include a diverse population, with only patients with obvious contraindications excluded. Broadening inclusion criteria could enable the findings to be more generalized to the population likely to receive the product post-marketing. Using a range of doses in Phase III trials would characterize better the relationship between exposure and the resulting clinical benefit and risk.

Potential interactions (drug–drug, drug–demographic, drug–disease, drug–food and drug–dietary supplement) should be addressed during controlled trials and specific safety studies. It is recommended that the potential for the following serious safety effects be assessed as part of all drug development programmes:

- QTc prolongation
- Liver toxicity
- Drug–drug interactions
- Polymorphic metabolism

Temporal associations between drug exposure and AEs are seen as critical to risk assessment, as they provide clues for determining whether the AE was related. Time-to-event analyses are appropriate for clinically important events that occur on a delayed basis and AEs that occur at initiation of treatment but diminish in frequency over time.

Patient subgroups

The summary of product characteristics (SPC) or product labelling will be primarily based on the results of the Phase III studies. The inclusion and exclusion criteria in Phase III protocols should, therefore, reflect the intended labelling for the new product. If all patients over 65 have been excluded from the pre-marketing trials then they should be excluded in the SPC. At least two specific subsets of patients will require specific monitoring:

- Elderly patients.

- Patients in whom disease will modify absorption, distribution, metabolism or excretion of the drug, though these tend to be the very patients who are excluded by the protocol in randomized clinical trials (Riegelman, 1984).

If the drug is intended for chronic usage, then a minimum of 100 patients should be followed up for 1 year. However, if a subgroup of 100 patients shows no serious AE, then how certain can one be that no serious ADR will occur in that subgroup in subsequent use?

The following simple rules calculate the risk for different size subgroups:

- Rule 1 – if none of n patients shows the AE then we can be 95 per cent confident that the chance of the event is at most 3 in n (i.e. $3/n$). The two corollaries for this rule are:

- Rule 2 – for the 99 per cent confidence interval the figure is 4.6 (i.e. $4.6/n$).

- Rule 3 – for the 99.5 per cent confidence interval the figure is 6.9.

The aptly entitled paper 'If nothing goes wrong is everything all right', which contains these rules, is worth reading (Hanley and Lippman-Hand, 1983). For any material change in risk discovery the increase in size of the denominator should be in the order of magnitudes (i.e. 1000, 10 000, 100 000, etc.).

Idänpään-Heikkilä (1983) said that Phase III studies lasting 2 weeks or less uncover the most frequent and the acute ADRs, but that for ADRs with longer latent intervals these trials need to be extended to 3 months. There will still be some important ADRs that will only be detected in studies lasting 6 months. All long-term studies are dogged with increasing numbers of withdrawals, and the protocol must make sufficient provision for a determined effort to establish their fate. The diminishing numbers can give a false impression of the incidence of ADRs with a long latent period, and life table analysis should be used to cope with this situation (O'Neill, 1988). The advantages put forward for the method are:

- It permits estimation of the cumulative ADR rate over a specific time interval.

- It handles losses from observation adequately.

- It allows determination of whether a time-specific ADR is occurring at a constant, decreasing or increasing rate.

- It may allow combining safety data from more than one clinical trial. Severe and easily recognized ADRs will be as easily detected in uncontrolled as in controlled studies (Idänpään-Heikkilä, 1983).

Controlled trials

Protocol

The protocol needs to consider all aspects of the clinical trial and it is useful to use a checklist to make certain that all the essentials have been considered. The following are the questions concerning ADRs that should be considered when writing the protocol. A safety monitoring evaluation plan should be in place before the start of any clinical trial.

Aim

- Do the aims of the study accurately describe the purpose of the trial as far as ADRs are concerned?

- Can estimates of the expected incidence of death and serious AEs in the study population, based on the disease and/or concomitant medications used to treat the disease, be provided?

- Any death or serious AEs that exceed these estimates would presume a drug relatedness and require notification of the regulatory authorities; remember fialuridine (Nickas, 1997).

Patient selection

Does the selection of patients bias the study as far as ADRs are concerned?

- Have patients who have previously had one of the trial drugs been excluded? If not, how will they be dealt with? There is more likely to be a problem in comparative controlled trials in chronic diseases where the alternatives are the new drug and the standard therapy. A patient who has already had the standard therapy without any problem is very unlikely to have an ADR in the study, whereas the patient who had developed an ADR while previously on the standard therapy will be excluded from the study. The statistical analysis of the trial results can weight the effect of previously having the standard against not having had it. Exclusion of these patients from the study could have an adverse effect on trial recruitment. The CRF must, therefore, have a space with the questions 'Has the patient ever had any of the trial medications? If so, with what result?' In hospitals there has been inadequate history of ADRs taken (Cook and Ferner, 1993; Shenfield *et al.*, 2001).

- Has the background noise been reduced to a reasonable level?

- Does the choice of investigator or hospital bias the selection of patients as far as type, severity or resistance to treatment of the target illness?

- If the target illness is chronic, then will the clinical features and relevant laboratory investigations be shown to be stable before the study?

- Are the inclusion and exclusion criteria at the right level so that the trial results can be extrapolated to a reasonable population of patients on the drug (e.g. women of childbearing age, etc.).

Trial design

Features to consider include the following:

- If the underlying disease is likely to produce AEs that might be confused with drug toxicity, then consider the use of a formal control group.

- If the study is not double-blind, will the lack of blindness bias the occurrence/collection of AEs in favour of one of the trial drugs?

- Will the known ADR of the trial drugs unblind the study? If so, how will this problem be overcome? Any controlled clinical trial where the type A ADRs of the drugs might allow the patients or investigator to identify which drug they are taking should be assessed for maintenance of blindness (see 4th edition).

- The protocol should state under what circumstances the treatment code can be broken by the investigator for medical emergencies.

- Does the consent form adequately represent the risks of the study?

- Does the protocol detail notification of serious AEs to the trial Ethics Committee/ Institutional Review Board (IRB)?

- Should a Data Monitoring Committee be used and how should it operate (Ellenberg *et al.*, 2002)? See also Chapter 11.

Concurrent therapy

Factors to consider include:

- What concurrent therapy should be permitted or forbidden?
- Is sufficient provision made for recording of concurrent therapy on the CRF?
- With the increasing number of drugs changing from prescription-only medicines (POM) to over-the-counter (OTC) drugs there should be special provision made to record all OTC drugs.
- Herbal remedies.

Baseline characteristics

It is important to document any characteristic that might be important in the analysis or assessment of any associated factors of a TESS. These may involve areas that are very sensitive for the patient, who may be reluctant to mention them spontaneously or even if prompted. They include:

- OTC products.
- Herbal medicines.
- Other alternative or complementary treatments, e.g. reflexology, aromatherapy, vitamins, etc. In 1997 42 per cent of the American population used alternative medicines (Eisenberg *et al.*, 1998).
- Alcohol consumption. Abnormal liver function tests (LFTs) during a study may be related to alcohol excess or abuse. The use of the Alcohol Use Disorders Identification Test (AUDIT) is probably sufficiently sensitive (89 per cent) and specific (91 per cent) if a cut-off score of >8 is used (Hearne *et al.*, 2002). Moderate alcohol consumption in elderly patients is associated with an increased risk of ADRs (Onder *et al.*, 2002).
- Mental problems.
- Sexual orientation. This is sensitive and its documentation will only be necessary in a very relevant indication.

The patient should be asked to give consent that their GP be contacted to enquire whether there is any reason known to him/her why the patient should not be entered in the study.

Adverse events (symptomatic)

Questions to ask include:

- Have the AEs to be collected been defined?

- How are the AEs to be collected:

  (i) Diary card.

  (ii) Questionnaire with or without analogue scale. Has the questionnaire been validated? (Offerhaus, 1979).

  (iii) Checklist.

  (iv) Standard question. Is the wording in the protocol and CRF?

  (v) Quality of life?

  (vi) Other?

- Does the protocol require the investigator to investigate fully all AEs, including seeking the aid of specialists where necessary? There is sometimes failure of companies to follow up serious AEs sufficiently. It is vital to obtain all the data that must be collected and would help decide on the cause of the AE.

- Does the protocol request the physician to make any interim diagnosis or drug attribution before breaking the drug code?

- Does the protocol allow for a sample of blood to be taken for drug levels in the case of serious AEs?

- Does the protocol inform the investigator that all serious AEs must be notified immediately to the company?

- Does the CRF allow sufficient space and require sufficient details for assessment of all types of AE?

- Does the protocol request full follow up on patients who have had a serious AE, stopped a trial drug due to an AE, or who have a laboratory abnormality or an AE at the last visit while on the drug?

- Does the protocol require full details of treatment of any AE to be recorded?

- Is the frequency of trial visits adequate to pick up the AEs and is the timing of the post-study visit suitable considering the disease and the drug?

- Who is to assess the causality of the AE?

- How are the AEs to be analysed and compared? Clinically only? Statistically? If the latter, then how?

Adverse events (asymptomatic)

Questions to ask are:

- Do the laboratory and other objective investigations cover potential ADRs?

- Is the frequency of sampling adequate and has a post-study sampling been agreed?

- How is the handling of patients with asymptomatic abnormal laboratory investigations to be dealt with (Sackett and Gent, 1979; DeMets *et al.*, 1980):

    (i)   By repeating tests?

    (ii) By further confirmatory tests?

    (iii) By clinical examination?

    (iv) By dechallenge?

    (v)   By rechallenge?

- How are the laboratory examination results to be assessed:

    (i)   According to the normal laboratory range as normal or abnormal?

    (ii) By the clinician and/or company physician?

    (iii) Clinically as well as statistically?

- Will the samples be analysed centrally in a multi-centre trial? If analysed in the hospital where the trial takes place, has the laboratory been approached? Have the details of storage and transport been decided? See Chapter 5.

Withdrawals

How are withdrawals to be investigated/followed up to make certain that the cause was not drug intolerance? Other questions to consider are:

- Is there a financial disincentive for the investigator to follow up withdrawals (i.e. withdrawals not paid for)?

- Is there provision for following up patients who change GP or move, so that they can be contacted for long-term follow up?

- If the study is in the UK and is long term, have arrangements been made with the NHS Central Register in Southport for patients to be flagged so that deaths will be identified (Cancer Research Campaign Working Party, 1980)?

- Is there a procedure for follow up of withdrawals?

Third-party 'interference'

Have sufficient arrangements (e.g. provision of a letter to be held by the patient) been made to ensure cooperation with the management of the patient during the trial, but outside the confines of the trial? Relevant factors to consider are:

- Provision for notification of trial with request to GP for cooperation.

- Provision for possible emergency admission to another hospital.

- Recording the use of OTC products by the patient .

- Provision of a card for the patient giving details of the trial and contact telephone numbers/addresses, requesting information from any doctor consulted.

General

What is the possibility that the trial will fulfil its aim regarding ADRs (i.e. what is the size of the type 2 error)? This involves considering:

- What incidence of adverse reactions (95 per cent confidence limits) appearing with only one of the comparative drugs could be detected?

- Can measurable safety outcomes be defined (e.g. a laboratory value above a defined point)?

- What difference in incidence of AEs in the investigational drug group compared with the control group, or the expected incidence of AEs from previous epidemiological studies, would the trial detect?

- Has it been agreed that adequate space will be given to the reporting of AEs in any subsequent papers (Ioannidis and Lau, 2001), including statements about the power of the study?

- Will all patients who have been randomized and taken even a single dose be analysed and accounted for as far as AEs are concerned (May *et al.*, 1981)?

- Since all pre-marketing studies have some risk to the patient, all studies need to be monitored for any undue risk and in studies of any length the possibility of interim analysis must be considered. The protocol should clearly specify safety variable outcomes that could necessitate patient discontinuation from the study or complete study termination (Enas *et al.*, 1989).

- There has been increasing use of CROs for carrying out part of the development of a drug and also an increase in the licensing out of products to other manufacturers. Inadequate preparation for these multiple sources of AE data can result in chaos when finally it is all put together for a licence application. Some form of template is necessary to develop a detailed agreement covering AE collection, processing, distribution and reporting (Fieldstad *et al.*, 1996; Society of Pharmaceutical Medicine, Pharmaco-vigilance Group Working Party, 1998).

Uncontrolled trials

These may vary from the use of the drug by a physician in a single patient resistant to other therapy to relatively large-scale dose–titration studies. All these studies should be governed by a protocol. All patients must be accounted for and detailed records kept (as for controlled studies).

From the point of view of ADRs, uncontrolled trials pose several problems:

- Without a control group the AEs that are symptoms alone and can occur in normal persons without drugs often cannot be attributed to the drug.

- Since the type of patient admitted to the study may not be tightly controlled, patients are entered with disease or complications other than the target disease, giving rise to the difficulty in deciding whether an AE is due to the natural course of the concurrent disease (or a complication) or to the drug.

- Concurrent therapy is often permitted in these uncontrolled studies and therefore attribution of AEs to the investigational drug may be difficult.

- The consent form, if it lists potential ADRs, may well bias reporting of AEs (Levine, 1987; Myers *et al.*, 1987).

An unaccountable fatal outcome occurring in an early phase uncontrolled study may, quite unjustly, be attributed to the drug and all further studies stopped or delayed. The practice of allowing investigators involved in controlled trials to use the drug in an uncontrolled study must be strictly limited and the investigator must be prepared to monitor the patients as strictly as if in a formal controlled trial. All AEs, no matter how trivial, must be documented and the pharmaceutical company notified of any serious AE without delay. This can be done using either a specifically designed record card, which is returned at regular intervals, or by the use of a standard AE form, which is returnable immediately after the event has occurred. The latter has the advantage that the event report is not delayed until the main CRF is returned.

Recording adverse events in clinical trials

From the point of view of recording AEs the essential division is into serious or non-serious. It is unusual that non-serious AEs or symptoms can be causally related to the drug on an individual basis; however, they can be grouped together and their incidence compared statistically in treatment groups. Clinicians are only likely to supply very limited information concerning non-serious events, and an extensive AE form may be inappropriate. A delay until the CRF is returned to the company may be important for non-serious AEs if they have caused the drug to be stopped and there is a possibility that they are causally related. They may need to be assessed individually for causality and more detailed information will be required. There are unlikely to be many similar serious AEs in the two treatment groups and they will, therefore, not be suitable for statistical comparison. The withdrawals possibly due to the drug should probably be notified to the company when they occur and, therefore, before the patient finishes the study. They will require subsequent follow up.

Non-serious adverse events

These are AEs that do not satisfy the definition of serious. These can be recorded on a special form, and the date of onset, duration, frequency, severity (mild, moderate or severe) and outcome should be noted. These will be assessed when the CRF is returned. The investigator must be encouraged to give full descriptions of these events, as a single word is not usually sufficient. Where the event comprises one or more symptoms with little objective data to back it up, it becomes very important for the investigator to record the patient's own description on the CRF. The diagnosis that the investigator makes should be recorded in their own words.

Serious adverse events

Serious AEs should be recorded on a serious AE form, and a copy despatched immediately to the company. The investigator must record all serious AEs, regardless of causality, but should be asked to make a causality judgement while blind to treatment. For serious AEs the seriousness and courses of action open may demand that the code be broken and the initial causality judgement may need to be changed once the results of all tests are known. These cases must be followed up by the company. The latter must be emphasized, because otherwise the investigator may delay sending the form until he has more information, and there is always a difficulty in deciding whether to notify a serious AE as soon as the possibility arises or to wait until all the data are available and thus establish a causal relationship (Dangoumau et al., 1978; Boisseau et al., 1980).

Follow up

Follow up is vital in order to obtain:

- Causality assessment.
- Response to dechallenge and possibly to rechallenge.
- Further investigations that would help in causality assessment, but may not be required for the patient's clinical management.
- Final outcome.

Follow up may also allow the trial monitor to help the investigator by giving previous experience with the event or suggesting reduction of dosage rather than stoppage for type A reactions.

The response to follow up requests from companies is often very poor, and this is true for Europe, USA and Japan. Some companies state that if there is no response to a follow up then it should be repeated either once or twice, but it is important to explain what information is needed and why it is needed. There is no reason to accept an inadequate reply, since investigators are under contract to the company and it should have been specifically referred to in the protocol. There are several points that should be considered:

- A *local* company physician could indicate what examinations are likely to have been done and what details should be available for each AE.

- A specific questionnaire may be advisable for certain areas, e.g. liver, haemolysis, kidney, thrombocytopenia and dermatology. See Bénichou's *Adverse Drug Reactions* (see Bibliography).

- If allergy is likely to have been involved, consider using the ENDA Drug hypersensitivity questionnaire (Demoly *et al.*, 1999).

- Consider extra payment for time spent investigating really important cases.

- Request photocopies of hospital records where applicable.

- If an AE falls outside the expertise of the investigator request him to ask the appropriate specialist to give an opinion at the company's expense.

- A site visit by a company physician can be very effective.

- The communications line may be long: HQ drug safety → HQ clinical research → local company clinical research → local company drug safety → ? CRO → local clinical research associate (CRA).

- The follow up may need to continue if the results of dechallenge and rechallenge are to be collected, or if the event is prolonged and it is necessary to continue until complete resolution.

Should withdrawals due to adverse events be notified before the end of a trial?

One can question the advantages of using solely the serious criteria as a reason for immediate notification. Drug withdrawals due to AEs may indicate too high a dosage regimen and need further investigation before further patients are recruited.
  Withdrawals due to AEs may be for several reasons:

- The patient or physician may have thought the AE to be due to the drug.

- The patient or physician may have thought the AE was not due to the drug, but that the AE made continuing with the drug undesirable (e.g. if the AE was renal impairment from natural causes, treatment with a renally excreted drug may be inappropriate).

- The physician may not know the cause of the event and, therefore, has stopped all treatments.

- The patient might have had several different signs and symptoms, but only one of these might be the actual reason for stopping the drug.

- The drug may have been ineffective.

- The dosage of the drug may be incorrect. This may be due to poor prescribing or the Investigator's Brochure (IB) gives a dosage regimen that is too high.

If type A ADRs due to an incorrect dose for an individual patient cause a patient to withdraw from a Phase II study, their notification at the end of the study may be too late for a change in dose for Phase III studies. This may be particularly relevant to indications requiring long-term therapy. Similarly, notification during Phase III studies would allow studies at the correct dose to run in parallel so that early in the post-marketing phase a lower dose would be available. It would also be sensible to take blood for drug levels in any patients complaining of type A events during Phase I and Phase II studies.

Incorrect dosage at marketing requiring change after marketing

Patients can experience ADRs that may have been preventable if a better estimation of the dose at marketing had been possible.

1. Post-marketing dosage changes over the period 1982–2000 showed 115 changes – 39 per cent increases (predominatly in the 1980s) and 61 per cent decreases (later on, mostly post-1993) (Heerdink *et al.*, 2002).

2. Of 499 new medical entities (NMEs) approved by the FDA between 1980 and 2000, 354 were evaluable; of dose changes with 73 NMEs, 58 were safety motivated (79 per cent). 'Post-marketing changes to labelled dosage regimens may reflect suboptimal drug development'. 'The rate of these changes is greater for newer drugs than older drugs' (Cross *et al.*, 2002).

3. Of drugs approved in the USA since 1979, 20 per cent required dose reduction after approval (Bashaw, 1992).

The reasons put forward were:

- The dose is commonly fixed at the level that has been shown to be effective in 90 per cent of the population *provided that the unwanted effects at this dosage are considered acceptable*. In 25 per cent of patients a smaller dose will be effective.

- Digit preference (e.g. a correct dose of over 50 mg may be rounded up to 100 mg).

- To avoid dose titration (Herxheimer, 1991; Venning, 1991).

- Once Phase III studies have started at the wrong dose, repeating the studies at the correct dose would produce an unacceptable delay in the Marketing Authorization Application (MAA)/NDA.

- 'The common practice of selecting the highest possible dose for use in large trials may result in an unacceptable incidence of unwanted and potentially serious adverse outcome', e.g. Hirudin (Conrad, 1995).

- Effective low doses determined in pre-marketing studies or in post-marketing studies are often omitted from the Physicians' Desk Reference (Cohen, 2001).

Effects of drugs on skilled performance

All new drugs should be tested for effects on the CNS at some stage (Jackson, 1990). The danger of drugs affecting car driving ability has attracted more attention in recent years. The use of medicinal drugs such as benzodiazepines and tricyclic antidepressants has been shown to more than double the risk of involvement in traffic accidents resulting in injuries (Ray *et al.*, 1992; Neutel 1995; Barbone *et al.*, 1998). In the EU, traffic accidents result in 50 000 fatalities and 1.5 million injuries each year, with a total cost of more than €70 billion (Cornelissen, 1997). The contribution of medicines to these figures is substantial, since an average of 10 per cent of the adult population is frequently using impairing medicinal drugs. At a very conservative estimate, if 10 per cent of the adult population is driving under the influence of impairing medication at twice the risk of being involved in traffic accidents, then those drugs are causing 4500 deaths, 135 000 injuries and €6.3 billion damage to the European society each year (De Gier, 1995).

Determination of a drug's effect on psychomotor performance can be derived from experimental psychopharmacology (Ramaekers, 2003). This discipline has made tremendous contributions to the development of relatively safer drugs for drivers. The methods used ranged from psychometric test batteries (e.g. the Digit Symbol Substitution Test) to psychomotor tests (e.g. reaction time, tracking, and Critical Flicker Fusion) and cognitive tests for measuring mnemonic functions. But more importantly, the simulation of real-life performance in driving simulators, closed-course driving and actual driving tests in real traffic conditions revealed the impairing properties of medicinal drugs, especially when compared with the impairing effects of alcohol in various blood concentrations. Although many studies are conducted with healthy volunteers not suffering from illnesses that might impair performance, the comparative data from studies with patients revealed that both volunteers and patients experience similar side effects of psychoactive drugs (Van Laar *et al.*, 1992; O'Hanlon, 1995; Ramaekers *et al.*, 1997).

Information concerning the increased potential for crash risk as a consequence of using potentially hazardous medicines must be meaningfully communicated to patients. The simplest way to achieve this would be by means of clear warning labels on the package. Most EU member states, however, do not require exterior warnings on packaging, and patients are informed about impairing effects only by the patient information leaflet. Since 1992, European legislation has required warnings regarding the ability to drive or use machines, written in lay language, to be part of the content of the patient drug information leaflet (Council Directive 92/27/EEC).

European Union 'Note for Guidance'

A warning system based on consensus among scientists was introduced in 1991 (Wolschrijn *et al.*, 1991); the major improvement of the system was its scheme for categorizing drugs according to their potential for impairing driving skills. The European authorities adopted a Note for Guidance for the, SPC(III/9163/90-EN, final approval by the CPMP on 16 October 1991).

In 1998, a survey was conducted to determine how responsible regulatory authorities in the different European countries have reacted to this Note for Guidance (De Gier, 1998a,b). The report of survey findings highlights that the European Ministers of Transport resolve that EU member states should encourage the systematic printing of a warning symbol on the packaging of medicines likely to impair driving (ECMT/CM93/5/Final). The Note for Guidance provides the framework needed to categorize drugs in order to provide three different warning symbols reflecting the following categories of Article 4.7 of the SPC 'Effects on ability to drive and use machines', on the basis of:

- the pharmacodynamic profile, reported ADR and/or

- impairment of driving performance or performance related to driving, the medicine is:

    1. presumed to be safe or unlikely to produce an effect;

    2. likely to produce minor or moderate adverse effects;

    3. likely to produce severe effects or presumed to be potentially dangerous.

For situations 2 and 3, special precautions for use/warnings relevant to the categorization should be mentioned.

Procedures for assessing warnings and guidelines for allowing categorization

Generally speaking, the drug regulatory authorities review the data provided by the drug manufacturers and assess whether these data support statements in the SPC. There are no criteria stipulating the number of reports or the kind of tests that are needed as a basis for their assessment; it is a case-by-case assessment. Furthermore, the methodology of experimental research on drug effects is still poorly described, although adequate descriptive information exists based on the consensus of scientific opinion.

Some harmonization has been achieved, e.g. in the provision of a specific Note for Guidance on the SPC of benzodiazepines as anxiolytics; the recommendation for information to be contained in the warning about the effects of these drugs on the ability to drive and use machines has been standardized. It offers no opportunity, however, for distinguishing between various benzodiazepines when data from experimental and/or pharmaco-epidemiological research demonstrate different behavioural toxicities. Unfortunately, this situation has not been recognized by the drug regulatory authorities as being an obstacle to accurate categorization. Hence, it is recommended that better guidelines be established to assist drug manufacturers to select appropriate drug testing methodologies and to reconsider the use of standard information for the warning section in the SPC.

A major problem in the categorization of drugs may be the lack of support from pharmaceutical companies that have to submit the relevant data. Even if a standardized methodology is applied to test a drug's impairing properties, there is still likely to be debate about the meaning of results. If a drug has been found to be impairing, then the issue will be whether it will be assigned to a different category than non-impairing drugs of the same therapeutic class.

Some drug regulatory authorities have indicated that experimental research alone is not sufficiently convincing evidence to support the formulation of different warnings. They have suggested that revision of the warning system should be based on results obtained from studies of large populations who have used the drugs. They propose that the study investigators should assess the risk potential of accident involvement for each individual drug. It is unclear whether there will be a need for the European Medicines Evaluation Agency (EMEA) to provide specific expertise in this area. Although regulatory authorities may feel much more comfortable selecting their own experts, some would welcome the specific expertise provided by EMEA. It is recommended that EMEA initiate an investigation to decide whether or not it should coordinate large-scale, case controlled pharmaco-epidemiological surveys. These would use existing databases in different EU member states to determine the relative risks of traffic accidents for users of all drugs identified as potentially dangerous.

Opportunities to improve warnings

A categorization system could improve the effectiveness of warnings, compared with the long lists of side effects that are currently provided as warnings. The new European Guideline on this subject (III/5218/97, final approval September 1998) provides an opportunity to improve the readability of the label and patient information leaflets with specific guidelines for certain categories of medicinal drugs. Clear statements are prescribed, and pictograms may be used as an additional measure if they make the message clearer to the patient.

There are current movements towards categorization systems for the purpose of improving warnings in at least five EU member states: Belgium, Germany, the Netherlands, France and Spain. Belgium was the first country that officially introduced the categorization system in April 1999, at the time that the Traffic Law was changed into a 'zero tolerance' law for illicit drugs (Charlier *et al.*, 1999). Medicinal drugs were not included in this new law, but the Belgian Minister of Transport considered these to be dealt with by preventive measures, such as prescribing and dispensing guidelines and a clear patient information leaflet. Furthermore, professional organizations in these countries have applied the same system in their efforts to support physicians and pharmacists in selecting relatively safer drugs for patients who drive.

The categorization system was originally proposed in 1991 by a group of international experts who wanted a system allowing healthcare providers and patients to understand more easily the severity of impairment by medicinal psychotropic medicines (Wolschrijn *et al.*, 1991).

In 2001, Spain became the second country in Europe to introduce an official categorization system for drugs having a potentially dangerous effect on driving (Del Rio Garcia, 2001).

In order to make the users of the categorization system aware of the meaning of each category, a comparison with the effects of alcohol, which are well known, was suggested by researchers in experimental psychopharmacology in the Netherlands, based on the views on test validation expressed several years ago (O'Hanlon *et al.*, 1986). Data collected in experimental research, in which over-the-road driving tests have been applied with most frequently used medicinal drugs and alcohol (as 'calibration'), have allowed researchers to interpret weaving effects by any drug as equivalent to that produced by a particular blood alcohol concentration (see Table 4.3).

Table 4.3   Categorization of warnings

Category	Impairment description for medicinal drugs	Comparison with blood alcohol concentration (BAC)
I	Presumed to be safe or unlikely to produce an effect	Equivalent to BAC < 0.5 g/l ($<0.05\%$)
II	Likely to produce minor or moderate adverse effects	Equivalent to BAC $0.5-0.8$ g/l ($0.05-0.08\%$)
III	Likely to produce severe or presumed to be potentially dangerous	Equivalent to BAC > 0.8 g/l ($>0.08\%$)

The most important advantage of the three-tier system over 'older' dichotomous drug class-based systems or systems based on quotations of long lists of side effects is the focus on the least impairing medications in each therapeutic class. Since these initiatives will have an impact on the views of patients, physicians and pharmacists, it would be advisable for them to be in accordance with present European Directives and Guidelines aimed at improving the readability of labels and patient information leaflets. Categorization and warning symbols, based on scientific consensus, have been shown to be feasible. By investigating the acceptance of a new warning symbol among patients, healthcare providers and drug manufacturers, the drug regulatory authorities could become more proactive in response to the actual needs of those who use the information presented.

Special subgroups

Children

Most drugs prescribed for children have not undergone extensive clinical trials in children, particularly in children under 2 years of age. Only between 20 and 30 per cent of approved drugs are labelled for paediatric use. Consequently, much drug prescribing in children is so called 'off label' use. The EMEA in October 2002 published a concept paper on the conduct of pharmacovigilance for medicines used by children (CPMP/PhVWP/4838/02), this identified the key issues as:

- Childhood diseases may be qualitatively and quantitatively different from adult diseases.

- Efficacy in children cannot always be assumed from adult efficacy data.

- Children may have different pharmacokinetics and dynamics to adults and, therefore, have particular vulnerability to ADRs.

- Children may have different drug metabolism, and consequently a different drug interaction profile compared with adults. Owing to specific ethical considerations, drug metabolism data in children may be very sparce at the time of registration.

- Children are growing and may, therefore, be susceptible to developmental disorders, as well as delayed ADRs not seen in adults.

- Certain ADRs may only be seen in children.

- Lack of clinical trials in children limits the safety data available.

- Lack of kinetics data may lead to under- or over-dosing in some age groups.

- Under-dosing may result in lack of benefit or development of resistance.

- Over-dosing may result in an increase of type A reactions.

- Lack of appropriate formulations may lead to incorrect dosing and use of products of less controlled quality.

- Children may be more susceptible to ADRs from specific excipients.

- Medicines used off-label may have inadequate product information to support safe use in children.

The EU guidance for clinical investigation of medicinal products in the paediatric population is ICH 11 (CPMP/ICH/2711/99); this has been followed in 2002 by a consultation document, *Better medicines for children, proposed regulatory actions on paediatric medicinal products*. In the USA, guidance for industry is also based on ICH E11, *Investigation of medicinal products in the paediatric population*, which was published in December 2000. There is the paediatric exclusivity provision of the FDA Modernization Act of 1997, which encourages paediatric studies by extending patent protection. This was followed by the FDA's Paediatric Rule, requiring paediatric studies starting in December 2000, but this was challenged in the courts and the FDA has issued a 'Call for Comments' on whether the rule needs to be changed.

The five age groups in ICH E11 are:

- pre-term newborn infants (born at <36 weeks gestation);

- term newborn infants (age 0 to 27 days);

- infants and toddlers (age 28 days to 23 months);

- children (age 2 to 11 years);

- adolescents (age 12 to 16–18 years, dependent on region).

The four groups of medicinal products are:

- To treat diseases in adults and children for which treatment exists.

- To treat diseases in adults and children that have no current treatment.

- To treat diseases that mainly affect children or are of particular gravity in children or have a different natural history in children.

- For diseases only affecting children.

On the whole, the adult experience of dose–effect relationships will provide a framework for dose titration and ADR monitoring. In other circumstances the medicinal product should be contraindicated for children until further data are available after initial marketing authorization (Jeffreys, 1995).

A survey of new molecular entities approved by the FDA from 1984 to 1989 showed that 80 per cent had no information regarding paediatric use (Roberts, 1996), and this continued in 1992 (Kearns, 1996). Drugs for use in children may be accompanied by problems not seen in adults or cause ADRs that are more frequent than in adults, e.g. antibiotic toxicity in neonates (sulphonamides, chloramphenicol), hepatotoxicity with sodium valproate and Reye's syndrome with aspirin use for viral infections.

The metabolism of drugs differs in young children. The activity of many P450 enzymes is reduced in the neonatal period and the variation in maturation of different enzymes makes it difficult to predict dosage requirements accurately at different ages. Glucuronidation is a major process of drug elimination in adults, but this is significantly reduced in neonates. Renal excretion is impaired in the first few weeks of life. After the neonatal period, renal function is normal (Choonara *et al.*, 1996). See also Chapter 2.

Suggested further reading includes Leary (1991), Kearns (1996) and ABPI (1996).

The elderly

Patients over 65 years of age comprise about 14 per cent of the population in most industrialized countries but they consume nearly 35 per cent of the drugs (Avorn, 1997). The EU/ICH E7 guidelines are provided in *Note for Guidance on Studies in Support of Special Populations: Geriatrics* (CPMP/ICH/379/95). The usual definition of elderly is over 65 years of age, but the FDA definition is over 60 years. There is a threefold increase in the incidence of ADRs in patients over 60 years compared with patients under 30, and 1 in 10 hospital admissions of older patients are for ADRs (Swafford, 1997).

The healthy old person does not seem to be more susceptible to ADRs compared with the young, but as a group the elderly have many factors predisposing them to ADRs.

Concomitant disease   Increased morbidity means that the elderly are often taking several drugs. Drug expenditure for the elderly accounts for 40 per cent of UK drug expenditure (O'Brien, 1995). There is also a parallel increase in the use of OTC drugs, resulting in an increased chance of drug interactions. The elderly are also targeted by manufacturers of alternative medicines.

Altered pharmacokinetics   Although drug absorption does not change, the drug distribution depends on the lean/adipose body mass ratio, and this declines with age. Protein-bound drugs are distributed differently due to reduced serum albumin concentration. Drugs excreted via the kidneys tend to have a lower clearance rate due to a decline in renal function. The hepatic blood flow and liver mass decline with age and oxidative metabolism may be impaired, although CYP4502D56 does not appear to change with age alone. See Chapter 2.

Altered pharmacodynamics   Beta blockers have less clinical effect for a given concentration in the elderly, but the elderly are more susceptible to the sedative effects of benzodiazepines. Anticoagulants are more likely to cause bleeding. In general, the elderly have less effective homeostatic mechanisms (e.g. temperature and blood pressure control) (Beard, 1991; Pollock, 1996).

Poor compliance   This may be partly due to polypharmacy, poor sight or failing memory.
    If a product is likely to be used by the elderly then studies need to be performed, especially if the following factors are present:

- a low therapeutic index

- the drug is excreted renally

- there is a possibility of interactions

- there are problems with drugs of the same class

- deterioration in organ function, which may affect pharmacokinetics or pharmaco-dynamics.

Interaction studies are usually recommended with the following groups of drugs:

- digoxin and oral anticoagulants

- hepatic enzyme inducers

- drugs metabolised by cytochrome P450 enzymes

- other drugs likely to be used with the investigational drug.

See O'Brien (1995).

Inclusion of elderly patients in clinical trials

- Any drug likely to be used by elderly people should be included in pre-marketing studies with an age distribution comparable to that anticipated in routine use.

- Pre-marketing evaluation should include assessing whether important age-related differences exist in efficacy and toxicity.

- Since unexpected differences may emerge in effectiveness or ADRs when a drug is used by large numbers of elderly patients, especially those too frail to be included in trials, plans for post-marketing surveillance (PMS) should be required at the time a drug is approved (Avorn, 1997).

Suggested further reading is Kitler (1989).

Pregnancy

Approximately 35 per cent of pregnant women in the UK take some drug during pregnancy, and this includes about 9 per cent who take OTC products (Rubin, 1995). The figure for the USA in 1993 was 68 per cent (Rubin *et al.*, 1993), for Italy 80 per cent in 1995 (Maggini *et al.*, 1997), and in 1996 for Brazil 94.6 per cent (Fonseca *et al.*, 1997). The animal toxicology will probably be the only evidence for or against teratogenicity until the drug is on the market, and from then on the evidence will be anecdotal unless large-scale epidemiological studies are undertaken. In the UK, the background incidence of major malformations is about 2.3 per cent at birth, rising to 4.5 per cent by 5 years of age. The incidence of spontaneous abortions in clinically recognized pregnancies is 10–20 per cent (Lack *et al.*, 1968). Drugs and chemicals together are thought to account for only about 4–6 per cent of malformations with the cause of 65–70 per cent unknown (Wilson, 1977). All drugs given to the mother, except high molecular weight compounds such as insulin and heparin, can cross the placenta.

Many physiological changes that may affect drug levels occur during pregnancy, including:

- Increased plasma, extracellular fluid, and fat stores

- Increased hydroxylation capacity by steroids, which may alter metabolism

- Albumin binding and binding to specific receptors may be altered

- The 40–50 per cent increase in glomerular filtration rate (GFR), which may affect drug excretion

- Gastrointestinal absorption of oral preparations may be impaired (Redmond, 1985)

The risks of drug use in pregnancy have been classified. The European SPC Guideline states that the following should be mentioned:

- Facts on human experience and conclusions from preclinical toxicity studies that are of relevance for the assessment of risks associated with exposure during pregnancy.

- Recommendations on the use of the medicinal product at different times during pregnancy in respect of gestation.

- Recommendations on the management of the situation of an inadvertent exposure, where relevant.

Examples of wording are provided in an appendix of the European SPC Guideline.

The US pregnancy categories are given in 21 CFR 201.57, *Specific Requirements on Content and Format of Labelling for Human Prescription Drugs*, and are summarized as follows:

A – Studies in pregnant women have not shown that (drug) increases the risk of foetal abnormalities if administered during the first (second, third, or all) trimesters of pregnancy. If this drug is used during pregnancy, the possibility of foetal harm appears remote.

B – Reproduction studies have been performed in animals at doses up to x times the human dose and have revealed no evidence of impaired fertility or harm to the foetus. There are, however, no adequate and well-controlled studies in pregnant women.

C – (Drug) has been shown to be teratogenic in species when given in doses x times the human dose. There are no adequate and well-controlled studies in pregnant women. (Drug) should be used during pregnancy only if the potential benefit justifies the potential risk to the foetus.

D – (Drug) can cause foetal harm when administered to pregnant women.

X – See Contraindications. (Drug) may cause harm when administered to a pregnant woman.

In Australia the guidance is:

A – Drug taken by many pregnant women with no harmful effects.

B1 – Limited human exposure shows no increase in harmful effects. Animal studies show no harmful effects.

B2 – Limited human exposure shows no increase in harmful effects. Animal studies inadequate or lacking.

B3 – Limited human exposure shows no increase in harmful effects. Animal studies show evidence of foetal damage.

C – Human studies may have shown harmful effects, but no malformations. Effects may be reversible.

D – May cause human foetal damage or malformations.

X – Should not be used during pregnancy, due to harmful effects.

The proposal to increase the number of women in clinical trials may result in more pregnancies in the early stages of a drug's development. Since there is a 3 per cent chance of major abnormalities in live births (DeLap et al., 1996) there will be the possibility that mothers with babies with abnormalities will sue the company.

In June 2001 the CPMP published two concept papers on 'The development of notes for guidance on the use of medicinal products during pregnancy: need for post-marketing data' (CPMP/EWP/PhVWP/1417/01) and on 'Risk assessment of medicinal products on human reproductive and development toxicities: from data to labelling' (CPMP/SWP/373/01).

Pregnancy registries

The goal of pregnancy registries is to provide clinically relevant human data that can be used in a product's labelling to provide useful information for treating and counselling patients who are pregnant or planning to become pregnant.

The criteria for selecting drugs for a pregnancy registry are:

- Issues arising from conduct of animal studies.

- Expectation of AEs during pregnancy based on structure–activity relationships.

- Findings of concern from case reports in the literature or identified from PMS.

- Expectation of high use pattern in women of childbearing age.

- Treatment needed for conditions associated with high morbidity or mortality.

- Inability to discontinue treatment ethically during pregnancy (e.g. new drugs in epilepsy where there is a two to three times greater incidence of malformations, mostly due to older drugs; Craig and Morrow, 1997).

A pregnancy registry is desirable for a drug when:

- Inadvertent exposures in pregnancy are likely to be common, for instance when a drug has a high likelihood of use by women of childbearing potential.

- It presents special circumstances, such as the potential for infection of mother and foetus by administration of live, attenuated vaccines. See FDA Guidance for Industry, Establishing Pregnancy Exposure Registries, August 2002.

Examples of pregnancy registries   These include:

- National birth defects registries (Schardein, 1993).

- UK National Teratology Information Service, which is part of the European network of teratology information services (Bateman and McElhatton, 1997).

- International Clearing House for Birth Defects Monitoring Systems, which covers Australia, France, Israel, Italy, Japan and South America, is referred to as the MADRE project (malformation drug exposure surveillance), and has been collecting cases since 1990.

- The Pegasus project – all pregnancies in Munich – 14 000 births per year and 85 per cent of women used at least one drug during pregnancy (Hasford, 1996; Cornelia *et al.*, 1997).

Suggested further reading is Mitchell (2000).

The Investigator's Brochure

Under the Code of Federal Regulations on Food and Drugs, Title 21, part 312.55 it is a requirement that all investigators are given an Investigator's Brochure (IB). The International Conference on Harmonization (ICH) *Guideline for Good Clinical Practice* (GCP) E6, 1996 defines the IB as 'A compilation of the clinical and non-clinical data on the investigational product(s) which is relevant to the study of the investigational product(s) in human subjects'. In the safety section of the IB, 'Tabular summaries of ADRs for all the clinical trials would be useful. Important differences in ADR patterns/incidences across indications or sub-groups should be discussed'. There is no mention of AEs. 'Guidance should be provided on the recognition and treatment of possible overdose and ADR that is based on previous human experience and on the pharmacology of the investigational product'; see also Chapter 9, ICH E6 – Good clinical practice.

The IB should provide a description of the possible risks and ADRs to be anticipated on the basis of previous experiences with the product under investigation and with related products. Klincewicz *et al.* (2001) have reviewed and discussed the regulations and guidelines concerning the safety sections of the IB.

Updating the Investigator's Brochure

The IB should be updated at least annually, but the frequency will depend upon whether there is any relevant new information (ICH E6). There have been some instances where the IB has not been updated during clinical studies (Mikhail, 1993). The question on how often the IB should be updated is difficult. It is easy to say that this should be whenever there is any relevant new data. In between regular updates a letter can be sent to all investigators and the Ethics Committees announcing any serious AEs, etc. (Mikhail, 1993). Since the term 'expected' refers to its mention in the IB, some companies take the view that the more AEs that are put in the IB the less they will need to report. The ICH recommend that the IB is kept current (e.g. through amendments/attachments), particularly for medically important safety data (ICH E6). The aim should be to have a single IB for use in all countries with regular updates, including anything relevant from new animal studies.

Unblinding

The importance of maintaining blindness as to the study drug is that it maintains the integrity of the study, and this approach is often emphasized by statisticians. However, ICH E2A advises that the blind should be broken for serious, unexpected ADRs; see Chapter 9. This is encouraged by authorities such as the UK MHRA and is usually done by Drug Safety staff, but without unblinding others involved in the study. The problem with this approach is that the frequency of the ADR in a large study might reach proportions that require further rapid action. The advantages of unblinding to facilitate expedited reporting are that it:

- allows ongoing safety evaluation of the product in development;

- facilitates updating of the IB;

- avoids need to update safety database after the study is complete;

- avoids expedited reporting of placebo/comparator cases;

- meets regulatory requirements.

Gait and Goldsmith (2000) argue that the ICH recommendation is not appropriate and that routine alerting should be based on submission of blinded, serious, unexpected related cases. It is recommended that the ICH E2A guideline should be followed unless the regulatory authorities, Data Safety Monitoring Board (DSMB) and Independent Ethics Committees/ IRBs have agreed otherwise before the study starts.

Clinical study reports

These are governed by the *Structure and Content of Clinical Study Reports* (ICH E3, 1995) and CPMP guidelines *Note for Guidance on Structure and Content of Clinical Study Reports* (CPMP/ICH/137/95).

The safety evaluation is considered on three levels:

- the extent of exposure (dose, duration and number of patients);

- the more common AEs;

- serious AEs and other significant AEs.

Three kinds of analysis and display are called for:

- Summarized data using tables and graphical presentations.

- Listings of individual subject data; for AEs these should include the subject identifier, age, sex, weight, severity, dose, seriousness, time to onset, action taken, outcome, causality assessment, concomitant treatment, etc.

- Narrative descriptions of events of particular interest.

Large studies will require detailed analysis of subgroups, whereas small studies may only require minimal analysis. The study report is best written by the person who has been dealing with the AEs during the clinical trial and who is familiar with the protocol and the data.

For further reading on this subject, see Gait *et al.* (2000).

Pooling of safety data

Many clinical trials are too small to reveal differences in AE rates between the investigational drug and controls, and even the larger studies are unlikely to be large enough to show differences in subgroups of patients. Pooling of safety data is required to maximize the usefulness of the total exposure to a new drug. Where possible, this should be done as the development programme progresses, not just at the end. Anyone dealing with pooling of data should be familiar with the *Guidelines for the Format and Content of the Clinical and Statistical Sections of New Drug Applications* from the Centre for Drug Evaluation and Research, FDA, Department of Health Sciences, July 1988. The relevant section is 'Integrated Summary of Safety Information'.

Before writing an Integrated Safety Summary it is useful to read a series of four papers published in the *Drug Information Journal* (Skinner, 1991; Garvey, 1991; Lineberry, 1991; Temple, 1991b).

More recently, the ICH have developed Multidisciplinary Topic M4 on the format and preparation of the Common Technical Document (CTD) to harmonize applications that will be submitted to regulatory authorities (ICH, 2002). This includes the Clinical Overview (module 2.5) and Clinical Summary (module 2.7), within which are the Overview of Safety (2.5.5) and Summary of Clinical Safety (2.7.4). Sub-headings are:

2.7.4.1   Exposure to the drug

2.7.4.1.1   Overall safety evaluation plan and narratives of safety studies

2.7.4.1.2   Overall extent of exposure

2.7.4.1.3   Demographic and other characteristics of study population

2.7.4.2   Adverse events

2.7.4.2.1   Analysis of adverse events

2.7.4.2.1.1 Common adverse events

2.7.4.2.1.2 Deaths

2.7.4.2.1.3 Other serious adverse events

2.7.4.2.1.4 Other significant adverse events

2.7.4.2.1.5 Analysis of adverse events by organ system or syndrome

2.7.4.2.2   Narratives

2.7.4.3   Clinical laboratory evaluations

2.7.4.4   Vital signs, physical findings and other observations related to safety

2.7.4.5   Safety in special groups and situations

2.7.4.5.1   Intrinsic factors

2.7.4.5.2   Extrinsic factors

2.7.4.5.3   Drug interactions

2.7.4.5.4   Use in pregnancy and lactation

2.7.4.5.5   Overdose

2.7.4.5.6   Drug abuse

2.7.4.5.7   Withdrawal and rebound

2.7.4.5.8   Effects on ability to drive or operate machinery or impairment of mental ability

2.7.4.6   Post-marketing data

The aim of pooling data is:

- to evaluate serious AEs too rare to be seen in each individual study;

- to discover whether any particular subgroup is more susceptible to an AE.

Analysis of subgroups that have not been defined prior to the study (so called 'data dredging') should not be performed as a part of efficacy analysis but is essential for safety analyses. However, when 'subgroups defined by the data are generated by the study results: often an effect is so suggested and then confirmed with statistical significance on the same data set' (Scott and Campbell, 1998). Ideally, any 'subgroup ADRs' found by this method should be confirmed by a subsequent study, as well as by group causation methods.

The first aim is subject to the total number of patients receiving the drug while the second depends upon looking at those subgroups of patients by variables. These may be patient variables:

- age
- sex
- weight
- race, country or centre
- concomitant disease (e.g. renal failure)
- indication and severity
- alcohol intake and smoking

drug variables:

- dose
- formulation
- frequency of administration
- route
- duration
- comparative therapy
- concomitant therapy
- blood/plasma level

or trial variables:

- type of study (controlled, uncontrolled or named patients)

- method of collection of AEs (diary card, checklist, questionnaire, general question or spontaneous reporting).

There are two approaches to the examination of the pool by variables: pool all studies and a heirarchical approach.

Pool all studies

This is only suitable if the variables that one wishes to examine are similarly represented in all studies (e.g. age, sex) and the studies are similar in design. With this approach the effect of small subgroups may be swamped by the majority of the patients (Figure 4.3).

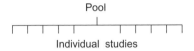

Figure 4.3   Schematic representation of 'pool all studies'

Hierarchical approach

If some studies have a common characteristic then they form a subgroup, which may have a different ADR pattern from the remainder of the studies. The first step is to look at the drug and indication concerned and then to list the variables, starting with those that are likely to have the greatest effect down to those not expected to have an effect. The former should be at the top of the hierarchical tree and the latter at the bottom. For example, one might expect more AEs in trials against an active drug control rather than one against placebo, since only mild disease cases are likely to be in the latter, and uncontrolled studies may contain patients not acceptable in controlled studies (which have stricter inclusion and exclusion criteria). Groups with a concentration of one variable that may show differences could be, for example, as shown in Figure 4.4. Groups of variables that need to be considered are:

- Patient – Race or nationality (Joelson *et al.*, 1997); concomitant disease (e.g. renal failure with a drug excreted renally); indication; drug; dose/blood level; duration; route.

- Trial – collection of AEs by questionnaire/checklist (these should always be analysed separately).

- Country – despite the ICH it is not possible to eliminate national medical characteristics from influencing clinical trials. A survey in Japan found that there was a different attitude to the USA and Europe in regard to: entry criteria, prohibited concomitant

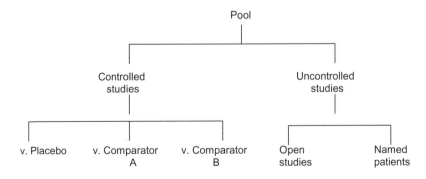

Figure 4.4   Schematic representation of hierarchical approach

drugs, informed consent and completion of CRFs (Ono *et al.*, 2002). Investigators in Japan have little incentive to perform clinical trials as they are not paid for this work (Miyazaki and Saito, 2002). The frequency of ADRs in Japan was significantly greater than in the USA and the EU (Homma *et al.*, 1994). In France and Germany the sales of drugs are twice as high as in the UK or USA, and so there is likely to be under-reporting of concomitant medication (see Chapter 1). Patients in eastern Europe tend to be more compliant in taking medication because of the culture in those countries, whereby the 'doctor knows best' (Neal, 2001). In any country where this paternalistic culture is present the patients may be reluctant to complain of AEs.

Using the above example as an illustration, the process of combining the studies starts at the roots of the hierarchical tree. If there is more than one placebo-controlled study then the incidence rates and the types of AEs are compared and if they are similar they can be combined. If they differ, then the trials are examined to see if there is another variable that might be responsible for the difference (e.g. one study, unknown to the company, had used a questionnaire and had thereby increased the incidence rate of all ADRs). If no explanation is forthcoming then the data are combined and a note made of the discrepancy. It may be that a similar discrepancy will be noted in other studies and point to a variable not previously considered. This process of comparing and then combining is continued to the top of the tree. When a definite difference is identified and the responsible variable found, then this group may be left out of the final pooling and treated separately. Those variables not examined on the way up the tree are examined in the complete pool of the data for any common AEs. The way in which this will be done will depend upon the variable and size of the pooled data (e.g. age may be looked at by decades or divided into below 65 years and above 65 years).

The analysis of healthy volunteer studies can be carried out in the same way and may give an early indication about which variable will be important for the analysis of patient data. However, volunteer data should not be pooled with patient data.

The advantages of the hierarchical approach are:

- Analysis can frequently be started earlier (i.e. when a subgroup is complete, rather than waiting for the whole database to be available).

- The effect of variables not apparent from analysing the whole database may be discovered.

- The incidence rates are likely to be more accurate, since variation due to a known subgroup will be excluded.

Serious adverse events

Owing to the small size of the pool of patients treated before Marketing Authorization, serious AEs are likely to be rare; and even with a database of 4000 patients, in some indications there are only likely to be a few serious AEs. Therefore, a meaningful comparison with a control group will probably not be possible. This generalization does not apply to potentially toxic drugs, such as cancer chemotherapy, and will of course depend upon the background noise from the disease being treated. If the AEs are type B events then the denominator must only include those patients who have taken the drug for a sufficient length of time, which is usually more than 5 days.

Withdrawals

All withdrawals should be listed with their cause. Those due to adverse effects of treatment should be treated similarly to serious AEs; this includes those withdrawn due to abnormal laboratory tests.

Deaths

All deaths should be listed and assessed as for serious AEs, and compared with the number of deaths expected in the study population. They should be examined for any common variables.

Incidence rate

The crude incidence rate is the number of subjects with the AE divided by the number exposed to the drug. In pre-marketing clinical trials the numerator is assessed by the collection of AEs and the number of each AE on the investigational drug is compared with the number on placebo to get the relative risk compared with placebo. Note, however, that it is the relative risk of that AE, not ADR. This will be dealt with further later, but first it is necessary to look at the problems collecting the numerator, the AEs.

The numerator

The incidence rate of AEs will depend upon the method used for their collection. Presuming that an AE occurs in a patient whilst on the investigational drug or placebo, there are numerous factors that will influence whether or not it is analysed at the end of the clinical trial.

- The patient experiencing an AE may not remember it, depending upon its severity, or may presume that it is nothing to do with the drug and, therefore, not report it, or may be too embarrassed to report it if it concerns a 'taboo' area. If it is severe and the patient thinks that it is due to the drug, then the patient may stop the drug and not report back to the doctor, thereby becoming a 'withdrawal'.

- The doctor may not allow a patient to report the AE if he is hurried or has a brusque manner. The doctor may not record the AE if he or she does not think that it is due to the drug, despite the protocol's exhortations.

Other methods, such as diary cards, questionnaires and checklists, collect a different set of the AEs that actually occurred to the patient; therefore, it is therefore not possible to mix them together to calculate an incidence rate.

Let us presume that all of the AEs are collected by spontaneous reporting and a standard question and that the AE we are concerned with is 'headache'. A decision must be made about whether it is better to calculate the numerator as the number of patients complaining of headache during the trial or whether the number of headaches per patient or both is needed (Cato *et al.*, 1983). Looking first at the 'number of patients complaining of headache'. Unfortunately, patients on placebo may 'catch' the same type of AE as the patients on active drug, and this will distort the analysis. Presuming that the headache has occurred as part of flu and has been reported, then the doctor may record it as: headache; headaches, fever and general aches; headaches, fever, general aches: diagnosis flu; or just flu or 'viral infection'. So the same patient may have different words recorded, depending upon the investigator, as follows:

- headache
- headache, fever and general muscular aches
- flu or viral infection.

When it comes to analysis of the AEs the method of counting is important. Grouping of symptoms when they have different mechanisms or aetiologies is wrong in the first instance. A drug-related effect may be drowned by unrelated events with different mechanisms. The other end of the scale, where the AEs are split into very small groups using the patient's actual words, is too far in the other direction, for instance counting separately right- and left-sided headaches. These processes are sometimes referred to as 'lumping and splitting'. The degree of grouping must make clinical sense, having the same mechanism or pathology (i.e. events that probably represent the same phenomenon). This is best done by scanning all the AEs to see whether there is a natural clinical grouping. The same symptom complex in many cases may represent a new ADR and should be counted separately from those cases with just a single symptom. So there may be headaches occurring in three categories:

- headaches alone
- headaches with other symptoms
- headaches as part of a diagnosis.

This makes it important that the investigator is instructed to group concurrent signs and symptoms together and give a diagnosis where possible. There is nothing to prevent grouping the first two categories together if, separately, they are equally represented in both the investigational drug group and the control group. The next hurdle is the classification of the AE using a dictionary. If different coders classify the same event under different terms then the incidence rates will of course be incorrect. The bigger the study, the bigger the problem. See also Chapter 12.

In large-scale placebo-controlled studies there is a problem with the number of different types of AE; there can easily be over 100 different types of event. When these are compared statistically between the investigational drug and the control group using $p < 0.05$ there are likely to be several statistically different results purely by chance. One of the solutions to this problem of multiple comparisons has been to adjust the p value required for each comparison so that the overall value remains at $p < 0.05$ (e.g. Bonferroni inequality) (Dunnett and Goldsmith, 1981). This sacrifices some sensitivity for specificity. Another approach is to use $p < 0.05$ for each comparison, realizing that there will be 1 in 20 false positives, but using it to generate hypotheses rather than test them (Enas, 1991). Hence, if formal testing is performed, then the nominal significance level should be used to flag the AE without adjustment in order to maximize power (Phillips *et al.*; 2000); see also Chapter 6. Further examination of the clinical details may then provide data to prove or rebut the hypothesis, e.g. common clinical characteristics, time to onset, etc.

So far there is the presumption that the unit of time for the event to occur has been short and constant (i.e. the same number finished the study as started). This is very rarely true. In this circumstance the crude incidence rate is satisfactory, but in longer studies there are likely to be withdrawals; this will alter the denominator and perhaps the numerator. If it is presumed that satisfactory statistical significance has been shown between the incidence rate in the investigational drug group compared with the control group, then the attributable incidence rate for the drug-related event should not be arrived at solely by subtracting the placebo rate from that of the active group, but should be given with confidence intervals. If specific ADRs have a negligible background incidence with objective data then it is possible to calculate an ADR incidence rate, but these are extremely rare.

The denominator

The total denominator in UK licence applications (1987–1989) varied from 43 to 15 962; median 1528 (Rawlins and Jefferys, 1991). The numbers of patients included in studies before MAA/NDA appear to be increasing substantially. A study of 15 products in the USA from 1994 to 2000 gave the figures shown in Table 4.4.

Table 4.4 Mean and median total number of subjects per application for biopharmaceuticals, new medical entities and new active substances (Reichert, 2001). Reproduced by permission of Drug Information Association

Products	Years	Number	Mean	Median
Biopharmaceuticals excluding recombinant protein products	1994–2000	12	1014	960
Biopharmaceuticals including recombinant protein products	1994–2000	15	5160	1007
New medical entities	1998	17	5697	4325
New medical entities	1999	19	4980	5435
New active substances	1995–1999	23	4478	NA

Incidence rates with confidence intervals only apply to the group of patients tested, and it may not be possible to extrapolate this to the general population or to a subsection of that population. Pre-marketing clinical trials have rigorous exclusion criteria, often excluding the very old, the young, those who are pregnant, those with concomitant disease and those with abnormal laboratory tests.

Having established that the investigational drug has a certain incidence rate of AEs (with confidence intervals), within the trial groups there may be subgroups with very large differences in incidence rates varying from almost 0 per cent to 100 per cent. These must, therefore, be looked at as well as the factors that govern them. Many factors or variables need consideration, not all being relevant for all studies. These include:

- Patient factors – age, sex, weight, race, country or centre, concomitant disease, indication, severity, alcohol and/or tobacco usage.

- Drug factors – dose or blood level, formulation, route of administration, duration, comparator therapy and concomitant therapy.

The number of patients in each subgroup may be so small that the power of the study is insufficient to show any differences and, therefore, it will be necessary to pool experience from as many of the pre-marketing trials as possible. However, this may still leave many subgroups inadequately represented.

During the pre-marketing studies, serious AEs will have been notified rapidly whilst the minor AEs will accumulate slowly as the studies progress and the CRFs are returned to the sponsor. At any one time the numerator for the serious AEs will be known accurately, but there will be only an estimate of the total denominator until the end of the study.

As already mentioned, many subgroups will not have been exposed to the drug by the time of marketing, and life table analysis will be required for exposures of different durations. The time to onset of a type A ADR depends upon the pharmacokinetics of the drug. If the various factors in the pharmacokinetic equation remain equal, then all the patients who are going to have a particular reaction should have had it by the time that the steady state has been reached for a particular tissue, the incidence rate after that time becoming low. However, for type B ADRs, depending upon hypersensitivity, the chance of hypersensitivity occurring before 5 days of treatment at the first exposure to a drug is low and then increases after the first week. These ADRs with a varying hazard rate should use the number of patients exposed for a sufficient length of time as a denominator. On the other hand, there are other ADRs with an almost constant hazard rate (e.g. thromboembolism with oral contraceptives), and under this circumstance the denominator is patient weeks/months.

Although an incidence rate for common type A AEs can be given for the investigational drug and possibly for placebo or standard drug from the clinical trial data, rare type A or B ADRs may be absent or only present in ones or twos in the whole trial programme. In this case, the small denominators for placebo and/or comparator drug will not allow a valid comparison, and a cohort study of historical controls will often be necessary to establish the background incidence in the population (Guess, 1991, 1994).

Final analysis of data

The global index of safety

This method uses a group of specialists who assign scores, 1–5, rating the 'severity' of each type of event. It was used for an antipsychotic drug for schizophrenia (Sacristan *et al.*, 2001). The acknowledged limitations of this method mean that it cannot be recommended.

Suggested method

The first essential is to have the resolve to find any ADRs present. Although the main aim will be to establish the presence of type A reactions, the data may contain individual type B ADRs. The grouping of trials in preparation for the final analysis, as described in the 4th edition of this book, may suggest areas for special attention. When all the data from pre-marketing studies are available they must be analysed by a blend of statistical and group causality techniques.

Statistical (descriptive): the incidence of each AE with the investigational drug is compared with the control. Since there may be over a 100 different types of AE in the database, every 100 comparisons should produce five significant differences at the $p = 0.05$ level purely by chance, i.e. very sensitive. Therefore, a further statistical comparison should be done using a technique to account for these multiple comparisons, e.g. Bonferroni, i.e. more specific. This will result in three groups.

Group 1 contains those AEs where there is no significant difference between the patient incidence in the investigational drug group and any control group. It is unlikely that any of these will prove to be a true ADR.

Group 2 contains those AEs where there is a statistical difference, which disappears when account has been taken of the multiple comparisons. These may include ADRs, but it is not very likely.

Group 3 contains those AEs where there is a statistical difference after allowance has been made for multiple comparisons. These are likely to be ADRs.

The next step is to look at Group 3 AEs for evidence of other clinical, demographic and laboratory differences between the events occurring in the investigational drug group and the control drug group; this may help to confirm or refute a causal relationship:

- Are there *a priori* hypotheses from drugs of the same class, animal or human pharmacology, animal toxicology, concurrent disease or disease characteristics, analysis of individual studies or individual cases during clinical development?

- Are there demographic differences (age, sex, race, nationality, etc.)?

- Is there a dose relationship?

- Is there temporal clustering related to the expected time to onset of the particular event, i.e. five times the half-life? Consider a statistical comparison for that time period (hazard function).

- Are there differences in the AE: severity, concurrent medication, associated symptoms, associated laboratory abnormalities, course of AE including withdrawals?

- Is there investigator causality?

- Is there biological plausibility?

This should then be repeated with Group 2 events. Further statistical analysis may be appropriate, e.g. event incidence for AEs that recur during treatment.

In Group 1 there may be a rare ADR. There may be a few extra events in the investigational drug group but not reaching the level of significance. These may include type B reactions or interactions with other drugs or diseases.

Finally, a decision should be reached as to whether a certain event is an ADR or not, and for ADRs whether any particular group is susceptible.

Inadequate reporting of safety data from clinical trials

It is essential that whoever is responsible for the safety aspects of a trial ensures that all the appropriate measures are included in the protocol and that the findings are included in the clinical study report. A survey of 192 published randomised drug trials in seven different indications (total 130 074 patients) showed that the quality and quantity of safety reporting to be variable and largely inadequate (Ioannidis and Lau, 2001). Severity of AEs and laboratory-determined toxicity was adequately defined in only 39 per cent and 29 per cent of reports respectively. Only 46 per cent of trials stated the frequency of specific reactions for stopping treatment due to toxicity, and the median space allocated to safety results was only 0.3 of a page.

Another survey of 185 clinical trials showed that 14 per cent made no mention of ADRs; 32 per cent could not be fully evaluated, either because numbers were not given for each treatment arm (52 per cent) or because a generic statement was made without full details (48 per cent). Details as to how clinical events had been recorded was given in only 15 per cent of cases, and similar details on patient symptoms in 17 per cent of trials. Only 49 per cent stated how severity had been defined. The median amount of space used for safety data in the results and discussion sections was 5.8 per cent (Loke and Derry, 2001).

Seventeen licensing applications for drugs used for post-menopausal hormone therapy were obtained from the Finnish Drug Agency, despite opposition from some pharmaceutical companies. They were examined for cardiovascular and thromboembolic events or superficial phlebitis. The trials and their reporting of unanticipated AEs were mostly inadequate. Many trials were of very short duration, the methods by which AEs were monitored and how reasons for withdrawals were assessed were unclear, and sometimes reporting was superficial. Adverse effects resulting in withdrawals, or the group in which withdrawals occurred, were not always reported. Examples of superficial reporting included 'one death, unrelated to treatment' (the reason was not specified) and 'one cancer' (type unspecified); a common statement was that 'there were no (serious) adverse effects'. How this conclusion was obtained was usually unclear, as was whether the fate of all patients allocated was known and whether only events thought to be drug related were included. In one application, a trial report stated that 'during the study, four serious adverse experiences, all in the placebo group, were reported'. Only when looking through the detailed tables did the reviewers find three cases of cardiovascular events in the hormone group. Either the authors regarded cancer but not angina or palpitations requiring hospital treatment as serious, or the summary text was purposefully misleading (Hemminki and McPherson, 2000).

Common errors made in reporting safety information (Ioannidis and Lau, 2002) are:

- Not reporting any safety data at all.

- Making only vague statements, such as 'the medication was well tolerated'.

- Not specifying a breakdown of events per study arm.

- Lumping different kinds of adverse effects under broad categories.

- Not providing severity, or lumping together numbers for different severity levels, and failing to define the scales used for categorizing severity.

- Giving p-values for comparison of events without numbers per severity level.

- Reporting only the most common events.

- Not providing information on AEs that lead to discontinuation of treatment.

- Providing data on subgroups without that for the total population.

- Over-interpreting the absence of adverse effects for small sample sizes.

- Reporting events without proper data on the observational unit.

Possible solutions for the improvement of the study of AEs associated with highly active antiretroviral therapy in AIDS have been proposed by Carr (2002). These include developing regulatory guidance and consensus methods, active reporting of AEs and a greater number of patients.

Conclusions

As far as ADRs are concerned, the clinical trial programme for a new drug needs to be based on the known problems found with similar drugs and the results of animal studies. The results of the healthy volunteer studies need to be assessed carefully for potential ADRs and then interpreted with previous findings from the animal studies. Each clinical trial will contribute information concerning the ADR profile of the drug, and each study protocol should be considered carefully in order to make the most of the drug exposure. The overall development programme plan must be balanced, such that questionnaires and checklists are used at the right stage with sufficient numbers of patients in order to have a reasonable chance to distinguish between the investigational drug and its controls.

The early clinical trials should be designed to distinguish the ADRs of the new drug from those of placebo-treated patients where this is possible. Later clinical trials will concentrate on comparisons with its potential competitors. Certain clinical trials may be allotted the task of monitoring for specific ADRs.

All patients in clinical trials should be asked a standard open question to elicit AEs at each study visit and given the opportunity to reply. Adverse symptoms should be followed up by clinical examination and/or investigations to search for objective confirmation. In those cases where the drug is withdrawn, the results of dechallenge should be observed, preferably without addition of other treatment either in substitution for the original drug or for treatment of the AE. Any investigations found to be abnormal at the time of the AE should be repeated. Uncontrolled studies before marketing should be restricted and should be documented and monitored as closely as the normal double-blind randomized clinical trials.

Whoever is responsible for the analysis of safety data should be able to review the protocols and have an input into their design with future safety analyses in mind. There will be many reasons why the clinical trials cannot be completely standardized, but there should be a 'by default' standard trial protocol that can be altered when necessary. The aim should not be to have completely standardized protocols, but to have them consistent: i.e. using standard safety modules where possible, and where this is not possible making certain that the analyses will not be made more difficult. This is especially true of uncontrolled trials, where a standard protocol can often be used. Similarly, named patients can still follow a standard protocol designed solely for that purpose. Uncontrolled studies should not be an opportunity for investigators to follow their own whims.

Future aspirations

These include:

- More attention to the lowest effective dose.

- Removal of legal restriction on access to company pre-marketing data to enable further research similar to that of Hemminki and McPherson (2000).

- Reappraisal of the pros and cons of measuring various laboratory parameters.

- Improvement in individual case follow-up.

- More information on the preferences of regulatory authorities as to the quantity, quality and presentation of safety data for the MAA/NDA.

- Better publication of information on adverse effects in clinical trial publications.

Acknowledgements

We are grateful to Dr Andrew Lockton for his contribution to the section on Phase I studies and to Dr Han de Gier for contributing the entire section on the 'Effects of drugs on skilled perfomance' and finally to Dr Marianne Keisu for her helpful comments.

References

ABPI/British Paediatric Association (1996). *Licensing Medicines for Children*. Association of the British Pharmaceutical Industry, ISBN 09500491 74.

Adamson H, Jacobs A and Warrington S (1998). Normal values for electrocardiogram intervals in young healthy subjects. *Int J Pharm Med* **12**: 289–291.

Aitken RCB (1969). Measurement of feelings using analogue scales. *Proc R Soc Med* **62**: 989–993.

Altman LK (2001). FDA faults John Hopkins over process in fatal asthma study. *New York Times*, 3 July.

Avery CW, Bertram PL, Allison B and Mandell N (1967). Systematic errors in the evaluation of side effects. *Am J Psychiatry* **123**: 875–878.

Anon. (1985). (Leader) Death of a volunteer. *Br Med J* **290**: 1369–1370.

Avorn J (1997). Including elderly patients in clinical trials. *Br Med J* **315**: 1033–1034.

Barbone F, McMahon AD, Davey PG *et al.* (1998). Assocation of road-traffic accidents with benzodiazepine use. *Lancet* **352**: 1331–1336.

Barrington P, Bowden MW and Dewland PM (1990). Arrhythmias in the normal heart. In *7th International Conference on Pharmaceutical Medicine*. Abstract 24-5108.

Bashaw ED (1992). Application of clinical pharmacological tools to facilitate clinical drug development. In *DIA Conference, Methods and Examples for Assessing Benefit/Risk and Safety for New Drug Application*, 20–21 July.

Bateman DN and McElhatton P (1997). National system for monitoring all drug use in pregnancy already exists. *Br med J* **314**: 1414–1415.

Beard K (1991). Special considerations in the assessment of adverse drug reactions in the elderly. *Pharm Med* **5**: 37–48.

Benjafield J and Adams-Webber J (1976). The golden section hypothesis. *Br J Psychol* **67**: 11–17.

Bernheim JL (1994). The clinical activity biases on the estimation of attributable drug side-effects. In *European Medicines Research, Perspectives in Pharmatoxicology and Pharmacovigilance*, Fracchia GN (ed.). IOS Press: 310–321.

Boisseau A, Begaud B, Albin H and Dangoumau J (1980). Evaluation d'un diagnostic d'effets indesirables des medicaments avec un recul de six mois. *Thérapie* **35**: 577–580.

Borghi C, Pallavivi G, Comi D, Lombardo M *et al.* (1984). Comparison of three different methods of monitoring unwanted effects during antihypertensive therapy. *Int J Clin Pharmacol Ther Toxicol* **22**(6): 324–328.

Brown JS, Kaitin KI, McAuslane N, Thomas KE *et al.* (1996). Population exposure required to assess clinical safety: report to the International Conference on Harmonization Working Group. *Drug Inf J* **30**: 17–27.

Bulpitt CJ and Fletcher AE (1990). The measurement of quality of life in hypertensive patients, a practical approach. *Br J Clin Pharmacol* **30**: 353–364.

Busto U, Sellers EM, Naranjo CA, Cappell H *et al.* (1986). Withdrawal reaction after long-term therapeutic use of benzodiazepines. *N Engl J Med* **315**: 854–859.

Cancer Research Campaign Working Party (1980). Trials and tribulations: thoughts on the organisation of multicentre clinical studies. *Br Med J* **281**: 918–920.

Carlsson AM (1983). Assessment of chronic pain: 1. Aspects of the reliability and validity of the visual analogue scale. *Pain* **16**: 87–101.

Carr A (2002). Improvement of the study, analysis, and reporting of adverse events associated with antiretroviral therapy. *Lancet* **360**: 81–85.

Cato A and Cached L (1988). How to deal with a sudden, unexpected death in clinical studes. In *Clinical Trials and Tribulations*, Cato AE (ed.). Marcel Dekker.

Cato AE, Cook L, Starbuck R and Heatherington D (1983). Methodologic approach to adverse events applied to Bupropion clinical trials. *J Clin Psychiatry* **44**(5, Sect. 2): 187–190.

Charlier CJ, Grenez OE, Maes VA, Smet HC *et al.* (1999). Invloed van geneesmiddelen op de rijvaardigheid [Impairing effects of medicinal drugs on driving performance]. Belgian Institutue for Traffic Safety (BIVV): Brussels.

Charlton R (2000). Research: is an 'ideal' questionnaire possible? *Int J Clin Pract* **54**(6): 356–359.

Choonara I, Gill A and Nunn A (1996). Drug toxicity and surveillance in children. *Br J Clin Pharmacol* **42**: 407–410.

CIOMS (1983). *Safety Requirements for the First Use of New Drugs and Diagnostic Agents in Man.* Council for International Organisation of Medical Sciences: Geneva.

Cohen JS (2001). Dose discrepancies between the *Physicians' Desk Reference* and the medical literature, and their possible role in the high incidence of dose-related adverse events. *Arch Intern Med* **161**: 957–964.

Conrad KA (1995). Clinical pharmacology and drug safety: lessons from hirudin. *Clin Pharmacol Ther* **58**(2): 123–126.

Cook M and Ferner RE (1993). Adverse drug reactions: who is to know? *Br Med J* **307**: 480–481.

Cornelia IRL, Kipferler P and Hasford J (1997). Drug use assessment and risk evaluation in pregnancy – The PEGASUS-project. *Pharmacoepidemiol Drug Saf* **6**(Suppl 3): S37–S42.

Cornelissen PAM (1997). A shared responsibility. Welcome address at the *Symposium on Road Safety in Europe*, European Parliament, 14 October, Brussels.

CPMP (1997). Points to consider: the assessment of the potential for QT interval prolongation by non-cardiovascular medicinal products. *EMEA*, December, (CPMP/986/96).

Craig JJ and Morrow JI (1997). Register of women who take drugs during pregnancy has been set up. *Br Med J* **314**: 603.

Croog SH, Levine S, Testa MA, Brown B *et al.* (1986). The effects of anti-hypertensive therapy on the quality of life. *N Engl J Med* **314**: 1657–1664.

Cross J, Lee H, Westelinck A, Nelson J *et al.* (2002). Postmarketing drug dosage changes of 499 FDA-approved new molecular entities, 1980–1999. *Pharmacoepidemiol Drug Saf* **11**: 439–446.

Dangoumau J, Evreux JC and Jouglard J (1978). Methode d'imputabilite des effets indesirables des medicaments. *Thérapie* **33**: 373–381.

Darragh A, Lambe R, Kenny M and Brick I (1985). Sudden death of a volunteer. *Lancet* **1**: 93–95.

Davidson CS, Leevy CM and Chamberlayne EC (eds.) (1979). Fogarty conference. *Guidelines for Detection of Hepatotoxicity due to Drugs and Chemicals.* USA Department of Health Education and Welfare (NIH publication number 79-313).

De Gier JJ (1995). Drugs other than alcohol and driving in the European Union. *Tech Report HP 95-54.* Institute for Human Psychopharmacology, University of Limburg, Maastricht, The Netherlands.

De Gier JJ (1998a). Survey on warning systems for medicinal drugs affecting driving performance. *Tech Report DGC*: 98-02. Institute for Human Psychopharmacology, University of Maastricht, The Netherlands.

De Gier JJ (1998b). Drugs and driving research: application of results by drug regulatory authorities. *Hum Psychopharmacol Clin Exp* **13**: S133–S136.

DeLap RJ, Fourcroy JL and Fleming GA (1996). Fetal harm due to paternal drug exposure: a potential issue in drug development. *Drug Inf J* **30**: 359–364.

Del Rio GMC, Alvarez Gonzalez FJ, Gonzalez Luque JC (2001). Guía de prescripción farmacológica y seguridad vial. Dirrección General de Tráfico, Madrid.

DeMets D, Friedman LM and Furberg C (1980). Counting in clinical trials. *N Engl J Med* **302**(16): 924–925.

Demoly P, Kropf R and Pichler WJ (1999). Drug hypersensitivity: questionnaire. *Allergy* **54**: 999–1003 (requests for copies to demoly@montp.inserm.fr).

DePonti F, Poluzzi E and Montanaro N (2000). QT-interval prolongation by non-cardiac drugs: lessons to be learned from recent experience. *Eur J Clin Pharmacol* **56**: 1–18.

De Vries BM, Hughes GS and Huysen LS (1991). Screening for illicit drug use in drug development studies. *Drug Inf J* **25**: 49–53.

Dimenas E, Dahlof C, Olofsson B and Wiklund I (1989). CNS related subjective symptoms during treatment with β adrenoceptor antagonists (atenolol and metropolol) two double-blind controlled studies. *Br J Clin Pharmacol* **28**: 527–534.

Donovan S, Mills J, Goulder MA, Dumelow NW *et al.* (1996). Electronic patient diaries: a pilot study. *Appl Clin Trials* **5**: 40–49.

Downing RW, Rickels K and Meyers F (1970). Side reactions in neurotics, 1: a comparison of two methods of assessent. *J Clin Pharmacol* **10**: 289–297.

Dunnett C and Goldsmith C (1981). When and how to do multiple comparisons. In *Statistics in the Pharmaceutical Industry*, Buncher CR and Tsay JV (eds). Marcel Dekker: 397–432.

Eisenberg D, Davis R, Ettner S, Appel S *et al.* (1998). Trends in alternative medicine use in the United States, 1990–1997. *J Am Asoc Med* **280**: 1569–1575.

Ellenberg SS, Fleming TR and DeMets DL (2002). *Data Monitoring Committees in Clinical Trials.* Wiley: Chichester.

Emanueli A (1984). A simple algorithm for assessing causality of adverse reactions. *Drug Inf J* **18**: 303–306.

Enas GG (1991). Making decisions about safety in clinical trials – the case for inferential statistics. *Drug Inf J* **25**: 439–446.

Enas GG, Dornseif BE, Sampson CB, Rockhold FW *et al.* (1989). Monitoring versus interim analysis of clinical trials: a perspective from the pharmaceutical industry. *Control Clin Trials* **10**: 57–70.

Fairweather WR (1996). Integrated safety analysis statistical issues in the assessment of safety in clinical trials. *Drug Inf J* **30**: 875–879.

Fayers PM and Jones SDR (1983). Measuring and analysing the quality of life in cancer clinical trials. A review. *Stat Med* **2**: 429–446.

FDA (2002). The clinical evaluation of QT/QTc interval prolongation and proarrhythmic potential for non-antiarrhythmic drugs. *Preliminary concept paper*, 15 November; revised 28 January 2003.

Fieldstad LM, Kurjatkin O and Cobert BL (1996). A template for adverse event reporting in licensing agreements. *Drug Inf J* **30**: 965–971.

Finney DJ (1965). The design and logic of a monitor of drug use. *J Chron Dis* **18**: 77–98.

Fisher S, Bryant SG and Kluge PM (1987). Detecting adverse drug reactions in post-marketing surveillance: interview validity. *Drug Inf J* **21**: 173–183.

Fonseca M, Freitas A, Pfafffenbach G and Mendes GBB (1997). Drug use in pregnancy: a pharmacoepidemiological study. Late breaker abstract. In *13th International Conference on Pharmacoepidemiology*, 24–27 August, Florida, USA.

Friedman LM, Furberg C and Demets DL (1985). *Fundamentals of Clinical Trials*, 2nd edition. PSG Publishing Company: 270.

Gait JE and Goldsmith D (2000). Should serious adverse events requiring expedited regulatory reporting be unblinded? *Int J Pharm Med* **14**: 37–39.

Gait JE, Smith S and Brown SL (2000). Evaluation of safety data from controlled clinical trials: the clinical principles explained. *Drug Inf J* **34**: 273–287.

Garvey TQ (1991). Can there really be an integrated safety summary? *Drug Inf J* **25**: 501–511.

Goldberg LI, Besselaar GH, Arnold JD, Lamberger L *et al.* (1975). Phase I investigations. *Clin Pharmacol Ther* **18**(5): 643–646.

Grant S, Aitchison T, Henderson E, Christie J *et al.* (1999). A comparison of the reproducibility and the sensitivity to change of visual analogue scales, Borg scales and Likert scales in normal subjects during submaximal exercise. *Chest* **116**(5): 1208–1217.

Guess HA (1991). Pharmacoepidemiology in pre-approval clinical trial safety monitoring. *J Clin Epidemiol* **44**(8): 851–857.

Guess HA (1994). Premarketing applications of pharmacoepidemiology. In *Pharmacoepidemiology*, 2nd edition, Strom BL (ed.). Wiley: Chichester; 353–365.

Guyatt GH, Townsend M, Berman LB and Keller JL (1987). A comparison of Likert and visual analogue scales for measuring change in function. *J Chron Dis* **40**: 1129–1133.

Hagman M, Jonsson D and Ilhelmson L (1977). Prevalence of angina pectoris and myocardial infarction in a general population sample of Swedish men. *Acta Med Scand* **201**: 571–577.

Hanley JA and Lippman-Hand A (1983). If nothing goes wrong, is everything alright? Interpreting zero numerators. *J Am Med Assoc* **249**: 1743–1745.

Harry JD, Baber N and Posner J (1995). HIV screening in healthy volunteers. *Br J Clin Pharmacol* **39**: 213.

Hasford J (1996). Drug utilization during pregnancy and its effects on fetal outcome. The Pegasus Project. Abstract. In *1st Congress of the European Drug Utilization Research Group. Rational Drug Use in Europe. Challenges for the 21st Century*, 27–30 June.

Haverkamp W, Breithardt G, Camm AJ, Jansen MJ *et al.* (2000). The potential for QT prolongation and pro-arrhythmia by non-anti-arrhythmic drugs: clinical and regulatory impllictions. Report on a policy Conference of the European Society of Cardiology. *Cardiovasc Res* **47**: 219–233.

Hearne R, Connolly A and Sheehan J (2002). Alcohol abuse: prevalence and detection in a general hospital. *J R Soc Med* **95**: 84–87.

Heerdink ER, Urquhart J and Leufkens HG (2002). Changes in prescribed drug usage after market introduction. *Pharmacoepidemiol Drug Saf* **11**: 447–453.

Hemminki E and McPherson K (2000). Value of drug-licensing documents in studying the effect of postmenopausal hormone therapy on cardiovascular disease. *Lancet* **355**: 566–569.

Herxheimer A (1991). How much drug in the tablet? *Lancet* **337**: 346–348.

Higginbotham FM and Rolan PE (1997). Clinical pharmacology studies in women of child-bearing potential. *Int J Pharm Med* **11**: 7–9.

Homma M, Hirayama H and Ichikawa K (1994). Studies on requirements for the assessment of clinical safety in nonsteroidal anti-inflammatory drugs. *Drug Inf J* **28**: 413–418.

Hounslow NJ, Tamarazians S, Wisema WT, Mann S *et al.* (1987). Use of a visual analogue meter. *Br J Clin Pharmacol* **23**(1): 117–118.

Huskisson EC (1974). Measurement of pain. *Lancet* **2**: 1127–1131.

Huskisson EC and Wojtulewski JA (1974). Measurement of side effects of drugs. *Br Med J* **2**: 698–699.

ICH (2002). M4 – Organisation of the Common Technical Document for the Registration of Pharmaceuticals for Human Use.

Idänpään-Heikkilä J (1983). *A Review of Safety Information Obtained from Phase I, II and III Clinical Investigation of Sixteen Selected Drugs*. USA Department of Health and Human Services, Public Health Service Food and Drug Administration.

Ioannidis JPA and Lau J (2001). Completeness in safety reporting in randomised trials: an evaluation of 7 medical areas. *J Am Med Assoc* **285**: 437–443.

Ioannidis JPA and Lau J (2002). Improving safety reporting from randomised trials. *Drug Saf* **25**: 77–84.

Jackson D (1990a). The assessment of tolerance and side-effects in non-patient volunteers. In *Early Phase Drug Evaluation in Man*, O'Grady J and Linit OI (eds). Macmillan: 197.

Jackson D (1990b). The assessment of tolerance and side effects in non-patient volunteers. In *Risk Factors for ADR – Epidemiological Approach*, Weber E, Lawson DH and Hoigne R (eds). *Agents Actions* (Suppl 29): 199.

Jaeschke J, Singer J and Guyatt GH (1990). Comparison of seven-point and visual analogue scales. *Control Clin Trials* **11**: 43–51.

Jagathesan R, Lewis LD and Mant TGK (1995). A retrospective analysis of the prevalence of HIV seropositivity and its demographics in the normal healthy volunteer population of a phase I clinical drug study unit. *Br J Clin Pharmacol* **39**: 463–464.

Jeffreys DB (1995). Children in research: ethical and practical issues. In *DIA Conference, Future Outlook for New Pharmaceuticals Post-1995*, 2–5 April.

Joelson S, Joelson IB and Wallander MA (1997). Geographical variation in adverse event reporting rates in clinical trials. *Pharmacoepidemiol Drug Saf* **6**(Suppl 3): S31–S35.

Johnson-Pratt LR and Bush J (1996). Activities of the pharmaceutical industry relative to the FDA gender guidelines. *Drug Inf J* **30**: 709–714.

Jones DR, Fayers PM and Simons J (1987). Measuring and analysing quality of life in cancer clinical trials: a review. In Aaronson NK and Beckmann J (eds). *The Quality of Life of Cancer Patients Monograph Series of the European Organisation for Research on Treatment of Cancer (EORTC)*, **17**: 41–62.

Joyce CRB, Zutshi DW, Hrubes V and Mason RM (1975). Comparison of fixed interval and visual analogue scales for rating chronic pain. *Eur J Clin Pharmacol* **8**: 415–420.

Kalra L, Jackson SHD and Swift CG (1993). Assessment of changes in psychomotor performance of elderly subjects. *Br J Clin Pharmacol* **36**: 383–389.

Karch FE and Lasagna L (1977). Toward the operational identification of adverse drug reactions. *Clin Pharmacol Ther* **21**(3): 247–254.

Kearns I (1996). Introduction: drug development for infants and children: rescuing the therapeutic orphan. *Drug Inf J* **30**: 1121–1123.

Kitler ME (1989). The elderly in clinical trials: regulatory concerns. *Drug Inf J* **23**: 123–137.

Klareskog L, Moreland L, Cohen SB, Sanda M *et al.* (2001). Global safety and efficacy of up to five years of Etanercept therapy. *Am Coll Rheumatol*: Abstr 150.

Klincewicz SL, Clark JA and LaFrance ND (2001). A review and analysis of key regulations and guidelines concerning the safety sections of the Investigator's Brochure. *Drug Inf J* **35**: 347–355.

Kramer MS and Hutchinson TA (1984). The Yale algorithm. *Drug Inf J* **18**: 283–291.

Lack I, Record RG, McKeowen T and Edward JH (1968). The incidence of malformations in Birmingham 1956–59. *Teratology* **1**: 263–280.

Lapierre YD (1975). Evaluation des effects secondaire chez les neurotics. Un essai avec les mesoridazin et le placebo. *Can Psychiatr Assoc* **26**: 60–61.

Larson SK, Elwin CE, Gabrielsson J, Paalryow L *et al.* (1982). Do teratogenicity tests serve their objective? *Lancet* **2**: 439.

Lasagna L (1981). Bias in the elucidation of subjective side effects. *Br J Clin Pharmacol* **11**: 111S–113S.

Lasagna L (1984). Techniques for ADR reporting. In *Detection and Prevention of Adverse Drug Reactions*, Bostrom N and Ljungstedt N (eds). Almqvist and Wiksell International: Stockholm; 146.

Leary PM (1991). Adverse reactions in children, special considerations in prevention and management. *Drug Saf* **6**(3): 171–182.

Levine MAJ, Bennett K, Grace E and Tugwell P (1990). Development of a disease specific adverse drug effects index. Abstract. *J Clin Es Pharmacoepidemiol* **4**: 127–128.

Levine RJ (1987). The apparent incompatibility between informed consent and placebo-controlled clinical trials. *Clin Pharm Ther* **42**: 247–249.

Lewis RV (1987). Quantifying side-effects of β-blockers; the role of visual analogue scales. *Hum Toxicol* **6**: 195–201.

Lewis RV, Jackson PR and Ramsey LE (1984). Quantification of side-effects of β-adrenoceptor blockers using visual analogue scales. *Br J Clin Pharmacol* **18**: 325–330.

Lewis RV, Jackson PR and Ramsay LE (1985a). Side-effects of β-adrenoceptor blocking drugs assessed by visual analogue scales. *Br J Clin Pharmacol* **19**: 255–257.

Lewis RV, Jackson PR and Ramsay LE (1985b). Measuring β-adrenocoptor blocker side-effects by visual analogue scales: reproducibility of scoring. Proceedings of the BPS, 10–12 April 275.

Lewis RV, Jackson PR and Ramsay LE (1985c). Measuring side-effects of β-adrenoceptor antagonists: a comparison of two methods. *Br J Clin Pharmacol* **19**: 826–828.

Lineberry C (1991). Approaches to describing common adverse events in the integrated safety summary. *Drug Inf J* **25**: 493–500.

Loke YK and Derry S (2001). Reporting of adverse drug reactions in randomised controlled trials – a systematic survey. *BioMed Central Clin Pharmacol* **1**: 3 (http://www.biomedcentral.com/1472-6904/1/3).

Lundberg RK (1980). Assessment of drugs' side-effects: visual analogue scale versus checklist format. *Percept Motor Skills* **50**: 1067–1073.

Lundström S (1993). Electronic patient diaries. *Appl Clin Trials* **2**(5): 35–37.

Maggini M, Raschetti R, Di Giovambattista G and Rossi A (1997). A population based study on drug use during pregnancy. *Pharmacoepidemiol Drug Saf* **6**(Suppl 2): 591.

Malik M and Camm AJ (2001). Evaluation of drug-induced QT interval prolongation *Drug Saf* **24**(5): 323–351.

Mashford ML (1984). The Australian method of drug-event assessment. *Drug Inf J* **18**: 271–273.

Maxwell C (1978). Sensitivity and accuracy of the visual analogue scale: a psycho-physical classroom experiment. *Br J Clin Pharmacol* **6**: 15–24.

May GS, Demets DL, Friedman LM, Furberg C *et al.* (1981). The randomised clinical trial: bias in analysis. *Circulation* **64**(4): 669–673.

McCormack HM, Horne JDeL and Sheather S (1988). *Psychol Med* **18**: 1001–1019.

McKenzie R, Fried MW, Sallie R, Conjeevaram H *et al.* (1995). Hepatic failure and lactic acidosis due to fialuridine (FIAU), an investigational nucleoside analogue for chronic hepatitis B. *N Engl J Med* **333**: 1099–1105.

Mehlman PT, Highley JD, Faucher P, Lilly AA *et al.* (1994). Hepatitis B outbreak in a drug trial unit; investigation and recommendation. *Commun Dis Rep Rev* **1**: R1–R5.

Mikhail M (1993). The importance of the investigator's brochure. *Appl Clin Trials* **2**(6): 56–58.

Mitchell AA (2000). Special considerations in studies of drug-induced birth defects. In *Pharmacoepidemiology*, 3rd edition, Strom BL (ed.). Wiley: Chichester; 749–763.

Miyazaki K and Saito H (2002). Sponsors' experiences with site management organizations in Japan. *Drug Inf J* **36**: 763–768.

Myers MG, Cairns JA and Singer J (1987). The consent form as a possible cause of side-effects. *Clin Pharm Ther* **42**: 250–253.

Naranjo CA, Busto U and Sellers EM (1980). A reliable method for estimating the probability of adverse drug reactions. *Clin Pharmacol Ther* **27**: 274–275.

Neal H (2001). The contract research organization perspective: audits in central and Eastern European countries. *Drug Inf J* **35**: 475–480.

Neutel CL (1995). Risk of traffic accident injury after a prescription for a benzodiazepine. *Ann Epidemiol* **5**(3): 239–244.

New Zealand Hypertension Study Group (1979). A multicentre open trial of labetalol in New Zealand. *Br J Clin Pharmacol* 179S–182S.

Nickas J (1995). Adverse event data collection and reporting: a discussion of two grey areas. *Drug Inf J* **29**: 1247–1251.

Nickas J (1997). Clinical trial safety surveillance in the new regulatory and harmonization environment: lessons learned from the 'Fialuridine crisis'. *Drug Inf J* **31**: 63–70.

Nony P, Boissel JP, Girard P, Lion L *et al.* (1994). The role of an initial single-blind placebo period in phase I clinical trials. *Fundam Clin Pharmacol* **8**: 185–187.

Norrby SR and Pernet AG (1991). Asssessment of adverse events during drug development: experience with temafloxacin. *J Antimicrob Chemother* **20**: 111–119.

Oates JA (1972). A scientific rationale for choosing patients rather than normal subjects for phase I studies. *Clin Pharmacol Ther* **13**(5), Pt 2: 809–811.

O'Brien A (1995). Licensing of drugs for the elderly. *Pharm Med* **9**: 185–190.

Offerhaus L (1979). Guidelines for evaluation of antihypertensive drugs in man. *Eur J Clin Pharmacol* **16**: 427–430.

O'Hanlon JF (1995). Zopiclone's residual effects on psychomotor and information processing skills involved in complex tasks such as car driving: a critical review. *Eur Psychiatry* **10**: 137S–144S.

O'Hanlon JF, Brookhuis KA, Louwerens JW and Volkerts ER (1986). Performance testing as part of drug registration. In *Drugs and Driving*, O'Hanlon JF and De Gier JJ (eds). Taylor & Francis: London; 311–330.

Onder G, Landi F, Vedova CD, Atkinson H *et al.* (2002). Moderate alcohol consumption and adverse drug reactions among older adults. *Pharmacoepidemiol Drug Saf* **11**: 385–392.

O'Neill RT (1988). Assessment of safety. In *Biopharmaceutical Statistics for Drug Development*, Peace KE (ed.). Marcel Dekker: New York; 543–604.

Ono S, Kodama Y, Nagao T and Toyoshima S (2002). The quality of conduct in Japanese clinical trials: deficiencies found in GCP inspections. *Controll Clin Trials* **23**: 29–41.

Orme M, Harry J, Routledge PA and Hobson S (1989). Healthy volunteer studies in Great Britain: the results of a survey into 12 months activity in this field. *Br J Clin Pharmacol* **27**: 125–133.

Parrott AC and Hindmarsh I (1978). Factor analysis of a sleep evaluation questionnaire. *Psychol Med* **8**: 325–329.

Peat M, Ellis S and Yates RA (1981). The effect of level of depression on the use of visual analogue scales by normal volunteers. *Br J Clin Pharmacol* **12**: 171–178.

Phillips A, Ebutt A, France L and Morgan D (2000). The international Conference on Harmonization Guidelines 'Statistical principles for clinical trials'. Issues in applying the guideline in practice. *Drug Inf J* **31**: 331–348.

Pollock B (1996). Clinical relevance of pharmacogenetic variations for geriatric psychopharmacology. *Drug Inf J* **30**: 669–674.

Powell JR (1986). Healthy volunteers, risk and research. *Drug Intell Clin Pharm* **20**: 776–777.

Ramaekers JG (2003). Performance and behavioural effects of medicinal drugs. In *Medico-legal Aspects of Drugs*, Burns M (ed.). Lawyers & Judges, Publishing Company: Tuscon, AZ; 169–213.

Ramaekers JG, Ansseau M, Muntjewswerff ND, Sweens P *et al.* (1997). Considering the P450 cytochrome system as determining the effects of antidepressants and benzodiazepines on the actual driving performance of outpatients suffering from major depression. *Int Clin Psychopharmacol* **12**: 159–169.

Rawlins MD and Jefferys DB (1991). Study of UK product licence applications containing new active substances, 1987–9. *Br Med J* **302**: 223–225.

Ray WA, Fought RL and Decker MD (1992). Psychoactive drugs and the risk of injurous motor vehicle crashes in elderly drivers. *Am J Epidemiol* **136**: 873–883.

Ramsay LE and Yeo WW (1995). ACE inhibitors, angiotensin II antagonists and cough. *J Hum Hypertens* **9**(Suppl 5): 551–554.

RCP (1986). A report of the Royal College of Physicians. Research on healthy volunteers. *J R Coll Physicians London* **20**(4): 243–257.

Redmond GP (1985). Physiological changes during pregnancy and their implications for pharmacological treatment. *Clin Invest Med* **8**(4): 317–322.

Reichert JM (2001). Clinical development of therapeutic medicines: a biopharmaceutical versus pharmaceutical product comparison. *Drug Inf J* **35**: 337–346.

Reidenberg MM and Lowenthal DT (1968). Adverse non-drug reactions. *N Engl J Med* **279**(13): 678–679.

Reigelman R (1984). Clinical trials. *Ann Intern Med* **3**: 455.

Rickels KR and Downing RW (1970). Side reactions in neurotics. II: can patients judge which symptoms are caused by their medications. *J Clin Pharmacol* **10**: 298–305.

Roberts R (1996). Studies in pediatrics: special issues. In *DIA Conference, Assessing Safety of Investigational Drugs*, 15–16 April.

Royle JM and Snell ES (1986). Medical research on normal volunteers. *Br J Clin Pharmacol* **21**: 548–549.

Rubin JD (1995). *Prescribing in Pregnancy*, 2nd edition. British Medical Journal Publishing Group: London; 1–2.

Rubin JD, Ferencz C and Loffredo C (1993). Use of prescription and non-prescription drugs in pregnancy. *J Clin Epidemiol* **46**(6): 581–589.

Ruskin A (1985). Working causality algorithm for drug–death association. In *The Detection of New Adverse Drug Reactions*, Stephens MDB (ed.). Macmillan Press: London; 235.

Sackett DL and Gent M (1979). Controversy in counting and attributing events in clinical trials. *N Engl J Med* **301**(26): 1410–1412.

Sacristan JA, Gomez JC, Badia X and Kind P (2001). Global index of safety (GIS): a new instrument to assess drug safety. *J Clin Epidemiol* **54**: 1120–1125.

Sanchez J, Costa A, Fresquet A, Abadia S *et al.* (1994). HIV screening 'healthy volunteers' and ethical committees. *Br J Clin Pharmacol* **37**: 469.

Schardein JL (ed.) (1993). *Chemically Induced Birth Defects* 2nd Edition. Marcel Dekker.

Scott E and Cambell G (1998). Interpretation of subgroup analyses in medical device clinical trials. *Drug Inf J* **32**: 213–220.

Scott J and Huskisson EC (1976). Graphic representation of pain. *Pain* **2**: 175–184.

Scott J and Huskisson EC (1979). Accuracy of subjective measurements made with and without previous scores: an important source of error in serial measurements of subjective rates. *Ann Rheum Dis* **38**: 558–559.

Shenfield GM, Robb T and Daguid M (2001). Recording previous ADRs – a gap in the system. *Br J Clin Pharmacol* **51**: 623–626.

Sibille M, Deigat N, Olagnier V, Vital-Durand D *et al.* (1992). Adverse events in phase one studies: a study in 430 healthy volunteers. *Eur J Clin Pharmacol* **42**: 389–393.

Sibille M, Deigat N, Janin A, Kirkessazi S *et al.* (1998). Adverse events in phase I studies: a report on 1015 healthy volunteers. *Eur J Clin Pharmacol* **54**: 13–20.

Simpson RJ, Tiplady B and Skegg DCG (1980). Event recording in a clinical trial of a new medicine. *Br Med J* **280**: 1133–1134.

Skegg DCG and Doll R (1977). The case for recording events in clinical trials. *Br Med J* **2**: 1523–1524.

Skinner JB (1991). On combining studies. *Drug Inf J* **25**: 395–403.

Society of Pharmaceutical Medicine, Pharmacovigilance Group Working Party. (1998). Monitoring drug safety in commercial licensing situations in Europe: a commentary. *Int J Pharm Med* **12**: 55–70.

Spilker B (1984). *Guide to Clinical Studies and Developing Protocols*. Raven Press: 45.

Steare SE and Morganroth J (2002). A rational approach to the planning and analysis of electrocardiogram safety data in clinical trials. *Int J Pharm Med* **16**: 133–140.

Stephens MDB (1984). Assessment of causality in an industrial setting. *Drug Inf J* **18**: 307–313.

Stephens MDB (1988). Clinical trails – the post treatment visit. *J Clin Res Drug Dev* **2**: 193.

Stinson JC, Pears JS, Williams AJ and Cambell RWF (1995). Use of 24 h ambulatory ECG recordings in the assessment of new chemical entities in healthy volunteers. *Br J Clin Pharmacol* **39**: 651–656.

Stone DH (1993). How to design a questionnaire. *Br Med J* **307**: 1264–1266.

Swafford S (1997). Older people take too many drugs. *Br Med J* **314**: 1369.

Tanser PH, Campbell LM, Carranza J, Karrash J *et al.* (2000). Candesartan cilexetil is not associated with cough in hypersensitive patients with enalapril-induced cough. *Am J Hypertens* **13**: 214–218.

Temple RJ (1991a). Access, science, and regulation. *Drug Inf J* **25**(1): 1–11.

Temple RJ (1991b). The regulatory evolution of the integrated safety summary. *Drug Inf J* **25**: 485–492.

Thompson M, Haynes WG and Webb DJ (1993). Screening for human immuno-deficiency virus: a survey of British clinical pharmacology units. *Br J Clin Pharmacol* **36**: 293–301.

Turner WM (1984). The Food and Drug Administration algorithm, Special Workshop, Regulatory. *Drug Inf J* **18**: 259–266.

Vandenburg MJ (1987). Difficulties of a visual analogue scale in the assessment of angina. *Br J Clin Pharmacol* **23**(i): 109–110.

Van laar MW, Volkerts ER and Van Willigenburg APP (1992). Therapeutic effects and effects on actual driving performance of chronically administered buspirone and diazepam in anxious outpatients. *J Clin Psychopharmacol* **12**: 86–95.

Venning GR (1991). How much drug in the tablet. *Lancet* **337**: 670.

Vickers J, Painter MJ, Heptonstall J, Yusof JMH *et al.* (1994). Community Disease Report. Hepatitis B outbreak in a drugs trial unit. Investigation, recommendations. *Commun Dis Rep CDR Rev* **4**: R1–R5.

Vomvouras S and Piergies AA (1995). Gender differences in study events during Phase I trials. *Clin Pharmacol Ther* **136**: PI-3.

Wagner AK, Kosinski M, Kellar S and Ware JC (1994). Influence of a patient completed symptom checklist on the subsequent reporting of AE in a clinical trial interview. Abstract 53A. *Control Clin Trials* **15**(35, Suppl).

Wallander AM-A and Palmer LS (1986). A monitoring system for adverse drug experience in a pharmaceutical company – the integration of pre and postmarketing data. *Drug Inf J* **20**: 225–235.

Wallander M-A, Dimenäs E, Svärdsudd K and Wiklund I (1991). Evaluation of three methods of symptom reporting in a clinical trial of felodipine. *Eur J Clin Pharmcol* **41**: 187–196.

Wallander M-A, Lundberg P and Svärdsudd K (1992). Adverse event monitoring in clinical trials of felodipine and omeprazole. *Eur J Clin Pharmacol* **42**: 517–522.

Weber JCP (1984). Epidemiology of adverse reactions to non-steroidal anti-inflammatory drugs. In *Advances in Inflammatory Research*, Vol. 6, Rainsford KD and Velo GP (eds). Raven Press: 1–7.

Weissman L (1981). Multiple dose phase I trials. Normal volunteers or patients; one viewpoint. *J Clin Pharmacol* **21**: 385–387.

Welch V, Singh G, Strand V, Fries J *et al*. (2001). Patient based method of assessing adverse events in clinical trials in rheumatology: the revised Stanford toxicity index. *J Rheumatol* **28**: 1188–1191.

WHO (1979). *Handbook for Reporting Results of Cancer Treatment*, Offset Publication no. 48. WHO: Geneva.

Wilson JG (1977). Teratogenic effects of environmental chemicals. *Fed Proc* **36**: 1698–1703.

Wolschrijn H, De Gier JJ and De Smet PAGM (1991). Drugs and driving: a new categorization system for drugs affecting psychomotor performance. *Tech Report*. Institute for Drugs, Safety and Behavior, University of Limburg, The Netherlands.

Woodworth TG, Furst DE, Strand V, Kempeni J *et al*. (2001). Standardizing assessment of adverse effects in rheumatology clinical trials. Status of OMERACT toxicity working group March 2000: towards a common understanding of comparative toxicity/safety profiles for antirheumatic therapies. *J Rheumatol* **28**: 1163–1169.

Yuen WC, Peck AW and Burke CA (1985). The subjective effects of dextromethorphan, codeine and diazepam in healthy volunteers. In *Proceedings of the British Pharmacological Society* 10–12 April; 290.

Zarafonetis CJD, Riley PA, Willis PW, Power LH *et al*. (1978). Clinically significant events in a phase I testing program. *Clin Pharmacol Ther* **24**(2): 127–132.

Zeally AK and Aitken RCB (1969). Measurement of mood. *Proc. Roy. Soc. Med.*, **62**, 993–996.

5

Clinical Laboratory Safety Data in Drug Studies

A. Craig

Introduction

Clinical laboratory measurements are an integral component of most drug studies for two major reasons, firstly to act as an efficacy endpoint in monitoring the success or otherwise of therapy and secondly to ensure patient safety on any new drug or reformulation. The pharmaceutical industry rarely employs physicians and scientists with expertise in clinical laboratory medicine. As such, there is a tendency for test selection, data-management and data interpretation to be based on historical knowledge. The industry rarely involves the clinical laboratory in study design, resulting in out-of-date parameters, with little appreciation of the limitation and advantages of specific test programmes.

In major clinical studies, the numerical element in a submission report may consist of 50 per cent laboratory data with many thousands of laboratory test results, which may increase to 80 per cent in phase 1, and early phase 2 studies. Thus, we are concerned with a vast volume of data, particularly related to the assessment of safety.

Why do we do laboratory tests?

- To provide information to support a clinical diagnosis.

- To extend a clinical diagnosis by offering information about causation.

- To indicate the presence of complications, including those due to treatment.

- To monitor prognostic information.

- To monitor the progress of the condition.

- To detect sub-clinical disease (screening).

Changes in serial results may be due to:

- the patient getting better

Stephens' Detection of New Adverse Drug Reactions Fifth Edition edited by John Talbot and Patrick Waller
© 2004 John Wiley & Sons, Ltd   ISBN: 0 470 84552 X

- the patient getting worse

- pre-analytical variation

- analytical variation

- biological variation

all of which demand considerable attention in any clinical study.

It is unfortunate that clinical laboratory systems evolved around automated analytical systems, which were designed for diagnostic and healthcare screening purposes. As such, these have tended to be used as basic screening procedures in drug-study safety monitoring. While it may have economical advantages to undertake a battery of health-care screening tests, is this really appropriate in drug studies? Should not greater attention be given to the chemical characteristics of the compound and the data available from pre-clinical toxicology studies to define the test requirements in later phases? Also, is it appropriate to employ identical tests at phase 1 similar to the later phases? In this respect, the most sensitive analytical procedures for the detection of toxicity should be employed as early as possible in development in order to eliminate compounds with a problem quickly rather than have this delayed to later phases with the resulting cost implications.

Efficacy testing differs significantly from safety monitoring, in that tests are being employed to demonstrate a change, which hopefully will occur in all subjects on active therapy. However, a full appreciation of the test limitations of the endpoint measurement is essential prior to statistical analyses, which must involve information from the clinical laboratory on analytical validation. Also, although analytical validation is a prerequisite, consideration must also be given to possible analytical method changes due to the drug or its metabolites. In safety monitoring, the data volume is large, and even in phase 3 studies only a few subjects may show toxicity effects, thus demanding critical examination of organ-specific tests.

Essentially, there are three different types of clinical laboratory providing services to the pharmaceutical industry. Local independent or hospital-based, central laboratory services and specialist core-research units, and all have a place in clinical studies. Over the last decade there has been favour in the use of centralized facilities, as these laboratories offer an all-encompassing service from study set-up and supplies, through analytical measurements to electronic data transfer to the sponsors facilities, and are compliant with the demands of good laboratory practices (GLPs). There is also demand from the pharmaceutical industry for central services to be provided on a global basis for consistency of data; but, as we shall see later, although global facilities are requested, *Homo sapiens* can hardly be considered to exhibit much degree of consistency. However, there will always be a requirement for local facilities, particularly when the study is concerned with acutely ill patients, e.g. myocardial infarction, stroke, etc., and test assessments are required immediately for patient care. Also, specialist analytical techniques, which may not always be available either locally or centrally, will demand the use of specialist core-clinical or bio-analytical laboratories.

The advantages of the central laboratory are:

- all-encompassing service

- one set of standards, units and reference ranges

- simplified data-management
- comprehensive range of tests
- uniform reporting and interpretation
- demonstrable quality and GLP compliance
- data and project management facilities
- monitoring facility for the sponsor.

The disadvantages are:

- no affiliation to local investigator
- lack of investigator confidence
- transport costs
- stability limitations and sample deterioration
- language issues.

The industry requirement for laboratory services from whatever sources include:

- comprehensive service – logistics, supplies, etc.
- analytical excellence and scientific excellence
- accreditation and documentation
- quality communication and response
- data management and electronic data transfer systems
- user friendly for investigators and monitors.

From this introduction, it should be apparent that the involvement of the clinical laboratory at an early stage would markedly enhance the completion of successful studies from the laboratory viewpoint and reduce potential problems related to logistics, test selection, data handling and interpretation.

Factors that influence interpretation of clinical laboratory data

Factors that may influence the interpretation of clinical laboratory results will be considered in the following sections:

- Pre-analytical factors
- Analytical standards
- Reference ranges and their value
- Intra-individual biological variation.

Pre-analytical factors

Table 5.1 details a short list of 'environmental' issues that can affect the interpretation of laboratory results, some of which are discussed below.

Table 5.1   A list of the important factors that may bear influence on data interpretation

Age/gender
Alcohol intake
Posture at sample collection
Circadian and seasonal variation
Diet
Drugs
Ethnic origin
Effect of exercise
Menstruation
Smoking
Stress

Age/gender

Many laboratory tests will show highly significant differences between male and female with or without changes over the growth life cycle.

Haemoglobin and most routine haematological measurements show little change with age, but there are significant differences between adult males and females. The haemoglobin reference range for males over 18 years of age is 13.5–18.0 g/dl, whereas females show a lower range at 12.5–16.0 g/dl and similar changes are noted with haematocrit and mean cell haemoglobin (MCH) levels.

Liver function tests do show minor changes with increasing age, with albumin lowering slightly from a mean value at the age of 30 years of 48 g/l to 44 g/l at 65 year of age. The enzymes aspartate aminotransferase (AST), alanine aminotransferase (ALT) and gamma glutamyltranspeptidase (GGT) all show slightly higher values for males. However, our own data in examining phase 1 normal volunteers has demonstrated a marked difference in females pre and post the age of 50 years, with the mean GGT enzyme activity changing from 14.5 to 21.6 IU/l. One of the major changes in liver enzymes is that of alkaline phosphatase (AP), which after a reduction from pre-pubertal level remains extremely stable for males. However, the female shows a highly significant difference pre- and post-menopause, with a mean change of 49.8 to 59.7 IU/l. We are now aware from measurement of specific bone AP that this increase is due predominantly to the bone isoenzyme.

Creatinine demonstrates a highly significant difference between males and females and a small increase with increasing age. The mean value for a male subject at the age of 50 is approximately 100 µmol/l and at the corresponding age in the female the value would be approximately 80 µmol/l

In terms of total cholesterol, there is a noticeable increase in males about the age of 30 with a mean increase from 4.7 to 5.5 mmol/l; thereafter there may be a slight increase or decline into the 65–70 age range. The female, on the other hand, shows a very significant difference pre- and post-menopause. The mean female total cholesterol in phase 1 volunteers <50 years of age was 4.71 mmol/l and it was 6.05 mmol/l in subjects >50 years.

Ethanol intake

The intermediate and long-term effect of ethanol ingestion was studied by Shaper *et al.* (1985), who compared occasional drinkers against subjects consuming more than six units daily in 7735 middle-aged men and demonstrated a 70 per cent increase in the mean gamma glutamyltranspeptidase and an 18 per cent increase in HDL-cholesterol, and smaller changes in uric acid and AST. Also, there was an increase in the red cell index of the mean cell volume (MCV) from 88 to 91 fl. Other changes in creatine kinase and electrolytes have also been noted.

Physicians are likely to identify only 20–50 per cent of patients with alcoholism attending medical centres, and this thus demands a high degree of clinical suspicion. Alcohol is, of course, metabolized rapidly, and its measurement in identifying the alcoholic is of little value. Although a number of new markers have been suggested and reviewed by Sharpe (2001), in essence GGT remains the most sensitive marker in conjunction with ALT and MCV. From a clinical trial viewpoint it is important to identify chronic alcoholics, as ethanol is a risk factor in certain diseases and there may be associations with various drug therapies that could result in adverse drug reactions.

Posture

Samples are usually obtained from a subject in either the supine or upright sitting position. In moving from the supine position to standing there is an efflux of water and filterable substances from the intravascular space to the interstitial fluid. One of the most significant changes is that of plasma active renin, which will show a mean of 22.5 µU/ml in the upright position changing to a mean value of 14.8 µU/ml when recumbent, with a similar change in aldosterone levels.

The non-filterable substances, such as proteins, cellular elements and compounds bound to protein, will increase in concentration by 8–12 per cent. We recently reviewed differences in subjects attending a phase 1 clinic for pre-study screening with the values obtained once the volunteer was selected. The volunteers attended for pre-study screen in the evening and the results were compared with the samples collected in the phase 1 unit when the volunteers were at rest, fasting and early in the morning. These results are shown in Table 5.2. Highly significant differences were noted in the measurements of total protein, albumin, calcium and neutrophils. These changes are undoubtedly due to the effect of posture, but other factors may also be contributing.

Prolonged use of a tourniquet in venesection will result in elevated concentrations of albumin, cholesterol and calcium, and excessive use will show changes in erythrocyte enzymes, which are at much higher levels of activity than plasma and, on a similar basis, elevation of potassium. Ideally, minimum use of a tourniquet is recommended for reliable results.

Table 5.2 Mean changes in clinical laboratory measurements from pre-study screen through baseline in 30 normal volunteers.

Test	Occasion		Significance
	Pre-screen	Baseline	
Total protein (g/l)	72.17	67.29	<0.001
Albumin (g/l)	44.26	40.81	<0.001
Calcium (mmol/l)	2.502	2.473	<0.001
White cell count (10^9/l)	7.61	5.76	<0.001
Neutrophils (10^9/l)	4.54	2.98	<0.001
Lymphocytes (10^9/l)	2.2	1.96	<0.05
Triglycerides (mmol/l)	1.53	1.11	<0.05
Alkaline phosphatase (IU/l)	56.4	50.58	<0.05

Circadian and seasonal variation

Many biochemical compounds show significant variation over a 24 h period, of which the most pronounced is that of the adrenal steroid cortisol. Figure 5.1 shows mean data from a group of 20 males from which samples were taken every 20 min over a 24 h period. These measurements were carried out using an old method; although there may be changes in the magnitude of units with newer methodology, the pattern over the 24 h period will be identical. With current radioimmunoassay the reference range for samples collected between 07:00 and 08:30 is 200–700 nmol/l, whereas samples collected in the afternoon or evening will have a reference range of 140–400 nmol/l, there being only minimal crossover.

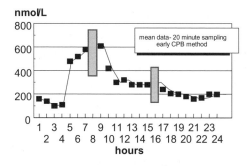

Figure 5.1 Diurnal variation of serum cortisol. Mean data from 20 individuals sampled at 20 min intervals over a 24 h period. The boxes show the calculated reference ranges at 8am and 4pm

The pituitary hormones are released in a pulsitile fashion under the control of the hypothalamus, but some also demonstrate a diurnal variation. Thyroid stimulating hormone shows a distinct sleep–wake pattern with the highest levels being found overnight. One of the most pronounced sleep–wake patterns is found in the secretion of growth hormone, and Figure 5.2 shows the typical changes in this hormone.

In a study by Pocock *et al.* (1989), noticeable changes in some safety profile biochemical markers were recorded over the period from 09:00 until 18:00. Triglycerides increased by

Serum hGH (mU/l)

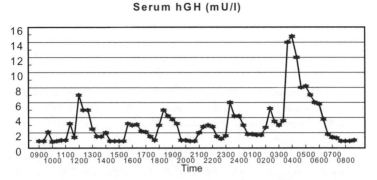

Figure 5.2   Human growth hormone changes over a 24 h period. From Saini *et al.* (1991), reproducibility of 24-hour serum growth hormone profiles in man, *Clinical Endocrinology*. Reproduced by permission of Blackwell Publishing

some 30 per cent over the time period irrespective of food intake. Similarly, inorganic phosphate increased by 20 per cent but this increase is abolished by fasting. Potassium showed an increase of 0.3 mmol/l and creatinine showed a slight reduction. There was a noticeable fall in bilirubin over the time period. These data are shown in Figure 5.3.

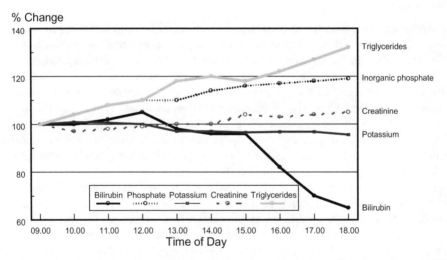

Figure 5.3   Diurnal variation of some biochemical markers. Reproduced from Pocock *et al.* (1989), *Journal of clinical Pathology* **42**: 172–179, with permission from the BMJ Publishing Group

In addition to changes within the 24 h clock, there are also significant seasonal differences in some measurements. Whilst we would expect to find changes in vitamin D between summer and winter, due to sunlight levels, in terms of tests in safety profiles, cholesterol has been shown to differ significantly. Rastam *et al.* (1992) reported that cholesterol values in males are 2.6–6.3 per cent higher in winter than summer, with the corresponding figures for females being 1.0–4.6%. Using the National Cholesterol Educational Programme upper limit guideline of 6.2 mmol/l, 25.4 per cent of men were above this level in winter, whereas only 13.5 per cent met the cutpoint in summer.

Therefore, attention to sample collection times is an important issue in data interpretation.

Diet

Prolonged fasting of 48 h duration will increase glucagon and decrease insulin levels. Owing to the increase in fat metabolism, ketone bodies will be found in blood and urine, and plasma glucose levels drop. Bilirubin, triglycerides and non-esterified fatty acids will all be elevated.

A meal high in fat content will increase the value of plasma alkaline phosphatase, presumably due to the intestinal isoenzyme. A diet high in protein will show an increase in urea and uric acid, with little change in creatinine.

Drugs

The possible effect of drugs on clinical laboratory measurements is beyond the scope of this presentation. For a review of this issue, readers may find the publication of Siest and Gaiteau (1988) of help in this direction.

Ethnic origin

The difference in race related to disease and biochemical measurements requires a lengthy review. Thus, this will be limited to a few general comments on chemical markers. Cholesterol values in the Japanese population tend to be lower than the equivalent levels in the Western population. The black african native show higher levels of immunoglobulins. There are highly significant differences in the enzyme creatine kinase between Afro-Caribbean, Asian and Caucasian populations (Sherwood et al. 1996). Alpha-fetoprotein, used diagnostically in the detection of spina bifida and Down's syndrome, shows major difference between Caucasian and Asian populations. Also, there are genetic differences regarding the African population, as they show a significant neutropenia in comparison with the Western population (Shaper and Lewis, 1971).

With our increasing knowledge of pharmacogenetics and associated cytochrome P450 enzyme systems, there is a much greater awareness of the effects of race on metabolic systems, and particularly in relation to the metabolism of drugs. The cytochrome P450 enzyme group located in the liver is involved in the metabolism of many therapeutic agents. There are about 200 CYP enzymes, which can result in individuals being classified as slow, intermediate and ultra-fast metabolizers with significant differences in therapeutic effects and toxicity when standard drug regimes are employed. Although some 80 per cent of the population on this planet are slow metabolizers, there are highly significant differences between races. CYP2C19 deficiency is found in 2–6 per cent of Caucasians, but in 19–25 per cent of Asians, which accounts for reduced rates of metabolism in these populations. Some 7 per cent of the Caucasian population are ultra-fast metabolizers of CYP2D6 with a prevalence of up to 29 per cent ultra-fast metabolizers in Africans. Consequently, individuals who differ in genetic make-up may not respond to a standard regime of drugs. Thirty per cent of the population do not respond to beta-blockers, with a similar percentage in respect of statins, and it has been reported that over 50 per cent of the population show a poor response to tricyclic antidepressants.

This brings into question a number of issues. How can we justify a global database in clinical studies with such a diverse worldwide population? It is now considered that by 2005, genotyping will be a routine procedure prior to prescribing many drugs; how will the clinical laboratories meet this inevitable challenge?

Exercise

The effect of exercise, whether on trained athletes or untrained individuals on biochemical and haematological tests is well defined. Intensive or sustained exercise induces 'sports anaemia' (Radomski *et al.*, 1980); however, even a short period of exercise has been shown to increase haemoglobin and leucocyte counts, which may take several days to return to baseline levels. Strenuous exercise may lead to dramatic increases in growth hormone, cortisol and the catecholamines, but these are usually of short duration and the values rapidly return to normal. There is also a highly significant increase in plasma lactate, which may influence acid–base balance, and rapid changes of short duration in antidiuretic hormone. More important is the release of muscle enzymes, in particular creatine kinase, which may take some 6–7 days post-exercise to return to basal levels; this is a point well worth noting in healthy volunteers taking part in phase 1 studies.

Menstruation

There are dramatic changes in hormones and steroids during the different phases of the normal menstrual cycle, and Figure 5.4 shows an example of the changes in pituitary follicle stimulating hormone (FSH) and ovarian 17β-oestradiol. These, together with other hormone changes, can elicit effects on body temperature, electrolytes and water balance. FSH offers one of the most discriminating tests of the perimenopausal period, with a marked increased secretion rising to extremely high levels, as shown in Figure 5.5.

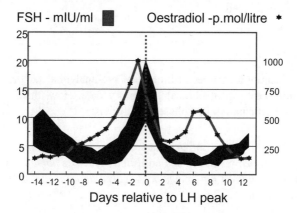

Figure 5.4   The changes in FSH and 17β-oestradiol during the normal menstrual cycle

Smoking

Tobacco smokers have a raised concentration of carboxyhaemoglobin, of the order of 8 per cent in comparison with 1 per cent in non-smokers. It has also been suggested that smokers

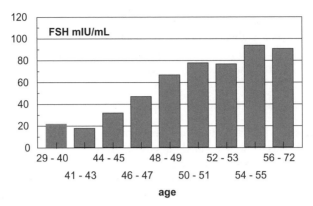

Figure 5.5   The change of FSH on entry and progression into the menopausal period. From Craig and Guilford (1993), *British Journal of Clinical Research*. Reproduced by permission of PJB Publications Ltd

have an increased level of plasma cortisol and catecholamines, leading to increases in non-esterified fatty acids.

Over the last few years there have been several studies that show increased concentrations of the acute phase reactants fibrinogen and C-reactive protein in smokers, and this may well account for the added cardiovascular risk in this population.

Stress

Psychological stress appears to cause an increase in plasma catecholamines resulting in an elevation of non-esterified fatty acids (NEFAs). Plasma cortisol, prolactin and growth hormone are increased in stressful situations, including phlebotomy, and the peripheral white cell count can also be increased.

So what is a normal volunteer?

The points above illustrate a number of biological pre-analytical factors that may have an influence on the interpretation of clinical laboratory data. How, then, might we define a normal volunteer for participation in a phase 1 study? As:

'A 20–40 year old, who does not drink alcohol or smoke, is unstressed, does not participate in heavy sport, resides at sea level in a moderate climate, has limited stress or sexual activity, lies flat on his or her back, eats a normal diet and is preferably of Western European nationality'

Sample collection procedure

Many of the points relating to sample collection procedure, e.g. posture, tourniquet use, and time of phlebotomy, have been covered in the above section. Moving now to the actual sample collection, most central laboratories will provide all necessary material for venesection, together with tube labels and comprehensive instructions on the procedure.

In the UK, two popular systems for blood collection are employed. Becton Dickinson Vacutainers or Sarstedt Monovette. Both companies provide an extensive range of blood collection containers, including tubes suitable for trace metals, containing special preservatives such as Aprotinin, and also for paediatric samples.

In diagnostic pathology testing there is a need for complex collection systems depending on the analyses being undertaken; therefore, comments on this section will be limited to the tests normally included in standard safety testing profiles.

Stability

There are considerable data available on the stability of safety profile tests. In terms of clinical chemistry measurements, our own laboratory has shown little change in the safety profile tests up to 96 h after collection. Some minor loss of ALT and AST activity is noted, but this is less than 10 per cent up to 96 h post-collection providing that the sample is treated as recommended. There is no apparent change in other enzymes, such as AP, GGT or creatine kinase. Whole blood samples for clinical chemistry will be unsatisfactory within a very short time due to leakage of the high concentration of potassium and phosphate and the activity of lactate dehydrogenase, ALT and AST for erythrocytes.

Up to 30 per cent of blood samples from general practice have raised potassium levels, and about 50 per cent of these are due to the sample being left overnight without separation of the red blood cells (Johnston and Hawthorne, 1997). Cooling these samples in a refrigerator accelerates the rate at which potassium leaks from the red cells.

Table 5.3 shows the results of samples from a single individual taken in duplicate in which analysis was carried out immediately on one sample and the second sample stored at 4 °C, then separated from the red cells the following day and analysed. The changes in AST, ALT, potassium and phosphate are significant, with the second sample results being above the upper limit of the reference ranges. Glucose measurement was carried out on the serum sample, and virtually all the glucose had been utilized by the continuing metabolism of

Table 5.3 Comparison of samples for biochemistry and haematology analysed within 2 h of collection against samples left untreated, separated the following day and analysed. Values in italics show highly significant differences

	Immediate	After 24 h
Haematology		
WBC (10^9/l)	9.0	8.5
RBC (10^{12}/l)	4.6	4.7
Hb (g/dl)	14.6	14.6
PCV (fl)	46.6	47.3
MCV (pg)	*96.7*	**105.4**[*]
MCH (g/dl)	30.3	30.2
MCHC(10^9/l)	31.4	29.6
Platelets(10^9/l)	304	280

(continued)

Table 5.3 (*continued*)

	Immediate	After 24 h
Clinical chemistry		
AST (IU/l)	*15*	*57*
ALT (IU/l)	*21*	*27*
AP (IU/l)	197	201
GGT (IU/l)	27	30
Bilirubin (μmol/l)	6.7	5.8
Glucose (mmol/l)	*5.6*	**0.3***
Urea (mmol/l)	7.0	7.5
Sodium (mmol/l)	142	145
Potassium (mmol/l)	*4.4*	**6.6***
Chloride (mmol/l)	109	101
Phosphate (mmol/l)	*1.1*	**2.9***
Creatinine (μmol/l)	*114*	*150*
Uric acid (μmol/l)	311	317
Calcium (mmol/l)	2.41	2.46
Total protein (g/l)	70	70
Albumin (g/l)	47	48
Cholesterol (mmol/l)	7.9	8.0

*Highly significant changes.

the red cells. The MCV increases cannot be controlled, as within 6 h of sample collection the red blood cells will show swelling in size. Although there is adequate evidence for the stability of the clinical chemistry safety tests, much of this is derived from normal levels of test concentrations. The stability of test concentrations in grossly abnormal situations, e.g. obstructive jaundice with highly raised levels of bilirubin, AP, and GGT, needs further assessment.

Table 5.4 Factors that can result in false positive and negative results

Albumin	+	Prolonged application of tourniquet
Bilirubin	−	Prolonged exposure to light
Bicarbonate	−	Prolonged exposure to air
Calcium	+	Prolonged application of tourniquet
	−	Use of wrong container – EDTA
Creatinine	+	Raised plasma acetoacetic acids
Glucose	+	Not fasting
	−	No fluoride preservative
Phosphate	+	Prolonged contact with RBC
	+	Haemolysis
Potassium	+	Use of wrong container – EDTA
	+	Haemolysis
Sodium	+	Contamination from IV fluids
	−	High glucose pulls sodium into cells
	−	Hyperlipidaemia
Triglycerides	+	Not fasting

Many specialist tests will demand specific collection methods, and it cannot automatically be assumed that all tests will be stable if stored at temperatures of -20 °C or below. The slow migrating lactate dehydrogenase, predominantly of liver origin, is unstable at $+4$ °C and below, and some enzymes, such as alanine aminopeptidase in urine samples, will demand the use of ethylene glycol to stop the samples freezing, which destroys this enzyme. Table 5.4 details a number of situations that result in falsely measured safety profile test results.

Analytical variation

The variability of an analytical measurement surrounding a value is extremely small in respect of the tests performed in safety monitoring with modern instrumentation. Generally, laboratories undertake two types of quality control programme to monitor performance: internal and external assessments.

Internal quality control (IQC) is usually carried out with lyophilized human serum available from laboratory suppliers. Generally, two levels of control are provided: within and outside the reference interval. Initially these samples are analysed within and between different analytical batches to establish the mean value for each measurement and the two standard deviation (2SD) distribution. These data are then incorporated into the laboratory data-management system. The quality control samples are treated identically to patient samples on every analytical run and the data-management system will accept or reject the batch analyses based on Westgard rules; see Westgard *et al.* (1981) and www.westgard.com/mltirule.htm.

The recommended Westgard rules generally applied are as follows:

- If both result within 2SD range, then **issue report**.

Reject if:

- One result exceeds 3SD.
- Both results exceed the same 2SD limit.
- Each result exceeds a different 2SD limit.
- The same material exceeds the same 2SD in a previous batch.
- The last 12 consecutive results are on the same side of the mean, rather than showing an equal distribution on both sides of the mean when the distribution is plotted graphically.

Thus, having established the rules and data within the laboratory data-management system, the computer will determine the acceptability of the performance. Table 5.5 shows a typical set of statistics from within the reference range quality-control sample over a period of 6 months.

There is no doubt that with each passing year the analytical precision of IQC improves, and this is closely monitored by laboratories to ensure reliable data on patient results. However, it must be remembered that as the acceptable data are extrapolated on 2SD ranges then at least 5 per cent of batches will be rejected on a statistical basis. Also, it is important

Table 5.5 The coefficient of variation, and 95 per cent confident limits for a mid reference range quality control sample showing the analytical variation surrounding the mean values. (With permission from Pivotal Laboratories, York)

Test	Value	CV (%)	−2SD	+2SD
AST	30	2.70	28	32
ALT	27	3.40	25	29
AP	158	2.20	151	165
GGT	48	2.60	46	50
Bilirubin	14	5.30	13	15
Glucose	3.1	1.20	3.0	3.2
Urea	5.2	1.50	5.0	5.4
Sodium	138	0.60	136.3	139.7
Potassium	4.5	0.60	4.4	4.6
Chloride	104	0.70	102.5	105.5
Creatinine	96	2.70	90.8	101.2
Uric acid	330	1.50	320	340
Calcium	2.52	1.60	2.44	2.60
Total protein	67	1.70	64.5	69.1
Albumin	37.4	1.40	36.4	38.4
Cholesterol	5.19	1.80	5.00	5.38
Thyroxine	105	3.20	98.3	111.7
WBC	6.7	2.30	6.4	7.0
RBC	4.22	1.10	4.1	4.3
HB	133	0.90	130.6	135.4
MCV	81.5	0.70	80.4	82.6
Platelets	202	5.50	179.8	224.2

to remember that it is the IQC that is the deciding factor on the release of the clinical laboratory report.

Concurrently, clinical laboratories participate in national and international external quality control (EQC) programmes in which samples are forwarded from a central source to many laboratories. A description of these complex and highly professional systems is outside the scope of this chapter. In the UK-NEQAS (www.ukneqas.org.uk) programme the result of the test is compared with the consensus mean for the method group, the variance and bias determined on the sample, and over a period of the last 10 quality control samples. Also, the programme incorporates tests of reproducibility and recovery of test material.

As EQC is based on consensus mean data; anything that would change in the technology or reagents employed by a large number of participating laboratories might result in a distortion of the statistics. Thus, the performance of the laboratory in both IQC and EQC must be examined independently.

Reference ranges

The subject of reference ranges is worthy of a separate review, and books are available on this topic (Grasbeck and Alstrom, 1981). There are a number of important issues that require comment at this stage. In the pharmaceutical industry the terminology of 'normal' ranges is still widely applied, and even when substituted with the word 'reference' in many cases the two are treated identically. The implication is that there is a gap between two populations, one healthy and the other diseased. This is not the case, and there is considerable overlap in the two populations.

Schneider (1960) concluded, 'the routine assessment of individual laboratory tests by reference to conventional population-based normal ranges, should no longer remain an accepted automatic practice'. The International Federation of Clinical Chemistry (IFCC) comments that a reference range merely serves as the basis for a more or less intuitive assessment of the biological information given by an observed value. The IFCC has laid down extensive guidelines on the collection of data to obtain the reference interval, which includes the segmentation and selection of the population, which should be greater than 120 estimates. The reference interval is then calculated by taking 95 per cent of the estimates and applying 90 per cent confidence limits at each end of the interval. At this stage, perhaps an example will illustrate the calculation. Table 5.6 shows the results of bone-specific AP measurements on 253 peri- or post-menopausal women with a median age of 50 years (95th percentile ranges 43–54 years).

Table 5.6 The statistics of bone-specific AP on 253 peri-menopausal women

Number	253
Minimum value	6
Maximum value	32.7
Mean	13.8
Standard deviation (SD)	4.36
−2SD	5.06
+2SD	22.5
Median	13.1
2.5th percentile	7.42
97.5th percentile	23.1

Examination of these data show the lowest estimate as 6 U/l, yet the 2SD lower range is 4.36 U/l, clearly implying that the distribution is not Gaussian (equal distribution of data frequency on both sides of the average value). Thus, prior to determining any calculation of the reference range, it is well worth plotting a frequency histogram in order to examine the distribution visually or preferably assess the asymmetry of these data by use of coefficients of skewness and kurtosis. Generally, biological compounds show a distinct shift to the right, as the distribution is not a random error. The results of the above data are shown in Figure 5.6 and confirm the skew to the right. Thus determination of the reference interval is not an easy exercise demanding careful use of statistics.

The resulting calculation of the reference interval on the bone-specific measurements on this study gave a lower limit of 7.42 with a 90 per cent confidence interval of 6.1–7.9 and at the upper limit a value of 23.1 with a 90 per cent confidence interval of 21.4–27.8

The basic problem with clinical studies is that, in terms of safety testing, we are looking at high volumes of data in which we are endeavouring to determine whether there is any adverse clinical laboratory event occurring. Thus, sensitivity is of course an important issue. Here, we are faced with the fact that there is no gap between healthy patients and those

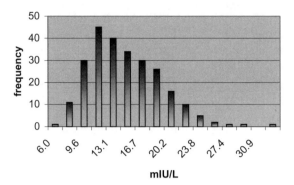

Figure 5.6 Data from normal healthy women aged 48–56 years for the measurement of bone-specific AP showing the skewed nature of the distribution

suffering from disease. Indeed, in all situations there is a considerable crossover between these two populations. Considering that moderately sized trials may consist of 500 patients with sampling on five occasions and with safety profiles consisting of 40 test measurements, the number of estimates approaches 100 000 test results. Assuming that there is total independence in the measurements, then on the basis of pure statistics one would expect $(1 - 0.95^{40})$ that there is an 87 per cent chance that one result would be outside the reference interval. However, we are aware that there is an association between different test measurements, e.g. haemoglobin has a relationship to PCV, MCV, MCHC, and in terms of chemistry GGT relates to AST, ALT, AP, etc. Thus, these measurements cannot be considered as independent. It has been estimated that, in a profile of 40–50 tests, statistically there is a chance that five results will be outside the reference interval. Now, ideally what the industry requires from laboratory testing is that all results should be normal; but, based on statistics, this will be impossible.

Figure 5.7 shows the likely crossover of a laboratory test with a population of healthy and diseased individuals. From this type of presentation we can determine the sensitivity and specificity of a particular test in assessing a diseased state. For example, consider the presentation in respect of glucose measurements from normal and diabetic populations.

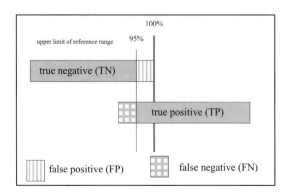

Figure 5.7 The influence of changing the reference range levels on false negative and positives

Increasing the effective reference range from 95 per cent of the population (black line) to 100 per cent (grey line) will enhance the sensitivity of the test, but with a resultant decrease in specificity and a greater number of false negatives. It is important, therefore, that the 95 per cent reference range be employed to maintain specificity.

Finally, many of the comments above relate to small changes outside of the reference ranges, which is naturally important in a drug study, where early warning of possible toxicity is important. However, the greater the distance from the upper or lower reference interval the greater is the likelihood of pathophysiology.

It is in the area of reference ranges that we encounter the major difference in the requirement between diagnostic pathology and the needs of the pharmaceutical industry in safety testing. Diagnostic pathologists are content to employ reference ranges based on 95 per cent of data from normal populations. However, as defined above, this results in a considerable number of single test results demanding clinical review in safety testing. In order to alleviate the number of so-called abnormals, a variety of approaches have been used. These include the increase of the 95th per cent percentile range to 99.7 per cent and also the application of multiplication factors to the upper and lower limit of the reference interval. As can be seen from Figure 5.7, whilst this may result in a lower number of 'abnormals' in safety profiles, it correspondingly alters the specificity of the analyte for the detection of disease with an increase in the false negative component.

For an excellent review of reference intervals, the definitive publication by Whitehead *et al.* (1994) in examining haematology and clinical chemistry data from some 80 000 subjects attending the BUPA screening programme should be consulted.

Intra-individual biological variation

In addition to the pre-analytical factors discussed above, there is an additional variation within any individual, as all biological compounds oscillate to a smaller or greater extent around an intrinsic homeostatic set-point. Williams *et al.* (1970) demonstrated that for many biochemical constituents the standard deviation of individual mean values was considerably greater than the average standard deviation of interpersonal fluctuations.

One of the early references to day-to-day variation was by Winkel *et al.* (1974), but a current listing of the intra- and inter-individual biological variation as a coefficient of variation for over 250 blood components can be found at http://www.westgard.com/ biodatabase1.htm (Rius *et al.*, 1999) Within the individual the mean variation surrounding a result is termed the *intra-individual biological variation*, and the difference in the set-points between different individuals is termed *inter-individual biological variation.*

In clinical studies we are looking at safety tests to monitor potential toxicities, and it is apparent that the use of the broad-spectrum population-based reference range does not offer the most sensitive assessment. What, then, is the alternative? For many years in diagnostic clinical chemistry we have employed the smallest significant difference (SSD) or critical difference (CD) for assessing changes in results from the same individual on different occasions. The clinician, looking at his patient reports, examines the changes in values against baseline reports to determine if there has been a significant difference in the analytical results due to time, therapeutic response, etc.

An original article in the *British Medical Journal* in 1989, discussing the interpretation of laboratory results, drew attention to the use of intra-subject variation and its relevance in clinical decision making (Fraser and Fogarty, 1989), and the value of this measurement in clinical trial safety profiles was reported by Craig (1994). The use of this parameter thus treats the individual as his or her own reference point and offers greater sensitivity than broad-spectrum reference ranges.

The calculation of the SSD is based on the following formula:

$$\text{SSD} = \sqrt{\text{CV}_{\text{av}}^2 + \text{CV}_{\text{libv}}^2} \times 2.77$$

where CV_{av} (%) is the coefficient of variation of the analytical variation and CV_{libv} (%) is the coefficient of variation of the intra-individual biological variation; the equation is multiplied by 2.77 standard deviations to provide the 95 per cent confidence limits.

The SSD is similar in health and in stable chronic disease, and Fraser (1993) showed that the average within-subject variation in healthy elderly people and younger adults is similar and that there is no apparent variation with different ethnic groups. Thus, it is possible to build a significant database on biological variation.

Table 5.7 details the SSD of the tests normally employed in standard safety profiles. These data were obtained from the Westgard database on the intra-individual biological variation and recalculated using information of analytical variation and 95 per cent confidence limits. In a comparison with our own unpublished SSD values. There is a very close agreement.

Table 5.7 The calculated SSD values for the tests normally encountered in clinical trial safety profiles. The intra-individual biological variation being obtained from Westgard

Test	SSD (%)	Test	SSD (%)
AST	33.0	Calcium	7.2
ALT	64.4	Phosphate	24.3
AP	17.4	Total protein	8.8
GGT	34.6	Albumin	8.7
Bilirubin	62.7	cholesterol	17.4
Glucose	14.0	HDL-cholesterol	21.5
Urea	34.3	Triglycerides	60.6
Sodium	2.6	Thyroxine	18.8
Potassium	13.4	WBC	31.7
Chloride	3.8	RBC	9.4
Creatinine	14.1	Hb	8.1
Uric acid	24.2	Platelets	29.5

A good example of the benefit of using the SSD is shown in Figure 5.8. This shows the reference range for serum creatinine and the SSD at 14%. Assuming that a subject enters at clinical trial with a baseline value of 80 µmol/l and the creatinine level increases by twice the SSD, then the result would still be within the reference range, yet it would have shown a highly significant difference from the subject's baseline.

Although there will always be a need for population-based reference ranges, these should be restricted to preselection of patients and incorporated into investigator reports. In terms of data analyses and information on trends during clinical studies, the SSD offers a more meaningful and sensitive measurement.

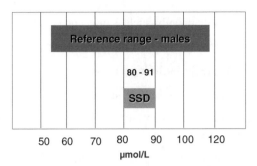

Figure 5.8 The effect of the SSD value on serum creatinine with a baseline level of 80 μmol/l in comparison with the assay reference range

Safety testing in drug development

The issue of clinical laboratory testing programmes in clinical trials is complex. It is important to appreciate that the most sensitive procedures should be employed as early as possible in clinical development. To reach phase 3 in the development programme and identify toxicity is expensive. Thus, at phase 1 and 2, careful selection of the correct tests is mandatory. The selection of the most appropriate tests should be based on information on the compound and details of the pre-clinical toxicology data.

There is a tendency in the industry to look at tests as individual entities related to specific biological functions, e.g. the relationship of calcium in bone metabolism. However, as calcium is in part bound to protein, any alteration in the protein concentration will significantly alter the serum calcium value. Thus, we can now consider calcium changes related to bone and protein metabolism, but also add that, as the kidney is involved in retaining calcium, pathophysiology of the renal mechanism will have an influence on the serum calcium result, and as the parathyroid glands produce the appropriate hormone to maintain calcium balance, a much broader picture is presented. Therefore, in the examination of abnormal results it is inappropriate to place too much credence on a single test measurement.

Rather than use an alphabetical listing of the safety tests, it is considered more convenient to group these as organ-related tests. First, we discuss aspects of Renal tests, e.g. urea, creatinine, creatinine clearance, uric acid, serum Cystatin C, β2-microglobulin, urinary N-acetyl-β-D-glucosaminidase (NAG), urinary microalbumin, electrolytes and glucose. The section on bone test then follows, and covers calcium, inorganic phosphate and new bone markers. Next, the section on liver tests includes discussion of enzymes, bilirubin, total protein and albumin, and prothnombin (PT) time. The lipids and lipoproteins section discusses the various forms of cholesterol and triglycerides. The various thyroid hormone screening tests are then mentioned. Finally, in the haematology section the discussion centres around the tests for hamoglobin, haematocrit, mean cell volume, mean cell haemoglobin, and various red and white cell count measures.

Renal

The kidneys can be considered as the controller of homeostatic mechanisms with the following major functions:

- Excretion of nitrogenous compounds, such as urea and creatinine.

- The retention of amino acids, glucose and other important compounds.

- The retention of bicarbonate for buffering purposes.

- The maintenance of electrolyte and water balance.

- Endocrine activities related to calcium, erythropoietin and renin–aldosterone axis, and the antidiuretic hormone (vasopressin).

Urea

- Urea is the major end product of nitrogen metabolism derived from protein and amino acids and is excreted in urine at high concentration.

- Its measurement may not always be due directly to renal impairment, as blood pressure and volume results in a low cardiac output with retention of urea.

- There is no significant difference in the values from males and females, but there is an increase with increasing age. Young healthy adults will show a value of about 4.0 mmol/l, which will increase to 7.0 mmol/l over the age of 65 years, presumably due to diminishing renal function in elderly subjects.

- In the USA the same measurement is undertaken but it is termed blood urea nitrogen (BUN). This is identical to blood urea but with the result expressed in terms of the nitrogen content (molecular weight 28) as opposed to the whole urea molecule (molecular weight 60). As different units are used to convert BUN to urea, the following formula applies:

$$\frac{BUN}{2.8}(mg/dl) = Blood\ urea\ (mmol/l)$$

The *reference range* is 2.5–6.8 mmol/l.

Low values are rare, but they may be seen in starvation and in conditions characterized by anabolic demand, such as pregnancy, malabsorption and severe liver damage.

High values occur in dehydration, acute and chronic renal disease, recent high protein intake, and decrease in effective circulating volume.

Creatinine

- Creatinine is a waste product of muscle metabolism that is excreted at a relatively constant rate in each individual. For this reason, urine measurement, e.g. of drugs, is usually expressed in terms of drug concentration per gram of creatinine.

- The measurement of creatinine is superior to urea, but nevertheless has limitations as a test of renal function. The reason for this is that there will be a reduction in the glomerular filtration rate (GFR) to less that 60 ml/min (normal 120 ml/min) prior to any increase in serum creatinine being apparent.

- Essentially, creatinine concentration is directly related to body weight.

- Males tend to have higher values in comparable age ranges than females, due to the relative difference in muscle mass.

- Dietary protein does not influence creatinine to the same extent as urea.

- Some compounds interfere in its measurement, including acetoacetic acids, ascorbic acid, bilirubin and glucose in high concentration.

Reference range: 70–120 µmol/l. Both males and females show an increase with increasing age, and the female values tend to be lower than the male by about 12–15 per cent.

Low levels may be found in severe muscle wasting and occasionally during pregnancy.

High levels can be found in renal functional impairment, obstruction of the urinary tract, and may be encountered in acromegaly and hyperthyroidism.

There is a very large list of drugs, particularly antibiotics and chemical compounds, that are known to be nephrotoxic.

Creatinine clearance

- As mentioned above, the serum creatinine does not show significant changes until the creatinine clearance as a measure of glomerular filtration is about 40 per cent of normal. Therefore, the measurement of the GFR provides a much greater sensitivity of renal impairment.

- Although there are sophisticated measurements of GFR, in the clinical environment creatinine clearance is generally adequate.

- The full creatinine clearance demands the collection of a timed 24 h urine specimen with a sample for serum creatinine, which is inconvenient for subjects in clinical trials.

- For a prompt determination of the predicted creatinine clearance suitable for monitoring potential drug toxicities, the formula reported by Cockcroft and Gault (1976) using only the serum creatinine is of considerable value. The formula has been modified by a number of workers to include body surface area (BSA) as an additional parameter, but the basic formula is:

$$\text{Predicted clearance (ml/min)} = \frac{[140 - \text{age}] \times \text{weight (kg)} \times k}{72 \times \text{Serum creatinine (µmol/l} \times 0.0113)}$$

where $k = 1.0$ for men and 0.85 for women.

Reference range: creatinine clearance values decline with increasing age and the clearance levels are lower in females. Using the above formula and correcting for BSA, the following creatinine clearance values (ml/min) apply:

	Males	Females
Adults to 30 years	60–130	55–120
Adults to 50 years	55–110	50–90
Adults to 80 years	40–79	38–62

Uric acid (urate)

• The major clinical laboratory interest in urate is in the identification of subjects with gout, when monosodium urate crystals penetrate the joints.

• Approximately 75 per cent is excreted in the urine and the remainder destroyed by gut bacteria.

• In the kidney, urate is filtered and fully reabsorbed in the proximal tubule, and thus the urate in urine is derived from excretion from the distal tubule.

Reference range: 220–450 µmol/l.

Low values are of no clinical significance, although it has been reported in Wilson's disease and some neoplasms.

Raised values are seen in renal failure, as well as in toxaemia of pregnancy, liver disease and sarcoidosis. Conditions that result in an increase in turnover of cells, such as pernicious anaemia, radiotherapy, polycythaemia, may all show elevation in uric acid. Also, increased levels can be found after exercise, and in hypothyroidism and hypoadrenalism.

A number of drugs are known to increase the plasma urate concentration, including diuretics, catecholamines, salicylates and ethambutol.

Serum cystatin C

• Simonsen *et al.* (1985) reported on the values of cystatin C as a measure of GFR, and since that time there has been increasing popularity in the measurement of this serum protein.

• It is produced in all nucleated cells, freely filtered in the renal glomeruli and almost completely reabsorbed in the proximal tubule.

• Serum cystatin C is an effective measure of GFR and avoids the need for the collection of 24 h urine samples.

• The values are not influenced by non-renal factors, such as muscle mass and protein intake.

- The value of the measurement and a comprehensive review of the reference ranges was recently published by Finney *et al*. (2000).

reference range: the reference range which applies to both sexes, is 0.5–1.1 mg/l.

β2-Microglobulin

- This is a 99 amino acid polypeptide present on the surface of nucleated cells and bound to class 1 HLA antigens. Over half the serum concentration originates from the lymphocytes.

- In normal subjects it is synthesized constantly at a concentration of 150 μg/24 h and eliminated exclusively through the kidneys and reabsorbed in the proximal tubules. In kidney disease, a comparison of the blood and urine results will help identify the source of damage. In glomerular disease the levels increase in blood and decrease in urine, whereas in tubular disease the urine concentration increases and the blood level falls.

- Increased serum levels may result from induction of autoimmune systems, high cell turnover or reduced GFR.

- Increased urine levels are encountered in renal impairment, usually prior to creatinine changes.

Reference range: normal serum concentrations are 0.7–3.0 mg/l; normal serum concentrations are 0.7–3.0 mg/l; normal urine concentrations are <20 mg/l.

Urinary N-acetyl-β-d-glucosaminidase (WAG)

- NAG has its origin in the epithelial cells of the proximal tubule which contain a large number of lysosomes, and due to its sizeable molecular weight (130 000) NAG cannot appear in the glomerular filtrate if the glomerular membrane is intact.

- NAG in urine is widely used for the assessment of renal disease and the detection of nephrotoxicity, particularly as related to hypertension, diabetes, arthritis, urinary tract infections, and to nephrotoxic drugs and environmental pollutants, many of which are attacked by lysosomes or by destruction of the cells in the proximal tubule.

- The enzyme is stable up to 50 °C for reasonable time periods, but owing to the nature of urine it is recommended that analysis takes place as soon after collection as possible. For short delays the sample can be collected with 0.1–0.3 per cent boric acid as a preservative.

- The second void sample of the day is preferred, and the enzyme can be measured in serum as well as urine.

reference range: urine NAG is usually expressed as μmol/h/mmol of creatinine and the reference range in that format is 7–28 μmol/h/mmol creatinine.

Urinary microalbumin

- The measurement of urinary microalbumin is of considerable interest as a sensitive marker of renal dysfunction, particularly in relation to diabetic nephropathy.

- Owing to the fact that type 2 diabetes is increasing in prevalence, and also that diabetic patients' lifespans are increasing, this disease now represents the most common single cause of end-stage renal dysfunction.

- About 30 per cent of patients of type 1 and 2 diabetes develop nephropathy.

- There are major racial differences in the prevalence of diabetes.

- The earliest clinical evidence of nephropathy is the appearance of abnormal concentrations of urinary microalbumin.

- Microalbuminuria in diabetic subjects reflects the presence of glomerular involvement in early renal damage, but recent studies have shown that there is also a tubular component to the renal complications. Indeed, it may well be that tubular involvement precedes glomerular changes.

- The measurement can be carried out on a random, overnight or 24 h collection of urine samples, but it is generally performed on a random sample with the result expressed in terms of creatinine.

Reference range: normal   <30 µg/mg of creatinine
microalbuminuria   30–300 µg/mg creatinine
albuminuria   >300 µg/mg creatinine

Electrolytes

Although the measurement of electrolytes is concerned primarily with mineral and water balance, owing to the close association with the renal endocrine systems, in particular the renin–aldosterone axis, the electrolytes may also be considered as tests of kidney function.

Sodium This is the principal biological cation and is strongly related to the extra-cellular osmolality and volume. There is a close association between sodium and body water.
Reference range: 135–145 mmol/l.
Low levels are found after severe ingestion of water, such as in fluid replacement following sweating, diarrhoea, vomiting and diuretic abuse. Dilutional hyponatraemia may occur in cardiac failure, liver failure, nephrotic syndrome and due to changes in the posterior pituitary antidiuretic hormone.
Raised levels are found in conditions related to water loss in excess of salt loss, as found dehydration and hyperminalocorticoidism.

Potassium   This is the major intracellular cation and has a pronounced effect on nerve and muscle membrane activity.

Reference range: 3.5–5.4 mmol/l.

Low levels: are found in conditions of gastrointestinal loss, such as diarrhoea, certain renal tubular defects and overactivity of the adrenal cortex. Hypokalaemia can cause muscle weakness. Drugs such as diuretics frequently result in low potassium levels and the adrenergic beta agonists may cause hypokalaemia to such an extent as to result in cardio-vascular effects.

Raised levels may be found in conditions of excessive cell destruction, acute and chronic renal dysfunction and with the administration of potassium supplement therapy. In markedly increased hyperkalaemia there is a significant risk of cardiac arrest. Haemolysis and marked thrombocytosis may cause falsely elevated results. Spironolactone, tetracyclines and some antineoplastics agents may results in elevated potassium values.

Glucose

Although glucose deserves a devoted section, because the kidney is strongly involved in maintaining a normal blood glucose level it is included here for convenience.

- Blood glucose level is a controlled balance between the amount entering circulation and that being removed by metabolism. It can be considered as a metabolic fuel and is dependent on diet, absorption, insulin from the pancreatic beta cells, glucagon from the pancreatic alpha cells, adrenaline, adreno-corticotrophic steroids and liver and muscle metabolism.

- Under normal circumstances glucose should not appear in urine, as all glucose in the glomerular filtrate is reabsorbed in the proximal tubule by active transportation. However, the active transportation is rate limiting and when the blood glucose attains a level of greater than 180 mg/dl (10 mmol/l) it exceeds the rate-limiting capacity and glycosuria results.

Reference range: there is a small but significant difference between the glucose concentration in whole-blood and serum due to the difference in the water content of the two fluids. To obtain whole-blood glucose samples it is essential that the collection tube includes a glycolytic inhibitor and fluoride/oxalate tubes are normally employed. Serum can satisfactorily be used providing that the sample is centrifuged and the serum separated within 1 h of collection. The fasting ranges are

whole blood	3.3–5.5 mmol/l
serum	3.8–6.0 mmol/l

As it is not always possible to obtain fasting samples from subjects in clinical studies, the *non-fasting reference range* employed is 3.7–7.8 mmol/l.

Low levels may be found in insulin overdose, insulin-secreting tumours (insulinoma) starvation, severe exercise, hypothyroidism and Addison's disease (adrenocortical hypoplasia).

Raised levels are usually found in diabetes mellitus, hyperthyroidism, Cushing's disease (adrenocortical hyperplasia) acromegaly and post-vascular accidents.

Type 2 diabetes is on the increase in all countries, as sadly are the complications (both macro-vascular and micro-vascular) of the disease. Statistics from the USA in 1998 showed that 10.3 million people were diagnosed as diabetic and additionally there are probably 5 million undiagnosed. It has been estimated that by the year 2025 some 5 per cent of the worldwide population will have type 2 diabetes, offering a challenge to the industry for new products and to the diagnostic business for much improved testing programmes.

Although self-testing of glucose levels can now be performed accurately by patients, this merely represents glycaemic control at a single point in time. This must be supplemented by more long-term glucose control with the use of haemoglobin A1c, and the assessment of macro- and micro-vascular testing to monitor and prevent diabetic complications.

Bone

Bone is living connective tissue comprising of an organic protein and the inorganic mineral hydroxyapatite. Some 90 per cent of the organic protein is type 1 collagen derived from the triple-helical procollagen molecule. The collagen molecule is cross-linked at both the C and N terminals to other type 1 collagen strands, forming the basic fabric and tensile strength of bone tissue. The cross-linking is accomplished by pyridinoline and deoxypyridinoline (DPD) as a result of condensation of lysine and hydroxylysine residues on adjacent collagen molecules.

Bone is constantly undergoing a process of remodelling which includes a degradation stage of bone resorption by the action of osteoclasts and a building stage of formation mediated by the action of osteoblasts.

During the resorption of collagen, both free and peptide-bound DPD is released together with both C- and N-terminal telopeptides (CTx and CNx). These peptides are specific fragments of type 1 collagen and for bone resorption.

Osteocalcin comprises 10–25 per cent of the non-collagen protein in bone and is specific to this tissue source. Osteocalcin is involved in bone formation by binding calcium to γ-carboxyglutamic acid residues. The enzyme AP is involved in bone formation and is thought to indicate the activity of the osteoblast. Although this enzyme is present in serum from both bone and liver, the bone-specific isoenzyme can be measured as a separate entity.

Calcium

- Calcium is widely distributed in both intra- and extra-cellular fluids and is concerned with bone formation and coagulation; it is a necessary activator for many enzymes.

- Plasma calcium levels are controlled by the level of parathyroid hormone (PTH) secreted from the parathyroid glands by its action on the kidney, bone and the gut via 1:25 dihydroxycholecalciferol (vitamin D3). Calcitonin from the C cells of the thyroid gland decreases osteoclastic activity and has the opposite effect from PTH.

- Approximately half of the plasma calcium is bound to protein, predominately albumin, and only the unbound (free ionized) calcium is physiologically active.

- PTH acts to stimulate the action of osteoclastic bone resorption, releasing calcium into the extra-cellular fluid, and decreases the renal tubular reabsorption of phosphate and increases the reabsorption of calcium. The control of the PTH secretion is dependent on a feedback mechanism of the free ionized plasma calcium level.

- As 50 per cent of calcium is bound to albumin any change in the concentration of this protein will significantly alter the calcium level, and most laboratories will include a correction for the protein difference. The formula for correction is:

$$\text{Corrected calcium} = \text{Measured Ca}^{2+} + \{0.02 \times [40 - \text{albumin concentration (g/l)}]\}$$

Reference range: 2.25–2.65 mmol/l (uncorrected). There is a slight difference between the sexes with males showing higher values, due presumably to the slight difference in albumin between males and females.

Low levels may be found in vitamin D deficiency, renal insufficiency, acute pancreatitis, low protein levels, hypoparathyroidism and prolonged anticonvulsant therapy.

High levels may be encountered in primary hyperparathyroidism, bone metastases, malignancy, hyperthyroidism, Paget's disease and acromegaly.

Inorganic phosphate

- Phosphorus is present as inorganic salts of phosphoric acid, and organic esters of glycerophosphate, nucleotide phosphate and lipid phosphorus.

- The erythrocytes are rich in phosphorus, the whole-blood concentration being about 10 mmol/l in comparison with plasma of about 4 mmol/l. Thus, any haemolysis of the samples renders it unsuitable for this measurement.

- Approximately 80 per cent is located in bone. It has a vital role in the transfer of energy.

- Phosphate is excreted by the kidney following glomerular filtration and tubular reabsorption. The latter process is inhibited by PTH, increasing phosphate excretion.

- As mentioned previously, inorganic phosphate levels increase significantly during the day and immediately after a meal there is a decline in phosphate due to the increase in insulin.

Reference range: 0.8–1.3 mmol/l.

Low levels are found in hyperparathyroidism, acute alcohol toxicity, hypokalaemia, malabsorption and hyperinsulinaemia. Antacid overuse and exercise may also demonstrate hypophosphataemia.

Raised levels are encountered in hypoparathyroidism, renal failure, thyrotoxicosis myeloma and excess vitamin D intake.

New bone markers

In terms of bone resorption, it is impossible to choose the single best collagen degradation marker. The publications from each diagnostic company inevitably favour their own product. Nevertheless, in terms of monitoring changes, in post-menopausal subjects on oestrogen or alendronate therapy all show significant changes, and these occur much more rapidly than bone mineral density measurements. Kyd *et al.* (1999) reviewed the clinical usefulness of DPD, CTx and NTx in patients on alendronate and showed that CTx and NTx were more sensitive than DPD, but that only baseline DPD showed an association with the bone mineral density measurement after 1 year. In clinical studies, sponsoring companies should communicate with the analytical laboratory to determine the most appropriate marker. Table 5.8 lists a number of the markers that are currently available.

Table 5.8   New bone markers for the determination of bone resorption and formation

Name	Diagnostic supply company
Bone resorption	
Deoxypyridinoline (free lysyl-pyridinoline) DPD	Metra (Quidel)
N-terminal telopeptide (NTx)	Ostex (Osteomark)
C-terminal telopeptide (CTx)	Osteometer (Crosslaps)
Bone formation	
Bone-specific AP	Hybritech, Quidel
Osteocalcin	Many diagnostic companies
Carboxyterminal propeptide of collagen (PICP)	Orion, Quidel

Similarly, in terms of bone formation marker, it is now generally considered that both bone-specific AP and osteocalcin should be employed.

   Osteoporosis is a common condition that can lead to fractures with a decreased quality of life. A woman's lifetime risk of fractures is 40 per cent whereas a man's risk is 13 per cent (Delmas and Fraser, 1999). Caucasians and Asians are the two ethnic groups with the highest risk of fractures (Lau and Cooper, 1996). The condition affects more than 25 million of the US population and results in 1.5 million fractures annually, and this is likely to increase with the increase in population age. The worldwide cost of osteoporotic fracture treatment is enormous and represents a challenge to the industry for efficacious therapeutic products and for the diagnostic clinical laboratory towards greater efficiency in testing programmes.

Liver

- The liver is located in the right hypochondrium and is the largest organ in the body, accounting for 5 per cent of body weight. It has little connective tissue but is highly vascular and metabolically extremely active. In the normal situation, 10–15 per cent of the total blood volume is in the liver and acts as a vascular reservoir.

- Roughly 80 per cent of blood entering the liver is venous blood from the portal vein, thus providing the liver with first choice of all material in the intestine. The remaining 20 per cent is arterial blood from the hepatic artery.

- The functions of the liver are principally bile production, protein, carbohydrate and lipid metabolism, ketone body formation, vitamin storage and inactivation of steroids, drugs and pharmacological agents.

- The functional unit in the liver is the hepatic lobule, a hexagonal arrangement of plates and layers of hepatocytes radiating outwards from a central vein in the centre of the lobule. Within the lobule are the sinusoids, consisting of endothelial cells and hepatocytes, similar to the structure in Figure 5.9.

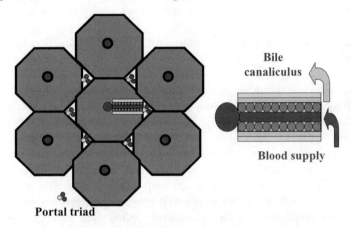

Bile
canaliculus

Blood supply

Portal triad

Figure 5.9   An outline of the structure of the liver lobule and sinusoids

'Liver' enzymes

- Although there are many enzyme measurements that can be undertaken to determine hepatitic dysfunction, these tend to be limited to AST, ALT, GGT and AP. It is important to remember that changes in liver enzymes often, but not always, indicate liver involvement. For example, elevation of AP may be due to bone disease or hyperthyroidism, and changes in the measured activity of AST and ALT to myocardial damage and the influence of muscle damage or exercise.

- GGT and AP are membrane-bound enzymes, ALT is located in the cell cytosol and AST in both the cytosol and the mitochondria, which may explain the variable pattern of enzyme changes found in different liver pathologies, dependent of the severity of the liver damage. Also, the enzyme activity within the cell is extremely high relative to the level encountered in plasma. The ratio of AST in the erythrocyte relative to plasma is 15:1, but in liver and heart cells it is approximately 8000:1.

- The classification of liver disease is complex, and the enzyme activities will change significantly over the course of a disease; thus, serial enzyme measurement may be required to attain a diagnosis.

- There are a large number of drugs, toxins and foodstuffs that can induce hepatic lesions, resulting in varied symptoms and enzyme profiles. In terms of drugs, it has been recorded that 5 per cent of all reported adverse events are associated with hepatic dysfunction or injury, and that 2–3 per cent of all hospital admissions are due to adverse drug effects linked with a hepatic reaction. Therefore, the detection of liver disease at an early stage is of overriding importance, both in diagnostic pathology and in the assessment of drug-induced reactions.

Gamma glutamyltranspeptidase   GGT is an enzyme present in kidney, liver and pancreas but with little activity in other organs. Its measurement is particularly sensitive to liver cell damage and cholestatic situations.

Reference range: 8–55 IU/l, but the distribution shows a marked skew to the right.

Low levels are of no significance.

High levels The greatest increase occurs in liver cell obstruction and malignancy (hepatoma and cancer of the pancreas). It is a useful marker for metastasis from breast and colon.

It is also raised in cirrhosis, hepatitis and infectious mononucleosis. Fatty liver (as in obesity and badly controlled diabetes) may give elevated values, and enzyme induction with a number of the anticonvulsant drugs (e.g. phenytoin and phenobarbitone) also shows raised enzyme activity.

GGT is particularly sensitive to alcohol toxicity and may show significant increases in persons who have more than three units of alcohol per day. In a recent review of old and newer biochemical markers for the detection and monitoring of alcohol abuse (Sharpe, 2001) concluded that GGT continues to remain the test combining the greatest convenience and sensitivity for monitoring alcohol, particularly when used in conjunction with AST, ALT and the MCV.

Aspartate aminotransferase and alanine aminotransferase

- Both enzymes are located in many tissues, but predominantly in the hepatocytes, myocardial cells, erythrocytes and skeletal muscle cells.

- AST has a bias toward myocardial cells and ALT towards liver cells, and thus the relative ratio of the enzyme activities are important in establishing the source of tissue damage.

- Moderate increases in both enzymes (less than 1.5 times the upper limit of the reference range) may be normal for the individual, due to ethnic origin or body mass index.

- In testing liver enzymes we are endeavouring to determine hepatocellular injury or cholestasis, and serial measurements may be required to confirm a diagnosis. Drugs that are hepatotoxic in certain individuals may give rise to significantly different pictures including cholestasis, viral-type hepatitis and often a mixture of both.

Reference range: ALT: 5–50 IU/l.

Low values are rare and of little significance.

High values are found in hepatitic cirrhosis, but the levels may only be moderately increased. Viral hepatitis can give markedly increased levels up to several thousand units. In chronic hepatitis, varying enzyme activity may be encountered, dependent on the stage of the disease. Cholestatic jaundice gives moderately raised levels, as can muscular trauma, including severe exercise and *in vivo* and *in vitro* haemolysis. In myocardial infarction there will be increased plasma levels, usually less in magnitude than AST. Drugs such as heparin, salicylates, opiates, tetracycline and isoniazide have been known to give asymptomatic rises in aminotransaminases.

Reference range: AST: 4–40 I U/l.

Low values are rare and of little significance.

High values of the order of 100–700 I U/l are found in myocardial infarction, and generally lesser levels in congestive cardiac failure. Similar increases are seen in cirrhosis and chronic alcohol toxicity, but may be variable. In viral hepatitis, markedly increased plasma levels are noted. Trauma, including surgery and muscular disorder, can give elevated levels, and phenothiazines, erythromycin, methyldopa, halothane and anabolic steroids are known to increase the AST and ALT levels.

Alkaline phosphatase

- AP is present in most tissue sources, particularly in the osteoblasts of bone, the biliary canaliculi in the liver, intestine, renal proximal tubules, and the placenta.

- In the normal adult non-pregnant serum the major contribution of the enzyme is from liver and bone.

- Convenient and reliable methods are now available for the measurement of bone-specific AP.

- The interpretation of abnormal AP activity must be examined in conjunction with other liver function tests.

Reference range: 70–250 IU/l (extremely dependent on method employed).

Low values are rare but may be encountered in children with growth hormone deficiency, severe anaemia and in congenital defects in phosphate metabolism.

High values may be found in a variety of clinical conditions:

- Bone disease, including rickets, osteomalacia, Paget's disease and secondary malignancy of bone.

- Hyperparathyroidism with bone involvement.

- Marked increase may be found in osteogenic sarcoma, a malignant tumour of the osteoblast.

- In liver disease the levels are increased moderately in acute hepatitis (usually less than threefold from the upper limit of the reference range). Infective mononucleosis with liver involvement can increase the AP by about five times, and in biliary cirrhosis and cholestasis marked increases may be found (10–15 times).

- Hyperthyroidism may show a slight elevation, as will samples from subjects in late pregnancy.

A large number of drugs have been implicated in cholestasis and hepatocellular toxicity. From a cholestatic aspect these include androgens, oestrogens, sulphonamides, tricyclic antidepressants, anticoagulants and diuretics; from a hepatocellular toxicity aspect these include aspirin, paracetamol, phenytoin and many antibiotics, in particular isoniazide. Therefore, considerable care and emphasis is necessary in all clinical studies in the interpretation of the liver enzymes.

Bilirubin

- The life span of erythrocytes is approximately 120 days; thereafter, they are broken down by the reticuloendothelial system, resulting in the release of haemoglobin. After the removal of the iron component for re-use, bilirubin is formed.

- The bilirubin formed is loosely bound to albumin and is transported to the liver, where it is conjugated. In normal circumstances the unconjugated portion represents the largest portion of the total bilirubin and is termed pre-hepatic or *indirect* bilirubin. Conjugation is accomplished in the liver with uridyl diphosphate glucuronyl transferase, rendering bilirubin water soluble, and is termed *direct*, which is then transported in bile.

- In the intestine bilirubin is degraded to stercobilinogen and a portion reabsorbed into the liver via enterohepatic circulation as urobilinogen to be excreted in urine. As the conjugated bilirubin is water soluble it can, therefore, be excreted by the kidneys, but in normal subjects the concentration in urine is extremely small, but it may be detected by dipsticks if the urine sample is concentrated.

- As the secretion of conjugated bilirubin into the bile is very rapid in comparison with the conjugation stage, healthy persons have almost no detectable plasma conjugated bilirubin.

- Most clinical laboratories define the upper limit of normal for total bilirubin as about 20 µmol/l, with no difference in the sexes. In our own laboratory we have isolated a database of subjects participating in phase 1 studies and found a significant difference between males and females; whereas the value of 20 µmol/l is acceptable for females, this range requires extension to 28 µmol/l for normal healthy fasting males. It has been suggested that this may be due to a partial defect in the conjugation enzyme, and be classified as Gilbert syndrome. However, without adequate proof of a conjugation defect this may simply be a difference between the sexes and can be classified as unexplained mild hyperbilirubinaemia.

Reference range: Males, 2–28 µmol/l; females, 2–20 µmol/l.
High values of bilirubin may be encountered in three circumstances:

- Pre-hepatic (haemolytic) – increased breakdown of RBCs, in excess of the conjugation limit, as in haemolytic anaemia, pernicious anaemia, neonatal jaundice and haemoglobinopathies.

- Hepatic – liver cell damage (acute, chronic, fatty liver hepatitis), intrahepatic obstruction, infective mononucleosis, chemical toxicity and Gilbert's disease.

- Post-hepatic – obstruction of the main bile ducts, whether due to stone, tumours, cancer at the head of the pancreas or biliary inflammation.

Reference range: urinary bilirubin, <3.5 mmol/l.
Reference range: urinary urobilinogen <17 mmol/L.
For an up to date assessment on the evaluation of liver chemistry tests, the American Gastroenterological Association Clinical Practice Committee report is well worth reviewing (Green and Flamm, 2002).

Total protein and albumin

- Plasma proteins are formed mainly in the liver, and albumin is quantitatively the most important, representing about 50 per cent of the total protein.

- Plasma proteins consist of a complex mixture of transportation agents, enzymes, coagulation factors, immunoglobulins, glycoproteins and lipoproteins, and there are over 100 individual plasma proteins, many at extremely small levels of concentration.

- As such, therefore, the measurement of total protein and albumin may be consider as a screening test.

- Further investigation usually commences with the application of protein electrophoresis, which separates the protein into the following fractions: Albumin, $\alpha 1$ globulins (predominantly $\alpha 1$ antitrypsin), $\alpha 2$ globulins (predominantly $\alpha 2$ macroglobulin and haptoglobin), β globulins (mainly complement and transferring), γ globulins (predominantly immunoglobulins).

Reference range: total protein, 64–82 g/l; albumin, 36–50 g/l. There is a slight but significant difference between the sexes (mean male value 45 g/l; mean female value 42.2 g/l). There is also a decline in albumin with increasing age, a point worthy of note with compounds which bind to albumin.
Low values may be found in nephrotic syndrome, glomerulonephritis, malabsorption and malnutrition.
High values may be found in dehydration, chronic liver disease, certain neoplasia, collagen disease and many other conditions.

Prothrombin time

- The hepatocytes synthesize most of the coagulation factors, of which factor II is PT.

- PT and factors VII, IX and X are vitamin K dependent.

- Therefore, measurement of PT may be considered as a liver function test; however, in this respect, other biochemical tests are considerably more sensitive.

Reference range: the results of PT should be reported in relation to the International Normalized Ratio (INR). This is the ratio of the patient's PT to mean PT reference range for the particular laboratory raised to the power of the International Sensitivity Index (ISI) provided by the reagent manufacturer.

A prolonged PT value may be found in

- inadequate vitamin K intake

- poor fat absorption

- liver damage due to impaired synthesis of PT complex factors

- hypofibrinogenaemia

- drug therapy, such as aspirin, anti-histamines and non-steroidal anti-inflammatory drugs.

In endeavouring to differentiate liver hepatocellular damage from cholestasis, the changes in various measurements shown in Table 5.9 may be of help.

Table 5.9   The different responses of liver function tests in hepatocellular damage and cholestasis. The ULRR factors (upper limit of the reference range) are for guidance only, as these will vary considerable during the progress of the diseases

	Cholestatic	Hepatocellular
ALT	Normal to slight increase, usually $<\times 5$ ULRR	Increased, usually $>\times 5$ ULRR
AST	Normal to slight increase, usually $<\times 3$ ULRR	Increased, usually $>\times 3$ ULRR
AP	$>3\times$ ULRR	$<3\times$ ULRR
GGT	Increased	Increased
Cholesterol	Slight increase	Normal or lowered
PT after vitamin K	Response	Nil

Lipids and lipoprotein

In a recent assessment in our laboratory of cholesterol values from volunteers accepted into phase 1 studies there were 336 males with a median age of 31 years (18–50) and 222 female subjects with a median age of 49 years (32–62). The calculated reference range employed in the laboratory is 2.9–7.3 mmol/l.

The males showed nine of the subjects with a cholesterol level greater than 7.3 in the range of 7.4–10.4 mmol/l. However, when the earlier desirable upper limit of cholesterol at 6.2 mmol/l was employed, 43 (13 per cent) of the males showed raised values. It is now being recommended that the desirable limit should be set at 5.6 mmol/l, if not lower.

The females showed 17 (7.6 per cent) of the subjects with values greater than 7.3 mmol/l in the range of 7.4–9.6 mmol/l. On using the desirable level of 6.2 mmol/l, 60 (27 per cent) of the volunteers demonstrated raised values. As the age range for the female population covered the peri- and post-menopausal period, these results were not unexpected.

Screening of the population will yield a number of asymptomatic subjects with markedly elevated total cholesterol values worthy of further investigation, and thus the inclusion of this measurement in pre-study safety profiles is essential.

- Dietary lipids are absorbed from the small intestine after emulsification with bile salts synthesized from cholesterol. The emulsification renders the lipids accessible to pancreatic lipase, liberating free fatty acids.

- Triglycerides are formed by esterification of three different fatty acids with glycerol and a portion of the fatty acids remains free as NEFAs.

- Phospholipids are also formed, containing phosphate in a nitrogeneous base in place of one of the fatty acid residues.

- Cholesterol derived from the mevalinate pathway is the precursor of bile acids, steroids, lipoproteins and vitamin D. In plasma about 60–70 per cent of the cholesterol is esterified with fatty acids to form cholesterol esters.

- The major lipoproteins are complex molecules of triglycerides and cholesterol surrounded by phospholipids, cholesterol esters and different proteins, termed apolipoprotein.

- The content of the various lipoproteins varies considerably, as shown in Table 5.10.

Table 5.10   The varying compositions of lipids in lipoprotein

Complex	Source	Electro-phoresis mobility	Protein (%)	Major protein	Triglyceride (%)	Phospho-lipid (%)	Cholesterol ester (%)	Cholesterol
Chylomicrons	Intestine	Origin	1–2	A, B	85–88	8	3	1
VLDL	Liver	Pre beta	7–10	B, C, E	50–55	18–20	12–15	8–10
IDL			10–12	B, C, E	25–30	25–27	32–35	8–10
LDL	VLDL	Beta	20–22	B	10–15	20–28	37–48	8–10
HDL2	Liver and	Alpha	33–35	A, C, E	5–13	26–43	20–30	5–10
HDL3	Intestine	Alpha	55–57	A, C, E	3–13	26–46	15–30	2–6

- *Chylomicrons* are the transporters of lipids from the intestine to all cells. In the capilliaries and adipose tissues the triglyceride component is removed by the action of the lipoprotein lipase enzyme.

- *Very low density lipoprotein* (VLDL) transports lipids from the liver to the cells and the fatty acid component is released for re-use, similar to the chylomicrons.

- *Intermediate density lipoprotein* (IDL) in the absence of metabolic disease is found in plasma at very low concentration and is considered a precursor of LDL.

- *Low density lipoprotein* (LDL) is the primary carrier protein for cholesterol for delivery to all tissues. Insulin and triiodothyronine (T3) increase the binding of LDL to cells, whereas glucocorticoids have the opposite effect. This may be an explanation for the hypercholesterolaemia associated with the uncontrolled diabetic and in subjects with hypothyroidism.

- *High density lipoprotein* (HDL) is the transporter of cholesterol from the cells to the liver. There are sub-fractions of HDL classified as 1, 2 and 3, which vary in composition. It has been suggested that HDL3 is static and HDL2 a dynamic parameter and that up until the menopause females tend to show higher HDL2 levels than males of similar ages.

- The measurements undertaken tend to be limited to triglycerides, total cholesterol, HDL and LDL fractions and in specific cases the inclusion of apolipoprotein A and B. Total cholesterol is of limited value in the assessment of coronary risk.

- Serum cholesterol levels are not altered significantly after a fatty meal, whereas triglycerides demand that the patient fasts for 12 h prior to sample collection.

- Both LDL and HDL show a reduction in levels during the day, but with post-prandial measurements using modern technology the changes during the day are unlikely to alter the clinical diagnosis.

Reference ranges: for all lipoproteins these need to be confirmed with the analytical laboratory.
Total cholesterol (mmol/l)

Age	Males	Females
<25–35	3.7–7.4	3.3–6.5
36–50	4.0–8.0	3.8–7.5
51–70	4.2–8.6	4.7–9.0
>70	3.7–8.8	4.5–9.0

LDL (mmol/l): males, 2.2–5.4; females, 2.3–5.8.

HDL (mmol/l): males, 0.7–1.9; females, 0.9–2.5.

Triglycerides (mmol/l); males, 0.3–3.6; females, 0.2–2.9.

Low total cholesterol levels may be found in

- severe liver damage
- hyperthyroidism
- malnutrition
- chronic anaemia.

Raised total cholesterol levels are used for the assessment of coronary risk and also in secondary hypercholesterolaemia, including

- hyperlipoproteinaemia

- biliary obstructure

- nephrotic syndrome

- hypothyroidism

- diabetes mellitus.

Low levels of HDL may be seen in

- obesity

- starvation

- lack of exercise

- smoking

- diabetes mellitus

- and a number of familial lipid disorders.

Raised levels of HDL may be seen in

- vigorous exercise

- moderate alcohol consumption

- insulin therapy

- a number of genetic abnormalities.

   The risk of atherosclerosis and coronary heart disease is associated with high levels of LDL, whereas HDL is inversely correlated to risk, and high concentrations may be considered as cardio-protective. A number of factors must be given attention in the collection of samples for lipoprotein assessment, including avoidance of alcohol for 4–5 days prior to sample collection, standardized posture at phlebotomy by sitting for 15 min, minimal use of a tourniquet and treatment must not be based on a single result.

Thyroid

The incidence of hypothyroidism in the world population is high, with estimates from the USA of 6–7 million. This figure refers to overt hypothyroidism and does not include the fact that the condition develops slowly. Screening to assess sub-clinical hypothyroidism will demonstrate a significant increase in this incidence figure. It has been suggested that worldwide some 200 million people may be affected by thyroid abnormalities.

   Elderly people, especially women, experience the highest incidence The Merck Manual of Geriatrics quotes a prevalence of 2–5 per cent of the population over the age of 65 years with overt disease, increasing to 5–10 per cent with the inclusion of the sub-clinical condition assessed by thyroid test measurements.

   With the life span of the worldwide population increasing and more clinical trials being carried out on the elderly the inclusion of thyroid tests in pre-screen safety profiles is essential to avoid on-study clinical issues due to this endocrine abnormality.

The inclusion of endocrine topics is outside the scope of this chapter, but some comment on thyroid is considered to illustrate feedback mechanisms:

- The thyroid cubical epithelium cells trap iodide from the circulation, which is initially linked to the amino acid tyrosine. In the thyroid gland this is converted to *triiodothyronine* (T3) and *tetraiodothyronine* (*thyroxine*; T4) and stored in a colloid with protein as *thyroglobulin*.

- The thyroid gland is part of the hypothalamic–anterior pituitary–thyroid axis and the control of the thyroid hormone secretion is exerted by the classical negative feedback system.

- Thyroid-releasing hormone (TRH) from the hypothalamus stimulates the release of the thyroid-stimulating hormone (TSH) from the anterior pituitary, which stimulates thyroid hormone release. As the blood concentration of the T4 from the thyroid increases, this inhibits both TSH and TRH, leading to a shutdown of thyroid activity, as shown in Figure 5.10.

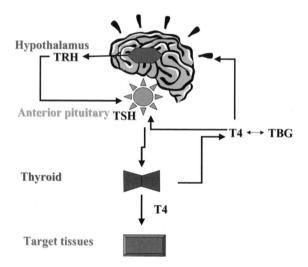

Figure 5.10 The feedback system of the hypothalamic–pituitary–thyroid axis

- Thyroid hormones (T4 and T3) are poorly soluble in water, and more than 99 per cent of the circulating hormones in blood are bound to a carrier proteins, particularly the thyroid-binding globulin and to a lesser extent the thyroid-binding pre-albumin, albumin and lipoproteins.

- T3 and T4 are carried by the blood to all body tissues. T4 is converted in the cells to T3, which binds to receptors in the nuclei to increase messenger RNA and hence protein synthesis. This results in an increase in oxygen consumption, heat production and increased metabolism.

- A normal thyroid output is required for normal growth.

- Owing to the high binding of the hormone to the thyroid-binding globulin, which is increased during pregnancy, hepatitis and with oestrogen-related drugs, the value of the total T4 is limited. Thus, the measurement of free T4 is preferred.

- TSH has a major benefit in hypothyroidism, in that it is increased usually prior to any obvious clinical signs of the disorder and hence is a valuable screening procedure.

Reference range: TSH, 0.3–5.0 mIU/l; free T4, 9.0–25.0 pmol/l; Free T3, 3.0–8.5 pmol/l.

Interpretation

- In hypothyroidism, the TSH results may be markedly elevated (>50 mIU/l) and the free T4 value is low. In borderline cases the free T4 may be normal, but the TSH is usually raised.

- On thyroid replacement therapy TSH should be the measure employed to monitor success of therapy

- In hyperthyroidism the TSH is low and, although sensitive methods are available, the diagnosis is usually confirmed by an elevated free T4.

- In hypopituitarism, both of the hormones will be reduced.

- Considerable care is required in the interpretation of thyroid function tests due to changes in the concentration of the thyroid-binding globulin. Increased levels of the protein may be congenital, due to high concentrations of oestrogen, hepatitis and influence by a number of drugs. Low levels of thyroid-binding globulin may be encountered in subjects on androgens, glucocorticoids and in clinical nephrotic syndrome and cirrhosis.

Haematology

Haematology is the study of the blood cells to determine normal haemopoiesis and/or the diagnosis of blood diseases. However, as is characteristic of most laboratory measurements the basic haematology profile is merely a screening procedure. In the event of any abnormality being identified, then much more rigorous testing of the bone marrow and associated biochemical markers is needed.

Blood is a specialist fluid tissue concerned predominantly with the transport system. The average volume is 5.6 l, representing about 8 per cent of body weight. Some 45 per cent of whole blood is cellular and 55 per cent plasma. Plasma is 93 per cent water, with the remaining solid content being mainly albumin.

The cellular content consists:

red blood cells $(4.1–6.5 \times 10^{12}/l)$

platelets $(250 - 500 \times 10^9/l)$

white blood cells $(4 - 11 \times 10^9/l)$.

For normal functional haemopoiesis, numerous substances are necessary. The kidney must secrete erythropoietin, which stimulates bone marrow cell production but also requires vitamin B12, thyroid and adrenal hormones, iron, copper, manganese, vitamin C, folic acid and the intrinsic factor secreted from the gastric mucosa.

The normal full blood count is accomplished with specialist analytical systems and includes the following measurements:

Haemoglobin (Hb, g/l)

Haematocrit (HCT or PCV, fl)

Mean cell volume (MCR, pg)

Red cell distribution width (RDW, %)

Mean cell haemoglobin (MCH, pg)

Mean cell haemoglobin concentration (MCHC, g/l)

Red cell count (RBC, $10^{12}/l$)

White cell count (WBC, $10^9/l$)

Differential white cell count (Diff WBC, $10^9/l$)

Haemoglobin

Haemoglobin is the protein that carries oxygen from the lungs to the tissues and in exchange carries carbon dioxide from the tissues back to the lungs. The molecule consists of four polypeptide chains, two α chains of 141 amino acids and two β chains of 146 amino acids. Each chain is conjugated with a haem group that binds the oxygen to ferrous ions.

Females have lower values than males, and although the molecular weight of haemoglobin is known, the SI unit has not been universally accepted.

Strictly, anaemia is defined as a decrease in total body red cell mass, but for practical purposes anaemia is usually defined by a haemoglobin value of <100 g/l.

Reference range: males, 135–180 g/l; females, 115–164 g/l.

Haematocrit

In the original technology the haematocrit was measured in a graduated tube filled with blood, which was centrifuged to pack the red blood cells. The percentage of packed cells is expressed relative to the total whole blood volume. With the analytical instrumentation now in common use the haemoglobin, red cell count and mean cell volume are measured and the other parameters calculated. In the case of the haematocrit this is obtained by multiplying the red cell count by the mean cell volume with results expressed in femtolitres.

Reference range: males, 0.40–0.54 fl; females, 0.37–0.47 fl.

Erythrocytes: red cell count

The erythrocytes are disc-shaped cells with a thick rim, and their major function is gas transportation and the maintenance of pH. Some of the 35 per cent cytoplasm is haemoglobin, and it also contains the enzyme carbonic anhydrase to convert carbon dioxide and water reversibly to carbonic acid.

Erythrocytes progress from blast cells in the marrow over a period of several days, then are released into peripheral circulation as reticulocytes. Within 24 h the reticulocytes change to erythrocytes and remain in circulation for about 120 days. Using special stains the reticulocytes can be determined; normally they represent only 1.5 per cent of the total RBC. The reticulocyte count can be considered as an index of bone marrow production. Increases are encountered in increased red cell turnover due to bleeding or haemolysis and in response to successful therapy in marrow deficiencies. A reduction in reticulocytes may be due to impairment in erythrocyte production, such as aplastic anaemia.

A drop in the RBC number causes hypoxaemia in the kidney, resulting in stimulation of erythropoietin which acts on the marrow to increase RBC production. Stimulus for erythropoiesis may also result from low levels of atmospheric oxygen, increased exercise activity and haemorrhaging.

Reference range: females $(3.9-5.6) \times 10^{12}/l$; males $(4.6-6.5) \times 10^{12}/l$.

Red cell indices

The red cell indices are sometimes referred to as absolute values and include MCV, MCH and MCHC, but the red cell distribution width should also be considered as an index.

Mean cell volume   The MCV defines the average volume of all the erythrocytes counted in an examination with the results expressed in femtolitres. After phlebotomy with the whole blood sample collected into EDTA containers the MCV will show an increase within 6–10 h. This is singly the most useful measurement, as it clearly classifies anaemias as microcytic and macrocytic (small and large volume cells) from normocytic cells.

Reference range: both sexes, 81–95 fl.

As the MCV expresses information on the average of the cell volume it is important to bear in mind that a normal MCV could be obtained but there might be an abnormal variation in the cell sizes. This is referred to as anisocytosis. The red cell distribution width RDW provides a measure of the dispersion around the mean cell population expressed as a percentage. The percentage is normally 11.5–14 per cent, and values greater than this indicate the degree of anisocytosis.

Reference range: both sexes, 11.5–14.5 per cent.

Mean cell haemoglobin   The MCH defines the *weight* of haemoglobin in the average red blood cell expressed in picograms. Since small cells have less haemoglobin than larger cells, variation in the MCH tends to follow the MCV.

Reference range: 26–32 pg.

Mean cell haemoglobin concentration   The MCHC defines the *amount* of haemoglobin in the average RBC compared with its size, with results expressed in g/l. As the red cells constitute about one-half of the whole blood and all the haemoglobin is located in the RBC, it would be expected that the MCHC value would be about twice the haemoglobin concentration.

Cells with low and high levels of MCHC are referred to as hypochromic and hyperchromic respectively.

Reference range: 300–350 g/l.

Anaemia   Anaemias are generally classified as microcytic or macrocytic (Figure 5.11).

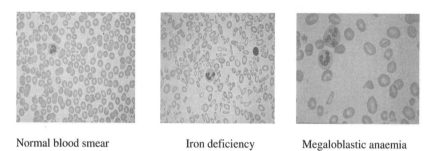

Normal blood smear   Iron deficiency   Megaloblastic anaemia

Figure 5.11   Typical stained blood smears showing normal, microcytic and macrocytic anaemias

The most common cause of microcytic anaemia is iron-deficiency due to blood loss from the stomach, intestine or excess menstruation. Defects in nutrition and or a lack of absorption, chronic inflammation, malignancy and thalassaemia may also cause an iron-deficiency anaemia.

Macrocytic anaemia causes are usually vitamin B12 deficiency, folate deficiency, alcohol abuse and liver disease. Of these the most important is pernicious anaemia, which results from the inability of the stomach to produce the intrinsic factor for the absorption of vitamin B12.

Haemolytic anaemia is due to a loss of RBC caused by an abnormally high rate of destruction due to inherited abnormalities, including red cell membrane defects, haemoglobin abnormalities as in thalassaemia and sickle disease, and metabolic disorders, such as glucose-6-phosphate dehydrogenase deficiency.

Aplastic anaemia is suppression of the blood cell formation in the bone marrow with a failure in the production of all types of cell. Most often aplastic anaemia occurs without any prior history and is termed idiopathic, but it may also be due to certain poisons, drugs, radiation and chemicals. There are a number of pharmaceutical products that have an association with aplastic anaemia in a minority of patients. These include chloramphenicol, non-steroidal anti-inflammatories, thyrostatics, psychotropics and some cardio-vascular drugs. However, it is sometimes difficult to confidently implicate medical drugs as the causative agent due to the idiopathic nature of the condition.

Polycythaemia is defined as an increase in total body erythrocyte mass – the opposite of anaemia. The blood volume is increased with hyperviscosity. It may occur due to abnormally low fluid intake or marked loss of fluid, secondary to defective saturation of arterial blood with oxygen at high altitudes or to a myeloproliferative disorder.

White blood cells

To consider the leucocytes as a group is of limited value, as each type of white cell has its own individual function; therefore, much greater emphasis should be placed on the absolute count for each of the different leucocytes. Traditionally, the differential white cell count expressed the values as a percentage, a practice that still continues and which is requested in many clinical studies. Fortunately, laboratories express the individual leucocytes in absolute values and, as an addition, the percentage figure may also be defined in the clinical laboratory report if required.

Reference range: both sexes $(3.5-11.0) \times 10^9/l$.

Granulocytes

The granulocytes include neutrophils, eosinophils and basophils, although it is questionable whether they should be grouped together.

Neutrophils In normal blood the neutrophils represent the largest population of the leucoctyes. They have a short life span of several days. They increase in response to bacterial infection, infarction, inflammation and acute body stress. Marked neutrophilia may indicate haematological malignancy. Smokers tend to have higher neutrophils than non-smokers, and corticosteroid therapy may increase the neutrophil count. Neutropenia is common in different ethnic groups, particularly Afro-Caribbean and Indian populations, and may be present in subjects on anticonvulsant and antithyroid therapy.

Reference range: $(2.5-7.5) \times 10^9/l$.

Eosinophils Increased eosinophils (eosinophilia) are found in allergic disorders and parasitic infestations. Other causes include rheumatoid arthritis, sarcoidosis, and acute rheumatic fever, and they may also increase in the resolution phase of infections.

Eosinopenia may occur in shock, major pyogenic infections, trauma, post-surgery and in response to corticosteroids, niacin (vitamin B3) and a number of other drugs.

Reference range: $(0.1-0.4) \times 10^9/l$.

Basophils The basophils represent a small concentration of the total leucocytes. If markedly increased then this may suggest myeloproliferative disease.

Other causes of basophilia include allergic reactions, ulcerative colitis, myxoedema, the therapeutic use of oestrogens, desipramine and antithyroid medication.

Reference range: $(0.0-0.2) \times 10^9/l$.

Lymphocytes Normally the lymphocytes represent about 35 per cent of the total leucocyte count. They originate from bone narrow, germ cell centres of lymph nodes and spleen. There are large and small varieties in peripheral blood and they have a life span of several months.

There are two varieties: T-lymphocytes react against foreign proteins, viruses, tissue transplants etc.; B-lymphocytes develop into immunoglobulins.

Lymphyocytosis occurs in viral infection, infective mononucleosis, infective hepatitis, chronic infections and thyrotoxicosis. Severe lymphocytosis may indicate lymphocytic leukaemia. A number of drugs can result in lymphocytosis, and these include haloperidol, phenytoin and niacinamide.

Lymphopenia is characteristic of AIDS patients, and can also occur in systemic lupus, renal failure and carcinomatosis.

Corticosteroids, lithium, niacin and ionizing radiation may result in lymphopenia.

Reference range: $(1.5–3.5) \times 10^9/l$.

Monocytes Monocytes share the same stem cell as neutrophils; they migrate into inflammatory sites and act as phagocytes under the influence of cytokines.

Monocytosis may be caused by chronic inflammatory processes, rheumatoid arthritis, Crohn's disease, tuberculosis and haematological neoplasms.

Monocytopenia is generally not a clinical problem.

Reference range: $(0.2–1.3) \times 10^9/l$.

Platelets (thrombocytes)

Thrombocytes are required for the maintenance of normal vascular endothelium. When vessels are damaged they act as a mechanical plug and by releasing serotonin, cause local vasoconstriction. They are essential for thrombin generation and release accessory factors for normal coagulation while also acting as phagocytes.

Thrombocytosis is seen in many inflammatory disorders, as well as in acute and chronic blood loss, after recent surgery, myeloproliferative disorders, haemolytic anaemia and post-exercise.

The most common cause of thrombocytopenia is small clots in samples for haematological assessments, but it is also found in megaloblastic and severe iron-deficiency anaemias, viral infections and aplastic anaemia. Non-steroidal anti-inflammatory drugs, diuretics and alcohol may also cause thrombocytopenia.

Screening for proper platelet function is best accomplished in conjunction with the bleeding time test.

Some drugs suppress the bone marrow, resulting in thrombocytopenia; however, in these circumstances there is usually a corresponding reduction in both white and red cells. Other drugs cause a production of antibodies, which attach to platelets leading to an isolated destruction of the platelet and is termed immune thrombocytopenia. The most common compounds related to thrombocytopenia are heparin, but quinidine, procainamide, carbamazepine and cimetidine have also been implicated.

Reference range: $(140–340) \times 10^9/l$.

Erythrocyte sedimentation rate and C-reactive protein

The erythrocyte sedimentation rate (ESR) measurement is carried out routinely on most hospital admissions. This simple laboratory test offers a measure of inflammation as an acute phase reactant. Elevated values are found in most inflammatory conditions, including bacterial and viral infections, tissue damage as a result of surgery, myocardial infarction, rheumatoid arthritis and certain malignancies.

ESR must be measured within hours, and thus is an unsuitable test in drug studies when samples are forwarded to central laboratories. Furthermore, ESR measurements are multifactorial and may be influenced by hypoalbuminaemia, hyperlipidaemia and severe anaemia. Also, there is a relatively slow response to clinical improvement.

C-reactive protein (CRP) is an unspecific marker of inflammation. As an acute phase reactant it responds similarly to the ESR test, but with a much more rapid response to inflammatory stimulation. The serum CRP levels will begin to increase within 6–12 h after the onset of inflammation. Also, an increase or decrease in the serum CRP concentration follows the changes in the clinical status of the patient much more rapidly than ESR changes; therefore, in monitoring the response to therapy CRP it has a major benefit. In certain inflammatory reactions a 1000-fold increase in CRP will be noted, offering much greater clinical sensitivity. CRP will also show increases in acute infection and in certain malignancies.

Reference range: in healthy non-smoking individuals the mean value is usually less than 1 mg/l, with an upper limit of 6 mg/l.

Urinalysis

Urinalysis performed by dipstick generally consists of the following assessments: pH, protein, blood, bilirubin, urobilinogen, glucose, ketones, nitrite and leucocytes.

pH

The pH of urine in healthy subjects is usually in the range of 4.5–7.8, but generally a much closer interval of pH 5.0–6.0 is found.

In the stomach, gastric acid is secreted in anticipation of a meal; however, there is an increase in blood pH known as the 'alkaline tide' after a meal, caused by bicarbonate ions being secreted into the extracellular fluid and then into venous blood that may result in post-prandial alkaline urine.

Acidic pH will be encountered in diabetic acidosis, in subjects on a high protein diet and in kidney failure, whereas alkaline urine may be found in severe potassium deficiency, diuretic treatment and vomiting.

Protein

The sensitivity of dipsticks is set to show negative values at concentration of <30 mg/dl.

Proteinuria can result normally during periods of stress and after physical exercise. Haemoglobin and vaginal secretion could well give positive readings.

In pathological conditions, raised urine protein levels may be found in renal disease, myocardial infarction, cardiac insufficiency, paraproteinanaemia and many other conditions.

In screening for diabetic microalbuminuria, even the trace readings on dipsticks do not provide adequate sensitivity.

Blood

Dipsticks will detect greater than 5 RBCs/μl and the test is specific for haemoglobin and myoglobin.

The principal causes of haematuria relate to the kidney or urogenital tract.

Haematuria is an important sign in glomerulonephritis, stone formation, tumours, intravascular haemolysis and during infections.

Myoglobulinuria is generally due to muscle injury or muscle necrosis and can be found in crush injuries.

Physical exercise can also give positive results.

Birlirubin

Normally bilirubin is undetectable, with adults excreting less than 0.1 mg/dl.

Values as low as 0.3 mg/dl will give a positive result.

The presence of bilirubin provides an early sign of jaundice, biliary stasis, or hepato-cellular damage, as in acute, chronic and alcohol hepatitis, liver cirrhosis and liver toxicity.

Urobilinogen

Normally, small amounts of urobilinogen are present and the dipstick test will detect concentrations greater than 0.4 mg/dl.

False negative results can occur in old samples and in samples exposed to direct sunlight. Drugs that colour urine can give false positive results.

Urobilinogen excess may be found when hepatitis, liver congestion, toxicity and liver tumours are present.

In situations of overload, such as in haemolytic anaemia, pernicious anaemia, and intravascular haemolysis, increases in urobilinogenuria will be found.

Glucose

The assessment of glycosuria probably led to the advent of urinary dipsticks, and these provide an inexpensive method for diabetic screening and self-monitoring.

Blood glucose values reaching the renal reabsorption threshold overspill into urine.

In fasting subjects' urine samples the levels are normally less than 20 mg/dl, and on random samples less than 30 mg/dl. The detection limit on dipsticks is normally set at 40 mg/dl.

Renal glycosuria may occur during pregnancy and when kidney function falls to 30 per cent or less of normal renal performance.

Ketones

The test detects acetoacetic acid and acetone, but does not detect β-hydroxybutyric acid. Values are normally less than 5 mg/dl and the detection limit of the dipstick is set at the 5 mg level.

Raised levels are found in diabetic ketoacidosis due to fatty acid metabolism acceleration in insulin deficiency.

Ketonuria of non-diabetic origin may be found in hunger states, patients on slimming diets, fever and in vomiting.

Nitrite

Most pathogenic bacteria have the ability to reduce nitrate (normally present in urine) to nitrite, and this forms the basis of the test.

Urinary tract infections are common and the spread increases with advancing years, particularly in the female.

False negatives may be found in strong diuresis, vegetable-free diets and in subjects being administered antibacterial therapy. This must be discontinued for at least 3 days prior to urinalysis for the test to be valid.

False positive results can occur when samples are left standing at room temperature for lengthy periods.

Leucocytes

The limit of detection is set at 10 leucocytes/μl for granulocyte esterase activity, and includes both intact and lysed cells. White cells in the range of 10–20/μl are classified as suspicious and levels greater than 20/μl are considered pathological.

False positive results may occur in excessive protein excretion.

Leucocyturia indicates the presence of inflammatory disease of the kidney and the urinary tract.

The great majority of positive findings are due to urinary tract infections, cystitis, pyelonephritis, glomerular disease and parasitic infestations.

All of the dipstick tests must be considered as preliminary screening procedures, and any abnormal result must be followed by microscopy of urine sediment and other appropriate blood measurements.

Test selection

Selection of the most appropriate clinical laboratory tests in drug studies is difficult to define, and that will vary dependent on the compound, data from pre-clinical toxicology studies and the phase of clinical development. In respect of the latter, it is important to remember that the most stringent testing should be undertaken at phase 1 to support early administration of the drug to humans. Thus, the most sensitive tests should be carried out as early as possible in the drug development to determine potential toxicities and so avoid substantially increased cost at the later phases of the drug programme. It is questionable, as to whether sufficient attention is devoted to the chemical structure of the compound and the pre-clinical data in clinical laboratory safety testing that could provide the necessary emphasis towards the most appropriate laboratory measurements.

Supplementing the above criteria will be the need for special testing dependent on the function of the new compound, and this will differ markedly from drug to drug. A definition of special measurements is beyond consideration in this section, but it is strongly recommended that these non-routine tests be discussed with the laboratory to ensure that the pre-analytical conditions are clearly met and the limitation of the procedure known.

If the range of laboratory investigations undertaken is the minimum possible for reasons of economy or endeavouring to minimize results outside the reference interval, then there will always be a possibility of a laboratory adverse event not being detected. It is well worth considering taking an additional sample of blood on all occasions and having this correctly stored by the analytical laboratory, which may then be used at a later date for other tests or for the confirmation of clinically significant abnormal results.

For general safety screening the tests shown in Table 5.11 are recommended as the minimum requirements, and these can be carried out on non-fasting patients.

In phase 1, additional sensitive tests of renal function should be given priority, including

Table 5.11   The recommended biochemical and haematological tests to be included in a general safety testing profile

Renal function and electrolytes	Urea
	Creatinine
	Uric acid
	Sodium
	Potassium
Glucose metabolism	Glucose
Bone and Protein metabolism	Calcium
	Total protein
	Albumin
Liver Function	Gamma glutamyltranspeptidase (GGT)
	Aspartate aminotransferase (AST)
	Alanine aminotransferase (ALT)
	Alkaline phosphatase (AP)
	Bilirubin
Lipid metabolism	Cholesterol
Thyroid function (pre-study)	Free thyroxine
	Thyroid-stimulating hormone (TSH)
Haematology	Haemoglobin
	Haematocrit
	MCH, MCHC and MCV
	Red cell count
	White cell count
	Differential white cell count
	Platelets
	C-reactive protein
Urinalysis	General screening dipstick

cystatin C as a measure of the GFR rate and NAG to assess renal tubular function, especially if there was any evidence of renal toxicity from animal studies.

Exclusion criteria and 'Panic levels'

To define pre-trial patient acceptance criteria is extremely difficult. At phases 1 and 2 the aim is to protect the safety of the patient by the exclusion of sub-clinical disease that might expose them to unnecessary risk. The aim is also to protect the drug by excluding patients with sub-clinical disease that might progress to overt disease during the study and be mistaken for a drug-induced effect. In phase 3 the patients are likely to have other diseases, and owing to the nature of the disease these patients may demonstrate clinical laboratory abnormal results. Furthermore, at phase 3 the monitoring of laboratory tests is undertaken to ensure that the drug is not affecting organ functions other than the target organ. Compiling these factors, to define values of acceptance is not an easy exercise.

Ideally, at phase 1 all results should be within the laboratory quoted reference ranges, particularly the measurements related to haematology, renal and liver function. As volunteers tend to be screened without any consideration being given to pre-analytical factors, any abnormality requires further sampling with attention being given to subject preparation and timing of phlebotomy.

In clinical laboratories, study coordinators and project managers need guidance on the interpretation of patient results. Table 5.12 lists the tests of a standard safety profile with detail of the reference ranges, a grey area of results requiring further investigation and 'panic' levels. These numerical values are based on clinical experience. The grey area defines test values marginally outside the reference range that demand confirmation for the subject to take part in phase 1 studies. The panic values assume that normal results were expected in the particular phase 3 study and refer to isolated single results, whereas the grey area values need to be examined with respect to organ-related tests. The information can be incorporated into the specific study database as alert ranges and used by study coordinators to contact the investigator immediately or, in his absence, the clinical project manager.

Table 5.12 A numerical guide to the necessary action when test results fall into the grey or panic areas

	Units	Ref. range	Grey area		Panic levels	
Haematology						
WBC	10^9/l	4.0–11.0	2.8	14.5	2	22
RBC	10^{12}/l	4.5–6.5	3.5	7.5	3	7.5
HB	g/dl	13.0–18.0	10	19	10	19
PCV	fl	40.0–54.0	32	60	30	65
MCV	pg	80.0–100.0	70	120	60	120
Platelets	10^9/l	150–400	130	500	100	650
Clinical chemistry						
AST	IU/l	13–40		80		80
ALT	IU/l	7–40		80		80
AP	IU/l	97–240		300		350
GGT	IU/l	3–38		80		120
Bilirubin	μmol/l	4.5–20		40		50
Glucose	mmol/l	3.8–6.0	3.0	8.5	2.5	12.5
Urea	mmol/l	2.9–7.3		8.5		11
Sodium	mmol/l	135–147	125	155	120	160
Potassium	mmol/l	3.8–5.4	3.0	6.0	2.5	6.2
Creatinine	μmol/l	83–127		170		170
Uric acid	μmol/l	220–450	150	650	150	650
Calcium	mmol/l	2.24–2.64	2.2	2.75	2.1	2.85
Total protein	g/l	59–79	50	85	50	
Albumin	g/l	38–50	28	58	28	
Cholesterol	mmol/l	3.1–7.5	2.3	8.0	2.3	9.0
Thyroxine	nmol/l	60–150	40	180	35	220

Harmonization of data from different laboratories

As mentioned previously, there are many occasions when local laboratories are used to support clinical studies. This is an obvious requirement when drug trials are being carried out on acutely ill subjects, such as patients with myocardial infarction, cerebral vascular accident, etc., but also a number of companies accept the resistance of investigators towards central facilities and use local-area laboratories. There is then a need to adjust the laboratory patient results from the various participating laboratories to attain a comparable structure of results in a single database.

There have been a number of reported procedures for 'normalizing' data (Abt and Krupps, 1986; Sogliero-Gilbert *et al.*, 1986; Chuang-Stein, 1992), all based on manipulating factors on the individual laboratory's lower and upper limits of the reference ranges being employed.

At this point it is important to appreciate that although the reference ranges used in central laboratories are accurately determined on a normal healthy population, and regularly reviewed and governed by standard operating procedures, this may not be the case with local laboratories, whose main interest is diagnostic pathology. Therefore, mathematical manipulation of patients' results based on lower and upper limits of reference ranges may not always be valid. Further, Groth and de Verdier (1993) commented on the transferability of clinical laboratory data, 'even with instruments of the same type and from the same manufacturer, and with identical reference materials for calibration, there may well be an inter-instrument difference that jeopardises the analytical goals'.

We were requested to review prolactin measurements undertaken as an efficacy marker and analysed by 14 different European laboratories. All the laboratories used their standard routine diagnostic kit for prolactin measurement. Five reported their results in ng/ml and the remaining laboratories reported in International Units as mIU/ml. However, different diagnostic manufacturer's kits were used and different international reference preparations were employed as calibrators and so the reference ranges varied dramatically. No amount of manipulation could ever harmonize these data, and as an efficacy marker, the results had to be discarded.

Dijkman *et al.* (2000) detailed the Virtual Central Laboratory (VCL) harmonization approach developed in the Netherlands, where samples are analysed in local laboratories and the patient results transferred electronically to the VCL data-management system. All participating local laboratories, irrespective of the instruments and technology employed, are provided with calibrators at the outset to determine conversion factors based on linear regression analyses to be incorporated into the data-management system. Concurrently, during the studies calibrator checks are included to ensure no deviations occur.

In our own laboratory, although a dedicated central facility, harmonizing data with different laboratories has had to be carried out in complex studies based in distant locations, including both efficacy and safety markers. The approach used in the Pivotal structure is carried out on randomly selected patient samples, usually 40 in number, shipped by courier immediately after collection and analysed in each laboratory at identical times on the same day. The statistical assessment includes calculation of the mean, median, confidence limits, paired *t*-test, the Passing and Bablok (1983) regression analyses and the Bland and Altman (1986) bias assessment. The regression equation is used to calculate any necessary correction factors to be applied to the participating laboratories, and the bias assessment used for confirmation.

To illustrate this structure, Figure 5.12 shows the results from two laboratories for serum creatinine determinations. Lab A, the reference laboratory, shows a mean value of 76.8 μmol/l and Lab B a mean value of 90.2 μmol/l. Application of the Passing and Bablok (1993) regression equation converts the results of Lab B to a mean value of 76.2 μmol/l.

The data from the Altman and Bland (1986) bias plots before and after the application of the regression equation are illustrated in Figure 5.13. The uncorrected data in the left-hand

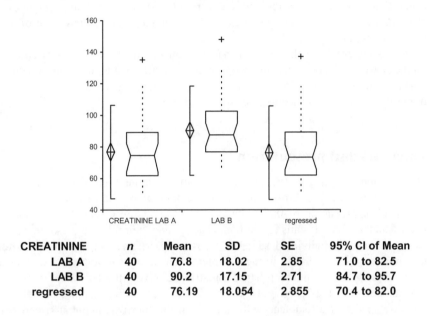

CREATININE	n	Mean	SD	SE	95% CI of Mean
LAB A	40	76.8	18.02	2.85	71.0 to 82.5
LAB B	40	90.2	17.15	2.71	84.7 to 95.7
regressed	40	76.19	18.054	2.855	70.4 to 82.0

Figure 5.12   The descriptive statistics of serum creatinine measurements performed in two laboratories, before and after the application of the Passing and Bablok (1983) regression equation

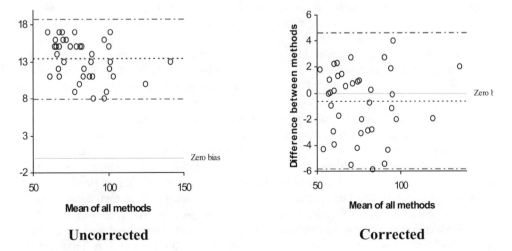

Figure 5.13   Shows the Altman and Bland (1986) plots of the serum creatinine measurements before and after the application of the regression equation

panel show a 13 per cent positive bias in the results from Lab B. After the application of the regression equation (right panel) all the results surround the zero line, demonstrating satisfactory correction. The maximum difference found after correction represented 6 µmol/l, which for creatinine is considered to be of little clinical significance.

The regression conversion of the data shown in Figure 5.13 can be applied to harmonize results for laboratory measurements carried out in difference laboratories. It must be appreciated that this type of correlation and correction study applies at a single point in time; therefore, to ensure that the parameters are maintained during the course of a study, meticulous IQC is mandatory.

It must be apparent from this section that harmonization of data requires cooperation between the analytical laboratories, the coordinating statistician, and the industry's biometric department if successful standardization of clinical laboratory results between different laboratories can be accurately accomplished.

Data analysis and presentation

The interpretation of efficacy data is generally not too large a problem, as it is usually directly compared with a control group and a definition of the efficacy is predefined. However, a full appreciation of the analytical limitations is an essential requirement, and although population-based statistics are mandatory and helpful it is also important to examine the change in individual subjects. Conversely, safety data present an extremely complex situation, as the change in measurement from normal to abnormal may occur in only a few subjects; thus, population-based statistics are of very limited value.

Two major points of confusion emerge. The first relates to the reference range, where it cannot be assumed that all subjects will fall within the 'normal' population and that the crossover between health and disease at the upper limit of the reference range has to be treated as a significant grey area. Also, the more subjects and tests that are included in a study the greater will be the likelihood of finding so-called abnormal results, and in new drug applications vast volumes of clinical laboratory data are included. The second issue relates to the fact that rarely do we find a single test result showing a clinically significant change as, in safety profiles, more that one test will usually be associated with a diseased state or an adverse drug reaction. Unfortunately, multivariate analyses of laboratory data using advanced software technology do not appear to help in this direction. For example, to combine the liver function tests of the aminotransferases, AP and bilirubin into a single database for interpretation only adds to the complications. Interpretation of laboratory reports and data still demands professional observation, which requires a combination of science, medicine, statistics and experience to derive any clinical significance on the testing.

A further complication lies in the fact that perhaps one investigator may find only one or two patients demonstrating minor changes in laboratory reports and considers these to be of little significance. However, there may be over 100 investigators all finding similar levels of the same abnormal results. Unless either the clinical laboratory with its total database or the sponsor is constantly monitoring these, early warning of possible toxicity may be missed.

With adverse events being the fifth major cause of death in hospitalized patients (Lazarou *et al.* 1998) and laboratory data playing an integral part in this process, it is important that laboratory safety analyses are given considerable attention at all stages of a trial. Generally, the clinical laboratory is unaware of who is on active drug and who is on placebo. Also, the laboratory has little patient case history information. Therefore, for the laboratory to help in interpretation will demand much closer involvement in the study. Nevertheless, the laboratory does have data on all patients in a particular study or centre and perhaps should be looking at providing interim interpretation on purely the laboratory data.

On many occasions I have been requested to evaluate clinical laboratory data, which is usually a mixture of both efficacy and safety measurements. As mentioned previously, efficacy is not a major problem and interpretation of the derived information is comparatively easy.

The structure below is a simplified approach using Microsoft Excel with Analyse-it (Leeds, UK; http://www.analyse-it.com) clinical statistical software as an example for formatting data, which can no doubt be transferred into more elaborate statistical packages.

Overall, clinical trial safety data is transferred into Excel electronically and using the pivot table facilities separate sheets are cut and pasted for each test using the test name, patient identifiers, occasions and results. These separate result sheets are sorted in increasing test result order in respect of the baseline sample and displayed as graphical presentations with high/low bars for the subsequent occasions. An example is shown in Figure 5.14, which provides a visual impression of the change in data over the study period. If required, the chart may be modified to include error bars based on the range of the SSD, which in the case of calcium is 7.2 per cent and thus highlight results outside this SSD parameter. From this the change from baseline is easily identified and any bias in the on-treatment samples noted.

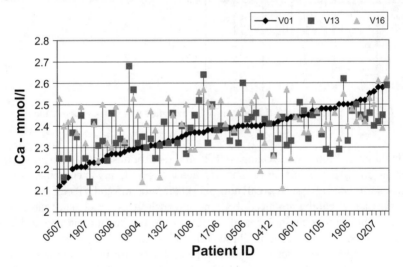

Figure 5.14 Calcium measurements in a clinical study with sampling at baseline (V01) and at 2 subsequent occasions (week 13 [V13] and week 16 [V16])

With the test results in Excel, it is a simple procedure to incorporate 'if functions' to highlight results above and below the reference interval and also results showing a significant change from baseline based on the SSD value.

An example of this is shown in Figure 5.15. The left-hand panel detailing the calcium values at baseline and two subsequent occasions. This panel may contain several hundred results, but by the application of 'if functions' and filtering, only those results outside the reference range can be viewed for assessment, as shown in the right-hand panel. Similarly, the application of the

Subject Id	V01	V13	V16	V01 RR	V13RR	V16RR	Normal %change	RVC
1904	2.21	2.45	2.49	L	N	N		12.7	raised
1907	2.21	2.25	2.32	L	N	N		5.0	
0305	2.23	2.14	2.07	L	L	L		-7.7	lowered
0307	2.23	2.42	2.41	L	N	N		8.1	raised
0906	2.23	2.31	2.24	L	N	L		0.4	
0905	2.24	2.33	2.5	L	N	N		11.6	raised
1708	2.26	2.24	2.32	N	L	N		2.7	
0308	2.27	2.46	2.3	N	N	N	ALL N	1.3	
1011	2.27	2.32	2.49	N	N	N	ALL N	9.7	raised
1709	2.27	2.34	2.39	N	N	N	ALL N	5.3	
0118	2.28	2.32	2.33	N	N	N	ALL N	2.2	
0115	2.29	2.68	2.48	N	H	N		8.3	raised
0912	2.29	2.57	2.53	N	N	N	ALL N	10.5	raised
0904	2.3	2.32	2.45	N	N	N	ALL N	6.5	
1704	2.3	2.35	2.14	N	N	L		-7.5	
2002	2.3	2.3	2.41	N	N	N	ALL N	4.8	
0908	2.31	2.34	2.47	N	N	N	ALL N	6.9	
2004	2.31	2.25	2.38	N	N	N	ALL N	3.0	
0110	2.32	2.31	2.16	N	N	L		-7.4	
0117	2.33	2.32	2.53	N	N	N	ALL N	8.6	raised
1902	2.33	2.46	2.45	N	N	N	ALL N	5.2	
0114	2.34	2.32	2.23	N	N	L		-4.9	
0902	2.35	2.4	2.41	N	N	N	ALL N	2.6	
0102	2.36	2.27	2.5	N	N	N	ALL N	5.9	
1008	2.37	2.39	2.29	N	N	N	ALL N	-3.5	
1009	2.37	2.45	2.29	N	N	N	ALL N	-3.5	
1702	2.37	2.52	2.56	N	N	N	ALL N	8.0	raised
1908	2.37	2.64	2.57	N	N	N	ALL N	8.4	raised
0311	2.38	2.32	2.51	N	N	N	ALL N	5.5	
1304	2.38	2.5	2.49	N	N	N	ALL N	4.6	
1706	2.38	2.38	2.35	N	N	N	ALL N	1.3	
2003	2.38	2.4	2.52	N	N	N	ALL N	5.9	
0103	2.39	2.39	2.41	N	N	N	ALL N	0.8	
1202	2.39	2.33	2.46	N	N	N	ALL N	2.9	
1402	2.39	2.37	2.38	N	N	N	ALL N	-0.4	
0410	2.4	2.32	2.46	N	N	N	ALL N	2.5	
0506	2.4	2.6	2.48	N	N	N	ALL N	3.3	
0602	2.4	2.43	2.38	N	N	N	ALL N	-0.8	
0807	2.4	2.44	2.51	N	N	N	ALL N	4.6	
1707	2.4	2.46	2.54	N	N	N	ALL N	5.8	
2001	2.4	2.35	2.19	N	N	L		-9.6	lowered
0306	2.41	2.43	2.32	N	N	N	ALL N	-3.9	
0412	2.41	2.41	2.55	N	N	N	ALL N	5.8	
1003	2.41	2.26	2.26	N	N	N	ALL N	-6.6	
0104	2.42	2.34	2.45	N	N	N	ALL N	1.2	
0204	2.43	2.44	2.11	N	N	L		-15.2	lowered
1201	2.43	2.31	2.57	N	N	N	ALL N	5.8	
0113	2.44	2.33	2.25	N	N	N	ALL N	-8.4	lowered
0601	2.44	2.44	2.44	N	N	N	ALL N	0.0	
1010	2.44	2.51	2.43	N	N	N	ALL N	-0.4	
0109	2.45	2.47	2.37	N	N	N	ALL N	-3.4	
0409	2.45	2.34	2.37	N	N	N	ALL N	-3.4	

Subject Id	V01	V13	V16	V01 RR	V13RR	V16RR	% change	RVC
0507	2.12	2.25	2.53	L	N	N	19.3	raised
0903	2.14	2.16	2.4	L	L	N	12.1	raised
0907	2.16	2.25	2.42	L	N	N	12.0	raised
0508	2.2	2.37	2.43	L	N	N	10.5	raised
0407	2.21	2.35	2.37	L	N	N	7.2	
1904	2.21	2.45	2.49	L	N	N	12.7	raised
1907	2.21	2.25	2.32	L	N	N	5.0	
0305	2.23	2.14	2.07	L	L	L	-7.7	lowered
0307	2.23	2.42	2.41	L	N	N	8.1	raised
0906	2.23	2.31	2.24	L	N	L	0.4	
0905	2.24	2.33	2.5	L	N	N	11.6	raised
1708	2.26	2.24	2.32	N	L	N	2.7	
0115	2.29	2.68	2.48	N	H	N	8.3	raised
1704	2.3	2.35	2.14	N	N	L	-7.5	
0110	2.32	2.31	2.16	N	N	L	-7.4	
0114	2.34	2.32	2.23	N	N	L	-4.9	
2001	2.4	2.35	2.19	N	N	L	-9.6	lowered
0204	2.43	2.44	2.11	N	N	L	-15.2	lowered
1503	2.48		2.46	N	L	N	-0.8	

Figure 5.15   The employment of 'if functions' to extract data with values outside the reference range and the SSD

SSD to highlight reference value changes (RVCs) can also be abstracted from the overall data to demonstrate changes of significance. There is then the opportunity to combine, by cutting and pasting, organ-related tests such as calcium, phosphate, albumin and AP, etc.

Also, shift tables can be produced from the spreadsheet. A simple shift table is shown in Table 5.13. This defines the number of test results below, within and above the reference range for each occasion in a study. These shift tables can be developed to a more complex form when there are a significant number of abnormal results, by illustrating the number of test results 25 per cent, 50 per cent and 100 per cent or greater than the upper limit of the

Table 5.13   A basic shift table of the calcium data showing the number of subjects in and outside the reference range on the different occasions

	Low	'Normal'	High
Baseline (V01)	11	64	0
Visit 13 (V13)	7	64	1
Visit 16 (V16)	8	66	0

reference range. It is also of help in interpretation to examine the number of subjects showing a change from within to outside the reference range between the baseline and the last visit, as demonstrated in Table 5.14, when the concern is the number of subjects with a change from normal to high.

Table 5.14 An example of a shift table to demonstrate the number of subjects showing a reference range change from baseline to final study visit

'Normal' to high	High to high
9	7
'Normal' to 'normal'	High to 'normal'
80	4

The basic statistical data can be obtained using Analyse-it and the information on the above calcium data is shown in Figure 5.16.

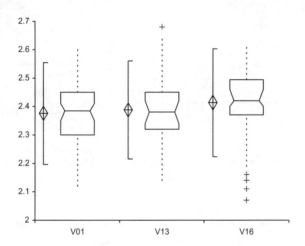

	n	Mean	SD	SE	95% CI of Mean
V01	76	2.376	0.1091	0.0125	2.351 to 2.401
V13	75	2.388	0.1051	0.0121	2.364 to 2.412
V16	75	2.413	0.1153	0.0133	2.387 to 2.440

Median	IQR	95% CI of Median
2.385	0.150	2.350 to 2.410
2.380	0.130	2.340 to 2.420
2.420	0.125	2.400 to 2.460

Figure 5.16 Basic statistical data obtained from Analyse-it software

Outliers can easily be identified from this, and both parametric and non-parametric information provided. Analyse-it can also be used to determine significance in these data, but in general these statistics can give misleading information. We have seen many occasions when the statistical difference is highly significant, yet from a clinical viewpoint is of dubious significance. Conversely, it is not uncommon for the statistics to show no significance in the data and yet reviewing individual patients may show major clinical differences.

Finally, Analyse-it offers a facility to determine agreement (or disagreement) between the baseline sample and subsequent occasions.

Figure 5.17 illustrates an example of the calcium data as both an x/y plot and a bias plot between baseline and visit 16. The bias data shows a mean difference of 0.037 mmol/l with the upper and lower dotted lines being the 95 per cent confidence limits. The calcium data used in the example are uncorrected for albumin concentration.

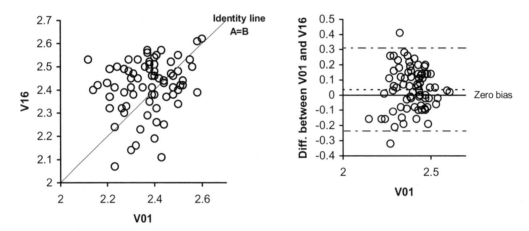

Figure 5.17   The x/y plot (left panel) and bias plot (right panel) between the baseline calcium levels and visit 16

This approach merely provides a tool to examine results outside of the reference range and the SSD and to obtain compiled statistical information on the laboratory test data. What is then required is a clinical assessment of the abnormal highlighted results. There is really no substitute for biochemists and haematologists experienced in the field of drug studies to help in the interpretation of laboratory safety data.

Conclusion

The views expressed in this chapter are those of the author and may contain some opinions not totally supported either by colleagues in Pivotal Laboratories or other central laboratories offering services to the pharmaceutical industry.

It must be remembered that laboratory medicine is not a static discipline. It is constantly changing with improvement in analytical procedures and technology. The pharmaceutical industry generally does not employ specialists in laboratory medicine and, therefore, there is a need for greater collaboration between sponsoring companies and the central laboratory to ensure success in the laboratory aspects of drug studies.

References

Abt K and Krupp P (1986). Pooling of laboratory safety data in multicenter studies. *Drug Inf J* **20**: 311–313.

Bland JM and Altman DG (1986). Statistical methods for assessing agreement between two methods of clinical measurement. *Lancet* **i**: 307–310.

Chuang-Stein, C (1992). Summarizing laboratory data with different reference ranges in multicenter trials. *Drug Inf J* **26**: 77–84.

Cockcroft DW and Gault MH (1976). Prediction of creatinine clearance from serum creatinine. *Nephron* **16**: 31–41

Craig A (1994). What reference range? *Clin Res Focus* **5**: 4–6.

Craig A and Guilford SA (1993). Endocrine assessment of the climacteric period in selecting patients for clinical trials. *Br J Clin Res A*, **4**: 1–9.

Delmas PD and Fraser M (1999). Strong bones in later life: luxury or necessity. *Bull World Health Org* **77**: 416–421.

Dijkman JHM, Scholten R and Craig A (2000). The Virtual Central Laboratory approach to the management of clinical laboratory data for clinical drug trials. *Eur Pharm Contractor* (May): 93–98.

Finney H, Newman DJ and Price CP (2000). Adult reference ranges for cystatin C, creatinine and predicted creatinine clearance. *Ann Clin Biochem* **37**: 49–59.

Fraser CG (1993). Age-related changes in laboratory test results. Clinical implications. *Drugs Aging* **3**(3): 246–257.

Fraser CG and Fogarty Y (1989). Interpreting laboratory results. *Br Med J* **298**: 1659–1660.

Grasbeck R and Alstrom T (eds) (1981). *Reference Values in Laboratory Medicine*. John Wiley.

Green RM and Flamm S (2002). AGA technical review on evaluation of liver chemistry tests. *Gastroenterology* **123**: 1367–1384.

Groth T and de Verdier C-M (1993). Transferability of clinical laboratory data. *Uppsala J Med Sci* **98**: 259–274.

Johnston JD and Hawthorne SW (1997). How to minimize factitious hyperkalaemia in blood samples from general practice. *Br Med J* **314**: 1200–1201.

Kyd PA, De Vooght K, Kerkhoff F, Thomas E *et al.* (1999). Clinical usefulness of biochemical resorption markers in osteoporosis. *Ann Clin Biochem* **36**: 483–491.

Lau EMC and Cooper C (1996). The epidemiology of osteoporosis. *Clin Orthpaed Relat Res* **323**: 65–74.

Lazarou J, Pomeranz BH and Corey PN (1998). Incidence of adverse drug reactions in hospitalized patients: a meta-analysis of prospective studies. *J Am Med Assoc* **279**: 1200–1205.

Passing H and Bablok W (1983). A new biometrical procedure for testing the equality of measurements from two different analytical methods. *J Clin Chem Biochem* **21**: 709–720.

Pocock SJ, Ashby D, Shaper AG, Walker M *et al.* (1989). Diurnal variation in serum biochemical and haematological measurements. *J Clin Pathol* **42**: 172–179.

Radomski MW, Sabiston BH and Isoard P (1980). Development of 'sports anaemia' in physically fit men after daily sustained submaximal exercise. *Aviat Space Environ Med* (Jan): 41–45.

Rastam L, Hannan PJ, Luepker RV, Mittelmark MB *et al.* (1992). Seasonal variation in plasma cholesterol. *Am J Prev Med* **8**(6): 360–366.

Ricos C, Alvarez V, Cava F, Garcia-Lario JV *et al.* (1999). Desirable specifications for total error, imprecision, and bias derived from biological variation. *Scand J Clin Lab Invest* **59**: 491–500.

Saini S, Hindmarsh PC, Matthews DR, Pringle PJ *et al.* (1991). Reproducibility of 24-h serum growth hormone profiles in man. *Clin Endocrinol* **34**: 455–462.

Shaper AG and Lewis P (1971). Genetic neutropenia in people of African origin. *Lancet* **7732**: 1021–1023.

Shaper AG, Pocock SJ, Ashby D, Walker M *et al*. (1985). Biochemical and haematological response to alcohol intake. *Ann Clin Biochem* **22**: 50–61.

Sharpe PC (2001). Biochemical detection and monitoring of alcohol abuse and abstinence. *Ann Clin Biochem* **38**: 642–664.

Sherwood RA, Lambert A, Newham DJ, Wassif WS *et al*. (1996). The effect of eccentric exercise on serum creatine kinase activity in different ethnic groups. *Ann Clin Biochem* **33**: 324–329.

Simonsen O, Grubb A and Thysell H (1985). The blood serum concentration of cystatin C as a measure of glomerular filtration rate. *Scand J Clin Lab Invest* **45**: 97–101.

Sogliero-Gilbert G, Mosher K and Zubkoff L (1986). A procedure for the simplification and assessment of lab parameters in clinical trials. *Drug Inf J* **20**: 279–296.

Westgard JO, Barry PL and Hunt MR (1981). A multi-rule Shewhart chart for quality control in clinical chemistry. *Clin Chem* **27**(3): 493–501.

Whitehead TP, Robinson D, Hale AC and Bailey AR (1994). Clinical chemistry and haematology: adult reference values. *BUPA Medical Research & Development Ltd*.

Williams GZ, Young DS, Stein MR and Cotlove C (1970). Biological and analytical components of variation in long-term studies of serum constituents in normal subjects. *Clin Chem* **16**: 1016.

Winkel P, Statland BE and Bokelund H (1974). Factors contributing to intra-individual variation of serum constituents: short-term day-to-day and within-hour variation of serum constituents in healthy subjects. *Clin Chem* **20**(12): 1520–1527.

6

Statistics: Analysis and Presentation of Safety Data

S. J. W. Evans

Introduction and background

All effective medicines have unwanted effects; it has been said that all medicines have two effects: the one you intend and one you don't want. The consequence is that there must always be a continuing assessment of the balance of the risks and benefits of all medicines. Statistical methods and statistical thinking contribute at all stages in the process of drug development. In this chapter, the statistical issues relating to detecting adverse drug reactions (ADRs), both in clinical trials and in observational data (including spontaneous ADR reports), will be considered. These adverse effects may be clinical diagnoses or the signs and symptoms that potentially lead to a diagnosis. They may also be the results of laboratory tests or investigations, e.g. of X-rays or electrocardiograms.

Many medicines are licensed on the basis of the effect on a surrogate variable for efficacy, whereas adverse effects are usually not surrogates but are responses of immediate clinical relevance to a patient. For example, a drug may be licensed on the basis of its effect on blood pressure or cholesterol level, although these variables are not in themselves of direct clinical importance to the patient. The clinically important effects are those of, for example, stroke or heart attack. Adverse effects are usually noticed as being effects of clinical relevance, though occasionally some are identified because the variable is being measured for other purposes (e.g. a rise in blood pressure or increase in QT interval).

The title of the chapter refers to 'safety data', but safety is really an issue of absence of harm, and most data are collected on the occurrence of adverse effects. Some discussion of how 'safety' can be presented and discussed in summarizing the knowledge about a medicine is included. The main focus of this chapter will be on the analysis of randomized clinical trials, observational studies and spontaneous reports. There are statistical and public health issues involved in balancing risk and benefits, but these will not be covered here (see Chapter 8). There are also statistical issues arising from toxicology studies and from early phases in clinical drug development programme, which will not be dealt with specifically (see Chapter 3).

Stephens' Detection of New Adverse Drug Reactions Fifth Edition edited by John Talbot and Patrick Waller
© 2004 John Wiley & Sons, Ltd   ISBN: 0 470 84552 X

The statistical effort in relation to randomized trials has, over the years, been mainly devoted to assessment of efficacy. Medicines are licensed on the basis of their quality, safety and efficacy. Very early testing of a new drug will check its safety in animals and many drugs fail to progress to testing in humans. The early phases of drug testing will look for major safety problems in humans, but the main statistical effort in the late phases is placed on efficacy. It is clear that there is no point in introducing a new drug unless it has some efficacy in treating the disease or condition for which it is to be used. Major improvements have been seen in the preparation of protocols, and there are detailed guidelines that deal with the statistical approach to the analysis of efficacy. The details on safety are much less. At the design stage of a trial a key factor is to ensure that the statistical power will be sufficient to demonstrate clinically relevant efficacy if it exists. Such power calculations do not usually take safety considerations into account explicitly. A particular problem when concluding that efficacy exists when it does not (type 1 error) is multiplicity. Modern protocols pre-specify efficacy outcomes to be studied so that the possibility of testing many of them and choosing the most extreme is removed. With safety, which is the absence of 'harm', it is usually impossible to pre-specify a particular variable or outcome as being 'of interest' – there are many possible variables, so the potential for finding false positive effects (type 1 errors) is high. If the rate of false positives is minimized, then inevitably the rate of false negatives is increased. When concerns have been raised through previous studies, including animal toxicology and general knowledge of pharmacology, then pre-specified outcomes should be included in the protocol.

Problems with clinical trials for detecting adverse reactions

The first problem is that the sample size will often be too low to detect adverse reactions that are, although relatively rare, of considerable clinical relevance. The typical pre-licensing phase 3 trial used for assessment of efficacy of a new drug will have from about 50 to about 500 patients per treatment arm. Occasionally there will be both smaller and larger trials, and more than one trial will usually be needed to obtain a marketing authorization. This leads to problems with important but rare adverse events (AEs).

The situation is shown in diagrammatic form in Figure 6.1: the horizontal axis shows the rate of an AE in the control group (as a proportion, e.g. 0.001 is 1 in 1000, 0.1 per cent) and the vertical axis shows the relative risk of that AE in a treated group, compared with the control, that can be detected using different sample sizes. Three lines are shown using sample sizes per group of 50, 300 and 2000 with 80 per cent power. The smaller sample sizes are chosen because they are typical in many trials used to demonstrate efficacy. The largest sample size is that typical of very large trials used to demonstrate important effects on clinical outcomes (such as myocardial infarction or death) in cardiology. The uppermost line obviously relates to the smallest sample size – it is only very large relative risks that can be detected with small samples. Figure 6.1 shows that with a small trial of 50 per arm, unless the proportion of patients with the adverse effect in the control group is at least 0.2 (20 per cent), then it is very unlikely that the trial will have sufficient power to detect a relative risk of at least four. With 300 per arm then the background rate in the controls has to be at least 10 per cent to have a reasonable power to detect a doubling of the rate. In most practical situations where the AE is occurring at 5 per cent or less in the control group, then only relative risks of at least five will be detectable as statistically significant. In many

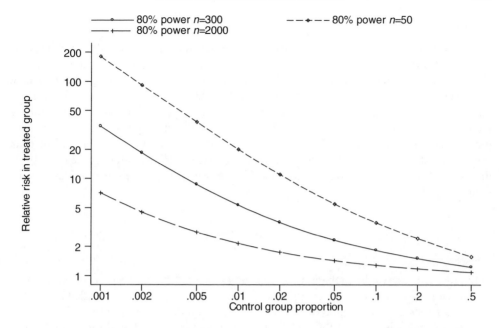

Figure 6.1 Relative risk detectable in studies of different size versus baseline rate of ADR

situations it is also clear that with important but rare ADRs the relative risks of 50 or 100 will be the only ones that can be detected in a single trial. In other words, only extreme levels of harm are detected in early trials, so that 'safety' is initially only the absence of extreme harm. Even with sample sizes of 2000 per group, detection of doubling of risks of 1 in 200 will not have good power.

This argument applies to a single adverse reaction. In practice, however, there is the potential for a large number of adverse reactions, so that the statistical analysis may need to take account of the problems caused by making multiple tests. The usual approach will result in adjustment to the significance test level so that the sample size necessary becomes very much greater. The use of adjustments will result in raising the rate of type 2 errors, i.e. real effects will tend to be missed. The need to combine data from several trials to achieve power is obvious and will be discussed later.

It is clear that, in typical phase 3 trials, the possibility of detecting even relatively frequent adverse reactions is small. It is important to use the most powerful statistical methods available to analyse information from such trials.

A further problem is that data on safety are reported erratically or unreported (Ioannidis and Contopoulos-Ioannidis, 1998). A more detailed investigation (Ioannidis and Lau, 2001) showed that the median amount of space on safety per article was less than one-third of a page and that less than half of reported trials gave specific reasons for the stopping of an individual's treatment. The quality varied by medical subject area, with a tendency for reports on treatments for arthritis and HIV to give more careful attention to safety than cardiovascular trial reports. This variation may in part be due to the extent and the perceived importance of the drug's expected toxicity.

Issues of multiplicity

As has been noted above, there are difficulties when several response variables are analysed and tested for statistical significance. The same underlying problem occurs whether significance tests or confidence intervals are used. In the context of checking whether a new medicine has efficacy, it is most important to be conservative in the analysis so as to minimize chance findings of apparent efficacy when there is truly no benefit from a medicine. If several statistical tests are carried out on different response variables, then the probability that at least one of them becomes significant rises with the number of tests carried out. If, for example, 10 tests are carried out, each using a significance level of 0.05, then if the tests are independent of one another the overall probability that at least one of them is significant is

$$1 - (1 - 0.05)^{10} = 0.4$$

In order to preserve the probability of concluding that a difference has occurred when no difference truly exists (a type 1 error), then the significance level can be divided by 10 (the number of tests carried out), so that each test uses a significance level of 0.005. Now, the overall probability is $1 - (1 - 0.005)^{10} = 0.049$ and the overall result still has a type 1 (false positive) error of approximately 0.05. This correction is called a Bonferroni correction. In practice, the various outcomes are not independent, so that the probability of finding at least one significant result is not as large as stated above. This also means that there is a tendency for a Bonferroni correction to overcorrect statistical tests; consequently, particularly when examining efficacy, other methods that are more powerful have been devised (Ludbrook, 1998).

The US Food and Drug Administration (FDA) have used rules (sometimes referred to as the Fairweather rules) that use 0.005 as the significance level for common tumours in toxicology testing in two-species–two-sex animal studies. They use 0.025 as the significance level for rare tumours, and note that the overall false positive rate is 10 per cent (Lin and Rahman, 1998). The consequence is that only extremely strong effects will be detected. This is part of the general problem of *multiplicity* that occurs in interpreting studies with many outcomes.

In the protocol, where efficacy is usually emphasized there is a pre-specified plan to study certain response variables. In studying new adverse reactions, no such pre-specified plan can usually be devised. The number of possible adverse effects is very large. There are also problems of how these effects are to be classified. In the medical dictionaries that are routinely used there are several levels of a hierarchy of terms, and at each level there are a number of terms used to group reactions. For example, in MedDRA there are 26 system organ classes, nearly 1700 high-level terms, and over 14 000 preferred terms (see Chapter 12). This means that any particular adverse reaction has problems of classification, and if even the coarsest classification level of system organ class is used then the potential for multiple significance tests is considerable. If AEs are classified at a high level, then grouping them may result in hiding a particular problem. There will always be a trade-off between grouping AEs in order to obtain sufficiently large numbers in any particular category and splitting them in order to find a specific problem. There is no general answer to this problem, since several classifications at different levels may need to be considered.

Analysis and presentation of data from trials

In a randomized trial comparing a new drug, in which new adverse reactions might be detected, there will be a comparator group that may be placebo or an active drug. In practice, during the development of a new drug, each AE of a serious nature will be examined individually to assess likely causality by staff from the company developing the drug. If necessary, new information will be released warning investigators of the possibility of this being an adverse reaction (see Chapter 11). The strength of the randomized trial is that causality can be inferred readily because randomization means that groups will, on average, be similar in all characteristics, both those observed and those unobserved. The statistical analysis can then be used to indicate that there is either a genuine effect associated with treatment or that an extremely unlikely chance effect has occurred. It is still possible that there are biases in execution of the trial, but these are less likely than in observational studies. When the control group is a placebo and evidence is convincing that an excess of the AE occurs in the new drug group, then this will be taken as strong evidence that it is causally related to the drug. The use of veiling (blinding), especially when it veils both patient and health professional who ascertains adverse effects, is very helpful in this context.

When the comparator group is an active drug, then the excess occurrence of an AE for the new drug will also be taken as evidence that this is an adverse reaction caused by the new drug. There are circumstances when the comparator drug is active and has a known adverse reaction, so occurrence of a similar rate of the AE will be taken as evidence that it is also an adverse reaction for this drug, though it might be the events are caused by neither drug.

For efficacy, as noted above, surrogate measures are often used; for safety data in respect of new ADRs, surrogate variables are rare. In many randomized trials there is monitoring of laboratory variables, such as liver function tests, that are used to check on safety (see Chapter 5). The analysis of these laboratory variables proceeds as for other continuous measurements used for efficacy. This should include analysis that allows for repeated measures over time. They do not themselves detect a new adverse reaction, but it is sensible to ensure that the most powerful statistical analysis is used so that if liver damage or renal damage starts to occur then this is detected at an early stage. The trend in population average values will often be a surrogate for infrequent larger changes that occur in individuals. It is sensible to look for trends in these measures rather than only to look for rates of occurrence of clinically relevant change in an individual, such as three times the upper limit of normal, or 10 times the upper limit of normal. The rates of clinically significant change are certainly important, but they may occur so rarely that statistical power is too low. Measures of efficacy are not taken as the rate of occurrence of a clinically significant change in an individual patient in blood pressure, but efficacy can be based on population changes. Statistical significance is too often used to substitute for clinical relevance in such situations. A similar argument should apply to liver function and other laboratory values measured for safety purposes. The rest of this chapter discusses binary data, i.e. whether an AE has occurred or not. A good description of issues relating to continuous data can be found in Chuang-Stein *et al.* (2001).

Statistical measures of the occurrence of adverse events

In the usual randomized trial where individuals are allocated to the new treatment or control in parallel groups, there are n_t participants in the treatment group who are followed and there are x_t participants who have a particular AE. The simplest measure of occurrence is the proportion of participants who have that event during follow-up, i.e. x_t/n_t. Similarly, with the same notation, the proportion in the control group who have that event will be x_c/n_c. There are standard statistical tests for the comparison of proportions, with the most obvious being a one degree of freedom chi-squared test or Fisher's exact test. These test the *null hypothesis* that the proportion with that AE is equal in the two groups. The null hypothesis is that the difference in proportions is zero. The data for the chi-squared test are laid out in a two-by-two table in Table 6.1.

Table 6.1   Occurrence of AEs by treatment group

	With AE	Without AE	Total
Treated	x_t	$n_t - x_t$	n_t
Control	x_c	$n_c - x_c$	n_c

Both the chi-squared and Fisher tests result in a statistical significance level (P value) that gives the probability of obtaining a difference in proportions as large as, or larger than the one observed when there is no true difference in the proportion. The measure of the magnitude of the difference between the treated and control groups may be given as a difference in proportions or as a relative measure. The difference in proportions is often expressed as a percentage, but proportion is the statistically preferred value.

The two obvious relative measures are the *odds ratio* (OR) and relative risk. The odds of the adverse event in the treated group are

$$x_t: n_t - x_t$$

and the odds in the control group are

$$x_c: n_c - x_c$$

Differences in odds do not have any obvious meaning, unlike their ratio, called the OR. This is

$$(x_t: n_t - x_t)/(x_c: n_c - x_c)$$

It is possible to take the *ratio* of the proportions rather than their difference, and this is then described as a *risk ratio* or *relative risk* (RR). For both these measures, the null value (no difference) is unity. The difference in proportions is sometimes described as the *risk difference,* or *absolute* difference in risk.

In public health terms it is always absolute differences that are important. A rate of an ADR of 1 in 1000 untreated patients compared with 2 in 1000 who are treated is a relative risk of 2. A rate of an ADR of 1 in 1 000 000 untreated patients compared with 2 in 1 000 000 is also a relative risk of 2, but the public health implications differ by a factor of 1000. Relative measures are more sensitive to causal effects; very high RRs (say >10) will usually be causal, but if the background rate is very low indeed then they may not result in major action being necessary. These considerations are very relevant to risk–benefit balance (see Chapter 8). The presentation of absolute effects of benefit have sometimes used what appears to be an absolute number, the NNT ('number needed to treat' in order than one treated person gets a benefit they would not otherwise have had). This is not an absolute number, it is the reciprocal of a difference in rates, so the time over which the outcome has been measured (often 1 year) needs to be given. 'NNT' is implicitly the NNT to obtain benefit. Some authors have used 'NNH' as the 'number needed to harm', but it should be 'NNT/H', i.e. the number needed to be treated so that one person gets a harm they would not otherwise have had.

To take a specific example from a large trial, the Women's Health Initiative (WHI) study (Rossouw *et al.*, 2002), the comparison between oestrogen + progestin (HRT for simplicity) with placebo for incidence of invasive breast cancer is shown in Table 6.2. Here, the proportions with breast cancer are $(166/8506) = 0.0195$ with HRT and $(124/8102) = 0.0153$ with placebo. The difference in proportions is 0.0042 (0.42 per cent). The odds of having breast cancer in the treated group were 0.0199 $(166/8340)$ and 0.0155 $(124/7978)$ in the placebo group. The odds ratio is 1.28, and the RR is 1.275. The simple chi-squared test here is 4.29 with a P value of 0.0384. It should be noted that it is always better to give exact P values rather than just, for example, <0.05. Fisher's exact test has a P value of 0.044. Usually, the chi-squared test will have a smaller P value than Fisher's exact test, particularly when there are small expected values for the chi-squared test, and the exact test is to be preferred.

Table 6.2 Occurrence of invasive breast cancer by treatment group in the WHI study

	With breast cancer	Without breast cancer	Total
HRT	166	8340	8506
Placebo	124	7978	8102

This illustrates that odds are always larger than proportions and that ORs are always further from the null value of unity than RRs. ORs have desirable mathematical properties and their use should be encouraged.

A confidence interval is a measure of the amount of statistical uncertainty around a value known as the *point estimate*. If a large number of 95 per cent confidence intervals (CIs) are constructed, then the true value of the parameter being estimated will be included within 95 per cent of such intervals. It is possible to construct CIs for summaries of data such as proportions, differences or relative risks. The CIs for the RR and OR are usually based on taking their logarithms and the CIs will be symmetric on a log scale. (The null value for log OR and log RR is zero.)

For the data from the WHI trial, the 95 per cent CI for the risk difference of 0.0042 is 0.00024 to 0.0082. This is an excess rate of 4 in 1000 patients who receive HRT and are followed up for an average of 5.2 years. This is an NNT/H of 250 for 5.2 years follow-up, i.e. an NNT/H of 1300 for one extra case of breast cancer per year over that first 5 years. The 95 per cent CI for the OR of 1.28 is 1.013 to 1.618. The 95 per cent CI for the RR of 1.275 is 1.012 to 1.606. None of these intervals (for the risk difference, OR or RR) contains the null value for the relevant summary (zero or one). This is consistent with the statistical significance tests that are taken to be statistically significant; the P value is less than 0.05. Rejection of the null hypothesis H_0 at an x per cent level and the $(100 - x)$ per cent CI excluding the value for the H_0 will usually be equivalent. Further details of how to calculate the statistical tests and confidence intervals are given in intermediate level textbooks in medical statistics (Altman, 1991) or in epidemiology (Rothman and Greenland, 1998).

Measures that take time into account

In the discussion above it has been assumed that each patient has been followed up until the end of the study, provided that the AE did not occur in that patient. In general this will not be true and the time that each patient is 'at risk' of having the AE will need to be taken into account. Even where there is a single dose, such as a vaccine, the follow-up period is still relevant. Immediate ADRs may not need to take time into account explicitly, but it is clear that the use of the word 'immediate' indicates that a time period over which ADRs are ascertained is relevant.

The usual summary used is to add up the total time at risk for each patient and sum that for the treatment and control groups separately. This then gives the total person time at risk for each group, usually expressed as say thousand person-years. Then, assuming that all the individuals did not have the AE at start of follow-up, the total number of those having the event during follow-up divided by the person-years gives the incidence rate. The ratio of incidence rates is referred to as a *rate ratio*.

In the WHI study there was a mean of 5.2 years of follow-up, so that in the HRT group there were 44 075 participant years (P-years) and in the placebo group there were over 41 289 P-years at risk: the rate per 10 000 person-years for breast cancer was 38 and 30 in the treated and placebo groups respectively. These are average rates over the follow-up period of the trial. The *rate ratio* is 1.27 (the same as the risk ratio to two significant figures). A risk has individuals as the denominators for the risks, whereas a rate has person-time as the denominator. Like the RR, the rate ratio is also described as a relative risk measure (Rothman and Greenland, 1998: 49).

It may be noted that the assumption made when using person-years as the denominator is that the risk of having an AE is constant at all times during the follow-up period. The risk per unit time is called the hazard rate, and using total person-years as the denominator assumes that this rate is constant over time. With some types of adverse reaction this assumption may be reasonable, but often this is not the case. For example, most hypersensitivity reactions are relatively rapid in onset and if they do not occur early in continuous treatment then their likelihood of occurring later is very much less. At the other extreme, any causal effect on cancer is likely to take at least a year, and more usually at least 3 years, before it could be detected. This is illustrated by the data shown in Table 6.3 taken from the WHI report (Rossouw *et al.*, 2002). A different assumption is that the *ratio* of the hazard rates in two groups is constant. This may be more realistic, and analysis methods that utilize this assumption are given below.

It could be argued that the expected effect of HRT on breast cancer should only start to appear after 2 to 3 years, so using the total person time as the denominator is very misleading. In the summary of trials submitted for licensing of a new medicine it is often found, that the total person time in the treated group across all the trials, or even the total number treated, is the denominator used in giving the rate of occurrence of AEs. This is

Table 6.3   Participant years, numbers of cases of breast cancer, rates and rate ratios by follow-up year and treatment group in the WHI trial

Year	HRT P-years	Placebo P-years	HRT BC[a]	Placebo BC[a]	HRT rate[b]	Placebo rate[b]	HRT/placebo rate ratio
1	8435	8050	11	17	13	21	0.62
2	8353	7980	26	30	31	38	0.82
3	8268	7888	28	23	34	29	1.17
4	7926	7562	40	22	50	29	1.72
5	5964	5566	34	12	57	22	2.59
6+	5129	4243	27	20	53	47	1.13
Total	44 075	41 289	166	124	38	30	1.27

[a] BC = number of cases of Invasive breast cancer.
[b] Rate per 10 000 participant-years.

rarely the best way of presenting or summarizing the data, and it must be treated with great caution. The correct ways of dealing with this issue have been set out (O'Neill, 1987) but are often ignored.

It is usually very much better to present the cumulative hazard of the AEs, and good examples are seen in Figure 6.2, regarding data from the WHI study (Rossouw *et al.*, 2002).

Figure 6.2 illustrates the cumulative risk (hazard) in each of the treatment groups for each of four classes of AE. At each time point when an AE occurs, the risk of occurrence is calculated based on the number of AEs occurring at that time divided by the number of participants at risk of having that event at that time. Those who have dropped out of the trial by that time point, for whatever reason, are not counted in the denominator. The method can also be used to examine benefits, and the original figure also showed benefit for two categories of clinical outcome: colo-rectal cancer and hip fracture.

The cumulative risk is obtained by calculating the probability of *not* having the event at that time point – this is sometimes referred to as the probability of 'survival'. This may be applied to AEs, though its original use was in looking at death rates. This cumulative 'survival' probability is obtained by multiplying the cumulative survival up to the previous time point by the current survival probability. The cumulative hazard is 1 − (cumulative survival). The process is started by assuming the survival probability at the start time is unity. The method is known as a Kaplan–Meier estimate of survival or cumulative hazard. Kaplan–Meier curves for AEs are best shown as cumulative hazard plots, as in Figure 6.2; this is a curve that goes upwards rather than the conventional survival curve, which goes downwards.

The calculation of the cumulative risk is simple and is given in most introductory medical statistics books, e.g. Altman (1991: 368).

The curves derived from the Kaplan–Meier method can themselves be misleading if too much attention is paid to the data at longer times. This is where the estimates are at their most uncertain, since the numbers 'at risk' may be rather small. Good practice truncates these curves so that data based on very few observations are not included. Figure 6.2 gives the numbers at risk (which is a good example to follow), but it can be seen that the numbers fall off after 4 years of follow-up, so that by year 6 of follow-up less than 25 per cent, and by year 7 less than 10 per cent of those randomized are at risk of having events.

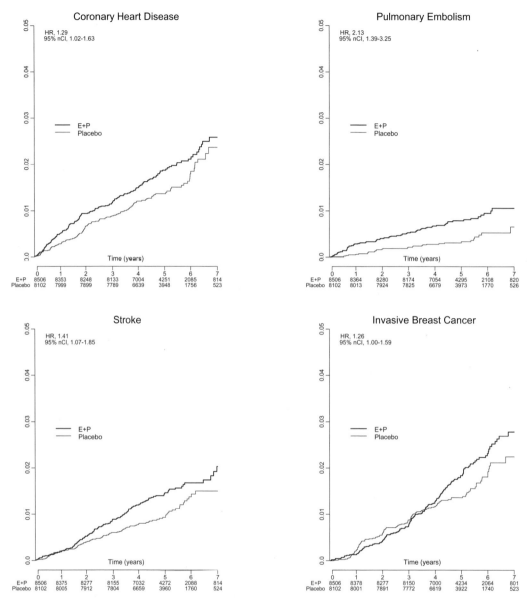

Figure 6.2   Examples of Kaplan–Meier estimates of cumulative risks (derived from Rossouw *et al.* (2002)

Statistical tests utilizing time since start of treatment

The Kaplan–Meier method does not directly provide significance tests or confidence intervals for comparisons between groups. It is possible to treat the data as comparisons of proportions as discussed above, but these do not take into account differences over time and do not fully utilize the data. The simplest method of comparing the curves is the log rank test (Peto *et al.*, 1977). Although the result of this test can be expressed as a chi-squared value, it is not the same as the simple chi-squared test presented above. The log rank test treats the data in a similar way to calculating a Kaplan–Meier estimate. At each time point where an AE (failure) occurs, it is assumed that the rate should be the same in the treated as in the control group. An overall rate across both groups is calculated so that an expected number of failures is obtained for each group at that time point. The cumulative difference between the observed number of failures (O) and the expected number (E) for the whole time period under consideration is obtained and $(O - E)^2/E$ can be compared with a chi-squared distribution on one degree of freedom for testing the difference between the curves. This is a test of the null hypothesis that the two curves are identical. It does not assume anything about the hazard rate itself – it does not have to be constant, but it does assume that the ratio of the hazards is always constant and equal to one. There are various subtle modifications of the log rank test that apply different weights to the information at the beginning of follow-up compared with that at the end of follow-up. Further details on survival analysis can be found in Collett (1994).

A more complex method for comparing time to event data is that known as proportional hazards regression or Cox regression. This, like the log rank test, compares an entire survival curve without making assumptions about the form of the hazard rate at any particular time, but it does assume that the ratio of the hazard rates between two groups is proportional at all times. This method can be used to adjust for other prognostic factors, as well as for making a comparison between a treated and a control group. It may be used both for data from randomized trials and observational cohort studies. The result of the Cox model is a hazard ratio, which is analogous to a relative risk averaged over all the time points considered. It also allows for a confidence interval around the hazard ratio to be calculated.

In the WHI study described above, the estimated hazard ratio for invasive breast cancer was 1.26 with 95 per cent CI 1.00–1.59, derived from a Cox model analysis. This is similar to the point estimate of relative risk calculated above as 1.28 with CI 1.01–1.61. The Cox model took into account the clinical centre where patients were being treated, age, prior disease and their treatment group in a simultaneous low-fat diet trial. These adjustments are usually less relevant in a clinical trial than in an observational study.

The log rank test and the Cox model can be described as semi-parametric. This is because they do not assume a parametric form for the hazard rate over time, but they both effectively assume proportional hazard ratios. It is possible to have fully parametric models that assume a particular form for the hazard rate. For example, the exponential model assumes a constant hazard rate. It is possible to allow for hazard rates that increase or decrease or are even J-shaped. Some of these methods are described by Collett (1994). There are also methods available for checking the assumptions of survival analysis and these should be used when examining the difference between groups in rates of occurrence of adverse outcomes.

When comparing rates with the number of cases with events as the numerator and person-time as the denominator, the basic assumption is that the number of cases follows a Poisson distribution. Analysis of these rates uses *Poisson regression*; see Clayton and Hills (1993). The results of these analyses can be expressed as incidence rate ratios.

The results from a Cox model analysis are always presented as relative measures of the effect rather than as absolute measures. It is not possible to obtain either absolute measures of rates or relative risks at a specific time point directly from the analysis. With parametric methods it is possible to obtain absolute measures, and this approach may therefore be used more often in the future.

Combining data from several trials: meta-analysis

A major problem with clinical trials is that they tend to be too small to detect uncommon or rare ADRs. There are obvious benefits to be gained from putting all the available information together to increase statistical power. In principle, this is more important for analysis of ADRs than for analysis of efficacy. However, most of the problems with trials are not solved by combining data. Important problems that remain relate to the classification of ADRs and in ensuring that all the relevant data have been captured. If the trials have excluded those likely to be treated in clinical practice then meta-analysis might give a false sense of reassurance. A major problem with the standard systematic review (the process of defining the problem, searching for all data and setting them out) is that the data may be derived from published papers. These are prone to 'publication bias' (Egger *et al.*, 2001). At the stage of applying for a marketing authorization for a new drug, both regulators and the company will have access to complete data on the drug prior to its being licensed. This means that there is no problem with 'publication' bias, since all the data are available (though unpublished at this stage).

The greatest strength of a meta-analysis of trials is that the results which are being combined are the within-study, between-treatment group differences. It means that the different studies themselves are not assumed to have similar results, but it is assumed that the between-treatment differences are relatively similar across studies. One of the consequences is that it is important that the scale on which the differences are measured shows consistency across studies. If the (absolute) baseline risk varies across studies, then it may be that the (absolute) risk difference differs markedly across studies, but the OR is consistent. Therefore, pooling the ORs across studies may be the best approach. Methods that assume the between-treatment differences are constant across trials are called *fixed-effect* models; where an allowance is made for some heterogeneity in the between-treatment differences, then these are called *random-effects* models. If the variation is very large, then even a random- effects model may not be sensible, and the very idea of combining disparate results should be questioned. The detailed statistical methods are beyond the scope of this chapter, but they may be found in Sutton *et al.* (2000) or Egger *et al.* (2001).

A frequently used but weaker, and in some instances flawed, approach to combining data is simply to add up the numbers across all trials of all the AE in the treated group divided by the number of patients randomized to treatment. The same is done for the control group and the overall rates compared between treated and control. In some instances this will give a similar result to a proper meta-analysis, but in most cases it will have less precision. This is particularly likely when there has been unequal randomization to treated and control in some of the trials, and such combination can be very misleading. Over- or under-estimation of between-treatment rates of events can occur. The method should not be used routinely.

A systematic review should be a routine part of the drug development process so that ADRs are able to be detected as far as possible (Koch *et al.*, 1993; Lee and Lazarus, 1997).

Analysis and presentation of data from observational studies

All the statistical methods that are used in clinical trials may be used in observational studies, but the interpretation is much less easy. Randomized controlled trials (RCTs) generally (but not inevitably) result in the formation of similar groups, so that 'like is compared with like'. In a particular trial there is no guarantee that the groups are similar, but the statistical significance test used to compare the overall results gives the probability that an observed difference results from chance imbalance in both measured and unmeasured prognostic factors. This does not relate to any tests comparing the measured prognostic factors, and it should be emphasized that tests comparing values at baseline are not generally sensible (Altman, 1998). In observational studies, groups can differ in relation to many factors other than the treatment comparison of interest; these include patient characteristics, follow-up, ascertainment of treatment or of medical outcomes. Some of the factors may not have been measured. This means that the differences observed may be due to chance or many other factors that could be systematically different, so the interpretation of statistical significance tests for observational studies does not have the same interpretation as in an RCT. Patients change treatments and the problems of classifying exposure when patients switch categories are considerable. This can be problematic in deciding whether an ADR is caused by the treatment a patient is receiving when the diagnosis is made, or whether some previous treatment led to the patient having symptoms that caused a change in medication, with these symptoms being a precursor of the disease that is only diagnosed later. For example, bleeding may lead to a patient changing from one HRT to another, and subsequently endometrial cancer is found. Is the cancer caused by the first or the second HRT, or by neither?

Bias can occur in trials, but it is much more of a problem in observational comparisons. When trying to assess whether a new drug is associated with an adverse reaction in an observational study, there will be a comparison of the rate of occurrence of the adverse effect between those exposed to the drug and a control group. Confounding occurs when a third factor is associated both with the treatment and with the adverse effect. For example, age will affect the rate of occurrence of many AEs (e.g. myocardial infarction), and if the treated group is older than the control group then age becomes a confounding factor. The problem of confounding hardly exists in trials because with randomization there is no tendency for any 'third factor' to be associated with treatment. Confounding has a major impact in non-randomized studies.

A major problem in drug safety is called 'confounding by indication'. This is a form of selection bias, also known as 'channelling'. It occurs when those who receive one treatment are more severe in their condition or, for other reasons, are at higher risk for the outcome being reported or occurring than those in the comparison group. The change to a second form of HRT can be a form of this type of bias. A study examining the differences between patients with arthritis prescribed a Cox-2 inhibitor and those not prescribed one provides an empirical example of this bias (Wolfe et al., 2002).

Methods for dealing with confounding

Confounding may be addressed in the study design or in the analysis. The general principle is to remove one of the two associations that give rise to confounding. First, the association of confounding factor(s) with the outcome and secondly the association of treatment with the confounding factor(s). If either of these associations is no longer present in the data as analysed, then confounding does not occur. This applies to the two main types of observational study, the case-control and cohort studies. In cohort studies, exposed and unexposed groups are followed and the rate of occurrence of the outcome is compared between the groups. In case-control studies the logic is reversed, and the comparison groups are formed of those who have had the outcome event and a similar group who have not had the outcome event. Then the previous exposure is compared in the two groups.

Design: matching to reduce confounding

Matching is frequently used in case-control studies to attempt to remove the association between the disease outcome and possible third factors that could also be associated with treatment. It has been routine to match on age and sex in case-control studies; and when studies are done in a database of general practice medical records, then matching by general practice has also been routine. This is usually done on a case-by-case basis (*individual matching*) or it may be done for groups of subjects (*frequency matching*). A full discussion of matching is given by Rothman and Greenland (1998). Here, it is made clear that matching does not reduce confounding unless the matching factor is also taken into account in the analysis. Matching may improve efficiency (statistical power) if the matching factor is a true confounder, but it may harm efficiency if it is not.

Overmatching has various effects. If a matching variable is associated with exposure but not disease then this usually results in loss of statistical efficiency but does not introduce bias. If matching is on a variable affected by exposure or by disease (or even worse, both) then bias can be introduced and the results become unreliable. Matching on symptoms or signs of disease is not advisable, because they can be associated with both the disease and the exposure under study, and hence the associations within the strata formed by the matching will be biased (Rothman and Greenland, 1998, 157).

In cohort studies, two groups of patients are followed up after receipt of treatment or the opportunity to receive it. The exposed group is compared with an unexposed group, which may be no treatment or an alternative treatment. They are each followed to see if an adverse effect occurs, with the methods of analysis very similar to those used in randomized trials. In order to deal with confounding, the objective is to make a comparison of similar groups. Matching may also be used in cohort studies. The details of analysis are complex, and the gains from matching are not great in many circumstances (Greenland and Morganstern, 1990).

Design: restriction

A variable that is constant within a study cannot be a confounder. Restricting a study to, say, only males means that gender cannot cause confounding. This means that the number of available subjects is markedly reduced, and it also causes difficulty for generalization of the results. The main use of restriction may be as part of a programme of studies when demonstration of an effect in, say, a high-risk group provides a basis for a wider study. A wider study of similar size would have greater variation and could fail to demonstrate an adverse effect.

Analysis: stratification to reduce confounding

An alternative approach to matching in the design can be used at the analysis stage by dividing participants into strata. The strata are defined by different levels of the confounding variable. For example, if age is a confounder then the data are split into several age bands so that comparisons between exposed and unexposed people within strata are made between those of similar age. The results are then combined across strata to give a single result that can be described as 'age-adjusted'. With this approach it is important to have sufficient strata so that within each stratum the rate of occurrence of the AE is consistent. Merely dividing the data into two strata will rarely be sufficient to adjust for confounding. Natural strata, such as hospital of treatment or general practice, are commonly used without there necessarily being strong evidence that such factors are confounders. Stratification may be by several different variables, with a consequence that, if many variables are used, the individual strata will contain few observations. This means that analysis methods for sparse data, such as Mantel–Haenszel, should be used. This treats the data within each stratum as a two-by-two table, obtaining ORs from the table and calculating a weighted average OR across all the strata, having weights that are proportional to the amount of information in each stratum (Rothman and Greenland, 1998).

Stratification can apply both to case-control and cohort studies. It is useful to examine the data with stratum-specific results, even if more complex analysis is used subsequently. Care must be taken not to overinterpret findings in one stratum compared with another, as variation is expected from one stratum to another just by chance.

For practical reasons, either relating to computing or to the cost of obtaining data, appropriate analysis to address confounding in a large cohort may be difficult. One approach used in these circumstances is to analyse a subset by forming a case-control study within a cohort. This is known as a *nested case-control* study, and has been much used within large databases such as the UK General Practice Research Database (Wood and Coulson, 2001).

Regression to reduce confounding

In most instances where there is a continuous confounding variable it is better to use a regression method to adjust for the confounding. There are two main approaches. First, the traditional method of adjusting for the effect of the confounding variable on the AE. This will usually involve logistic regression in a case-control study. In a cohort study, where the time taken for the AE to occur is analysed, then a survival analysis method such as proportional hazards regression is used. In all forms of regression analysis, issues such as linearity of effects and choice of which variables (called covariates) to include in the model lead to difficulties. The pre-specification of the analysis is not always done, so there is potential for finding the most 'interesting' results by doing very many analyses and reporting only one. A second and newer, perhaps controversial, method is to calculate what is called a *propensity score*.

Propensity scores

This method uses logistic regression to examine the factors that are associated with exposure to treatment. The propensity is a score that measures the probability of individuals with different characteristics using a drug, and is derived from the measured variables that are assumed to be associated with treatment. It does not necessarily assume that these factors are associated with the (adverse) effect being studied. Patients are then divided into strata based on their propensity score, or the propensity score is used in a regression model to analyse the occurrence of the AE. Adjustment using propensity score has some advantages, particularly when dealing with relatively rare AEs in observational data (Braitman and Rosenbaum, 2002). The precision of any regression equation is dependent on having a sufficiently large number of occurrences of the response variable. The numbers who are treated are usually very much larger than the number of occurrences of an adverse effect. This means that the equation relating a propensity score to the probability of treatment is able to be more precisely determined than an equation relating to the occurrence of the adverse effect (Wang and Donnan, 2001). This means that the method allows the association between treatment and a rare outcome to be modelled using many potential measured prognostic variables. It does not adjust for unmeasured variables that are not associated with the measured variables, but then no observational method is able to do that.

A recent example used propensity scores to allow for possible differences between a group treated with rifampicin and pyrazinamide compared with a control group receiving isoniazid (Jasmer et al., 2002). Treatment was given based on alternating weeks in treating latent tuberculosis infection. The outcome being studied was hepatotoxicity. There were 18 cases of grade 3 or 4 hepatotoxicity in 411 patients in the trial; 16 were in the combined treatment group and two in the control. The analysis stratified patients into five groups using the quintiles of the propensity score, to allow for possible differences between the groups. The crude OR was 8.5 (95 per cent CI 1.9–76.5), and adjusting for propensity the OR was 7.8 (1.7–71.3). In this study, little difference would be expected between the groups, but the method can be of considerable value. Further details may be found in Rosenbaum (2002).

Meta-analysis of observational studies

Systematic reviews with an accompanying meta-analysis are of greatest strength in the context of randomized trials; however, they can also have a place when examining observational studies. For example, meta-analysis has been used in the controversy over whether oral contraceptives containing desogestrel and gestodene have a higher rate of occurrence than those containing levonorgestrel (Hennessy et al., 2001; Kemmeren et al., 2001). In these examples the cohort and case-control studies were combined to obtain an estimated overall effect.

The chapter in Egger et al. (2001) on observational studies is of particular relevance to issues of safety. Brewer and Colditz (1999) give a summary of the potential for the use of meta-analysis in assessing ADRs and post-marketing surveillance. In the same issue, Temple (1999) discusses some of the limitations. Meta-analysis is highly relevant in the regulatory setting, when all safety data from randomized trials and observational studies of a new drug are available. There are obvious limitations from using only published papers, both because of the general problem of publication bias (where positive results are more likely to be published) and because of the poor quality of data reporting in relation to possible adverse reactions (Ioannidis and Lau, 2001).

There are methods for combining data from observational studies and including randomized trial data (Sutton and Abrams, 2001). Unfortunately, observational studies may each be subject to the same type of bias, and the usual problem of low statistical power may not be the main issue. Allowing for non-sampling errors will generally be necessary.

Use of statistical methods for signal detection with spontaneous reports

A major method of detecting new ADRs has been the use of spontaneous reports (SRs) of suspected ADRs coming from health professionals (and in some countries from patients). The 'Yellow Card' system in the UK has been one of the best known methods (Davis and Raine, 2002). Inferring causality on an individual basis for each report is rarely possible. It is sensible to use all the data coming from SRs, so that, even though the individual reports are not very reliable, taken as a whole they provide insight. The object in the first place is to detect a *signal* of a possible new ADR. Further detailed evaluation of the signal will then need to take place to test whether it is truly a real ADR, caused by the drug. The problem is that although there may be suspicion of an AE being caused by the drug, it is possible that the AE is merely part of the background – i.e. most diseases induced by drugs may also occur in the absence of any drug treatment. Statistical methods described below can help to sort the true ADRs from those that are just background.

The standard method for a long time was to take the rate of occurrence of the SRs and compare this with what might be expected as 'background'. The numerator in the rate is the number of reports and the denominator is the number of prescriptions. This has many problems: the denominator is only a variable proxy for numbers of users. It is also well known that SRs will usually be an underestimate of the true number of ADRs and the extent of this under-reporting is not known. The figures that are often quoted, such as 10 per cent of ADRs are reported, are not strongly evidence-based. Under-reporting is very variable and is dependent on factors such as the seriousness of the reaction. At best, a sensitivity analysis can be done to examine a plausible range of rates of SRs, but this is not usually helpful. The data on prescriptions may also be delayed in time, so that immediate assessment of a possible new ADR is also delayed.

Disproportionality methods

An alternative approach is to use the data on SRs without using prescription data. This is analogous to using a proportional mortality ratio, as is done in population epidemiology when accurate denominators are unavailable. The basic idea is to compare reports for a particular medical term, as the proportion of all reports, making the comparison between a particular drug and, for example, all other drugs in a database of SRs. This is illustrated in Table 6.4. The database may be the entire database for a country's regulatory authority, the worldwide database held by the World Health Organization (WHO), or it can be the database of a particular company. Many of the reports will be background, so that those that are caused by the drug are expected to occur at a higher rate with this drug than in the rest of the database. Various disproportionality methods have been described, and their utility has been reviewed by van Puijenbroek *et al.* (2002). They are described below.

Table 6.4   Spontaneous reports classified by reaction and drug

	Particular reaction	Other reactions	Total
Drug of interest	a	b	$a + b$
Other drugs	c	d	$c + d$
Total	$a + c$	$b + d$	

The ratio of the proportions has been described as a *proportional reporting ratio* (PRR; Evans *et al.*, 2001). The principle of the method was first suggested by Patwary (1969). It has been used by regulatory authorities and also by some companies. A closely related approach is to use the OR rather than the ratio of proportions. This has been referred to as a *reporting odds ratio* (ROR) and used initially for consideration of particular ADRs for evaluation rather than simply detection of a signal (Stricker and Tijessen, 1992; Egberts *et al.*, 1997; Moore *et al.*, 1997).

$$\text{PRR} = \frac{a/(a+b)}{c/(c+d)} \qquad \text{ROR} = \frac{ad}{bc}$$

The PRR and ROR will be approximately the same if $b \gg a$ and $d \gg c$, as will usually be the case.

The expected value in cell a, assuming that the proportion of reports for this reaction for this drug is the same as this reaction for all drugs, is obtained by

$$E = \frac{(a+c)(a+b)}{a+b+c+d} \qquad (6.1)$$

The observed count $O = a$. An alternative is to use all other drugs to determine the expected ratio, so

$$E = \frac{c(a+b)}{c+d} \qquad (6.2)$$

The analysis of the table should strictly be done on independent observations, so that the rates should use 'all *other* drugs' as the category, rather than 'all drugs'. If the size of the database is very large compared with the number of reports for the drug of interest, then including this drug's reports in the total will make virtually no difference to the result.

An alternative way of looking at this approach is comparing the number of observations of a particular drug–reaction combination O (cell a in Table 6.4) with the number expected (E), based on the row and column marginal totals. This is the way that the expected counts are derived for a chi-squared test. The generality of this approach will be discussed in another context below. The PRR is then simply O/E. It has been suggested that a cut-off of PRR = 2 or more, the number of reports for a particular drug–reaction combination >2 and a $\chi^2 > 4$ can be used to define a signal (Evans *et al.*, 2001). A $\chi^2 > 3.84$ is the exact value for a significance test at 0.05. This is then evaluated in further detail to see if there is evidence to suggest that the ADR is indeed causal. This approach will detect new ADRs and allow a focus on important signals when a large number of reports are received. However, the cut-off of PRR > 2 results in a large number of potential signals to be evaluated and higher cut-offs may be used.

There are a number of issues that need to be addressed when using disproportionality methods. The analysis can be performed at any level of classification. The dictionaries used for these classifications may have a fully hierarchical system, e.g. MedDRA (Chapter 12). The term actually recorded by a health professional is at a very low level in the hierarchy of terms, such as 'heart attack'. This will possibly have other synonyms, and the 'preferred term', at a higher level, might be 'myocardial infarction'. A still higher level term could be 'ischaemic heart disease', and the highest might be 'cardiovascular disease'. The problem is that the lower level of terms may not have many reports and there can be misclassification, so that a grouping at a higher level may be preferable in this context. Most usage of PRR methods has been at the 'preferred term' level, but this has the consequence that a large number of reports will be for a single reaction (at PT level)–drug combination. In a UK database of over 400 000 SRs, there are about 110 000 different drug–reaction combinations. About 70 000 of these only occur once in the database. There has been little work to show what is the most sensitive and specific level at which to detect new ADRs. It seems likely that the best strategy is to choose a level for maximum sensitivity, which will require a fairly high level, then to investigate in more detail those drug–reaction combinations that are suggestive of a signal. Any automated system should allow for searching for new ADRs at more than one level in the hierarchy. In a system for automatic screening, the only feasible drug comparator is all drugs; but, for a detailed investigation, other groupings, such as same class of drug or same indication, may provide insight.

The next problem is whether to adjust for other factors such as age and sex. There is no doubt that background events will be age and sex dependent, so that it is sensible to stratify the data by age and sex provided that age and sex are known for most of the reports. This approach has recently been used by the FDA (see DuMouchel method below). It is likely that, in some circumstances, this will increase sensitivity and specificity, but it is important that the method used works well with sparse data, since stratifying will mean that the numbers in each 2×2 table will tend to be small. It is also possible to adjust for other factors, such as calendar time. This latter factor is more relevant when scanning an entire database, but it is less sensible when using the method for monitoring new reports as they arrive.

A further issue is whether to use all reports or only those of a serious nature. The term 'serious' has been used to mean those events that result in hospitalization (or its prolongation), death, and congenital malformation. At the UK MCA the word 'serious' is used in the ADROIT database to refer to a set of terms that are regarded as being serious whether they have one of those outcomes or not. Other dictionaries have different thresholds for terms of a serious nature, such as 'critical terms' in the WHO dictionary. The MCA has used PRR methods for examining serious events as part of a prioritization approach. The most important ADRs from a public health perspective are the serious ones, but this does not mean that lesser terms can be ignored.

When examining a class of drugs, it is reasonable to look at the PRR for each drug separately, but great care must be taken in making between-drug comparisons. There can be biased reporting for a particular drug–reaction combination, but much biased reporting applies to all suspected reactions for a specific drug. This implies that using prescriptions as a denominator will be more biased than the proportional methods. It is possible to use a statistical test for differential effects between drugs of the same class, but the danger is that these will lead to 'over-interpretation', since the underlying data are not of a high quality. The coding of drugs according to the ATC classification allows for sensible objective grouping of drugs for signal detection purposes. It must be emphasized that this process is one of scanning for signals rather than demonstrating causality.

A more important problem occurs when there are a very large number of reports for a particular drug–reaction combination. This is likely to be a true ADR, but it can result in reducing the PRRs for other reactions for that drug, and reducing the PRRs for that reaction in other drugs. This is because the numbers in cell a become large for this drug–reaction combination; when another drug is examined for this reaction then the total in the database is inflated and no longer provides what may be regarded as 'background'. Similarly, the total of reports for this drug is then higher and the proportion of reports for other reactions is then less. This is illustrated by Figure 6.3 which shows the spectrum of the proportion of reports

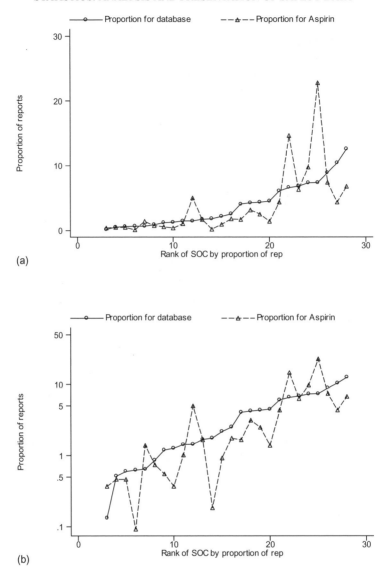

Figure 6.3   Percentage of reports in each system order class: (a) linear scale; (b) logarithmic scale

for aspirin, derived from the MCA's 'Foreign' database (i.e. reports sent by companies to the UK authority originating from outside the UK). A relatively smooth line is drawn giving the proportion of reports for the whole database as a reference. The horizontal axis has the type of ADR, and this is sorted in order of increasing frequency in the database. The numeric label is arbitrary. In Figure 6.3(a) it is shown on a linear scale and in Figure 6.3(b) it is shown on a log scale, so that the proportionate height of the point for aspirin and a particular reaction above the line for the database is a measure of the PRR. The very large number of reports of gastrointestinal bleeding reduces the PRR for other reactions. Incidentally, it is notable that there is a 'trough' for cardiovascular reactions, which might be expected in view of the known benefit of aspirin.

The remedy is to recalculate the PRRs, subtracting the data for the identified reaction from the entire database. This is not difficult for one particular instance, but it is difficult to do in a routine manner.

One statistical issue is whether the unit of reporting is taken as a report or as a reaction, since several reactions may appear on a single report. From a statistical point of view it is better to use a report as the unit, since there is possible dependence between reactions on the same report. However, precision is not the main requirement for a method of signal detection, and approximate answers will suffice. Apparent statistical precision is spurious, since sampling error is not the main problem; there are many biases in the data and their value is in signal detection, not in confirmation.

There is some potential for these methods to be used in assessing data from clinical trials. Control groups in trials can be a very useful source of the rate of occurrence of background AEs, and their potential has not yet been fully exploited.

A major problem with the PRR and similar methods (including ROR) occurs when the expected number is very small. This has two effects: first, the value of the PRR can be very high indeed with a small expected value; second, the PRR itself is not a reflection of how many reports have been received. Using a chi-squared test or a CI in combination with the PRR deals with this to some degree, but the chi-squared test (and CIs) will tend to be less than robust with very small expected values. A PRR of 200 is obtained with one report when 0.005 are expected and the same PRR occurs when 200 reports are observed with one expected. These have different implications for public health. The approaches discussed below seek to address this explicitly.

WHO Bayesian confidence neural network

This is a method based on the same principles described above but with more mathematical sophistication. It has been developed in Sweden and is in use by the WHO Centre for International Drug Monitoring in Uppsala, the Uppsala Monitoring Centre (UMC; Bate et al., 1998). It uses what is effectively $\log_2$ of the PRR and calls this the *information component* (IC). It also calculates a CI around the IC so that a signal is detected if the lower limit of the 95 per cent CI (using a log scale) is above zero. The method has been validated by examining signals that would have been generated in the period 1993–2000 and testing whether they were in standard reference texts, Martindale and the Physician's Desk Reference (Lindquist et al., 2000). The method showed a useful performance with 85 per cent negative predictive value and a 44 per cent positive predictive value. It was noted that there were 17 positive associations that could not be dismissed as false positive signals, even though they were missing from standard texts. The 'gold standard' is itself not truly a perfect standard and conclusions, therefore, must inevitably be limited.

A comparison between the Bayesian confidence neural network (BCNN) method and the PRR and ROR has been made by van Puijenbroek et al. (2002). This showed that each of the methods gives very similar answers when numbers of reports are greater than about three, but that, as expected, PRR and ROR are more unstable with small numbers of reports. They used the lower 95 per cent CI for the PRR, which is equivalent to using the PRR when chi-squared is statistically significant at the 5 per cent level, as discussed above.

The overall effect of the WHO method is similar to the PRR method used by the UK MCA, but based on a larger database derived from worldwide regulatory authorities. The

BCNN method has not generally been used with stratification of the data by age, sex and calendar period, though this would be possible.

DuMouchel method

The method that has been used in recent years by the US FDA is also a Bayesian method (DuMouchel, 1999). There is a public-domain version of the software that was used to carry out the analyses. It is similar to the PRR and other methods in utilizing the same type of 2×2 table, and emphasizes the O/E approach. However, it has some advantage in that it is less vulnerable to small values of the expected count than the other methods, especially the PRR and ROR.

The method involves one pass through the entire database of SRs of (suspected) ADRs to estimate the parameters of the Bayesian prior distribution of the number of reports for all the drug–reaction combinations (hence, it can be seen as a form of empirical Bayes rather than based on subjective prior probabilities). The second pass then determines the departure from what might be expected given the number of reports for this reaction in total and the number of reports for this drug in total. This departure is approximately proportional to O/E (the PRR) but shrinks the value towards unity, the null value, which makes a notable difference if the expected value is very small.

The assumption is that the prior distribution for the ratio of the observed counts in a particular drug–reaction combination to the expected counts is a mixture of two gamma distributions. Hence, the method is described as a 'gamma Poisson shrinker'. The result presented is the geometric mean of the empirical Bayes estimate of the posterior distribution of the 'true' PRR. This is given the symbol EBGM, and the value of this is used to rank drug–reaction combinations. It is also possible to calculate a standard error for this estimate, and, as with the WHO method, the lower 95 per cent confidence limit is used for signal generation purposes.

Figure 6.4 shows a plot of the values derived from the DuMouchel method against the PRR for a selection of potential signals from the MCA's ADROIT database. The symbol on the graph shows the number of reports for a particular drug–reaction combination. It shows that small numbers of observed reports can result in a high PRR (with a correspondingly very small expected number) but the EBGM is not as extreme. In most instances the number of reports is large enough not to make any notable difference, but with small expected numbers it is likely that the PRR will generate too many false positive signals. This is partly why the MCA have also used a cut-off requiring at least three reports for a drug–reaction combination.

Figure 6.4 shows that those drug–reaction combinations with small numbers of reports tend to move above a line of equality, and the EBGM shrinks them to much lower values.

The DuMouchel method is at its strongest in scanning an entire database to see if anything has been missed using the traditional case-by-case evaluation. It requires notable computer resources to carry out a regular monitoring of new reports, but this is not a major drawback since it is not difficult to run the whole process on a weekly or monthly basis.

There are new developments of DuMouchel's method to allow for examination of drug interactions that have been applied within the FDA (Szarfman et al., 2002). This is described as a 'multi-item gamma Poisson shrinker' (MPGS). The software for this method is available commercially. This is very elegant and obtains signal scores for pairs, triplets and higher-order multiple numbers of drugs used by individual patients. The other methods using SR

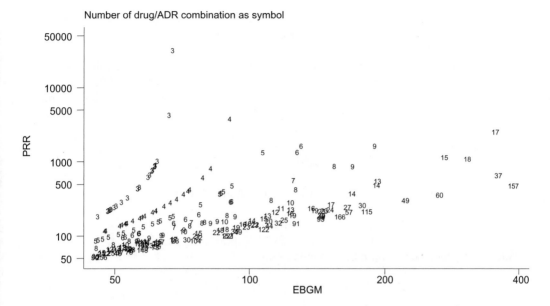

Figure 6.4 Proportional reporting ratio versus empirical Bayes geometric mean for data from UK ADROIT database

databases have used each drug–reaction combination as a single entity rather than taking into account the fact that there may be more than one drug mentioned on a report. The potential for automated scanning of databases to look for drug interactions is beginning to be used in the FDA and in other systems. For a good review of the application of Bayesian methods see Gould (2003).

Sequential probability ratio tests

It is possible to compare two hypotheses based on the likelihood of observing the data given each of the hypotheses. The comparison of the likelihoods can be done in a sequential way with accumulating data, and are called sequential probability ratio tests (SPRTs). These tests discriminate between two hypotheses in the most powerful way and have been used in sequential medical trials (Armitage, 1958). They are used in industrial statistics for monitoring processes and were developed during World War II but not published until afterwards by Barnard (1946) and Wald (1947) independently. Much work has been done on this and similar methods in the context of monitoring clinical trials as data on efficacy accumulate (Whitehead, 1997). A new application has been in monitoring death rates in medical practice (Spiegelhalter *et al.*, 2003). Here, it is suggested that these be applied to the problem of monitoring SRs to detect new ADRs.

The two hypotheses of interest are that the number of reports coming in for a particular drug and particular reaction is what is expected, i.e. the null, or alternatively that the number of reports is importantly divergent from the expected number. For example, the MCA has used a cut-off of two for PRRs, so a reasonable alternative hypothesis is to look for at least a doubling of the risk of a particular reaction.

The log-likelihood ratio (LLR) of the two hypotheses is calculated on the basis of accumulating data. This measures the relative likelihood of the two hypotheses given the data. It is for this process of dealing with accumulating data that this method is particularly suitable.

It is necessary to assume that SRs can be described using a Poisson model (which applies generally to counts of the number of events), and the alternative hypothesis is framed as the ratio of the rate for the observed to expected rate; in other words, effectively a relative risk (RR). The correct LLR to use, where O is the observed number of SRs for a particular drug–reaction combination and E is the number expected, is then

$$O \log(\text{RR}) - E(\text{RR} - 1)$$

If a doubling of risk is of interest, then RR $= 2$ and so the LLR becomes

$$O \log(2) - E$$

And so this suggests that for on-going monitoring

$$O0.69 - E$$

is calculated as the LLR, which can be checked against a cut-off value.

The value of E can be calculated from the existing SR database just as described for PRRs above, using Equations (6.1) or (6.2). In principle the value of E could be obtained from other means, such as data on morbidity in a population similar to that treated by the drug, but the most straightforward way is to use the SR database. The use of this method, stratified by age and sex or other factors, has not yet been fully developed and tested in practice.

The threshold values allowing for continuous monitoring are given in Table 6.5. For risks of false positives and false negatives of 0.05, then, the boundary is 2.94.

Table 6.5 Threshold values for a LLR for Poisson counts

Type 1 error (α)	Type 2 error (β)	LLR threshold
0.05	0.05	2.94
0.05	0.1	2.89
0.05	0.2	2.77
0.1	0.1	2.20
0.1	0.2	2.08

If a reaction has an extremely low background rate and occurs very rarely indeed, then E will be close to zero. With zero expected events, then, the threshold is crossed when $O0.69$ becomes >2.94, i.e. $O > 4.26$. This suggests that action should be taken when $O > 5$. This is a relatively conservative attitude towards false positive and false negative errors, and the most sensitive cut-off is when $O0.69 > 2.08$, in other words approximately $O > 3$. This could be seen as a statistical justification of the old threshold of more than three spontaneous reports being regarded as a signal. The problem with that approach was that it assumed an extremely low background rate for that medical event.

The use of the SPRT in signal detection is still being developed, but it can be seen to place more emphasis on the difference between the observed and expected than just on their ratio. The consequence is that, although the alternative hypothesis is effectively a PRR >2, the magnitude of the number of reports is a major factor determining the generation of a signal. At the same time, it is clear that in public health terms there is a need for different thresholds for different possible reactions. Phocomelia or aplastic anaemia may need only a single report associating their occurrence with a particular drug to be sufficient to require immediate detailed investigation and follow up. There is further work to be done in setting standards for such monitoring.

Summary and conclusions

Trials

Standard methods of analysis may be used in analysing occurrence of adverse effects. In general, for ADRs (binary data) it is best to use survival analysis and to show plots of cumulative hazard over time in order to allow for dropout from trials and effects of medicines that are not necessarily constant over time. When an ADR is associated with continuous laboratory measurements, analysis should examine trends, just as is done for efficacy variables, in addition to converting them to binary variables using a cut-off, such as three-times the upper limit of normal (see Chapter 5).

Very large trials are needed to allow statistical methods to demonstrate the existence of adverse reactions, unless they are very common. The use of meta-analysis of all the available trials does help to increase power, but even then the power may remain limited. The consequence is that observational studies will continue to be necessary for detecting most unexpected ADRs.

Observational data

Again standard methods can be used. Bias is likely to be greater than in RCTs, but careful design and analysis can give reliable answers, although small effects must always be treated with caution. Propensity score methods have utility, especially in cohort studies when analysing rare outcomes, and many important ADRs are very rare.

The problem of studying multiple outcomes has not been solved. It is possible to use adjustments that reduce type 1 errors, but these automatically increase type 2 errors. It has been argued by some epidemiologists that adjustment is unnecessary, (Rothman, 1990). It seems sensible to treat new and unexpected findings that are inconsistent with previous knowledge or with other data from within a single study with caution, but there is an argument for approaching analyses of variables that are used for safety with a precautionary approach while being more stringent when multiple outcomes are examined for efficacy. The very use of the word 'safety' (as opposed to 'harm', which is what is actually studied) implies an asymmetry. Patients need reassurance over safety (Chapter 16), and there is a need to ensure that issues of safety are not dismissed too readily. Some studies are set up to test hypotheses in regard to safety that have been generated by individual case reports; when the response variable of interest is pre-specified, the problem of multiplicity is reduced.

Spontaneous reporting

The detection of new adverse reactions will depend on careful recording by health professionals, both of drugs used and medical events. Their suspicions, and in some cases those of patients, are vital to early recognition. Statistical methods can aid this process, provided they are used effectively at all stages in drug development from pre-licensing through to post-marketing surveillance. Disproportionality methods, such as the PRR, are effective tools for the analysis of data from spontaneous reports of suspected adverse reactions. Their mathematical sophistication must not be allowed to give undue weight to poor quality original data. These measures are to be used as signals of potential hazards and should not be misinterpreted as proof of causality.

Ongoing monitoring of new drugs may be helped by a statistical method like the SPRT, which takes the repeated examination of data into account. Statistical methods can be improved and introduced to support the never-ending vigilance required to extend knowledge about adverse reactions to drugs. Such knowledge should always be considered provisional and be open to re-evaluation in the light of further experience.

Acknowledgements

I am grateful to Professor Stuart Pocock, who made many valuable comments on this chapter. I wish to thank Dr Raine and the UK MCA for permission to use data derived from the ADROIT database. Dr David Spiegelhalter suggested the use of SPRTs for Poisson counts in monitoring death rates.

I am also grateful to Roussow et al. for taking the time to supply a modified version of their original figure (Figure 6.2).

Stata software version 7 (College Station, Texas, USA) was used for calculating power for Figure 6.1, and for processing data to create other figures.

References

Altman DG (1991). *Practical Statistics for Medical Research*. Chapman and Hall: London.
Altman DG (1998). Covariate imbalance, adjustment for. In *Encyclopedia of Biostatistics,* Armitage P and Colton T (eds). Wiley: Chichester.
Armitage P (1958). Sequential methods in clinical trials. *Am J Public Health* **48**: 1395–1402.
Barnard GA (1946). Sequential tests in industrial statistics. *J R Stat Soc* (Suppl 8): 1–26.
Bate A, Lindquist M, Edwards IR, Olsson S et al. (1998). A Bayesian neural network method for adverse reaction signal generation. *Eur J Clin Pharmacol* **54**: 315–321.
Braitman LE and Rosenbaum PR (2002). Rare outcomes, common treatments: analytic strategies using propensity scores. *Ann Intern Med* **137**: 693–695.
Brewer T and Colditz GA (1999). Postmarketing surveillance and adverse drug reactions: current perspectives and future needs. *J Am Med Assoc* **281**: 824–829.
Chuang-Stein C, Le V and Chen W (2001). Recent advancements in the analysis and presentation of safety data. *Drug Inf J* **35**: 377–397.
Clayton D and Hills M (1993). *Statistical Models in Epidemiology*. Oxford University Press: Oxford.
Collett D (1994). *Modelling Survival Data in Medical Research*. Chapman and Hall: London.
Davis S and Raine J (2002). Spontaneous reporting – UK. In *Pharmacovigilance*, Mann R and Andrews E (eds). Wiley: Chichester.

DuMouchel W (1999). Bayesian data mining in large frequency tables. With an application to the FDA spontaneous reporting system. *Am Stat* **53**: 177–190.

Egberts ACG, Meyboom RHB, de Konig GHP, Bakker A, *et al.* (1997). Non-puerperal lactation associated with antidepressant drug use. *Br J Clin Pharmacol* **44**: 277–281.

Egger M, Davey Smith G, Altman DG (eds) (2001). *Systematic Reviews in Health Care. Meta-analysis in Context*, 2nd edn. British Medical Journal Books: London.

Evans SJW, Waller PC and Davis S (2001). Use of proportional reporting ratios (PRRs) for signal generation from spontaneous adverse drug reaction reports. *Pharmacoepidemiol Drug Saf* **10**: 483–486.

Gould AL (2003). Practical pharmacovigilance analysis strategies. *Pharmacoepidemiol Drug Saf* **12**: 559–574.

Greenland S and Morganstern H (1990). Matching and efficiency in cohort studies. *Am J Epidemiol* **131**: 151–159.

Hennessy S, Berlin JA, Kinman JL, Margolis DJ *et al.* (2001). Risk of venous thromboembolism from oral contraceptives containing gestodene and desogestrel versus levonorgestrel: a meta-analysis and formal sensitivity analysis. *Contraception* **64**: 125–133.

Ioannidis JPA and Contopoulos-Ioannidis DG (1998). Reporting of safety data from randomized trials. *Lancet* **352**: 1752–1753.

Ioannidis JPA and Lau J (2001). Completeness of safety reporting in randomized trials: an evaluation of 7 medical areas. *J Am Med Assoc* **285**: 437–443.

Jasmer RM, Saukkonen JJ, Blumberg HM, Daley CL, *et al.* (2002). Short-course rifampin and pyrazinamide compared with isoniazid for latent tuberculosis infection: a multicenter clinical trial. *Ann Intern Med* **37**: 640–647.

Kemmeren JM, Algra A and Grobbee DE (2001). Third generation oral contraceptives and risk of venous thrombosis: meta-analysis. *Br Med J* **323**: 131–134.

Koch GG, Schmid JE, Begun JM and Maier WC (1993). Meta analysis of drug safety data. In *Drug Safety Assessment in Clinical Trials*, Solgliero-Gilbert G (ed). Marcel Dekker: New York; 279–304.

Lee M-L and Lazarus R (1997). Meta-analysis of drug safety data with logistic regression. *Drug Inf J* **31**: 1189–1193.

Lin KK and Rahman MA (1998). Overall false positive rates in tests for linear trend in tumor incidence in animal carcinogenicity studies of new drugs. *J Biopharm Stat* **8**: 1–15 (see also discussion 17–22).

Lindquist M, Stahl M, Bate A, Edwards IR *et al.* (2000). A retrospective evaluation of a data mining approach to aid finding new adverse drug reaction signals in the WHO international database. *Drug Saf* **23**: 533–542.

Ludbrook J (1998). Multiple comparison procedures updated. *Clin Exp Pharmacol Physiol* **25**: 1032–1037.

Moore N, Kreft-Jais C, Haramburu F, Noblet C *et al.* (1997). Reports of hypoglycaemia associated with the use of ACE inhibitors and other drugs: a case/non-case study in the French pharmacovigilance system database. *Br J Clin Pharmacol* **44**: 513–518.

O'Neill R (1987). Statistical analyses of AE data from clinical trials. Special emphasis on serious events. *Drug Inf J* **21**: 9–20.

Patwary KW (1969). Report on statistical aspects of the pilot research project for international drug monitoring. WHO, Geneva.

Peto R, Pike MC, Armitage P, Breslow NE *et al.* (1977). Design and analysis of randomized clinical trials requiring prolonged observation of each patient. II. Analysis and examples. *Br J Cancer* **35**: 1–39.

Rosenbaum PR (2002). *Observational Studies*. Springer-Verlag: New York.

Rossouw JE, Anderson GL, Prentice RL, Kooperberg C *et al.* (2002). Risks and benefits of estrogen plus progestin in healthy postmenopausal women. *J Am Med Assoc* **288**: 321–333.

Rothman KJ (1990). No adjustments are needed for multiple comparisons. *Epidemiology* **1**: 43–46.

Rothman KJ and Greenland S (1998). *Modern Epidemiology*, 2nd edn. Lippincott-Raven: Philadelphia.

Spiegelhalter DJ, Kinsman R, Grigg O and Treasure T (2003). Risk-adjusted sequential probability ratio tests: applications to Bristol, Shipman, and adult cardiac surgery. *Int J Qual Health Care* **15**: 7–13.

Stricker BHCh and Tijessen JGP (1992). Serum sickness-like reactions to ceflacor. *J Clin Epidemiol* **45**: 1177–1184.

Sutton AJ and Abrams KR (2001). Bayesian methods in meta-analysis and evidence synthesis. *Stat Methods Med Res.* **10**: 277–303.

Sutton AJ, Abrams KR, Jones DR, Sheldon TA *et al.* (2000). *Methods for Meta-Analysis in Medical Research*. Wiley: Chichester.

Szarfman A, Machado SG and O'Neill RT (2002). Use of screening algorithms and computer systems to efficiently signal higher-than-expected combinations of drugs and events in the US FDA's spontaneous reports database. *Drug Saf* **25**: 381–392.

Temple R (1999). Meta-analysis and epidemiologic studies in drug development and postmarketing surveillance. *J Am Med Assoc* **281**: 841–844.

Van Puijenbroek EP, Bate A, Leufkens HGM, Lindquist M *et al.* (2002). A comparison of measures of disproportionality for signal detection in spontaneous reporting systems for adverse drug reactions. *Pharmacoepidemiol Drug Saf* **11**: 3–10.

Wald A (1947). *Sequential Analysis* Wiley: New York.

Wang J and Donnan PT (2001). Propensity score methods in drug safety studies: practice, strengths and limitations. *Pharmacoepidemiol Drug Saf* **10**: 341–344.

Whitehead J (1997). *The Design and Analysis of Sequential Clinical Trials*, revised 2nd edn. Wiley: Chichester.

Wolfe F, Flowers N, Burke TA, Arguelles LM *et al.* (2002). Increase in lifetime adverse drug reactions, service utilization, and disease severity among patients who will start COX-2 specific inhibitors: quantitative assessment of channeling bias and confounding by indication in 6689 patients with rheumatoid arthritis and osteoarthritis. *J Rheumatol* **29**: 1015–1022.

Wood L and Coulson R (2001). Revitalizing the General Practice Research Database: plans, challenges, and opportunities. *Pharmacoepidemiol Drug Saf* **10**: 379–383.

7

Causality and Correlation in Pharmacovigilance

S. A. W. Shakir

Introduction and historical background

Human beings have been concerned about causality, i.e. what causes what in this world and why, for a long time. With regard to health, for thousands of years, men and women attributed events, such as disease, to a variety of physical and conceptual 'causes', including natural phenomena, e.g. an eclipse, evil spirits or the wrath of the Gods.

The publication in 1638 of Galileo's book *Dascori* marks the beginning of the modern scientific era. In his book, Galileo introduced concepts such as description first, explanation second and that description could be carried out using the language of mathematics. Following Galileo, the most notable philosopher who wrote about causation was David Hume, the Scottish 18th century philosopher. In his major work *A Treatise of Human Nature*, Hume addressed a number of aspects related to causality, and many of the concepts that he proposed remain valid. One of his useful thoughts was that there is no such thing as an impression of a causal relationship. According to Hume, we can perceive by mere observation of *a* and *b* that *a* is above *b* or to the right of *b*. He held the view that when we say *a* causes *b*, we mean that *a* and *b* are constantly conjoined by fact, but not that there is some necessary connection between them. In Hume's view we have no other notion of cause and effect but that of certain objects, which have been always conjoined. Bertrand Russell adds that we cannot penetrate into the reason of the conjunction (*Russell on Hume*).

Although practical biomedical sciences tend generally not to be concerned during day-to-day work about causation with such philosophical rigour, the principles of causation must be taken into consideration in all work that examines interactions between events with regard to a possible cause and effect relationship. Francis Goulton, the inventor of finger-printing and cousin of Charles Darwin, measured the length of a person's arm and the size of that person's head and asked to what degree can one of these qualities predict the other. Goulton's experimental work, while technically simple, documented for the first time in the history of science that the correlation between two biological variables can be connected on the possible basis of measurement rather than human judgements, i.e. that the attribute to the correlation to variation of the two organs is partly due to common causes. This led Pearson

Stephens' Detection of New Adverse Drug Reactions Fifth Edition edited by John Talbot and Patrick Waller
© 2004 John Wiley & Sons, Ltd   ISBN: 0 470 84552 X

to state, 30 years later, that his interpretation of Goulton's work was that there was a category broader than causation, namely correlation, of which causation was only the limit. This new concept of correlation brought psychology, anthropology, medicine and sociology in large parts into the field of mathematical treatment. (Pearl, 2001)

In general, the two fundamental questions about causality are:

1. What experimental evidence is required for legitimate inference of a cause and effect relationship?

2. Given that we are willing to accept causal information about the phenomena, what inferences can we draw from such information and how?

Pharmacovigilance and pharmacoepidemiology are new scientific disciplines. In common with other biomedical sciences, causation is much harder to ascertain than correlation in these disciplines. There are many examples in biomedical sciences where correlations are generally accepted without full ascertainment of causality. For example, whilst science continues to work to identify the precise pathway of causation, to a patient and to society it is clear that the relationship between smoking cigarettes and lung cancer is accepted. Similarly, the relationship between the use of aspirin and the development of Reye's syndrome in children is generally accepted without full understanding of the pathophysiological mechanisms involved.

The notions of necessary and sufficient causes

The notions of necessary cause and sufficient cause are of interest in a number of applications, both in science and law. For example, oxygen is necessary for fire to set in a room; however, alone, oxygen is not sufficient for starting a fire and another action, such as striking a match, is needed to start a fire. This is very important in pharmacovigilance. For example, a person with partially patent coronary arteries may have no symptoms at rest but will get angina when exercising, with the development of severe anaemia or when receiving a medication that constricts the coronary arteries. Apart from very extreme levels, these three factors will not cause angina in a patient with fully patent coronary arteries. Therefore, the partial patency of the coronary arteries is a necessary but insufficient condition for the angina to occur. Since medicines are not always taken by people who are otherwise healthy, some people by the nature of their genetic constitution (which may affect the pharmacokinetic or pharmacodynamic responses to drugs) and patients with a previous medical history or other predisposing factors are more likely to experience some adverse drug reactions (ADRs) than people without such conditions. Awareness of the impact of such factors on the likelihood of developing specific ADRs is an important consideration in causality assessment.

Factors to be considered in causality assessment

In day-to-day medical practice, the boundaries between the concepts of a cause and a correlation are blurred; the word 'cause' is usually used somewhat loosely. This may have been driven by practical needs, since one of the reasons why patients consult doctors is to know what has caused their condition. Many patients are disappointed if the doctor does not provide them with a possible cause. For example, a patient with a rash may be understandably disappointed if his doctor tells him that he is unsure whether the cause of the rash is a viral illness or an allergy. For practical clinical purposes, lack of precision in the application of the concept of 'cause' may lead to no harm as long as there is awareness that, in most cases, the interaction between the presumed cause and effect is a relationship, which in some cases may be a strong relationship, but not a definite cause. Although this notion is true to some extent when dealing with ADRs, the distinction between a cause and correlation needs to be more precise. For example, as nearly every patient will get bradycardia with high doses of beta-blockers and since bradycardia is a common adverse reaction with therapeutic doses of beta-blockers, it is not unreasonable to say that beta-blockers cause bradycardia in many patients. Conversely, while it is accepted that prolonged use of hormone replacement therapy (HRT) is associated with slight increase in the incidence of breast cancer (Dixon, 2001), and therefore a small number of long-term users will develop this condition, it is more appropriate to describe the interaction as an association. The reason for the difference between beta-blockers and HRT is the difference in the level of the certainty and strength of the association, both of which are much greater for the former than the latter. These two examples are relatively easy to handle, because of the abundance of good quality relevant data; but this is not the case for many other adverse events with medicines.

The clinical diagnosis of suspected ADRs is not different from the clinical diagnosis of conditions caused by other environmental factors, such as microbial or physical agents. The diagnostic process follows the usual steps of obtaining history, conducting an appropriate physical examination, ordering appropriate investigations and sometimes using time as a diagnostic tool. Some 30 years ago Irey (1972) described comprehensively the diagnostic problems in drug-induced disease and proposed strategies to aid the diagnoses of these conditions. Much of what was proposed by Irey remains applicable. For example, the emphasis on time to onset, the differential diagnoses (of causes other than the drug), the selection of the responsible drug on the basis of the pattern of the event or by exclusion, and the emphasis on rechallenge and dechallenge are all aspects that remain valid and applicable.

Performing causality assessment in pharmacovigilance may involve making a decision based on the information in a single adverse event or suspected ADR report (or a series of such reports) on the relationship between exposure to a drug and the reported adverse event or the suspected ADR. While this process is generally referred to as causality assessment, it is in fact an assessment of possible relatedness between exposure to a medicine and an adverse event. This evaluation which is useful in pharmacovigilance and essential in clinical medicine is different from the broader process of assessing causality of adverse reactions on the basis of data from multiple sources (see p. 338). There are many similarities between the clinical diagnosis of suspected ADRs in individual patients and causality assessment of case reports in pharmacovigilance. The points that need to be considered in both include:

1.   The temporal relationship (time to onset)

The temporal relationship is perhaps the most important point to consider in assessing the relationship between exposure to a drug and a subsequent adverse event. Since most ADRs are 'Type A' (pharmacologically related) reactions, a plausible temporal relationship between exposure and the onset of the suspected ADR, taking into consideration the pharmacological characteristics of the drug, is normally the first point to consider in the assessment of causality. A causal relationship is supported when the onset of an ADR coincides with the expected peak tissue concentration of the drug. Conversely, in most cases doubt should be raised when the onset of an ADR bears no relationship to the pharmacological characteristics of the drug.

With regard to measurement of the time to onset, it important to consider the nature of the reaction. For short-term reactions, e.g. flushing with a calcium channel blocker, the relevant time to onset is the time between the last dose and the onset of the reaction. With long-term reactions, e.g. cataracts with systemic corticosteroids, the relevant period is the time between starting treatment and the development of the reaction.

2. The clinical and pathological characteristics of the events

Since ADRs are caused by definite pathophysiological mechanisms (although many are unclear at the time of assessment), conformity with the recognized clinical and pathophysiological patterns of the ADR is supportive of a causal relationship. For example, the clinical manifestations and laboratory abnormalities of patients with anaemia following the use of α-methyldopa are expected to be consistent with the diagnosis of haemolytic anaemia (a recognized association) and doubt about relatedness should be raised when other types of anaemia are attributed to the use of this product.

3. Pharmacological plausibility

Pharmacological plausibility is based on previous knowledge of the drug, including its pharmacodynamic and pharmacokinetic characteristics. It is self-evident that causality is supported for events that can be explained on the basis of the pharmacological characteristics of the suspect drug, e.g. when the occurrence of the event coincides with the expected peak concentration in the affected organ.

4. Existing information

Whether the event has been previously reported as an adverse reaction (in clinical trials and post-marketing). Although the Summary of Product Characteristics (SmPC), or the Investigator Brochure for products in development, includes a list of adverse events or suspected ADRs that have been previously reported, the search for important events may need to include prescribing and pharmacological information in other sources.

5. Concomitant medication

The role of concomitant medications and medications taken prior to the event that could have caused the event. In patients who are taking more than one drug, it is frequently difficult to decide which one is the more likely cause of the suspected ADR. All the points that need to be considered for causality assessment for the suspect drug apply to concomitant medications or drugs to which the patient was exposed.

6. Underlying and concurrent illnesses

Some events which are attributed to drug exposure may be simply manifestations of pre-existing conditions. Furthermore, patients with some diseases, e.g. AIDS, respond differently to drugs, with qualitatively and quantitatively different ADR profiles. Patients with some conditions may experience altered responses to medications, e.g. patients with heart failure may experience augmented responses to cardiovascular medications.

7. Dechallenge or dose reduction

Recovery after stopping the drug or dose reduction is important, particularly when the timing of the full recovery or improvement is consistent with the pharmacological characteristics of the drug. However, it is noteworthy that some events, e.g. deafness with aminoglycosides, are irreversible.

8. Rechallenge or dose increase

The occurrence of ADRs after dose increases or rechallenge is a strong indicator of causality, particularly if the onset of the suspected ADR is pharmacologically plausible. A note of caution is to resist temptation for using rechallenge as a diagnostic tool unless clinically warranted and informed consent has been obtained. There must a valid reason for the rechallenge and the practitioner and the institute must be trained and prepared for all eventualities, e.g. severe anaphylaxis and cardiac arrest.

9. Patients' characteristics and previous medical history

Previous medical history including previous history of drug allergies and the presence of renal or hepatic impairment can be very relevant in the diagnosis of suspected ADRs. For example, patients with atopy or a history of allergy to drugs are more likely to experience allergic ADRs. Female sex, low body weight, renal impairment and hepatic impairment are well known risk factors for ADRs (see Chapter 2).

10. Drug interactions

A plausible temporal relationship with the introduction or cessation of a concomitant drug with potential for interaction is an important consideration in causality assessment.

11. The quality of information in the report

Whereas minimal information is required for valid regulatory reports, causality assessment requires all the necessary data elements. In many cases in pharmacovigilance practice this can be obtained only after seeking detailed follow-up information from the reporter.

The clinical diagnosis of ADRs and causality assessment in pharmacovigilance require expertise that includes sound biomedical education and the ability to apply relevant clinical and pharmacological knowledge. Specifically, they require:

- Awareness that the event could be an ADR for one of the drugs that the patient is receiving. Therefore, practitioners and assessors should be aware of the common and serious ADRs for the medicines used, including their clinical patterns and other biological aspects.

- Access and ability to use information sources and they need to establish links with medical information departments or pharmaceutical companies for information on rare events or drugs with which they are unfamiliar.

- Basic knowledge of the pharmacokinetic (absorption, distribution, metabolism and excretion) and pharmacodynamic characteristics of the drugs used, as well as potential for drug interactions.

- Familiarity with special investigations that aid the diagnosis or monitoring of suspected ADRs, including their indications and limitations. Such investigations include measurement of drug blood levels, tissue biopsy, etc.

- Clinicians who are responsible for the management of patients with suspected ADRs must be trained to handle unclear situations. For example, if even after careful consideration it remains unclear which of several drugs that the patient is receiving is the most likely cause of a suspected ADR, then a strategy for stopping the drugs one at time and evaluating the response to dechallenge may be needed. This requires weighing the benefits gained from each drug with the detrimental effects of its withdrawal and the management of the consequences of these clinical decisions.

Methods for causality assessment

Many systems for causality assessment have been proposed. These have been mostly used during regulatory reporting by pharmaceutical companies, assessment by regulatory authorities or in academic research. According to Jones (2000), these systems can broadly be divided into three categories:

1. Unrestricted clinical evaluation/global introspection.

2. Algorithms, with or without scoring.

3. Bayesian probabilistic methods.

Each of these categories has advantages and disadvantages, as discussed below.

Unrestricted evaluation/global introspection

This is the most commonly used method by clinicians and by many pharmaceutical companies and regulatory authorities. Although the method is easy to apply and resembles the day-to-day medical practice with its 'common-sense' approach, it lacks transparency and is subject to the fallibility of human judgement. The method permits inconsistency, as well as missing or misinterpreting important points.

Structured algorithms with or without scoring

There are many structured or semi-structured algorithms for causality assessment. These range from simple flow charts (with or without scoring) to lengthy questionnaires with tens of questions that need to be analysed by powerful computers (Jones, 2000). The advantages of structured assessments include transparency and consistency. When a structured method for causality assessment is applied properly, no points are missed. A consistent method of assessment facilitates communication between healthcare professionals and aids documentation and audit. Disadvantages include reduced ability to apply clinical judgement and, with algorithms that include scoring, adherence to the scores in place of clinical judgement.

With regard to algorithms, one that has gained popularity in pharmacovigilance assessment is the system proposed by Naranjo *et al.* (1981), perhaps because of its simplicity;

see Table 7.1. At a clinical level, Sackett (1991) proposed a scoring system for deciding whether a treatment had caused an adverse effect in a particular patient that is more comprehensive than the system proposed by Naranjo *et al.* (1981).

Table 7.1   A scoring strategy for deciding whether this treatment caused that adverse effect in this particular patient (Naranjo *et al.*, 1981). Reproduced by permission of Elsevier Science (Mosby)

		Yes	No	Don't know
1.	Are there previous *conclusive* reports on this reaction?	+1	0	0
2.	Did the adverse event appear after the suspected drug was administered?	+2	−1	0
3.	Did the adverse reaction improve when the drug was discontinued or a *specific* antagonist was administered?	+1	0	0
4.	Did the adverse reaction reappear when the drug was readministered?	+2	−1	0
5.	Are there alternative causes (other than the drug) that could on their own have caused the reaction?	−1	+2	0
6.	Did the reaction reappear when a placebo was given?	−1	+1	0
7.	Was the drug detected in the blood (or other fluids) in concentrations known to be toxic?	+1	0	0
8.	Was the reaction more severe when the dose was increased, or less severe when the dose was decreased?	+1	0	0
9.	Did the patient have a similar reaction to the same or similar drugs in *any* previous exposure?	+1	0	0
10.	Was the adverse event confirmed by any objective evidence?	+1	0	0

Categorization of causality (relatedness) for individual suspected adverse drug reaction reports

There have been many classification systems proposed for causality (Stephens, 1988). The numbers of categories in these systems range from six (certain, probably, possible, unlikely, conditional/unclassified and unassessable/unclassifiable) in the World Health Organization (WHO) system (Edwards and Biriell, 1994) to three in the European A,B,O system (Meyboom, 1998). In general, the systems use modifications of the factors initially proposed by Irey (1972). The Drug Safety Research Unit (DSRU) in Southampton uses a modified version of the WHO system. The system used by the DSRU includes the five categories defined below, viz. probable, possible, unlikely, awaiting further information and unassessable. The only difference between the DSRU and the WHO systems is that the former does not include the category 'certain', because it is very unusual to be certain about causality from a single case report and the term probable is considered sufficient for events that may be categorized as certain in the WHO system.

1. *Probable*: a clinical event, including a laboratory test abnormality, that is well defined clinically and/or pathologically, occurring with a reasonable time sequence to administration of the drug, more likely to be attributed to the drug than to concurrent disease or other drugs and which follows a clinically reasonable response on withdrawal or dose reduction (dechallenge) or reintroduction of the drug (rechallenge) or dose increment.

Other supporting criteria for a probable case include laboratory investigations, such as high drug levels, or histological findings supportive of a drug-induced effect.

2. *Possible*: a clinical event, including a laboratory test abnormality, with a reasonable clinical and pathological definition (not a vague description of a clinical entity), occurring with a reasonable time sequence to administration of the drug but which could also be explained by concurrent disease or other drugs or chemicals. Information on other criteria, such as dechallenge, rechallenge and confirmatory investigations, may be either not fully available or inconclusive.

   Medical judgement is necessary to classify reports for which it is possible that the event was caused by the drug but another cause, e.g. an underlying illness is far more likely. These should normally be classified as 'unlikely'.

3. *Unlikely*: a clinical event, including a laboratory test abnormality, with a temporal relationship to drug administration that makes a causal relationship improbable or in which other drugs or underlying or concurrent diseases provide far more plausible explanations.

4. *Awaiting further information*: a clinical event, including a laboratory test abnormality, about which more data are essential for proper assessment or the additional data are under examination.

5. *Unassessable*: A report for which it was not possible to obtain the additional information necessary for an appropriate evaluation.

An important feature of post-marketing safety evaluation is the large number of reports, which even after follow-up remain with incomplete (sometimes with very limited) information. However, even with such limitations it is possible to assess individual reports to the five categories outlined above.

Bayesian probabilistic methods

In simple terms, the Bayesian approach to statistics is based on assigning a prior probability to the event under investigation. In drug safety, the prior probability of an adverse reaction is based on information obtained from pre-marketing clinical trials and epidemiological studies for patients with the underlying illness. That probability is then modified in the light of the information obtained from the new information. The revised probability is called the posterior probability (Kirkwood, 1994).

There has been long-standing academic interest in the application of Bayesian approaches to causality assessment (Jones, 2000), but the progress has not been as fast as the proponents of the methods would have hoped, nor have the methods been generally embraced by regulatory authorities or pharmaceutical companies. There are two main reasons for this:

1. While the Bayesian approach to statistics resembles, to some extent, human intelligence, the apparent complexity of its mathematics deters those unfamiliar with statistics.

2. Even with increasing availability of epidemiological and pharmacoepidemiological databases, background information for calculating prior probabilities is often either sparse or unavailable. Furthermore, pre-marketing data from clinical trials are mostly confidential between the pharmaceutical companies and regulatory authorities and are not available for the scientific community to be used for estimating the prior probability. Even when they are available, they may not be in a format that could be used for Bayesian evaluation of the causality of ADRs.

It is important that the Bayesian methods for causality assessment in pharmacovigilance continue to develop, because they could play an important role in the field.

When to assess causality (relatedness)

1. By the prescribing doctor or investigator for clinical research subjects.
    The clinical diagnosis of ADRs, which is usually performed in an unstructured way, is an exercise of causality assessment. With regard to clinical research, doctors participating in clinical trials are required, according to study protocols, to conduct causality assessment for all adverse events regardless of causation.
    The advantage of clinicians conducting causality assessment is that the practising doctor or the investigator has detailed knowledge of the patient's current condition(s), previous history, concomitant medications, etc., as well access to clinical documents and reports of investigations. The disadvantage is that clinicians may have not been trained to assess causality for ADRs and may apply an incomplete, incorrect or inconsistent approach.

2. When the report is initially received by the regulatory authority or a pharmaceutical company.
    Early assessment of causality aids classification of reports for processing, e.g. whether the report should be sent to regulatory authorities in an expedited manner. The disadvantage of such early assessment is that initial reports may include limited information and further follow-up information is required for proper evaluation. However, from time to time a need may arise to conduct causality assessment for medically important, serious and expected reports to assess their impact on the risk–benefit profile of the product. However, it is extremely rare that public health decisions are based on the information included in a single case report.

3. When follow-up information is received.
    The advantage is that causality assessment benefits from the maximum information that can be realistically obtained for an individual report. In nearly all circumstances the enhancement of assessment by the additional information compensates for the delay required to wait until all the necessary information for the evaluation is available.

4. At the time of signal generation.

5. At the time of investigating a safety issue or writing a periodic safety update report (PSUR).

Assessing causality from multiple information sources: the application of the Bradford-Hill criteria in pharmacovigilance and pharmacoepidemiology

Although the assessment of individual case reports or clusters of case reports is an important part of pharmacovigilance, drug safety signals and hypotheses are generated from several sources. In addition to spontaneous reports of suspected adverse reactions and published case reports, information sources for pharmacovigilance include animal studies, clinical pharmacology studies, clinical trials and pharmacoepidemiological studies. In an ideal world all generated signals would be evaluated and investigated further if necessary. Currently, this happens infrequently and usually in a limited way. Regulatory and clinical decisions are made on the data available at the time of evaluation. In 1998, the CIOMS IV Working Group raised concerns regarding the limitations and inconsistencies of safety evaluations by regulatory authorities of important drug safety issues such as product withdrawals (CIOMS, 1998). The CIOMS IV report provided pragmatic, yet comprehensive, and useful guidelines for safety evaluation. Together with earlier initiatives, this provides a good foundation to build on to improve safety evaluation, but the field requires further methodology, policy research and audit.

Although the safety of medicines must consider some specific issues, such as variation in compliance and drug interactions, the general principles that are used to study environmental hazards are applicable with some modifications. One of the most important papers published in the 20th century with thoughts on the epidemiological basis of disease causation was a summary of a lecture given by Sir Austin Bradford-Hill (who was then Emeritus Professor of Statistics at the University of London) entitled 'The environment and disease: association or causation' in 1965 (Bradford-Hill, 1965). In the introduction, he asked two simple questions: 'How in the first place do we detect the relationship between sickness, injury and conditions of work? How do we determine what is a physical, chemical and psychological hazard of occupation, and in particular those that are rare and not easily recognized?' Bradford-Hill described 'aspects' of an association that need to be considered before deciding on the most likely interpretation of its causation.

These aspects, listed in Table 7.2, are commonly referred to as the Bradford-Hill criteria for a causal association, and they have been used by epidemiologists and others when addressing causation of disease in a broad range of situations (Rothman and Greenland, 1998). In his lecture, Bradford-Hill described strengths and weaknesses of each of these aspects with regard to their contribution to an inference of causation. These criteria have

Table 7.2 The Bradford-Hill criteria

1.	Strength
2.	Consistency
3.	Specificity
4.	Temporality
5.	Biological gradient
6.	Plausibility
7.	Coherence
8.	Experimental evidence
9.	Analogy

been used to interpret evidence from pharmacoepidemiological studies. In the broader discipline of pharmacovigilance, consideration of these criteria, with modifications dictated by the nature of the data, can be very helpful in the interpretation of evidence from various sources at different levels. Shakir and Layton (2002) outlined thoughts on the application of Bradford-Hill's criteria to the evaluation of pharmacovigilance data with some examples.

Strength

Bradford-Hill stated that strong associations are more likely to be causal than weak associations. Weak associations are more likely to be explained by unrelated biases. For example, the association between smoking and lung cancer is so strong (studies show relative risks ranging between 10 and 30) that, even if some biases were operating, a shift of the association to non-causal is unlikely (Strom, 2000). In general epidemiology, a relative risk of <2 is considered to indicate a weak association (Strom, 2000). This is one of the major problems of pharmacoepidemiology, it is uncommon to find high relative risks (>2) for ADRs, particularly for serious ADRs, with marketed medicines, compared with placebo or with other products. In general, this is because medicines associated with a high incidence of serious ADRs would have been considered too toxic for marketing.

With regard to signal generation in pharmacovigilance, to complement qualitative methods, new approaches have been proposed such as proportional reporting rates (PRRs) (Evans *et al.*, 2001) and Bayesian confidence propagation neural network (BCPNN) (Bate *et al.*, 1998). In essence, these methods compare the proportion of a particular event reported for a drug with the whole database (which includes all or some of the other products monitored by the organization). A high PRR or information component (IC) in BCPNN suggests that an event has been reported more frequently than expected with the product and may indicate a safety signal. Although higher PRRs and ICs do not necessarily indicate a greater likelihood (Evans *et al.*, 2001) of causality, they do suggest stronger signals. It is possible to apply the Bradford-Hill strength criterion in signal generation in pharmacovigilance; for example, in a recent study using the WHO database of spontaneous reports of ADRs, BCPNN was used to examine the strength of the signals relating to heart muscle disorders with antipsychotic drugs (Coulter, 2001). Clozapine, an antipsychotic that had previously been reported to be associated with heart muscle disorders, had a much higher IC than lithium, a drug not known to be associated with such disorders. This example demonstrates the feasibility of applying the strength criterion in assessing the results of the quantitative methods for signal generation in pharmacovigilance.

Consistency

Bradford-Hill stated that repeated observations of an association in different populations under different circumstances provide additional support for a causal association. However, he cautioned that lack of consistency does not rule out a causal association, because some effects may be produced by the causes only in certain circumstances.

Because of the low relative risks of ADRs generally detected in pharmacovigilance and pharmacoepidemiological studies, the consistency of findings in different populations is highly important. For example, in studies conducted to examine the association between the use of the commonly called 'third-generation' oral contraceptives (OCs; gestodene and desogestrel) and deep-vein thrombosis, although the strength of the association in some of the studies may have been weak by conventional epidemiological standards (a relative risk between 1.5 and 2) (Hannaford, 2000), the consistency of the finding of a higher risk among users of the third-generation OCs in different populations utilizing different methods supports an inference of causation.

With regard to pharmacovigilance studies, reporting of a particular event in different populations is supportive of a true association. An example is the association between the antiepileptic, lamotrigine, and serious skin reactions (Stevens–Johnson syndrome and toxic epidermal necrolysis); this was strengthened by the fact that spontaneous reports were sent both from hospitals and the communities in several countries, and that cases were reported in clinical trials (Guberman *et al.*, 1999) and in a prescription-event monitoring (PEM) study (Mackay *et al.*, 1997).

The utilization of the Bradford-Hill consistency criterion (by conducting several studies with different methodologies in different healthcare systems to study the safety of a particular drug) is perhaps the most important approach to address any uncertainties resulting from the low relative risks that are commonly detected in pharmacoepidemiological studies.

Specificity

Bradford-Hill stated that a cause leads to a single effect, not multiple effects; but he cautioned that, although the concept of specificity is sometimes useful, it could be misleading.

In pharmacovigilance, specificity is important because drugs cause ADRs by specific mechanisms, which may or may not be known at the time of the enquiry. Associations between the use of some drugs and an increase in the incidence of cancer have been reported. For example, prolonged use of HRT is associated with a slight increase in the incidence breast cancer (Dixon, 2001). True associations such as this one are specific. In most circumstances it is not plausible that the use of a drug is associated with an increase in the incidence of multiple cancers. In the 1990s, a controversy was raised by a suggestion of an association between the use of intramuscular vitamin K in neonates and childhood cancer (Golding *et al.*, 1992). It is difficult to think of a mechanism by which a single injection of vitamin K can lead to increasing the likelihood of development of several cancers in childhood. Subsequent studies were more focused in studying the association between injectable vitamin K in neonates and specific cancers, e.g. acute lymphoblastic leukaemia (Ansell *et al.*, 1996). This demonstrates the need for specificity when considering a causal association in pharmacoepidemiology and pharmacovigilance.

Because of the incomplete information in many spontaneous reports, attention must be paid, by trying to obtain follow-up information, to ensure that the reports include sufficient information to enable a specific diagnosis. For example, if a drug is suspected to be associated with anaemia, then confirmation needs to be sought regarding the type of anaemia and whether there is consistency between the reported cases clinically and haematologically (with regard to the type of anaemia).

Temporality

Bradford-Hill stated that there is a necessity that cause precedes effect in time. This is very important in pharmacovigilance. Many ADRs occur in patterns based on relation to exposure, the pharmacological characteristics of the drug and host responses (Type A reactions). A consistent pattern with regard to temporal relationship is, therefore, very important in assessing the causal relationship between drug exposure and an adverse event or a cluster of events. The need for a plausible and generally consistent temporal relationship also applies to Type B (unpredictable) ADRs. Conversely, although an inconsistent pattern does not exclude a causal relationship, one should be doubtful of a possible causal relationship.

Studying temporal relationships in pharmacovigilance should take into account the effects of drug interactions (e.g. when the pharmacological plausibility that an ADR is related to a drug is supported by the timing of the introduction or stopping a concomitant medication) or the occurrence of illnesses (e.g. renal impairment) or a physiological state (e.g. dehydration).

Biological gradient

Bradford-Hill stated that a biological gradient as demonstrated by a dose–response curve is well known in epidemiology. It has been demonstrated in numerous studies that the number of cigarettes smoked and the number of years of smoking are directly related to the development of major smoking-related hazards (cancer of the lung and cardiovascular diseases) (Strom, 2000). However, care should be taken, because biological gradient can sometimes can be complex. For example, although it is well known that excessive drinking of alcohol is associated with detrimental dose-related effects, drinking small amounts of alcohol can be protective (Burns et al., 2001).

In pharmacovigilance, a causal association is supported when an ADR occurs in a dose-dependent manner, or from cumulative exposure over a prolonged period of time. There are many examples when causal association was supported by plausible dose relationships, such as the oestrogen content of the combined OC pills and deep-vein thrombosis (Inman et al., 1970) and the systemic effects of nasal and inhaled corticosteroids (CSM/MCA, 1998).

Plausibility

Bradford-Hill stated that biological plausibility of a hypothesis is another aspect to be considered for causal inference. He added that plausibility is an important concern that may be difficult to judge.

In pharmacovigilance, plausibility is easy when the mechanism is known, as in the case of non-steroidal anti-inflammatory drugs (NSAIDs) and gastrointestinal bleeding. However, it is difficult when the mechanism is unknown, as for many Type B ADRs. In such situations, an ADR may not be detected readily, e.g. the delay in the recognition of the association between the use of practolol and the oculomucocutaneous syndrome (Wright, 1975).

Research is needed to study whether the strength of plausibility can influence the levels of relative risk needed to accept an inference of causation, i.e. whether it possible with strong pharmacological plausibility to accept a lower level of relative risk as an indicator of causal association than when the plausibility is weak.

Coherence

Bradford-Hill defined coherence as the cause-and-effect interpretation whose data should not seriously conflict with generally known facts of the natural history and biology of a disease. The principle of coherence is useful in pharmacovigilance and pharmacoepidemiology. For example, the proposed possible association between a single intramuscular injection of vitamin K, the neonatal period and childhood cancers lacked coherence with the understanding at the time of the pathogenesis of cancer (Golding *et al.*, 1992). However, one has to keep an open mind regarding associations that are not coherent with contemporary knowledge, because understanding of the biological basis of ADRs often comes at a later stage.

Experimental evidence

Experimental evidence as a supporter of causal inference is self-evident. Studies in biological models, as well as in animal and human experiments, may all lend support to signals raised by pharmacovigilance. It is commonly necessary to conduct experimental studies to better understand the signals generated in pharmacovigilance and pharmacoepidemiology, e.g. when a drug interaction that was not previously evaluated is suspected.

Analogy

Bradford-Hill said that inventive scientists could find analogies everywhere. An analogy finds a source of more elaborate hypothesis about an association under study. As elsewhere in biomedical sciences, analogies can guide or mislead. For example, while cough has been reported in 5–20 per cent of patients who take angiotensin converting enzyme (ACE) inhibitors, the association between cough and angiotensin II (A_{II}) receptor antagonists, e.g. losartan and irbesartan, has no pharmacological plausibility (Hardman and Limbird, 2001). Therefore, in evaluating reports of cough with A_{II} antagonists, an analogy with ACE inhibitors is inappropriate.

Conversely, the analogy between COX-2 inhibitors and conventional NSAIDs with regard to the gastrointestinal safety profile continues to be appropriate until we fully understand the interaction between the pharmacological selectivity of the COX-2 inhibitors and their clinical effects.

Conclusion

The application of Austin Bradford-Hill's criteria for evaluating causal associations in pharmacovigilance and pharmacoepidemiology is very useful. This requires understanding of the general characteristics of pharmacovigilance data, e.g. under-reporting, misclassification and poor quality of information from third parties. Further work is required to propose ways to handle such limitations.

References

Ansell P, Bull D and Roman E (1996). Childhood leukaemia and intramuscular vitamin K: findings from a case-control study. *Br Med J* **313**: 204–205.

Bate A, Lindquist M, Edwards IR, Olsson S *et al.* (1998). A Bayesian neural network method for adverse drug reaction signal generation. *Eur J Clin Pharmacol* **54**(4): 315–321.

Bradford-Hill A (1965). The environment and disease: association or causation. *Proc R Soc Med* **58**: 295–330.

Burns J, Crozier A and Lean ME (2001). Alcohol consumption and mortality: is wine different from other alcoholic beverages? *Nutr Metab Cardiovasc Dis* **11**(4): 249–258.

CIOMS (1998). *Benefit risk balance for monitored drugs: evaluating safety signals.* Report of CIOMS Working Group IV, Geneva.

Coulter DM, Bak A, Meyboom RHB, Lindquist M, Edwards R (2001). Antipsychotic drugs and heart muscle disorder in international pharmacovigilance: data mining study. *BMJ* **322**: 1207–1209.

CSM/MCA (1998). The safety of inhaled and nasal corticosteroids. *Curr Probl Pharmacovig* **24**: 6.

Dixon JM (2001). (Editorial) Hormone replacement therapy and the breast. We should worry about the increase in the risk of breast cancer. *Br Med J* **323**: 1381–1382.

Edwards IR and Biriell C (1994). Harmonisation in pharmacovigilance. *Drug Saf* **10**: 93–102.

Evans SJW, Waller PC and Davis S (2001). Use of proportional reporting ratios (PRRs) for signal generation from spontaneous adverse drug reaction reports. *Pharmacoepidemiol Drug Saf* **10**: 483–486.

Golding J, Greenwood R, Birmingham K and Mott M (1992). Childhood cancer, intramuscular vitamin K, and pethidine given during labour. *Br Med J* **305**: 341–346.

Guberman AH, Besag FM, Brodie MJ, Dooley JM *et al.* (1999). Lamotrigine-associated rash: risk/ benefit considerations in adults and children. *Epilepsia* **40**: 985–991.

Hannaford P (2000). Cardiovascular events associated with different combined oral contraceptives: a review of current data. *Drug Saf* **22**: 361–371.

Hardman JG and Limbird LE (eds). (2001). *Goodman & Gilmans's The Pharmacological Basis of Therapeutics*, 10th edition. McGraw-Hill: 694–696, 828, 833.

Inman WH, Vessey MP, Westerholm B and Engelund A (1970). Thromboembolic disease and the steroidal content of oral contraceptives. A report to the Committee on Safety of Drugs. *Br Med J* **ii**: 203–209.

Irey NS (1972). Diagnostic problems in drug-induced diseases. In *Drug-induced Diseases*, vol. 4, Meyler L and Peck HM (eds). Excerpta Medica: Amsterdam; 1–24.

Jones JK (2000). Determining causation from case reports. In *Pharmacoepidemiology*, Strom BL (ed.). Wiley: Chichester; 525–538.

Kirkwood B (1994). *Essentials of Medical Statistics*. Blackwell Sciences: 73.

Mackay FJ, Wilton LV, Pearce G, Freemantle SN *et al.* (1997). Safety of long term lamotrigine in epilepsy. *Epilepsia* **38**: 881–886.

Meyboom RHB (1998). *Detecting Adverse Drugs Reactions*. The Netherlands Pharmacovigilance Foundation, LAREB, 's Hertogenbosch; 87–88.

Naranjo CA, Busto U, Sellers EM, Sandor P *et al.* (1981). A method for estimating the probability of adverse drug reactions. *Clin Pharmacol Ther* **30**(2): 239–245.

Pearl, J. (2001) *Causality reasoning and inference*, Cambridge University Press pp. xiii–xvi.

Rothman KJ and Greenland S (eds) (1998). *Modern Epidemiology*, 2nd edition. Lippincott Williams & Wilkins: 24–28.

Sackett DL, Haynes RB, Guyatt GH, Tugwell P (1991). Clinical Epidemiology: A Basic Science for Clinical Medicine. 2nd Edition. Lippincott-Raven: Philadelphia: 285.

Shakir SAW and Layton D (2002). Causal association in pharmacovigilance and pharmacoepidemiology. *Drug Saf* **25**(6): 467–471.

Stephens MDB (1988). The diagnosis of adverse medical events associated with drug treatment. In *The Detection of New Adverse Drug Reactions*, 2nd edition. Macmillan: 73–114.

Strom BL (2000). *Pharmacoepidemiology*, 3rd edition. Wiley: Chichester.

Wright P (1975). Untoward effects associated with practolol administration: oculomucocutaneous syndrome. *Br Med J* **i**: 595–598.

8

Managing Drug Safety Issues with Marketed Products

P. C. Waller and H. H. Tilson

Introduction

This chapter takes a practical look at the handling of post-marketing drug safety issues. The process of handling such issues is shown in Figure 8.1, and this forms the basis on which this chapter is structured.

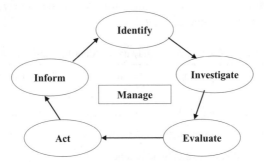

Figure 8.1 Process of handling a drug safety issue

There may be differences in the ways issues are handled, or perceived, depending on where one works (e.g. regulatory or industry setting) or where the issues emerge, since medical and regulatory contexts vary from country to country. However, for all of us the goal is the same, i.e. to protect patients, and the means of achieving this should converge from all directions. The broad aims of pharmacovigilance personnel are that any medicine should be used in a way that best balances its effectiveness with its safety. Where necessary, steps should be taken to improve safety and promote safe use by informing users, and engaging them promptly and effectively.

In order to meet the above aims, both regulatory authorities and companies need to work proactively and in partnership to identify and manage safety issues. With proper use of the systems available, many potential issues will be identified but only some of them will turn

Stephens' Detection of New Adverse Drug Reactions Fifth Edition edited by John Talbot and Patrick Waller
© 2004 John Wiley & Sons, Ltd   ISBN: 0 470 84552 X

out to be real and/or important. Judgements will need to be made, sometimes based on limited information, as to whether there is an issue in need of attention. When this is considered to be the case, it will be necessary to investigate it by assembling all the relevant evidence available and, sometimes, by designing specific new studies. Consideration will need to be given at an early stage to the possible outcomes, and specifically as to how safety might be improved. The output of the process will usually be a benefit-to-risk analysis, with proposals for changes in the recommendations for use of a medicine, with withdrawal on safety grounds being relatively unusual (Jefferys *et al.*, 1998). Communicating any necessary changes is a key issue in determining the effectiveness of the measures that are ultimately taken.

The first stage is the identification of a possible hazard. What is found depends on where and how you look, and this is the starting point for considering how to manage a drug safety issue.

Identification of drug safety issues

Assessment of drug safety involves bringing together all the available information from multiple sources. It begins with the basic pharmacological and pre-clinical studies and should continue until the end of potential sequelae of marketing exposure, a period that may span many decades. Potentially important drug safety issues can be identified at any stage of drug development. In the post-marketing phase they are particularly likely to be identified in the first few years after marketing, although new issues also arise with long-established drugs. There are several reasons why important drug safety issues may not be detected until after marketing, and these are listed in Table 8.1.

Table 8.1   Reasons why drug safety issues may not be identified until the post-marketing period

The ADR is rare and, therefore, undetectable until a large number of patients have been exposed to the drug

There is a long latency between starting the drug and development of the ADR

Subpopulations susceptible to the reaction have not been treated in large numbers

The drug has not been studied in normal clinical practice:
- Patients treated in clinical practice are likely to have different characteristics to trial patients (e.g. demography, other diseases, other medication)
- in clinical practice a drug is less likely to be used strictly in accordance with the prescribing recommendations by both doctors and patients, and with less monitoring

In order to ensure that safety problems that have not been recognized or fully characterized at the pre-marketing stage are handled promptly, proactive processes are required for screening emerging data for potential issues. At the stage of initial identification it is unusual for it to be clear-cut that the hazard is drug related, and this has led to the concept of 'signalling'. Alternative terms, which may be regarded as synonymous in this context, are 'alerting', 'early warning' and 'hypothesis generation'. A signal is simply an alert from any available source that a drug may be associated with a previously unrecognized hazard or that a known hazard may be quantitatively (e.g. more frequent) or qualitatively (e.g. more serious) different from existing knowledge. Spontaneous adverse drug reaction (ADR) reporting is the classic signalling system, and its major purpose is to provide early warnings of possible hazards. Indeed, a signal could be defined on the basis of single case reports, although the broader concept indicated above is preferred. Other than spontaneous ADR reporting, signals may come from studies of various types. The subsequent processes for assessment, investigation and possible action (see below) are required regardless of the type of data leading to identification of an issue.

Signals: where to look

Effective monitoring of drug safety requires a systematic approach in order to identify and use information from many sources, both published and unpublished, as it becomes available. Drug safety hazards post-marketing are most frequently identified from spontaneous reports or epidemiological studies, but they still may arise from clinical trials or even pre-clinical studies. Information from any of these sources needs to be evaluated and used to build a picture of the safety profile of drugs on a continuous basis. There are now many drug safety bulletins published, e.g. by regulatory authorities and the World Health Organization. These and other published sources need to be screened systematically and as carefully as any other data source by those involved in drug safety monitoring.

Whilst the utility of spontaneous ADR reporting schemes and formal studies in the identification of drug safety issues is well established, the large automated population-based databases containing prescriptions and outcomes, and disease registries for generating signals have been under utilized. Such databases can be screened for single cases of disorders likely to be drug induced. Alternatively, when adequate usage data are available, the frequencies of associations between drugs and medical events can be examined for differences from expected values. These methods might be able to detect signals missed by other approaches, and they are likely to be developed and used more in the future.

Signals: what to look for

Identifying signals is a selective process based on the apparent strength of the evidence and the potential importance of association. In practice, a signal is something that, if found to be drug related, would be considered clinically important and might impact on patient management or the balance of benefits and risks. What to look for depends on the type of data being used, which can be broadly divided into data from spontaneous reporting or from formal studies. Both types of data may be published or unpublished.

Spontaneous adverse drug reaction reporting data

The commonest source for identification of significant drug safety concerns arising with marketed medicines is spontaneous suspected ADR reporting. These are individual case reports from health professionals (and, in some countries, consumers and other third parties) of adverse events that the reporter considers *may* be related to the drug or drugs being taken. Reporters are not asked to provide all adverse events that follow drug administration, but to report selectively those they suspect were ADRs. There may be several reasons why a reporter suspects a drug may have caused an ADR, and these are summarized in Table 8.2.

Table 8.2 Reasons for suspecting a relationship between a drug and an adverse event

Reason	Requirement
Temporal association	Plausible temporal relationship between taking drug and development of the possible adverse reaction
Dechallenge	Relationship between discontinuation of the drug abatement of the possible adverse reaction
Dose–response	Relationship between dose and severity of the possible adverse reaction
Rechallenge	Recurrence of the possible adverse effect with reintroduction of the drug
Mechanism	Pharmacological or toxicological basis for anadverse reaction
Class effect	Knowledge that a similar drug or class of drugs produces this adverse reaction
Absence of alternatives	Lack of another explanation (e.g. other drugs and diseases) for the possible adverse reaction

None of these factors on its own (apart from the need for drug administration to precede the suspected ADR) is essential in leading to suspicion of a causal association; but, the more that apply, then the greater suspicion is likely to be. Greater suspicion does not invariably lead to greater likelihood of reporting, since knowledge of a mechanism and the effects of similar drugs may deter reporting.

One common feature of all spontaneous ADR reporting systems is underreporting. The possible reasons why an ADR may not be reported are well recognized: the 'seven deadly sins' (Inman and Weber, 1986). It is less clear which factors are, in practice, the most important, and this may vary between countries and over time. A figure of 10 per cent of ADRs being reported has been quoted, but the reality is likely to be that the level of underreporting is highly variable according to many factors, the most well recognized being as follows:

- seriousness of the reaction

- novelty of the drug

- whether or not the effect is recognized and has been publicized.

It is clear that appropriate feedback to reporters and specific measures to encourage reporting are an essential element of an effective approach. The latter comes into three categories as follows:

- promotion of the approach

- facilitation of reporting

- education about drug safety and the benefits of ADR reporting.

Inherent in any spontaneous ADR reporting system is a monitoring process that recognizes the dynamic nature of data. A prerequisite for an effective system is a database from which data can be retrieved in a format useful for screening. Regular and systematic review of what is new on the database in the context of what was there previously is needed. This is usually done by reviewing all the data for individual drugs or products looking for reactions of potential concern. However, an alternative approach is to bring together all the data for a particular ADR and review the drugs that have been suspected of producing the reaction and the numbers of cases. This approach is likely to be more useful to regulatory authorities than to companies, because they can cover all marketed medicines.

Spontaneous reporting systems exist throughout the developed world and in some developing countries. The World Health Organization maintains a database of worldwide spontaneous reports in Sweden (Uppsala Monitoring Centre, 1998). Screening of spontaneous ADR data needs to be performed on both a national and an international basis, and there should be a worldwide perspective to this function. Companies, operating locally, have to collect and act upon local data and adhere to local regulatory reporting obligations; furthermore, companies operating multinationally must collate worldwide data for their products in order to understand the evolving benefit to risk balance and act responsibly to protect the public health, as well as to meet statutory obligations for ADR reporting and periodic safety updates (see Chapter 9).

Utilizing spontaneous reporting data

In the context of spontaneous reporting, a signal is normally a series of cases of similar suspected ADRs reported by health professionals associated with a particular drug. A single case is not usually sufficient (Edwards *et al.*, 1990). When the ADR is a disease that is rare in the general population (e.g. aplastic anaemia, toxic epidermal necrolysis), a small number of cases associated with a single drug is unlikely to be a chance phenomenon (Begaud *et al.*, 1994), even if the drug has been used quite widely. In this situation, three cases may be considered a signal and five cases a strong signal.

The level of drug usage is vital in assessing the likely order of magnitude of frequency. However, it is not necessarily critical in determining whether or not there is a signal that needs to be evaluated. Likewise, the strength of evidence for the individual cases will be important to consider later; but, initially, the key issue is whether or not there is an 'unexpected' number of cases. If the event is common in the general population, then a large number of cases would be needed to raise a signal. A judgement has to be made from all the information available, which depends more on the apparent strength of the evidence than the number of reported cases.

A number of comparative methods are available for using spontaneous reporting data to generate signals. Calculating reporting rates based on usage denominator data (Speirs, 1986), either as prescriptions dispensed or defined daily doses, may enable a signal of an increased frequency of a particular ADR in comparison with alternative treatments to be derived. All spontaneous ADR reporting schemes are subject to a variable and unknown degree of underreporting, which means that such comparisons are crude. They need to be interpreted carefully, particularly if the drugs being compared have been marketed for different indications or durations, or if there has been significant publicity about the adverse effects of one of the drugs.

The other principal approach for making comparisons between drugs is to use the proportions of all ADRs for a particular drug that are within a particular organ system class of reactions (e.g. gastrointestinal or cutaneous). This is known as profiling (Inman and

Weber, 1986), a method that has an advantage over reporting rates in that it is independent of the level of usage. The data may easily be displayed graphically as ADR profiles. Related mathematical approaches have also been developed (see Chapter 6).

Drugs are authorized and used differently across the world, and even in neighbouring countries there are often major differences in clinical practice, reporting culture and labelling that may impact on ADR reporting. Whilst it is reasonable to review, for example, the number of cases of a possible reaction reported worldwide in the context of worldwide sales data, it should be recognized that the above differences and varying patterns of reporting across countries limit this approach. One approach to dealing with this is to focus particularly on the source of the greatest number of cases and to attempt to identify why it may have emerged from that source.

Formal studies

Although formal studies of drug safety have a particular place in the investigation of signals generated by methods such as spontaneous ADR reporting (i.e. hypothesis testing), they may also provide the initial evidence producing a drug safety concern. Such studies often start with efficacy rather than safety as the primary objective; but, if they have the potential to provide new safety data, then it is important that the emerging evidence is kept under regular review. In particular, it is vital to maximize the potential of studies to identify adverse effects, particularly if they are to expose large numbers of patients relative to exposure in previous studies. This should be achieved by ensuring that the design, methods and analyses facilitate safety assessment (e.g. by including comparator groups and measuring important outcomes) and by monitoring the data using a sequential approach that is specified in advance. In a randomized double-blind study, a safety monitoring group with access to the codes but no direct contact with investigators or other study personnel is essential. An analogous group is also desirable in open studies. It is important to define in advance the criteria that would lead to actions such as stopping the trial. If unexpected cases of an adverse outcome occur, then these need to be evaluated both individually and in the context of the frequencies in the different exposure groups. The advantages of the trial design (e.g. control groups, known denominators) and a statistical analysis should be fully utilized in judging whether or not a signal is present, and in assessing the likelihood of a causal association.

Processes for identifying drug safety hazards

In order to undertake the systematic approach to drug safety monitoring described above, systems and processes must be established to ensure that all the necessary information is brought together at a single point. For pharmaceutical companies this is recognized in European legislation through the establishment of a requirement for a qualified person for pharmacovigilance. Likewise, European regulatory authorities now have clear obligations to transmit data to companies and other authorities. Within a pharmaceutical company or regulatory authority there may be several groups dealing with data that are relevant to drug safety. Links between groups handling pre-clinical studies, clinical trials and pharmacovigilance data are needed, and effective communication between such groups is essential. Functional drug safety groups that review all safety data generated internally or externally are required to avoid issues being overlooked. Drugs or groups of drugs should have individuals assigned (physicians, pharmacists, scientists) who have a particular interest in the field and who take prime responsibility for reviewing emerging information and undertaking initial assessments.

Any group involved in drug safety should aim to identify an emerging signal rapidly. Once an issue has been identified, then information about it may be disseminated in many ways. It is important for both regulatory authorities and companies to be prepared to evaluate and manage issues regardless of the original source.

Once a signal has been identified from any source the next step is to perform an initial assessment. The main purpose of the initial assessment is to make a decision regarding whether or not the possible hazard requires detailed investigation. The key principles of the initial assessment are to review the strength of the evidence that indicates a possible drug-related hazard, consider how that evidence can be extended (e.g. by further analyses) and to consider the other evidence that is immediately available which may help to support or refute the hypothesis. There are four key issues that will determine whether or not a signal should be investigated further, as signified by the acronym 'SNIP':

- the *strength* of the signal;

- whether or not the issue or some aspect of it is *new*;

- the clinical *importance*, as judged by the seriousness of the reaction and severity of the cases;

- the *potential* for preventive measures.

The main factors influencing the assessment vary depending on the source of the signal and, in particular, whether it derives from spontaneous reporting or from a formal study.

Signals derived from spontaneous reporting

In many cases, the initial signal will consist of a case series of similar ADRs occurring with a particular medicine. The principal factors that need to be taken into account in the assessment of such signals are given in Table 8.3. Broadly, this consists of the details of the cases themselves and other evidence that may provide insights into the issue.

The cases producing the signal need to be reviewed individually. Evidence for causality in individual cases can be assessed by a number of methods (see Chapter 7). At this stage, further information on the cases may need to be obtained but could take some time to gather. The extent, methods, and substance of such follow-up need to be individualized to the specifics of the case and potential signal at hand (CIOMS Working Group V, 2001).

The need for follow-up does not, however, preclude an initial view as to whether the problem warrants further evaluation. A large number of poorly documented cases of an ADR that has important consequences for users (e.g. because they are serious and/or potentially preventable) will at least warrant consideration of other evidence whilst further information is being obtained. However, the greater the number of cases in relation to usage and the better documented they are, then the greater will be the need to investigate the problem fully. It is important to establish a case definition (e.g. liver injury) using standardized diagnostic criteria; CIOMS (1999) is a useful publication in this respect. The next step is identify those cases that fulfil the definition and which may provide reasonable

Table 8.3 Factors influencing the initial assessment of a possible hazard arising from a case series

Evidence to be considered	Underlying issue
1. *The cases producing the signal*	
Individual case assessment: temporal relationship, effect of dechallenge/rechallenge, alternative causes (see Table 8.2)	Causality
Quality of the information regarding cases	Documentation
Number of cases in relation to usage of the medicine	Frequency/reporting rate
Severity of the reactions	⎫
Seriousness of the hazard	⎬ Implications for patients and public health
	⎭
2. *Other evidence*	
Pharmacological or toxicological effects of the drug	Mechanism
Known effects of other drugs in the class	
Pre-clinical studies	⎫ Possible class effect
Clinical trials	⎬ Existence of other evidence that may support or
Epidemiological studies	⎭ refute the signal

evidence of a drug-related hazard (the cardinal cases). A view of the case series as a whole should be formed in addition to assessments of the individual cases. Depending on the quality of data, the same number of spontaneous reports and the same level of usage may provide good or poor evidence of a hazard. The key difference is often whether or not there are frequent alternative causes (these are often called 'confounding factors').

Consideration of alternative causes

Table 8.4 lists the explanations, other than a causal relation between suspect drug and event, that need to be considered. The most common alternative causes are concomitant medication and coexisting disease. In the first case, the adverse event is a reaction to a drug and the issue is which drug is implicated or sometimes whether there might be an interaction between two or more drugs. A common situation is that there is an alternative explanation because the patient was concomitantly exposed to a drug that is recognized to cause the ADR in question. An example might be a patient with schizophrenia taking chlorpromazine who is also given a new antipsychotic drug and develops hepatitis. The reporter may suspect

Table 8.4 Possible explanations for a reported ADR other than a causal relationship between suspect drug and the adverse event

Related to medication
    Single other drug – recognized cause
    Single other drug – unrecognized cause
    Combination of drugs (may include suspect drug)

Not an ADR
    Coexisting disease unrelated to indication for suspect drug
    Newly emerging disease
    Complication of indication for suspect drug

either of the drugs or both but is much more likely to report it if the new drug is suspected. Clearly, such a case of suspected hepatitis due to the new drug may not have been caused by it, but there are several reasons why it might have been reported. In some cases the reporter will have been unaware of the recognized ADR or the reporter may have had good reasons (perhaps relating to the temporal relationships of drug administration and the reaction, or response to dechallenge) for suspecting that the new drug is implicated.

The situation where the patient has been taking two or more medicines, none of which is recognized to produce the suspected ADR, is also common. Only one drug may be suspect – often because the event occurred shortly after its initial administration or because the drug is new – but sometimes all the drugs are listed as suspect. In these circumstances it may be possible to form a view of the most likely cause or combination of causes, based on pharmacology, temporal relationship and dechallenge. However, often no clear judgement can be made and formal studies are needed. This is particularly likely when patients start taking multiple drugs simultaneously, as in highly active anti-retroviral therapy.

Possible interactions are often particularly difficult to interpret when the signal arises from spontaneous reporting. The number of cases is usually very small and a watching brief would usually be an appropriate initial reponse in the absence of one or more of the following circumstances:

- there are several plausible cases;

- the reported cases provide objective evidence of interaction (e.g. repeated laboratory measurements during periods of single and dual drug exposure);

- there is a plausible mechanism, based on the known pharmacokinetics and pharmacody-namics of the drugs, that has not yet been investigated in formal interaction studies (in which case such studies should be initiated);

- the drug has a narrow therapeutic index and the suspected ADRs reported are serious.

Often, the major alternative explanation for one or more suspected ADR reports is that the event was not an ADR but was a naturally occurring disease that may or may not be related to the indication for the suspected drug. Since most ADRs are similar to diseases that occur naturally (a notable exception is fibrosing colonopathy with high-strength pancreatic enzymes (Smyth et al., 1995)), this explanation almost always requires considera-tion. A recent example for which the possible roles of drugs and underlying diseases is still not resolved is the occurrence of lipodystrophy and various metabolic abnormalities in patients treated for HIV infection.

Two important factors to take into account are the rarity of the disease in the population and whether or not the disease is related to any intercurrent illness, including the indication for the suspect drug. A series of cases of a rare disease (e.g. Guillain–Barré syndrome – a severe form of neuropathy that may sometimes be drug induced) occurring in relation to exposure to a particular drug is much stronger evidence of an association than a similar series of cases of a common disease (e.g. myocardial infarction). This does not mean that drugs are less likely to cause common diseases, just that such associations are harder to detect. When the suspected ADR is a complication of the underlying disease for which that drug was given, spontaneous reporting is likely to be unhelpful. Whilst it is possible that a drug may increase the risk of the complication developing (e.g. re-perfusion arrhythmias with streptokinase), data from a formal study measuring risk are almost invariably required in order to make a satisfactory judgement about the issue.

In some of the circumstances described above, information derived from a series of cases is, by its nature, unsuited for making the necessary judgements. In this situation, the possible implications for public health and the other evidence listed in section 2 of Table 8.3 are the key factors in determining whether and how to progress the issue. If the cases are scanty and most are associated with reasonable alternative explanations, then a watching brief is likely to be the most appropriate course. At the other extreme, a well-documented series of cases of a particular suspected ADR without obvious alternative explanation and/or with evidence of a possible mechanism should rapidly lead to consideration of both what further investigation may be warranted and what action is needed to minimize the risks. Many issues come between these extremes, and this requires careful consideration of evidence from various sources and of the possible ways in which any issue might be investigated further.

Signals derived from formal studies

There are many possible sources from which drug safety issues may arise (see above). Those that do not come from reporting of individual case reports derive from formal studies, usually either a clinical trial or an epidemiological study. Occasionally, however, new safety issues may arise with a marketed medicine as a result of pre-clinical (i.e. animal) data, examples being the possible carcinogenicity of carbaryl (Calman et al., 1995) and danthron (Committee on Safety of Medicines/Medicines Control Agency, 2000), or human volunteer work (e.g. interaction studies).

Signals derived from studies have the potential to be stronger than those derived from spontaneous reporting. This is because the design and analysis of the study may enable much better judgements about causality and frequency to be made (e.g. in the case of randomized, double-blind trials). However, at the stage of initial assessment there is often only one study available, and even if this has a strong design and apparently clear findings there is no certainty that it is providing the correct answer. Examples of formal studies with findings that seem likely to be false positives include those associating selegiline with increased mortality (Lees, 1995) and neonatal vitamin K with childhood cancer (von Kries, 1998).

The underlying issues listed in Table 8.3 are also pertinent to assessment of signals derived from a formal study. The frequency of the relevant event is likely to be the triggering factor, in that a greater frequency of the event relative to a comparator (either an alternative treatment or no active treatment) usually constitutes the signal. The assessment of increased risk depends on the quality of the study design and the statistical power of the analysis. Causality may be established by exclusion, as far as possible, of three major causes of false positive findings: chance, bias and confounding. The strength of the evidence for causality is a key consideration for an initial assessment. This approach to assessment of causality based on data from formal studies is summarized in Table 8.5 (see also Chapter 7). Finally, consideration must be given to the implications for patients and public health, taking particular account of the severity, seriousness and frequency of the outcome in the context of the disease being treated.

Table 8.5   Assessment of causality based on formal studies

Possible explanation	Key evidence to be considered
Chance	Levels of statistical significance and power of study Whether or not there was a prior hypothesis How many tests were performed?
Bias	Study design – how were patients allocated to treatments? How were the data on outcomes collected?
Confounding	What factors other than drug treatments could explain differences between groups? What steps have been taken to control for confounding in the design or analysis?
Causal	Extent to which chance, bias and confounding have been excluded as alternative explanations Availability of evidence from other sources that may support an association or explain it (e.g. a mechanism)

Bias and confounding

There are many types of bias that may affect the results of clinical trials and epidemiological studies. Bias is a systematic distortion of the findings by a specific factor and does not imply deliberate manipulation by the investigator (i.e. fraud). An example of bias is recall bias in case-control studies. Cases with a disease are often much more likely to recall exposures that may have led to their illness than controls who are not ill. Such a bias could be overcome by using an objective record of whether or not the patients were exposed, if available.

In general, clinical trials are less prone to bias because they tend to incorporate particular design features (e.g. prospective random allocation to treatments and double-blinding) for this purpose. Epidemiological studies observe patients treated in the 'real world' and the possibility of bias is ever present (Collet and Boivin, 2000). Nevertheless, such studies are important because:

- some issues cannot, in practice, be studied by controlled trials;

- bias can often be eliminated or minimized;

- 'real world' data are more generally applicable than those derived from clinical trials.

A confounder in an epidemiological study is a factor that is related to both the outcome and exposure of interest. An example of a confounder is smoking, which is related to both use of the oral contraceptive (OC) pill (smokers are more likely to use the pill than non-smokers) and an adverse outcome for which OCs may increase the risk (myocardial infarction). In a study of myocardial infarction and OC use it is essential to measure smoking status and to attempt to control for it. A study that did not do this could only be used to provide 'supportive' evidence of an association between OC use and myocardial infarction, since an increased risk in OC users could simply be a consequence of smoking.

Confounding can be controlled for in two broad ways: in the design by matching (ensuring through selection that cases and controls are similar for specified variables) or in the analysis by statistical adjustment of the data to account for any imbalances between groups which could impact on the results. When data have been adjusted for confounders it is important to take into account both the crude (i.e. unadjusted data) and the adjusted risks, but usually greater weight should be placed on the latter.

Overall assessment

The overall assessment of causality depends on the extent to which any alternative explanations have been excluded and also on the availability of other supporting evidence. Formal criteria for causality assessment, such as those described by Bradford-Hill (1965), are often hard to apply at the stage of the initial assessment. However, it may be possible to bring all the evidence from clinical trials or epidemiological studies together in a formal meta-analysis (Berlin, 2000). This will indicate the overall strength of the evidence for or against a causal association and the likely magnitude of the risk. Meta-analysis is an increasingly used and valuable technique that is well established in the field of randomized clinical trials but which is more controversial for epidemiological studies. When evaluating any meta-analysis it is important to consider whether all the available evidence has been included, the quality of that evidence, and whether significant heterogeneity between study populations limits the overall conclusions that can be drawn.

Signals arising from studies can sometimes be supported by data from spontaneous ADR reporting. Although the primary purpose is to provide signals, spontaneous reporting data can also be used for hypothesis strengthening and, in particular, for identifying risk factors in ordinary practice. If there are already a substantial number of cases, then the issue should have already been signalled, but sometimes the signals are missed or considered unassessable. Most signals derived from studies lead to a review of the available spontaneous reporting data, although absence, or near absence, of cases cannot be considered to refute a signal strongly. This is because spontaneous reporting systems may fail to signal some drug safety hazards (a notable example being the case of oculomucocutaneous syndrome due to practolol, many cases of which were reported retrospectively after the association was publicized in the literature).

The final step in the initial assessment is to consider the way forward. The key decision is whether simply to keep a watching brief or to gather further evidence proactively. The overall strength of the evidence for a hazard and its potential implications for the balance of risks and benefits are the principal factors that should underpin this decision. The process of further investigation is described in the next section.

Investigation

When the initial assessment has indicated that there is sufficient evidence of concern to warrant further investigation, detailed consideration should be given to the most appropriate means of resolving the outstanding issues. There is no standard recipe for this process, because every issue is different. The factors most likely to require clarification relate to causality, mechanism, frequency and preventability. Assessment of these issues may require new formal studies, but the hypothesis may be strengthened or weakened using immediately available sources of retrospective information such as epidemiological databases (Wood and Waller, 1996); see below. The principal epidemiological databases that are used for drug safety purposes, and their utility, are listed by Strom (2000). These databases have the potential to provide rapid answers to important questions, facilitating immediate risk management and the design process of definitive studies.

To address the key factors listed above may require laboratory, clinical or epidemiological studies. Detailed consideration of the first two are beyond the scope of this chapter, but the principles underlying the epidemiological approach will be considered in some detail.

Epidemiological studies of drug safety

The basic elements necessary for an epidemiological study of drug safety are:

- a record of drug exposure

- a record of outcomes

- access to detailed medical information about individual cases.

The first two elements may be held in the same database, designed as an automated medical record (as in the UK General Practice Research Database (GPRD) or one of the managed care or HMO databases in the USA), or in separate databases that are 'record-linked', e.g. one of the claims payment data sets. The key element of record linkage is the cross-identification of individuals in both databases so that exposures and outcomes are linked for individual patients. This is exemplified in the MEMO system based in Tayside, UK, where completely separate databases of encashed prescriptions and hospital discharge records are linked through a unique identifier known as the Community Health Index number (Evans and MacDonald, 2000).

Another approach which is well established in the UK, is prescription-event monitoring (PEM; Shakir, 2002), for which prescriptions are obtained from the Prescription Pricing Authority and used to create cohorts of patients exposed to new drugs. Event data are collected subsequently from general practitioners. PEM has also been shown to be feasible and useful in New Zealand (Coulter, 2002).

Even though no source of data is perfect, the quality and accuracy of the data are important considerations when setting up an investigation. The effect of random inaccuracies in the data will be a tendency to underestimate a true association. Inaccuracies in the data would generally have to be very marked to cause a true association to be completely missed, but the practical problem is that they might produce sufficient dilution of the association to lead to an uncertain result. Data inaccuracies will only explain an apparent positive association if they are gross or there is systematic bias present. A modest degree of inaccuracy in the data is unlikely to produce a positive finding when no such association exists.

Drug exposure data

The record of drug exposure in epidemiological studies is invariably imperfect. In the GPRD or one of the managed care databases in the USA, for example, it is a record that a prescription was issued by a doctor. In the MEMO scheme in Scotland, or one of the Pharmacy Benefit Management or claims payment datasets in the USA, it is a record that the prescription was encashed, which is likely to be substantially preferable. In a study in Tayside, UK, up to 15 per cent of patients did not cash the prescription issued (Beardon *et al.*, 1993). However, in neither case is there any certainty that the patient used the prescribed medicine as intended (Sackett *et al.*, 1986) – this can only be assessed by interviewing subjects or by monitoring compliance. The interview approach has some advantages (e.g. it can be applied to non-prescription medicines) but, because patients are generally not precise observers of their own behaviour, it is not necessarily more accurate than a prescription record. Furthermore, such data are potentially subject to systematic biases, notably recall bias (see above for explanation).

Outcome data

Similar issues arise regarding the quality and accuracy of the outcome data. It is usually considered necessary to verify outcomes held on a computer record by reviewing the medical records. This will eliminate basic data-entry errors and, to an extent depending on the outcome being studied and the diagnostic criteria used, improve the accuracy of the outcome data. It may also allow the time of onset of the disease to be clarified (it is important to know whether or not cases are 'incident' i.e. new) and better measurement of potential confounders. However, it should be recognized that there is also a disadvantage inherent in this process, which is that selection of the best-documented cases is being practised. There is, therefore, potential for selection bias and the incidence of the outcome is likely to be underestimated. It has been argued that these disadvantages may outweigh the benefits of case validation (Evans and MacDonald, 1997), and this is an issue that needs further research.

Selective use

A particular issue that arises in the design and interpretation of many epidemiological studies of drug safety relates to whether or not the drug of interest is being used selectively in patients who have different characteristics to those using the chosen comparator drug(s). It is well recognized that this is a common occurrence and that it may, in part, relate to marketing strategies. For example, claims that a non-steroidal anti-inflammatory drug has less gastrointestinal toxicity than others may lead to it being selectively used in patients with a history of such problems, a phenomenon known as channelling (Petri and Urquhart, 1991). The result in an observational study is that such a drug will apparently be associated with a higher risk of gastrointestinal toxicity than comparators. This is called 'confounding by indication'. It is analogous to an imbalance at baseline in a randomized trial. The most satisfactory way to deal with this problem is by adjustment for the relevant risk factors, but this is not always feasible, leading to difficulties in data interpretation.

Use of computerized databases

For reasons of cost and speed, epidemiological studies of drug safety are increasingly being based on data from computerized databases that have primarily been collected for another purpose (Jick *et al.*, 1991). Use of the databases listed by Strom (2000) has demonstrated the potential of this approach in the investigation of a wide range of drug safety issues. Both major types of epidemiological study design have been used, i.e. cohort and case-control designs.

In a cohort design, a defined population is followed forwards in time and the incidence of the outcome in question is measured and compared in individuals exposed or not exposed to the drug of interest. Both absolute and relative risks can be measured using this approach.

In a case-control design, cases of the outcome of interest are identified along with a group of controls drawn from the same population who do not have the outcome. Prior exposure to the drug(s) of interest is then compared in cases and controls. These studies provide measures of relative risk in the form of odds ratios, but they do not directly measure absolute risks. A further approach is for a case-control study to be 'nested' within a cohort design. This method has the advantages of both approaches, particularly if it used used to facilitate more detailed control of potential confounding than can be achieved in a complete cohort.

Initiating new studies

Study design is a key issue when initiating a new study for the specific purpose of further investigating a drug safety issue (i.e. hypothesis testing). Important specific issues that should be addressed are:

- clear specification of the hypothesis to be tested;

- achieving adequate statistical power to detect as significant clinically important risks compared with those attributable to therapeutic alternatives (a power calculation should always be performed);

- minimization of bias (primarily through processes for selecting subjects and collecting exposure and outcome data);

- control of confounding in the design (by matching) or analysis (by adjustment, normally using multivariate statistical techniques).

In addition to the study design, there are many logistic issues to be addressed regarding the processes for assuring the quality of the data and the validity of the study. Particular consideration should be given to potential ethical issues and to how the data are going to be monitored if the study is prospective. It is sensible for pharmaceutical companies to set up independent advisory boards to oversee such studies, and they are now becoming the norm for most studies that are relevant to drug safety.

Evaluation

When new data become available from purpose-designed studies they need to be considered and reviewed in the context of existing data. An assessment should be made as to whether and how the new evidence changes the previous evaluation, focusing particularly on the strength of the evidence for a drug-related association and possible approaches to prevention. In the latter respect, detailed analysis of the data to identify possible risk factors for the hazard is important. Suppose that a rare hazard has been identified along with several risk factors. It may well be that the benefits of the medicine are clearly sufficient to outweigh the hazard overall but not in particular individuals with risk factors for the outcome. An example of this would be venous thromboembolism (VTE) with hormone replacement therapy (HRT). The risk of VTE is two to three times greater in users than non-users of HRT (Castellsague *et al.*, 1998), i.e. there is an increased relative risk. However, the probability of VTE occurring in a healthy middle-aged women is small (the background absolute risk is about 1 in 10 000 per year) and the benefits of HRT to an individual in terms of symptom relief and protection against osteoporosis may be considerable. Patients with a high baseline risk of VTE, perhaps because they have previously had a deep venous thrombosis, will be subjected to the same increase in relative risk if they use HRT, but this represents a much higher absolute risk of VTE. Unless the benefits of the treatment are substantial, such a risk could outweigh the potential benefits to that individual.

The role of those involved in drug safety is to make recommendations that are justified by the scientific evidence and allow users to make informed decisions. A detailed approach to balancing risks and benefits of marketed medicines has been put forward by CIOMS Working Group IV (1998). Sometimes the balance of risks and benefits will be sufficiently clear-cut to allow firm recommendations (such as contraindications), whereas in other situations less directive advice will be warranted. There is no easy mathematical formula for determining the benefit–risk balance (as implied by the often used term 'benefit-risk ratio'), and in all cases a judgement is required. Such judgements are usually made by expert committees, which include practising clinicians and, in recent times, lay persons amongst the members. A possible thought process for judging the benefit–risk balance is as follows:

Risks	*Benefits*
Who is at risk?	Who may benefit?
Magnitude of absolute risk	Magnitude of expected benefit
Risks associated with alternatives	Benefits associated with alternatives

Benefit-to-risk balance
Is it reasonable to accept the risk(s) to gain the potential benefits?
If so, in what circumstances?

Before moving on, it is important to point out that these steps have been described in a simplified chronologic sequence: detect a signal, develop a hypothesis, explore the hypothesis, consider the action needed. In reality, each of these steps may require both reconsideration of prior thinking and anticipation of subsequent possibilities. In particular, the epidemiological study, here portrayed as 'hypothesis testing', may often be best considered proactively (i.e. before a signal has actually been detected), and put in place just in case it might be needed. The large linked databases are particularly well suited to such an approach, since they permit assembly of exposed cohorts at any time, including those already in the cohort and all those accruing during an ongoing period of study (N.B. the terms 'retrospective' and 'prospective' are not really appropriate under such circumstances to describe data collection; rather, they should be reserved for descriptions of study method, e.g. cohort study as a prospective design). Studies of 'banked' cohorts may then be tapped in the event of emergence of a signal or continued until, in the absence of a signal, it may be concluded that they are no longer needed.

The next section deals with how the evidence gathered in the processes described above can be used to take action that improves the safe use of medicines.

Action

When a drug safety hazard has been identified and sufficient information is available on which to base a judgement about the implications for users, the overall aim of promoting the safest possible use of the agent becomes foremost. A plan is required for providing appropriate information to health professionals and patients, so as to minimize the risk of the hazard. The urgency of implementation of this plan will vary depending upon the frequency and seriousness of the ADR and the place of the drug in clinical practice. An important principle is that, whenever the actions proposed may significantly alter prescribing, the necessary information needs to be made available rapidly. On rare occasions there is a need to withdraw the drug from the market on safety grounds. This invariably requires immediate actions by both the company and the regulatory authority in order to ensure users are informed and to recall distributed supplies of the drug. Even more rarely, there may be national circumstances that result in an action taken in one or a few countries but not all countries. In the case of major but non-global actions, such as withdrawal for safety reasons in a single country, clear explanations for the individual actions need to be provided to those not undertaking the action.

The nature of the action taken in response to a drug safety issue will depend on several factors, which are listed in Table 8.6. In terms of the hazard, the influencing factors here are much the same as the underlying issues in the initial assessment phase (see Table 8.3), but also included here should be consideration of the benefits of the drug in relation to alternatives and the nature of the disease being treated (CIOMS Working Group IV, 1998).

Table 8.6 Factors influencing the type of action taken and timing in relation to a drug safety issue

Seriousness of the hazard (i.e. its potential for a fatal outcome, or to lead to hospitalization or disability)
Frequency
Preventability
Nature of the disease being treated
Benefits of treatment with the drug
Availability of alternative treatments

An important aim is the provision of clear product information. Several sections of the product information may include vital information for safe use. These are listed in Table 8.7, with examples. Changes to product information need to be tailored to specific issues and placed in the context of the existing information. Key safety information should come first within a particular section and may need to be highlighted. The amount of information added should be proportionate to the importance of the issue and care must be taken to avoid duplication (cross-referencing between sections is preferable to repetition) or adding excessive information that does not aid the prescriber. Non-contributory information dilutes

Table 8.7 Sections of product information that may require amendment in response to a drug safety issue

Section	Examples
Indications/uses	Limiting the indications to particular conditions with the greatest benefits by removal of indications: (a) for which the benefits are insufficient to justify use; (b) for which use is associated with a greater risk of the ADR
Dosing instructions	Reductions in dose (may be applied to specific groups, e.g. the elderly); limitations on duration or frequency of treatment (especially for ADRs related to cumulative dose); provision of information on safer administration
Contraindications	Addition of concomitant diseases and/or medications for which the risks of use are expected to outweigh the benefits
Interactions	Addition of concomitant medications or foods that may interact; advice on co-prescription and monitoring
Pregnancy/lactation	Addition of new information relating to effects on foetus or neonate; revised advice about use in these circumstances based on accumulating experience
Warnings/precautions	Addition of concomitant diseases and/or medications for which the risks of use need to be weighed carefully against the benefits; additional or modified recommendations for monitoring patients
Undesirable effects	Addition of newly recognized ADRs; improving information about the nature, frequency and severity of effects already listed
Overdosage	Adverse effects of overdosage; management, including the need for monitoring

important messages and may increase the likelihood of the key facts being missed. The principles of how to address safety aspects of product information have been reviewed in detail by the CIOMS Working Group III (1995).

Actions to prevent adverse drug reactions and promote safer use of medicines

The types of action that may be taken vary according to the potential means of preventing the ADR. In particular, hazards may be minimized by recommending the targeting of the drug to patients least likely to be at risk of the ADR and/or by specifically contraindicating it in patients with identifiable risk factors. Many factors will have an impact on the potential for preventing ADRs. These relate to both patient and drug characteristics, and they are summarized in Table 8.8.

Dose and duration of treatment are often important issues in resolving drug safety issues, since the risks of many hazards are related to one or both of these parameters. It is quite common for dosage regimens to change during the post-marketing period in response to safety concerns, and many drugs have been initially recommended at doses higher than necessary (e.g. thiazide diuretics, prazosin, captopril). In re-evaluating dose in response to a safety concern, it is essential that consideration is given to the evidence for efficacy at lower doses. It is conceivable that reducing dose could lessen efficacy whilst having only a limited effect on safety. In theory, the balance of benefits and risks could be made less favourable, and empirical reductions of dose to levels that have not been shown to be efficacious are,

Table 8.8 Factors that may impact on the potential for prevention of ADRs

---

User characteristics
    Demographics: age, sex, race
    Genetic factors: polymorphisms (e.g. acetylator status)
    Concomitant diseases (e.g. impaired hepatic or renal failure)
    History of previous ADRs (e.g. allergy)
    Compliance

Drug characteristics
    Route of administration
    Formulation (e.g. sustained versus immediate release, excipients)
    Dosage regimen
    Therapeutic index
    Mechanisms of drug metabolism and route of excretion
    Potential for drug interactions

---

therefore, inappropriate. Limiting the duration of treatment is another potential action that requires consideration of the benefits and needs to be coherent with the therapeutic objective. For example, it may be a rational measure for antibiotic-related hepatitis when the risk increases with longer courses of therapy (e.g. with co-amoxiclav), but it would be a pointless move where chronic therapy is needed, such as with antihypertensive or antidiabetic drugs. On rare occasions reformulation has been a successful strategy, e.g. for a time-released formulation for a drug with a peak blood-level-related toxicity, such as bupropion.

Timing

An important consideration is how quickly information needs to be made available to users. A new life-threatening ADR, such as cardiac arrhythmias with terodiline (Rawlins, 1997), requires immediate communication, whereas the addition of a symptom that does not appear to be associated with serious consequences (e.g. nausea) to the undesirable effects section of the product information could be actioned at the next routine revision. Furthermore, in the latter case there may be no particular need to draw attention to the problem. Most issues come between these two extremes, and a judgement needs to be made about the speed of action and the most appropriate method of communication.

Changing product information

The identification of a new ADR or the accumulation of important new evidence about a recognized reaction leads to a need to make changes to the product information. Such changes may be initiated by the regulatory authority or the pharmaceutical company. Regardless of who proposes the changes, it is essential that there is exchange of information and discussion between the parties in order to attempt to reach agreement on the actions proposed and facilitate their rapid implementation.

When the regulatory authorities and companies are in broad agreement about the nature and impact of a drug safety issue, it is likely that negotiations regarding the details of necessary action will be successful and changes can be made on a voluntary basis. However, if the parties do not agree about the actions required, then authorities may exercise compulsory powers to remove a drug from the market or change the conditions of the authorization. Both companies and authorities normally try to avoid such procedures for safety issues, since they may involve unsatisfactory delays and limit the actions that can be taken until the outcome is known. When the issue has urgent public health implications the authority may act rapidly to withdraw the product(s) from the market.

Any change to product information that has significant safety implications should be actively drawn to the attention of the relevant health professionals, usually by circulating the new product information under cover of a 'Dear Doctor/Pharmacist' letter. Invariably, such changes also require production of new patient information and they may also require revision of the information on the packaging. When the changes being made are vital for ensuring patient safety they need to be implemented very quickly and it may be necessary to recall all old stock.

Safety issues affecting drug classes

Drug safety issues affecting a large class of drugs (such as the concerns about possible increased risk of VTE associated with the use of HRT) provide particular difficulties. In such cases it is important for information provided about the issue to be consistent unless there is clear evidence of a difference among products. There is less likely to be a place for individual companies informing users, particularly as this may lead to unwarranted differences in the information provided. In such circumstances communication may be best achieved via a drug safety bulletin or, if the matter is urgent, a 'Dear Doctor/Pharmacist' letter may be sent directly by the regulatory authority.

In summary, minimizing the risks of ADRs usually requires a variety of measures, and effective communication to professional and lay audiences. The latter issue is dealt with in the next section.

Communicating about drug safety

Introduction

Communicating information to users is a vital step in the process of handling a safety issue with a marketed medicine. Ultimately, the successful handling of a specific problem depends not only on making the right decisions, but also on presenting the proposed action in a way that leads users to react appropriately. In this section, the principles underlying successful communication in drug safety are discussed in terms of how to get across the right messages for the right audiences (e.g. health professionals, patients and the media) in the right way and at the right time.

Getting started

Once a decision has been taken on the appropriate action to reduce the risk from a drug safety issue, careful planning is required. This will include how and when action is to be taken and the optimization of communications to ensure that all those who need to know about the action are informed in a clear and timely manner. If the safety issue represents a major hazard to the public and significant action (such as when a product withdrawal) is planned, then it is essential to act quickly. A project team should be formed made up of a leader to oversee the planning and execution of communications and members with the necessary knowledge and experience of drug safety, communication and distribution networks. A communication plan will be drafted to make clear the key messages, the audiences to be targeted (and how to reach them), who is responsible for drafting documents, who should review them and who will sign them off. The plan should include dates and times for production of drafts, for initiating distribution and for communications being received. It should be reviewed regularly and may need to be changed in light of emerging events. Contingency for a major change in events, such as a leak of information to the media, should be included.

Getting the message right

The key requirements for a successful drug safety communication are summarized in Table 8.9, i.e. accurate, balanced, open, understandable and targeted. These can be recalled by the mnemonic 'ABOUT', as they are the considerations about which one can formulate the process. The proposed communication should be tested against these requirements by a review process that includes both individuals who are experts in the field and those who are generalists. Communications intended for patients should be written in plain language and reviewed by lay people. In the multicultural and diverse world-marketplace, making information available in the appropriate languages represents a growing challenge. In urgent situations it is vital to spend enough of the time that is available ensuring that these requirements are met.

Table 8.9 Key requirements for a successful drug safety communication (ABOUT)

Requirement	Comments
Accurate	Are the facts and numbers correct? Make sure you have included all the information that the reader needs to know
Balanced	Have you considered both risks and benefits; is the overall message right?
Open	Be honest about the hazard – don't hide or minimize it; make it clear what has led you to communicate now
Understandable	Keep it as straightforward as possible – the reader is more likely to respond appropriately if the message is simple and clear
Targeted	Consider your audience and their specific information needs

It is particularly important in any communication about drug safety to ensure that essential information is clearly conveyed and not obscured by other, less important information. The key facts and recommendations must be worded unambiguously and should be placed in a prominent early position, with use of highlighting.

Healthcare professionals

A model for a written communication to healthcare professionals is shown in Figure 8.2. The numbered paragraphs are intended to describe the content of the particular section rather than to be used as headings. The model should aid making the letter open and

---

IMPORTANT SAFETY INFORMATION

Dear Health Professional,

PRODUCT (Approved name): HAZARD DESCRIPTION

1. The problem

2. The evidence

3. Conclusions drawn from the evidence

4. Practical recommendations

5. Enclosures (if any)

6. Contact points

Signature

Figure 8.2 A model written communication to healthcare professionals

informative, and can be tailored to the specific issue. It is important for credibility that communications to health professionals are signed by a senior professional, such as the company Medical Director or the chair of an expert committee. One of the key aspects is to inform healthcare professionals of any action that they need to take. Simple instructions will help prevent unnesessary consultations and minimize further enquiries. Contact points should be given for the provision of further information. This is particularly important, as some individuals will not have understood the messages, some will want more information or access to the data leading to the action, others will want detailed advice on patient management and some will want to complain. Contact points should include a Website address, the number of a telephone helpline and an address for written correspondence.

Patients and the public

The key principles with patient information are that it should, in substance, be the same as the information provided to health professionals and it should be presented in language that they can understand. Good patient information adds to and reinforces the main issues that should be discussed between health professionals and patients, and does not make statements that could interfere with that relationship.

The media

Most important drug safety issues, and some less important ones, will receive attention in the media. Often, this will originate in medical journals with a scientific paper or news item forming the basis of subsequent television and newspaper coverage. The lay media have great potential influence on the perceptions of large numbers of users of medicines.

Furthermore, healthcare professionals may first hear about a drug safety issue through the media. Therefore, the media need to be handled with considerable forethought. It should be recognized that the immediate need of journalists is for a story that will interest their customers. The aim should be to provide them with the necessary facts and interpretation so as to give them maximum opportunity for balanced reporting. Unfortunately, a balanced perspective of risks and benefits may not lead to a newsworthy item, and journalists often tend to overrate anecdotal evidence (e.g. in putting emphasize on the problems experienced by a particular individual). Journalists' expectations may also be unrealistic in relation to the level of safety of medicines or the quality of the evidence suggesting harm. They can be expected to highlight disagreement amongst experts in the field or any other factor that increases the newsworthiness of the item. With these considerations in mind, a basic model for providing the media with information is proposed in Table 8.10.

Table 8.10   Basic model for providing information to the media

1. Nature of the problem: drug, hazard, precipitating factor(s)
2. Evidence for the hazard: strengths, weaknesses
3. What is being done: e.g. reviewing, investigating, new studies, changing labelling, etc?
4. What are the implications for (a) health professionals and (b) patients?
5. Overall balanced view of risks and benefits

Some journalists specialize in health and even in pharmaceutical reporting, and they may be more substantively orientated than some of their peers. On occasion it is possible to establish a long-standing respectful relationship with such professionals. This includes in-depth briefings about the broad and difficult challenges of risk identification and quantitation as well as the specifics of a particular safety issue. Such relationships, in turn, can result in opinion leadership and helpful public health communication during crises.

Professional organizations and patient representative groups

Professional organizations and patient representative groups offer both potential benefits and potential threats to a communication plan. Such organizations may be willing to contribute to the drafting of communication documents and in so doing improve them by offering perspectives that regulatory or company personnel do not have. They may give quotes relating to the action being taken, and these can then be used in media briefing and in response to complaints. These organizations may be prepared to help with the distribution of communications and, if they are adequately briefed (e.g. with a detailed 'question and answer' document), to handle some of the enquiries that inevitably follow communication about a major safety issue. Ideally, contacts with these organizations should also be built proactively rather than making first contact at the time of an urgent drug safety issue.

Distributing the messages

Healthcare professionals

It is essential to be clear which healthcare professionals need to know about the safety issue. Usually, all general practitioners will need to be informed, with hospital medical staff, hospital and community pharamcists and nursing staff being informed depending on the drug in question. Occasionally, when the safety issue relates to a drug only used by a small number of hospital specialists, it may be acceptable to target this specialist group, together with those pharmacists and nursing staff working in the relevant speciality. However, if there is any doubt as to whether generalists may be providing healthcare to those receiving the specialist treatment then a letter distributed widely is necessary.

Distribution lists can be accessed via commercial and professional organizations. Which to choose will depend on how the drug is used. Some commercial organizations also offer faxing services, which can be very useful when a leak has occurred or is likely to occur.

Information being distributed should also be added to the regulatory authority and company Websites. This also provides an opportunity to provide more detailed information (such as a summary of the data leading to the action and a 'question and answer' document) and linkage to other, related, refereed professional Websites.

Patients and the public

In certain situations, particularly if the hazard is potentially life threatening, it may be appropriate to include 'boxed warnings' on patient information leaflets and/or the packaging. An example of such a case is the contraindication to use of beta-blockers in patients with a history of asthma or bronchospasm, where it is vital that the patient does not use the product. Here, good patient information adds an extra safeguard in the event of a prescription being dispensed that would have potentially lethal consequences for the patient.

When information is provided to health professionals regarding an urgent drug safety issue that is likely to attract media attention, an information sheet that can be copied and given to patients may be of considerable value to practitioners.

It is increasingly likely that patients will first learn of a drug safety issue via the media. This reinforces the need to ensure that media briefing is clear and explains any action that patients need to take and provides contact points for further information. Telephone helplines may be very helpful for some major safety issues. They should be staffed by appropriately trained personnel who have access to comprehensive 'question and answer' documents. The Internet is a further medium for patients to achieve access to information, and for some patients this will be their first port of call. The many unrefereed sites on the Web make it increasingly important that company and regulatory Websites be accessible, widely available and attractive. They should include current, clear, and simple information about any emerging issue.

The media

Providing written information to newspapers and the makers of television programmes through a spokesperson should be the usual method of interaction, with informal conversations being best avoided. Interviews for television or radio may be requested, and careful consideration should be given to their potential benefits and harm in the context of the specific situation in question. Such interviews invariably have the potential to inflame an issue, but refusal to appear can also be damaging. If it is decided that the interview should be accepted, then it is important that the individual to be interviewed has both undertaken media training and is fully briefed about the issue, the key messages and the pitfalls likely to be encountered.

When it is predicted that a drug safety issue is likely to attract media attention and where there is considerable potential for unbalanced reporting likely to lead to patient alarm and possibly harm, it is usually best to adopt a proactive approach. One model is to set up a press briefing rather than awaiting enquiries from the press, so allowing you the opportunity to present the facts in a balanced way. An alternative is to hold a press conference backed up with a written briefing for journalists. A press conference requires considerable planning, but it will allow the facts to be clearly presented and allow journalists an opportunity to clarify issues they do not understand. When successful, a press conference can lead to journalists printing the exact messages you want the public and health professionals to receive. This may be achieved by using experienced staff to explain the facts and required action and backing it up through providing journalists with a written briefing.

Professional organizations and patient representative groups

At an early stage in the communications planning, a list of relavent professional and patient representative groups, together with named contacts and telephone and fax numbers, should be drawn up. If it is intended that these groups will have input to draft communications, help with distribution or take enquiries, then first contact will need to be made many days before communications 'go live'. If their input is not required then such organizations should at least be faxed, in confidence and for information, the letter being sent to healthcare professionals.

Timing the messages

Ideally, professional and patient organizations will be informed prior to all relevant healthcare professionals. In turn, relevant healthcare professionals will be informed prior to any media briefing, but this is logistically very difficult. Although the media will almost inevitably hear about a major safety issue before all relevant healthcare professionals have been informed, it is essential to try to put a mechanism in place for communicating with healthcare professionals before there is major media coverage.

Beyond communication: risk management

Historically, the tools for management of drug risks have been based in the product information and risk communication processes described above. However, recent developments, notably in the USA, warrant separate mention here. In addition to ensuring that all parties are aware of risks inherent with the drug, it is important that risks in the normal clinical use of medications also be understood and addressed. These activities to manage preventable risks range from efforts as traditional and straightforward as emphasizing in product information the need for monitoring of laboratory tests to detect possible adverse reactions as early as possible and react clinically (e.g. with dose reductions), to efforts as sweeping as restricting the use of products to specific providers or settings. One of the most widely accepted and best understood is the standing recommendation for liver function monitoring, e.g. with the anti-tuberculosis medication isoniazid. In patients who neither have symptoms of an underlying disease (their tuberculosis infection is asymptomatic) nor of drug toxicity (there are no symptoms associated with early hepatotoxicity), risk management entails careful, detailed explanations to physicians and, through them, to patients about the risk, their responsibilities to undertake regular checks, and also the provision of practical information about the frequency of monitoring, recommended tests and possible actions.

More extensive programmes to manage risk may be indicated, e.g. use of clozapine is associated with schemes for ensuring that haematological monitoring is performed in order to detect and prevent the consequences of agranulocytosis. In the USA, with the acne-control medication isotretinoin (Accutane), simple warnings by physicians, deemed sufficient elsewhere in the world, were clearly not working adequately to reduce the risks of pregnancy exposure and the known teratogenicity of the drug. Thus, the sponsor, in collaboration with the FDA, developed and launched a series of efforts that included a patient registry, informed consent forms, and detailed patient information materials.

These approaches are now termed 'risk management programmes' and they have recently been recognized as part of the drug approval process in the newly legislated Prescription Drug User Fee Act III. As now conceived, companies need to consider the spectrum of efforts that might be appropriate to ensure safe and effective use in the market place, and to commit, during the new drug approval process, to undertake and monitor such efforts following approval.

Ensuring that action to protect patients is effective

Perhaps the most important aspect of risk management is ensuring that any action taken to protect the public from a drug risk is effective. With the exception of when a drug is withdrawn from the market, all action on drug safety will aim to reduce rather than to eliminate risk. If the drug in question is of proven therapeutic benefit then this is entirely appropriate. However, simply adding warnings to product information, recommending monitoring or contraindicating an at-risk patient group, or even launching what may appear to be a more comprehensive 'risk mangement programme', may not adequately protect public health. It is important, therefore, to monitor that the actions have been effective and to continue to monitor the drug safety issue(s) on an ongoing basis. A list of possible methods of evaluation is given in Table 8.11.

Table 8.11 Possible methods of evaluating the effectiveness of actions taken

1. Communications. Have they been received and understood (using market research techniques)?
2. Prescribing. Extent to which it is consistent with revised recommendations in product information (using longitudinal patient databases)
3. Spontaneous reporting. Do serious cases continue to be reported? Do reported cases reflect contraindicated use?
4. Observation/formal study of prescribing and events. Has the action resulted in reduced morbidity/mortality from the ADR in practice (using longitudinal patient databases or epidemiological study)?

In the past, the number and nature of spontaneous reports received have been used as the main method of evaluating the effectiveness of action. However, because of various potential biases, this approach has significant limitations. An active public emphasis upon safety issues may result in increased reporting, whereas the existence of a formal program may be an excuse for underreporting. The extent and nature of these subtle biases are likely to be obscure. Thus, ideally, ADRs and other untoward events following use of the drug would be prospectively monitored. This might be done using a formal observational study or by monitoring prescribing and events in a longitudinal patient database such as the GPRD, or a managed care or claims payment database. However, the complexity and extensiveness of the risk management programme may require more elaborate hands-on survey and monitoring techniques, to observe whether each of the components is being executed effectively.

If there is evidence that the action(s) taken has not affected relevant measures of drug usage, or reduced the morbidity or mortality associated with the drug, then further action and communications will usually be necessary, or, in the extreme, the drug may be withdrawn.

Managing the process

At the heart of the process of drug safety management is the business of managing the processes, the centre of the circle (Figure 8.1). Those unfamiliar with this sector are often surprised by the extent to which these responsibilities are shared by industry and regulators.

The multinational pharmaceutical company is responsible for the safe and effective use of its products anywhere in the world where it markets or contracts to have them marketed. Although each company organizes this function in its own way, there are some general principles and common approaches. Multinational companies will, for example, create drug safety monitoring functions in each of their national affiliate companies, to ensure that any ADR reported to the company will be handled effectively. This will entail several steps: communication with the reporter to assure that the details necessary to understand the report have been received; recording and management of the information regarding the case; and, as appropriate, reporting to the local regulatory authority in the jurisdiction, transmission (often with translation) to the international headquarters offices, and associated data management and quality assurance functions. The international office, likewise, will require staffing, automation and technical support to receive, interpret, quality assure and, as necessary, provide consultation to the local partner to ensure the completeness and quality of each report. Centrally, the company will wish to maintain a professional staff to conduct ongoing review of the reports as they accrue and, as necessary, assure that the international immediate and periodic reporting requirements are all met. For questions about the safety of a company's product, or the efforts to monitor and manage its safety, the company is the repository of the greatest expertise. For larger companies, this requires staffing with physicians, nurses, pharmacists, informatics specialists and other professional staff, possibly numbering in the hundreds.

Regulatory authorities likewise require professional and technical staff competent to understand the impact and import of individual drug safety case reports and overall drug experience patterns. Their reponsibilities differ from those of the individual company. First, the responsibilities for the specifics of individual case work-up and aggregate analysis are generally those of companies; it falls to the regulator to ensure that these responsibilities have been fulfilled. In addition, of course, the regulatory authority will wish to have expertise and staffing adequate to perform the same safety review functions already described for the industry. Depending on the national context, the regulatory authority may be the primary recipient of ADRs (e.g. in the UK, where the majority of cases are reported directly to the national agency); in others, the primary agent for drug safety case management will reside with the industry (e.g. in the USA, where the majority of cases are reported directly to the companies). Each country's regulatory authority will organize its drug safety enterprise differently. However, they all share in common the need for expertise in medicine, pharmacology, informatics, epidemiology and regulatory science.

Audit

To ensure an efficient and effective system for handling drug safety issues, audit should be performed of all the steps in the process. Audit will include measuring performance against targets for data collection and processing, case management and clinical evaluation, signal generation and pattern evaluation, decision making, regulatory action and communication.

In general, each agent in the system, company and regulator alike, will wish to have its own internal system of audit, to ensure continuous quality improvement. In addition, however, regulators may elect, and in many countries are required by law, as part of their sector governance functions, to perform audits upon the regulated industry. In these instances, it is important that such audits be governed by common sense and focus upon auditing the steps and processes which will make a difference in the quality of the function, and not simply 'counting what's easy to count'.

Conclusion: some thoughts on the future

The methodologies underpinning pharmacovigilance have been developed over the last 30 years to a level that affords patients a reasonable degree of protection against unwanted effects of medicines. However, these still need to become more sophisticated to meet the challenges of the changing world of therapeutics. Innovative methodologies are also needed in order to enhance the capabilities of drug safety personnel to respond quickly to important issues. Technological advances, and the increasing availability of computerized databases that can be used to research drug safety issues, are providing new opportunities for better investigation and communication about drug safety.

Expectations of drug safety from both the professions and the public have increased over the past decade and are likely to continue to do so (Asscher et al., 1995). The primary consideration in this field must always be the well-being of patients using the medicine. When making decisions based upon analysis of benefit-to-risk balances, a fine line often has to be drawn between restricting the availability and choice and of achieving the proper balance between the benefits and the risks that inevitably accompany the use of any medicine.

Many uncertainties remain in the field. Whilst there is agreement on common practices, there is little research to document best practices. There is agreement on the need for proper staffing and resourcing, but there is little research to document the necessary competencies and expertise, much less appropriate training and accreditation for the professions involved. Whilst there is evolving agreement on harmonized practice, e.g. upon a timeline of 15 days for expedited reporting or 6 months for a periodic safety update, there have been few studies to demonstrate the value of such consensus.

In the future, improvements in the quality of the evidence, in the decision-making processes and in the tools used and competencies required to detect and manage risks are all possible (see Chapter 16). Further developments in standards and audit are required to cover the whole pharmacovigilance process, as are better measures of its success or failure. Scientific developments in various disciplines relevant to pharmacovigilance should be used to underpin these advances.

References

Asscher AW, Parr GD and Whitmarsh VB (1995). Towards safer use of medicines. *Br Med J* **311**: 1003–1005.

Beardon PHG, McGilchrist MM, McKendrick AD, McDevitt DG *et al*. (1993). Primary non-compliance with prescribed medication in primary care. *Br Med J* **307**: 846–848.

Begaud B, Moride Y, Tubert-Bitter P, Chaslerie A *et al*. (1994). False-positives in spontaneous reporting: should we worry about them? *Br J Clin Pharmacol* **38**: 401–404.

Berlin JA (2000). The use of meta-analysis in pharmacoepidemiology. In *Pharmacoepidemiology*, 3rd edn, Strom BL (ed.). John Wiley: Chichester; 633–659.

Calman K, Moores Y and Hartley BH (1995). Carbaryl. Department of Health PL CMO(95)4.

Castellsague J, Perez Gutthann S and Garcia Rodriguez LA (1998). Recent epidemiological studies of the association between hormone replacement therapy and venous thromboembolism. *Drug Saf* **18**: 117–123.

CIOMS (1999). Reporting adverse drug reactions – definitions of terms and criteria for their use. CIOMS, Geneva.

CIOMS Working Group III (1995). Guidelines for preparing core clinical safety information on drugs. CIOMS, Geneva.

CIOMS Working Group IV (1998). Benefit–risk balance for marketed drugs: evaluating safety signals. CIOMS, Geneva.

CIOMS Working Group V (2001). Current challenges in pharmacovigilance: pragmatic approaches. CIOMS, Geneva.

Collet JP and Boivin JF (2000). Bias and confounding in pharmacoepidemiology. In *Pharmacoepidemiology*, 3rd edn, Strom BL (ed.). John Wiley: Chichester; 765–784.

Committee on Safety of Medicines/Medicines Control Agency (2000). Danthron restricted to constipation in the terminally ill. *Curr Probl Pharmacovigil* **26**: 4.

Coulter DM (2002). PEM in New Zealand. In *Pharmacovigilance*, Mann RD and Andrews EB (eds). Wiley: Chichester; 345–361.

Edwards IR, Lindquist M, Wiholm B-E and Napke E (1990). Quality criteria for early signals of possible adverse drug reactions. *Lancet* **336**: 156–158.

Evans JMM and MacDonald TM (1997). Misclassification and selection bias in case-control studies using an automated database. *Pharmacoepidemiol Drug Saf* **6**: 313–318.

Evans JMM and MacDonald TM (2000). The Tayside Medicines Monitoring Unit (MEMO). In *Pharmacoepidemiology*, 3rd edn, Strom BL (ed.). John Wiley: Chichester; 361–374.

Bradford-Hill A (1965). The environment and disease: association or causation? *Proc R Soc Med* **58**: 295–300.

Inman WHW and Weber JCP (1986). The United Kingdom. In *Monitoring for Drug Safety*, 2nd edn, Inman WHW (ed.). MTP Press: Lancaster; 13–47.

Jefferys DB, Leakey D, Lewis J, Payne S *et al*. (1998). New active substances authorized in the United Kingdom between 1972 and 1994. *Br J Clin Pharmacol* **45**: 151–156.

Jick H, Jick SS and Derby LE (1991). Validation of information recorded on general practitioner based computerized data resource in the United Kingdom. *Br Med J* **302**: 766–768.

Lees AJ, on behalf of the Parkinson's Disease Research Group in the United Kingdom. (1995). Comparison of therapeutic effects and mortality data of levodopa and levodopa combined with selegiline in patients with early, mild Parkinson's disease. *Br Med J* **311**: 1602–1607.

Petri H and Urquhart J (1991). Channeling bias in the interpretation of drug effects. *Stat Med* **10**: 577–581.

Rawlins MD (1997). Predicting the future from lessons of the past. *Int J Pharm Med* **11**: 37–40.

Sackett DL, Haynes RB, Gent M and Taylor DW (1986). Compliance. In *Monitoring for Drug Safety*, 2nd edn, Inman WHW (ed.). MTP Press: Lancaster; 471–483.

Shakir SAW (2002). PEM in the UK. In *Pharmacovigilance*, Mann RD and Andrews EB (eds). Wiley: Chichester; 333–344.

Smyth RL, Ashby D, O'Hea U, Burrows E *et al.* (1995). Fibrosing colonopathy in cystic fibrosis: results of a case-control study. *Lancet* **346**: 1247–1251.

Speirs CJ (1986). Prescription-related adverse reaction profiles and their use in risk–benefit analysis. In *Iatrogenic Diseases*, 3rd edn, D'Arcy PF and Griffin JP (eds). Oxford University Press: Oxford; 93–101.

Strom BL (2000). How should one perform pharmacoepidemiology studies? Choosing among the available alternatives. In *Pharmacoepidemiology*, 3rd edn, Strom BL (ed.). John Wiley: Chichester; 401–413.

Uppsala Monitoring Centre (1998). A network for safety. WHO Collaborating Centre for International Drug Monitoring, Uppsala.

Von Kries R (1998). Neonatal vitamin K prophylaxis: the Gordian knot still awaits untying. *Br Med J* **316**: 161–162.

Wood SM and Waller PC (1996). Record linkage databases for pharmacovigilance: a UK perspective. In *Databases for Pharmacovigilance*, Walker SR (ed.). Centre for Medicines Research: Carshalton; 47–54.

9

Regulatory Aspects of Pharmacovigilance

B. D. C. Arnold

Introduction

Pharmaceutical companies have a responsibility to make the use of their medicines as effective and as safe as possible. Hence, companies need to conduct effective pharmacovigilance throughout the life cycle of all medicinal products, so that accurate, well-informed and up-to-date information is provided to physicians, pharmacists and patients. In addition, companies must keep regulatory authorities informed with regard to the ongoing safety profiles of their products so that the authorities can fulfil their own obligations to protect public health.

Each company should collect safety data on all of its products, from all available sources on a worldwide basis, and have appropriate evaluation and reporting mechanisms in place. However, the current diversity of regulatory requirements for reporting adverse drug reactions (ADRs) results in different authorities requesting that information from the same source be presented according to different inclusion criteria, formats and time intervals. Despite the best efforts of the Council for International Organizations of Medical Sciences (CIOMS) and the International Conference on Harmonization (ICH), it is evident that effort put into compliance with diverse ADR reporting requirements draws resources away from the medical evaluation of safety signals. Thus, a single set of standards for the worldwide communication of safety information is still required in order to facilitate a shift in emphasis away from the administration of safety data towards more cost-effective identification and evaluation of important safety signals.

Council for International Organizations of Medical Sciences

CIOMS is a non-governmental organization established in 1949 by the World Health Organization (WHO) and the United Nations Educational, Scientific and Cultural Organization (UNESCO), primarily to act as a forum for capturing and disseminating opinion on new

Stephens' Detection of New Adverse Drug Reactions Fifth Edition edited by John Talbot and Patrick Waller
© 2004 John Wiley & Sons, Ltd   ISBN: 0 470 84552 X

developments in biology and medicine, as well as in exploring their social, ethical, moral, administrative and legal implications.

In 1986, CIOMS initiated the 'CIOMS I' Working Group with the objective of standardizing expedited ADR reporting requirements. Subsequent CIOMS working groups have addressed a variety of safety-related topics, as follows:

I   International reporting of adverse drug reactions

Ia   Harmonization of data elements for electronic ADR reporting

II   International reporting of periodic drug-safety update summaries

III   Guidelines for preparing core clinical-safety information on drugs

IV   Benefit–risk balance for marketed drugs: evaluating safety signals

V   Current challenges in pharmacovigilance: pragmatic approaches

VI   Safety monitoring and evaluation during clinical trials.

Groups I–V have completed their activities and, with the exception of CIOMS Ia, have published their recommendations as CIOMS reports; CIOMS VI activities are ongoing. Each CIOMS Working Group report represents a significant milestone in pharmacovigilance. Groups I, II and V have contributed significantly to the harmonization of international ADR reporting requirements, and are described further below.

CIOMS I – International reporting of adverse drug reactions

The CIOMS I group was formed with the objective of developing an internationally acceptable method for manufacturers to report post-marketing ADRs rapidly and effectively to regulatory authorities. The group comprised individuals from regulatory authorities and pharmaceutical companies and issued its final report in 1990.

The group established the principle that serious, medically substantiated, unexpected ADRs should be regarded as the most important source of safety signals in marketed products, thereby warranting expedited data collection, evaluation and notification to authorities. This principle has survived reasonably well as international harmonization of reporting requirements has progressed, albeit with resistance to acceptance by some authorities.

The final report of the CIOMS I group contains several recommendations relating to conventions and definitions, report content and format. In due course, this established the CIOMS I form for worldwide expedited reporting.

Conventions presented by the CIOMS I group that have been carried forward into many ADR reporting regulations worldwide, include:

- A 'suspected reaction' means that a physician or other healthcare professional has judged it a reasonable possibility that an observed clinical occurrence has been caused by a drug.

- CIOMS reports are not required for 'events' or 'experiences' where causal judgement has not been made; the exception to this rule relates to spontaneous reports, which should always be regarded as suspected reactions.

- Companies should take local prescribing texts into account when determining whether a serious ADR is 'expected' or not for expedited reporting purposes.

- Recognizing that initial notifications of ADRs to pharmaceutical companies are often lacking in detailed information, CIOMS reports should be filed once they contain the following minimum standard of information:

  - an identifiable source

  - a specific patient

  - a suspected drug

  - a suspected reaction.

- Manufacturers should submit completed CIOMS I forms to regulatory authorities within 15 *working* days after initial receipt of information, thereby allowing companies sufficient time to collect reasonably detailed information on a case before notification and reducing the need for follow-up reports. Unfortunately, this concept has not survived intact, with regulatory authorities generally requiring expedited reports within 15 *calendar* days.

- The 'regulatory clock' should start once the company, or any part or affiliate of a company, receives sufficient information to qualify as a CIOMS report.

CIOMS II – International reporting of periodic drug-safety update summaries

The CIOMS II Working Group was convened with the objective of developing a model periodic safety update report (PSUR) that could serve as the basis for harmonizing international approaches to periodic reporting, and it issued its final report in 1992.

The CIOMS II Working Group established well-recognized standards for PSURs that have progressed through the European Union (EU) and ICH processes dealing with this topic. Although the CIOMS II recommendations have been superseded by the report format and content recommended in the ICH E2C guideline on this topic, the following principles established by the CIOMS II group merit recognition:

- PSURs should provide a critical review of safety information accumulated from various sources since the time of the previous review, and put this information into context against the earlier information.

- Each regulatory authority requiring a safety update should receive the same PSUR simultaneously.

- PSURs should represent routine compilations of safety information, so that both manufacturers and regulators can be reassured that pertinent safety data have been reviewed in a systematic manner.

- Cumulative data should only be required to place issues into context.

- PSURs should be based upon the drug substance under review and should include combination products, with reference to the active moiety; it may also be appropriate to differentiate formulations, routes of administration and indications within the same report.

- The timing of PSURs should be based on the international birth date (IDB), i.e. the date of first approval by a regulatory authority; the manufacturer's safety database should then be locked at six-monthly intervals thereafter, creating a series of 'official' data lock points.

- A cumulative series of six-monthly updates should suffice to meet the needs of those regulatory authorities that require annual, biennial or five-yearly PSURs.

In addition, the CIOMS II final report contains a useful example PSUR, containing an evaluation of two fictitious safety issues that arose during the period under review, evidently based on a 'real-life' situation and produced by an experienced drug safety organization. This example illustrated very well the level of critical evaluation that a company could reasonably apply during the production of a PSUR, and it is still relevant to this day when complying with global PSUR requirements.

CIOMS V – Current challenges in pharmacovigilance: pragmatic approaches

The CIOMS V Working Group was convened to consider practical proposals on a wide range of issues concerning pharmacovigilance and ADR reporting, including unresolved issues from previous CIOMS Working Groups, and it issued its final report in 2001.

Topics covered by the report include:

- Sources of individual case reports
  - consumer reports
  - published literature
  - the Internet
  - solicited reports
  - aspects of clinical trial reports
  - epidemiology – observational studies and use of secondary databases
  - disease-specific registries and regulatory ADR databases
  - licensor–licensee interactions
- Good case management practices
  - clinical evaluation of cases
  - assessing patient and reporter identifiability

- – criteria for assessments of seriousness and expectedness

- – case follow-up

- – narrative summaries

• Good summary reporting practices

- – PSUR content

- – frequency and timing of reporting

- – miscellaneous proposals for managing PSURs

• Determination and use of population exposure data

- – PSURs and exposure data sources

- – technical considerations

- – spontaneous reporting and patient exposure

- – examples of denominator determination and use

- – patient-exposure and measurements of risk

• Clinical safety reporting regulations

- – overview of current regulations

- – recommendations for change

Although only recommendations, it is evident that many of the proposals within this report will be considered under the ICH process and/or incorporated into local regulations. In addition, many companies have chosen to adopt several of the recommendations into daily working practice without the need for regulation to occur in support.

The International Conference on Harmonization

Origin and objectives

The ICH is a unique project bringing together regulatory authorities from three regions (EU, USA and Japan) with experts from the pharmaceutical industry. The process involves discussion of scientific and technical aspects of product registration, leading to recommendations that facilitate harmonization of requirements for product registration, thereby reducing the need to duplicate effort during the development of new medicinal products.

The terms of reference of the ICH were defined as follows:

• Provide a forum for constructive dialogue between regulatory authorities and the pharmaceutical industry regarding differences in the technical requirements for product registration in the EU, USA and Japan.

• Identify areas where modifications in technical requirements or greater mutual acceptance of R&D procedures could lead to more economical use of resources without compromising safety.

- Recommend practical ways to achieve greater harmonization in the interpretation and application of technical guidelines and requirements for registration.

Co-sponsors of the ICH are:

- European Commission (EC)
- European Federation of Pharmaceutical Industries and Associations (EFPIA)
- Ministry of Health, Labour and Welfare (MHLW), Japan
- Japan Pharmaceutical Manufacturers Association (JPMA)
- Food and Drug Administration (FDA), USA
- Pharmaceutical Research and Manufacturers of America (PhRMA).

In addition, the International Federation of Pharmaceutical Manufacturers' Associations (IFPMA) provides the ICH secretariat, and the WHO, European Free Trade Association and Canada have provided observers to the process.

Five ICH conferences have taken place to date:

- ICH1 November 1991, Brussels
- ICH2 October 1993, Orlando
- ICH3 November 1995, Yokohama
- ICH4 July 1997, Brussels
- ICH5 November 2000, San Diego.

The ICH6 meeting is scheduled for November 2003 in Osaka, Japan.

Clinical drug safety-related topics have been addressed at several ICH meetings, primarily in association with expedited and periodic reporting requirements as well as developing standards for the electronic communication of clinical safety data. Recently, the ICH Steering Committee initiated a second phase of drug safety-related activities at a meeting in Brussels (February 2002). Topics being considered under this phase include:

- An addendum to the E2C (PSUR) guideline
- ICH E2D – Post-approval Safety Data Management: Definitions and Standards for Expedited Reporting
- ICH E2E – Pharmacovigilance Planning

The addendum to ICH E2C has been completed and is now considered part of the ICH E2C guideline. At the time of writing, the E2D and E2E guidelines are in development and, hence, are not considered further.

The International Conference on Harmonization process

Expert working groups (EWGs), containing experts from each of the six ICH co-sponsors, provide technical advice to the ICH Steering Committee with regards to harmonization topics, with the objective of producing a guideline on their respective topic that then forms the basis for implementation within each ICH region. Each guideline passes through five stages ('Steps') from original selection of the topic through to legislated implementation:

Step 1 Selection of topic, preliminary discussions and preparation of a draft guideline

Step 2 Formal consultation with stakeholder organizations

Step 3 Consolidation of comments and preparation of a revised draft guideline

Step 4 Endorsement of the final draft by the ICH Steering Committee and 'sign-off' by the co-sponsors

Step 5 Incorporation into domestic regulations or other administrative procedures.

To date, there have been three 'Clinical Safety Data Management' EWGs addressing the following topics:

- E2A Definitions and standards for expedited reporting

- E2B Data elements for transmission of individual case safety reports (ICSRs)

- E2C PSURs for marketed drugs.

In addition, the ICH E1 guideline (Population exposure) defines the extent of population exposure needed to assess clinical safety during development of a new product and the ICH E6 Guideline (Good clinical practice) specifies some obligations relating to safety reporting during the conduct of clinical trials.

Two 'multidisciplinary' topics had clinical safety as one of their components, ICH M1 (Medical terminology for regulatory purposes) and ICH M2 (Electronic standards for the transfer of regulatory information and data). These topics were addressed by working parties, which then produced standards for adoption rather than specific guidelines.

International Conference on Harmonization definitions

Adverse event

The E2A and E6 guidelines indicate that an adverse event (AE) is any untoward medical occurrence in a patient or clinical investigation subject administered a pharmaceutical product, and which does not necessarily have to have a causal relationship with this treatment.

Hence, an AE can be any unfavourable or unintended symptom, sign, laboratory parameter or disease entity temporally associated with the use of a medicinal product, regardless of any causality assessment by either the reporting healthcare professional or company physician.

Adverse drug reaction

In the context of clinical investigations, the E2A guideline indicates that all noxious and unintended responses to a medicinal product relating to any dose should be considered as suspected ADRs.

The guideline signifies that the phrase 'responses to a medicinal product' means that a causal relationship between a medicinal product and an AE is at least a reasonable possibility. However, it then confuses matters by also indicating that an AE should be considered as an ADR if 'the relationship cannot be ruled out'. This leaves regulatory authorities and companies to interpret the definition of an ADR, for example:

- an AE could be considered an ADR if it is not possible to exclude totally that a causal relationship exists; or

- there needs to be a plausible reason as to why a causal relationship might exist for an AE to be considered as an ADR.

The first (more conservative) interpretation would mean that almost any AE having a temporal relationship to administration of an investigational product (i.e. virtually all of them) could be considered as an ADR. However, the second interpretation has further support within Section III.A.1 of the E2A guideline, which indicates that:

- all cases judged by either the reporting healthcare professional or the sponsor as having a reasonable suspected causal relationship to the medicinal product qualify as ADRs;

- the expression 'reasonable causal relationship' is meant to convey, in general, that there are facts (evidence) or arguments to suggest a causal relationship.

Regarding marketed products, the E2A and E6 guidelines both restate the WHO definition, indicating that an ADR is a response to a drug that is noxious and unintended and which occurs at doses normally used in man for prophylaxis, diagnosis or therapy of disease or for modification of physiological function.

Spontaneous reports are defined within the E2C guideline as any unsolicited communications to a company, regulatory authority or other organization that describe ADRs in patients and which do not derive from a clinical study or other organized data collection scheme. The E2A and E2C guidelines indicate that spontaneous reports from consumers or healthcare professionals should all be regarded as suspected ADRs. In contrast, guidance is lacking as to when a literature report qualifies as a suspected ADR.

Serious adverse event/adverse drug reaction

ICH E2A and E6 define an AE (or ADR) as serious if it:

- results in death

- is life threatening

- requires inpatient hospitalization or prolongation of existing hospitalization

- results in persistent or significant disability or incapacity

- is a congenital anomaly or birth defect.

In addition, the E2A guideline introduced the concept of 'medically important' AEs that should also be regarded as 'serious' even if they do not meet any of the above criteria (see below).

Death The ICH guidelines do not provide specific guidance on the interpretation of the criterion 'results in death', thereby leaving it open to interpretation by companies and regulators. For example, death is usually the outcome of an event that causes it and, in general, the cause of death would be regarded as the AE; one exception is 'sudden death', which should usually be regarded as the AE and 'fatal' as its reason for being 'serious'. In some countries (e.g. Germany and Sweden), the term 'unexplained death' may also be reported as a specific event, whereas in the USA all reports of death should be submitted to the FDA, even if the cause of death (i.e. the underlying AE) is unknown.

Life threatening The term 'life threatening' refers to an event where the patient was at *immediate* risk of death at the time of the event, not an event that might have caused death had it been more severe. For example, although pulmonary embolism has the potential of being life threatening in some circumstances, it should only be considered 'life threatening' if it was so severe in intensity that there was an immediate risk of the patient dying from the pulmonary embolism.

Hospitalization The term 'hospitalization' refers to the situation when an AE is associated with an unscheduled admission into hospital, for the purpose of investigating and/or treating the AE. For example, when administration of a drug results in thrombocytopenia, which then necessitates an overnight admission for bone marrow biopsy and platelet transfusion.

Usually, hospitalization that occurs on an elective basis should not be regarded as a serious AE. For example, when a patient is admitted into hospital for a scheduled cholecystectomy, for the treatment of pre-existing cholelithiasis, this would usually not be regarded as an AE *per se* and the fact that the patient is hospitalized is irrelevant. However, if the patient suffers an unexpected deterioration in their condition (e.g. development of acute cholecystitis) that requires hospitalization for urgent cholecystectomy, then a serious AE has occurred, even if it was considered unrelated to the drug therapy.

Further interpretation is required when the local medical environment is considered. The practice within many pharmaceutical companies is to consider any hospital stay exceeding 24 h as 'hospitalization'.

Disability or incapacity The term 'persistent or significant disability' is open to interpretation and requires judgement. In general, it should be regarded as any situation where an AE has a clinically important effect on the patient's physical or psychological well being, to the extent that the patient is unable to function normally.

Congenital anomaly Any congenital anomaly observed in a child should be regarded as a 'serious AE' when the mother (or father) was exposed to a medicinal product at any stage during conception or pregnancy.

Medically important adverse events   ICH E2A introduced the concept of 'medically important' AEs, which may also be known by the phrase 'required medical intervention'. The two terms should be regarded as synonymous, as both refer to events of clinical significance that might otherwise not be considered as serious if the other criteria are used but yet they may jeopardise the patient's health such that medical intervention is required to prevent one or more of the 'serious' outcomes. These situations should usually be regarded as 'serious', both in a clinical and a regulatory sense – this emphasizes that the determination of 'seriousness' should be a matter of clinical judgement rather than regulatory 'box ticking'.

For example, this might apply in a situation where a patient requires treatment in an emergency room for allergic bronchospasm but is not formally admitted, as such patients can be discharged home on a same-day basis. Other examples cited in the E2A guideline that should usually be considered as serious are blood dyscrasia or convulsions that do not result in hospitalization or development of drug dependency or drug abuse.

Unexpected adverse event/adverse drug reaction

ICH E2A and E6 indicate that an adverse reaction should be regarded as 'unexpected' if its nature or severity is not consistent with information in the relevant source documents, namely the company's Investigator's Brochure (IB) (investigational products) or local prescribing information texts (marketed products).

Reports that add significant information on the specificity or severity of a known ADR may also be considered as unexpected events, for example:

- a report of interstitial nephritis for a product that has a recognized association with acute renal failure;

- a report of fulminant hepatitis for a product that has hepatitis as a labelled ADR.

Unlisted adverse event/adverse drug reaction

An unlisted ADR is one whose nature, severity, specificity or outcome is not consistent with the information included in the 'Company Core Safety Information', itself a section of the company's core prescribing information text.

Although similar to the above definition of 'unexpected', the E2C guideline introduced the concept of 'unlisted' ADRs specifically for periodic reporting purposes. Hence, whereas 'unexpectedness' should be based on the relevant local prescribing text or IB and used for expedited reporting purposes, 'listedness' should be based on the company's 'core' prescribing text(s) and used only for periodic safety reporting purposes.

ICH E2A – Clinical safety data management: definitions and standards for expedited reporting

The E2A EWG was created to develop standards for the issue of expedited reports for development products. The resultant guideline reached Step 4 in October 1994 and has since been implemented, to a greater or lesser extent, within all three ICH regions.

The E2A guideline defines expedited reporting requirements for all ADRs relating to products under clinical investigation, including the investigation of new formulations or indications for products already on the market. The fundamental principle is that serious unexpected ADRs warrant expedited reporting to regulatory authorities, provided that they meet minimum criteria for reporting and include a causality assessment. This includes reports from the following sources:

- any clinical or epidemiological investigation, regardless of design or purpose
- post-marketing use
- published literature
- ADR registries generated by regulatory authorities.

In contrast, the E2A guideline indicates that expedited reports should not be necessary for:

- serious expected ADRs
- serious AEs from clinical investigations, which have been considered as unrelated to the study drug
- non-serious ADRs.

Reporting requirements

The ICH E2A expedited reporting requirements are summarized in Table 9.1.

Table 9.1   ICH expedited reporting requirements

Report	ADR type
7-day	Fatal or life-threatening unexpected
15-day	Serious unexpected

With regard to fatal or life-threatening unexpected ADRs, the sponsor should notify regulatory authorities as soon as possible, but no later than seven calendar days after first knowledge that a case qualifies. The initial notification may be made by telephone, facsimile or in writing. Within a further eight calendar days, each initial notification should be followed by a complete report, including relevant previous experience with the same or similar medicinal products and an assessment of the importance and implications of the findings. Other serious unexpected ADRs should be notified as soon as possible, but no later than 15 calendar days after first knowledge by the sponsor that the case meets the minimum criteria for reporting.

With regard to informing investigators, Independent Ethics Committees (IECs) or Institutional Review Boards (IRBs), the E2A guideline simply cross-refers to the ICH E6 guideline that discusses the need to provide new safety information to such parties (see below).

Minimum criteria for reporting

However a case report is submitted for expedited reporting, Attachment 1 of the E2A guideline details the data elements that should be included within a report:

- patient details

- suspected medicinal product(s)

- other treatment(s)

- details of the suspected ADR(s)

- details on the reporter of the suspected ADR(s)

- administrative and sponsor/company details.

In many instances, the information required for a final description and evaluation of a case report may not be available within the stipulated time frames for expedited reporting. Thus, the guideline indicates that initial reports should be submitted within the specified time frames provided that the following minimum criteria are met:

- an identifiable patient

- a suspected medicinal product

- an identifiable reporting source

- an event or outcome that can be identified as serious and unexpected

- a reasonable suspected causal relationship (for cases arising from clinical investigations).

Although a submitted case report may satisfy only these criteria, the sponsor of the clinical investigation is still obliged to seek follow-up information on the case and submit this as it becomes available.

Causality assessments

ICH E2A indicates that formal causality assessments are required for case reports arising from clinical investigations: all cases considered by either the reporting investigator or the sponsor as having a reasonable possibility of a causal relationship to the study drug qualify as suspected ADRs.

At present, a standard international nomenclature to describe causal relationships is lacking. As a result, pharmaceutical companies vary in their approach to causality (see Chapter 4). Several companies have opted to consider an AE as either 'suspected' or 'not suspected', in accordance with the concept that the phrase 'reasonable causal relationship' means that there are facts, evidence or other reasons to suggest a causal relationship. These companies then simply oblige their investigators to answer only 'Yes' or 'No' to an appropriately phrased question on causality.

Post-study events

When patients experience serious AEs after completion of their participation in a clinical trial and they report these events to the investigators that had cared for them, the E2A guideline advises that these reports should be considered as though they were study reports, even though they may not be entered onto the clinical trials database itself. Hence, for safety data management purposes, they still need causality assessments and a determination of expectedness.

Managing 'blinded' therapy cases

In the event that an ADR arises from a 'blind' clinical study, ICH E2A provides a lengthy consideration of the need to break the 'blind' for expedited reporting purposes. Although it is advantageous to retain the 'blind' for all patients prior to final study analysis, the E2A EWG recognized that breaking the 'blind' for a single patient usually has little or no implications for the conduct of the study or analysis of the final data. Hence, the guideline recommends that the 'blind' should be broken for individual cases that qualify for expedited reporting, although it should still be maintained for the individuals responsible for the analysis and interpretation of study results.

The guideline provides one exception to this rule. When a fatal or other serious outcome is the primary efficacy endpoint in a clinical trial, it is possible that the statistical integrity of the investigation may be compromised if the 'blind' is broken in advance of the final study analysis. In this instance, the guideline advises companies to reach agreement with regulatory authorities that such events should be treated as disease-related and not be subject to routine expedited reporting.

Reactions associated with active comparator or placebo treatment

The guideline indicates that serious unexpected ADRs, occurring in patients given active comparator agents as part of a clinical investigation, should be notified by the sponsor either directly to the appropriate regulatory authorities or to the product manufacturer. The sponsor is left to choose the recipient of the report.

The guideline also advises that events associated with administration of a placebo usually do not satisfy the criteria of a suspected ADR and, therefore, do not qualify for expedited reporting.

Expedited notification of other safety information

The E2A guideline indicates that there may be other situations that require rapid communication to relevant authorities, for example:

- an increase in the rate of occurrence of an 'expected' serious ADR that is judged to be clinically important;

- a significant hazard to the patient population, such as lack of therapeutic effect in patients with life-threatening conditions;

- a major safety finding from a newly completed preclinical study, such as a finding of positive carcinogenicity.

In these situations, the sponsor should apply medical and scientific judgement as to whether the information materially influences the benefit–risk assessment of the study drug or whether it is sufficient to consider changes in the conduct of the clinical trial.

ICH E2B – Clinical safety data management: data elements for transmission of individual case safety reports

Background

A variety of regulations require individual case reports to be transmitted between various interested parties:

- from reporting sources to regulatory authorities and/or pharmaceutical companies;

- between regulatory authorities;

- between pharmaceutical companies and regulatory authorities;

- within regulatory authorities or pharmaceutical companies;

- from regulatory authorities to the WIIO Collaborating Centre for International Drug Monitoring, Uppsala, Sweden.

Although transmission of this information has generally been paper-based, in recent years there has been increasing use of electronic media for this purpose, whether through on-line access, tape or file transfer. Hence, it has become necessary to develop an electronic format capable of accommodating database-to-database transmission and taking advantage of the definition of common data elements and standard transmission procedures. These have given rise to the development of the E2B and M2 EWGs respectively.

The E2B EWG had the objective of standardizing the data elements needed for the transmission of ICSRs, regardless of source and destination. The scope of this topic did not encompass the definition of database structures, the design of paper report forms, QC/QA aspects or technical security issues.

The E2B guideline reached Step 4 in July 1997 and has since formed the basis of schemes for the electronic communication of safety data, for expedited and/or periodic reporting purposes within all ICH regions.

Data elements

In essence, ICH E2B defines data elements that could be useful in the clinical assessment of an individual case report. They are sufficiently comprehensive to cover complex reports from most sources, different data sets and transmission situations or requirements. Equally, the guideline acknowledges that there are many case reports that lack a substantial number of data elements, and as such they would not be available for inclusion in a transmission. Hence, the guideline serves to provide data elements that might cover each conceivable circumstance.

The guideline has also accounted for the fact that the same data can be provided in different ways, e.g. age information can be sent as the date of birth and date of reaction/ event, age at time of reaction/event or patient age group according to the available information. In this example, age would be provided by the most appropriate set of data elements rather than including multiple elements or redundant data.

Although structured data are recommended for transmission between databases, the E2B guideline makes provisions for the transmission of some free-text items, including a free-text narrative summary, as safety databases often contain large amounts of unstructured data.

Minimum information

The E2B guideline supports the criteria specified by ICH E2A with regard to the minimum information required for an ADR case report. In addition, it indicates that any one of several data elements is considered sufficient to define an identifiable patient (e.g. initials, age, gender) or reporter (e.g. initials, address, qualification) and that the patient and reporter may be the same individual and still fulfil the criteria for minimum information.

In addition, the following administrative information is required as a minimum for an electronic report:

- sender identification

- report identification number

- date of receipt of most recent information.

Content of the data

The E2B guideline divides the data elements into sections pertaining to administrative and identification information (Section A) or information on the case (Section B).

Section A: administrative and identification information   This section contains information necessary for identifying the report, reporter and different persons or institutions involved in the processing of the report, as well as indicators of specific report management, divided into three subsections:

A.1 Identification of the case safety report

A.2 Primary source(s) of information

A.3 Information on sender and receiver of case safety report

Section B: information on the case   This section allows for the collection and transmission of comprehensive information on the case, whether as structured information or as free text in many instances, divided into five subsections:

B.1 Patient characteristics

B.2 Reaction(s)/event(s)

B.3 Results of tests and procedures relevant to the investigation of the patient

B.4 Medicinal product(s) information

B.5 Narrative case summary and further information

Parent–child reports

Although such events are uncommon, the E2B guideline makes specific provision for case reports that relate to ADRs in the offspring of parents taking a suspect drug. When a report concerns an ADR in a child (or foetus), the details of the child or foetus should be regarded as the primary information for Section B, i.e. the patient characteristics should describe the child or foetus, whilst the mother (or father) should be described in the parent-specific subsection.

If the ADRs occur in both parent and child or foetus, then a separate case report should be completed for each, together with appropriate cross-references between the two.

The management of case reports that relate to spontaneous abortions or miscarriages is specifically addressed within the E2B guideline. Section B.4 of the E2B guideline indicates that case reports relating to foetuses should only be recorded as such if they concern identified foetal abnormalities or death. This section also states that early spontaneous abortion, an event that occurs in a significant proportion of pregnancies, should be treated as a parent reaction.

ICH E2C – Clinical safety data management: periodic safety update reports for marketed drugs

The E2C EWG was formed with the objective of creating a guideline on the format and content of PSURs relating to marketed products, rather than investigational compounds. The guideline reached Step 4 in November 1996 and has been formally implemented within the EU and Japan. Although E2C has not yet been formally adopted in the USA, the FDA has accepted PSURs produced in accordance with E2C standards, subject to a waiver against the regulated periodic reporting requirements. More recently, they have issued a proposed rule indicating that formal implementation of E2C will occur in due course.

An addendum to E2C has recently been developed, reaching Step 4 in February 2003. The addendum takes into account issues arising from interpretation of the original E2C guideline by regulatory authorities and relevant recommendations from the CIOMS V report.

The E2C guideline and its addendum endorse the fundamental principle established in the CIOMS II report that all relevant safety information should be presented, together with a critical clinical evaluation, covering data sets that span 6-month intervals. However, the guideline does not specify the schedule for submission of PSURs, leaving it to be determined by local regulatory requirements.

General principles incorporated within the guideline and its addendum include the following:

- A single PSUR should cover all dosage forms, formulations and indications for a given pharmacologically active substance; separate presentations may be used within that PSUR for different dosage forms, indications or patient populations.

- Information on a combination product may be presented in a separate PSUR, with cross-reference to the single agent(s) PSUR(s), or as a subsection within one of the single agent PSURs.

- Cumulative data are only required with respect to information presented on regulatory status and the summary of serious unlisted ADRs; all other data presented within the report should be derived only from the period covered by the report

- The schedule for submitting PSURs should be based on the date of first market authorization for the product, i.e. the IBD, regardless of the dosage form, formulation or uses covered by the report; manufacturers are encouraged to synchronize national birthdates (i.e. the date of national authorization) with the IBD in order to facilitate the production of a single PUR that can be submitted to multiple regulatory authorities on a simultaneous basis

- Subject to discussion with the relevant regulatory authorities, the 'clock' may be restarted (i.e. return to a 6 month submission schedule) after important additions or changes in clinical use are approved, e.g.:

  - a new, clinically dissimilar indication

  - a previously unapproved use in a special patient population, such as children, pregnant women or the elderly

  - a new formulation or new route of administration

- The 'Company Core Data Sheet' (CCDS) should form the basis for determining whether an ADR is 'listed' or 'unlisted'; this should be used for inclusion of ADRs within the line listing, to determine whether clinically relevant changes have occurred to the safety profile of a product and whether there should be amendments to the relevant core prescribing text(s).

- The PSUR can refer to a lack of therapeutic effect in appropriate circumstances, e.g. with regard to medicinal products used in the treatment of life-threatening conditions.

Content of the report

Each PSUR should have 10 sections, namely:

1. Introduction
2. Worldwide market authorization status
3. Update of regulatory authority or market authorization holder (MAH) actions taken for safety reasons
4. Changes to reference safety information
5. Patient exposure
6. Presentation of individual case histories
7. Studies
8. Other information

9. Overall safety evaluation

10. Concluding statement.

Regulatory information

Each PSUR should be viewed as a 'stand-alone' document. Hence, the introduction to the report should place it in the context of previous reports and refer to associated products covered by separate reports (e.g. combination products).

Each PSUR should provide updates on the regulatory status of the product under review, including:

- a table indicating the worldwide marketing authorization status in all countries where a regulatory decision has been made about the product;

- an update of regulatory authority or MAH actions, with details on safety-related actions taken during the period under review and also since the data lock point.

For the 6-month and annual reports, the PSUR should use the version of the CCDS that was applicable at the start of the review period as the reference document and include it as an appendix to the report. If considered more practical, companies may use the CCDS that was in effect at the end of the reporting period for longer duration PSURs or Summary Bridging Reports. Whichever version of the CCDS is used as the reference document, this should be clearly stated within the text of the PSUR.

The report should indicate any changes made to the CCDS during the review period, together with a presentation of the modified sections. In addition, as there may be a delay between changing a CCDS and implementation of local label changes, the guideline recommends that each local operating company should provide a comment on any differences that exist between the CCDS and local safety information at the time of submitting the PSUR to their regulatory authority.

Patient exposure

The PSUR should provide an estimate of patient exposure covering the same period as the interval safety data. The report should describe the method used, such as:

- patient days
- number of prescriptions
- number of dosage units
- bulk sales (tonnage).

Whenever possible, the data should be provided by age and gender. If the PSUR includes data from clinical studies, then denominators from those clinical studies should also be provided.

Presentation of cases

The PSUR should incorporate data from all sources, including:

- direct reports to the company (spontaneous notifications, clinical studies, named-patient use);

- published literature;

- reports received from regulatory authorities;

- other sources, e.g. contractual partners, special registries, poison control centres or epidemiological databases.

Companies should use AE terms derived from their current terminologies in the line listings and summary tabulations. The usual practice is to include these at the preferred term level (or equivalent).

Line listings   Specific ADRs should be presented as line listings that provide key information on individual case reports, thereby allowing regulatory authorities to select case reports for which they may require further detail when evaluating safety signals generated by the report. The line listings should be limited to the interval data relevant to the period under review. Selection of the ADRs is dependent upon the source of each case (see Table 9.2).

Table 9.2   ADRs that qualify for inclusion in a PSUR line listing

Source of report	ADR type
Spontaneous	Serious (all) and non-serious unlisted
Literature	Serious (all) and non-serious unlisted
Clinical trial or post-marketing surveillance (PMS) study	Serious
Named-patient or 'compassionate' use	Serious
Regulatory authority	Serious

Case reports should be organized by body system. Individual patients should only feature once within the line listing; those presenting with more than one ADR should be placed within the body system appropriate to the most clinically serious ADR.

Full details of content and format of the line listing are provided within the ICH E2C guideline.

Summary tabulations   In addition to line listings, ICH E2C indicates that relevant safety information should also be presented as aggregate summary tabulations, organized by body system. This includes data from 'other sources' that may not have been presented in the line listings, e.g. non-serious listed spontaneous reports and serious ADRs from registries.

The E2C guideline provides a recommended format and indicates that there should be separate tabulations for:

- serious and non-serious ADRs

- listed and unlisted ADRs

- non-serious listed spontaneously reported reactions

- serious ADRs from 'other sources', sorted by source of information or country.

When there is a small number of cases, or the information is inadequate for any of the tabulations, a narrative description should suffice instead of a formal tabulation.

The data presented in the summary tabulations should be based on the interval data. However, a cumulative figure is required for serious unlisted ADRs, representing all cases reported to date, either in tabular form or as a narrative in the text of the report.

Analysis of individual case histories   The company may present brief comments on individual case reports, for example a discussion on particular serious or unanticipated findings. However, the section allowing for these comments should not be confused with the global assessment in the Overall Safety Evaluation (see below).

Studies

The PSUR should contain information on the design and results of all relevant company-sponsored studies analysed during the period under review that contain important safety information, including relevant epidemiological, toxicological or laboratory investigations. In addition, the PSUR should contain a description of all new studies, initiated or being planned during the period under review, with respect to the evaluation of any safety issue.

Reports in the published literature that contain important safety information, including relevant abstracts from meetings, should be summarized and the publication references given.

Other information

Any unusual lack of therapeutic effect regarding a product used to treat serious or life-threatening diseases should be described, especially if it might represent a significant hazard to the treated patient population.

Any important safety information received after the data lock point should be presented in a separate section within the PSUR, including significant new cases or important follow-up data.

Information on specific risk management programmes for the product should also be discussed in this section. Likewise, when a comprehensive safety or benefit–risk analysis has been conducted, a summary of the analysis should be included in this section.

Overall safety evaluation

The overall safety evaluation should contain a concise analysis of the data presented within the PSUR, including important safety information received after data lock or resulting from the cumulative summary tabulations of serious unlisted ADRs. This section should include the company's evaluation of the significance of the data and should highlight any new information on the following:

- change in the characteristics of listed reactions, e.g. severity, outcome, target population;

- serious unlisted reactions;

- non-serious unlisted reactions;

- increased frequency of listed reactions.

The information should be presented by System Organ Class (SOC) rather than by listedness or seriousness. Related terms, even if found in different SOCs, should be reviewed together for clinical relevance.

  In addition, the evaluation should address any issues that have arisen with regard to the following (including lack of significant new information):

- drug interactions;

- experience with overdose (deliberate or accidental) and its treatment;

- drug abuse or misuse;

- positive or negative experiences during pregnancy or lactation;

- experience in special patient groups (e.g. children, elderly, organ-impaired individuals);

- effects of long-term treatment.

Concluding statement

The PSUR should conclude by indicating which safety data are not in accordance with the previous cumulative experience and/or with the current reference core prescribing text. It should then specify and justify any action that is recommended or has been initiated by the company.

Summary Bridging Reports and Addendum Reports

The addendum to E2C introduced two new concepts, Summary Bridging Reports and Addendum Reports, following on from recommendations from the CIOMS V report.

  A Summary Bridging Report is a concise document integrating the information presented in two or more PSURs, to cover a specified period over which a single report is required by regulatory authorities, e.g. two consecutive 6-month reports for an annual report or 10 consecutive 6-month reports to make a 5-year report. The report should not contain any new data but should provide a brief summary bridging two or more PSURs in order to facilitate assessment of the appended PSURs by the authority.

An Addendum Report is an update to the most recently completed PSUR and should be used when a regulatory authority requires a safety update outside the usual schedule based upon the IBD, e.g. in support of a local product licence renewal in Europe more than 6 months after the data lock point of the most recent 5-year PSUR. The report should summarize the data received between the data lock point of the most recent PSUR and the regulatory authority's requested cut-off date. The report does not need to include an in-depth analysis of the additional cases, as these will be included in the next regularly scheduled PSUR.

Full details on the content and format of Summary Bridging Reports and Addendum Reports are provided in the CIOMS V report and the addendum to ICH E2C.

ICH E6 – Good clinical practice

Good clinical practice (GCP) is a standard for the design and conduct of clinical trials, providing assurance that the data and results are accurate and credible, and that the rights and confidentiality of trial subjects are protected. The E6 EWG issued a guideline for GCP that reached Step 4 in May 1996. The guideline has since been adopted in all three ICH regions, as well as other countries, e.g. Australia and Canada.

Obligations of the investigator

In addition to complying with applicable local regulatory requirements, the E6 guideline indicates that investigators should report all serious AEs immediately to the sponsor, except for those AEs that are exempted by the trial protocol or other trial documentation, e.g. the IB. In addition, AEs and/or laboratory abnormalities identified as critical to the safety evaluation should be reported to the sponsor in accordance with reporting requirements and time limits specified within the protocol. The investigator should also provide the sponsor and the IEC/IRB with any additional requested information on reported deaths, e.g. autopsy reports.

Obligations of the sponsor

The E6 guideline indicates that, in addition to complying with applicable regulatory requirements, the sponsor should notify promptly all concerned investigators, institutions and regulatory authorities of any finding that could adversely affect the safety of subjects participating in the clinical investigation or impact upon the conduct of the trial or alters the IRB/IEC's approval/favourable opinion to continue the trial.

Investigator's Brochure

The IB serves three functions:

- present clinical and non-clinical data relevant to the study of the investigational product in human subjects, thereby facilitating the investigators' understanding of the benefit– risk of the proposed trial;

- detail specific safety monitoring procedures required during the course of the trial;

- serve as a reference document for sponsors when determining the 'expectedness' of an AE report for regulatory reporting purposes.

The ICH E6 guideline contains a recommended Table of Contents and suggestions for the content of each section of an IB. In particular, Section 6 of the IB should provide information on the safety experience in humans, including tabular summaries of ADRs from all clinical trials conducted to date and a discussion of any differences in pattern/incidence across indications or sub-groups. It should also provide a description of the possible risks and ADRs anticipated on the basis of prior experience with the investigational product and related products.

Section 6 should also present any significant information from marketed use in those countries where the product has been granted a marketing authorization, including relevant safety and efficacy information from the current core prescribing text(s) for that product.

ICH M1 – Medical Terminology Expert Working Group

Medical terminologies are required so that the *verbatim* terms used by reporters to describe AEs can be classified into a smaller number of clinically meaningful terms, whilst preserving some semblance of the original reporter's intended description. This facilitates searches for related terms when evaluating specific safety issues as well as the preparation of line listings or summary tabulations for periodic reports.

Although various terminologies have been available for use for many years (e.g. COSTART, WHO-ART, ICD-9 and various company terminologies), many of the existing terminologies have been criticized for their lack of specificity, limited retrieval options and inability to handle complex combinations of signs and symptoms effectively. Hence, no medical terminology was accepted on a worldwide basis for regulatory reporting purposes.

In 1994, ICH formed the M1 Medical Terminology EWG as a multidisciplinary initiative with the objective of developing a single medical terminology that can be used for international regulatory purposes. They utilized the MEDDRA terminology, originally developed by the UK Medicines Control Agency (MCA), as its basis; eventually the new terminology became known as MedDRA (Medical Dictionary for Regulatory Activities). MedDRA was developed on the understanding that it should have relevance to all areas of drug and device regulation, i.e. not just for ADR reporting. Specific goals for its development included:

- ensure worldwide use through collaboration with and participation of stakeholders in its development;

- build from existing terminologies to maximize compatibility;

- provide mechanisms and structures that would facilitate translation into different languages;

- ensure long-term maintenance of the terminology beyond its initial implementation.

The ICH Steering Committee approved the M1 recommendations in July 1997. Thereafter, production versions were produced that included all COSTART, WHO-ART, J-ART, HARTS and relevant ICD-9-CM terms. This allowed all data previously coded using one of these terminologies to be capable of direct one-to-one matching with MedDRA terms (see Chapter 12 for further information).

Use of MedDRA for adverse drug reaction reporting

The FDA uses MedDRA in support of its AERS safety database. At present, it is not mandatory that a company pre-codes case reports in MedDRA before electronic notification to the FDA, whether for expedited reports or periodic safety updates.

Within the EU, MedDRA is used in support of the EudraVigilance database. With effect from January 2003, companies have been required to use MedDRA for pre-coding medical terms used when expedited reports are submitted electronically to the European Agency for the Evaluation of Medicinal Products (synonym: European Medicines Evaluation Agency; EMEA) and EU member state authorities. It is possible that the mandated use of MedDRA for other aspects of regulatory submission (e.g. clinical trial reports, periodic safety updates, marketing authorization application (MAA) submissions and product information) may follow in due course.

Within Japan, the MHLW issued guidance on the use of MedDRA in 1999, allowing companies to use MedDRA in support of ADR reporting, Japanese prescribing information texts, Japanese new drug application documentation and re-examination packages. In May 2002, the MHLW announced its plans for electronic ADR reporting, with initial implementation scheduled for October 2003 and becoming mandatory in due course, at which time the use of MedDRA in support of electronic ADR reporting will also become mandatory.

ICH M2 – Electronic standards for the transfer of regulatory information

The M2 EWG (Electronic standards for the transfer of regulatory information – ESTRI) was established in 1994 in order to define electronic standards that would facilitate electronic communication of clinical safety data between regulatory authorities, the pharmaceutical industry and other interested parties. The group planned to select standards from those already available in this field and recommend those that would have broad acceptance, be able to evolve with the development of technology, and that would be independent of the technical infrastructure used by a sender, receiver or vendor, thereby facilitating practical implementation in each ICH region.

The project includes the verification of procedures for consistent, accurate transfer of information, as well as the evaluation of encryption technologies and key certification procedures for the transfer of regulatory information.

Tests have been conducted to define logical electronic communication standards, to ensure the integrity of information and data exchange between companies and authorities. Tests have also involved the transfer of encrypted and non-encrypted files between a number of international centres.

As a result, the M2 EWG has made a series of recommendations relating to:

- implementation of electronic standards for the transfer of regulatory information and data (ESTRI)

- the Core Standard Set

- use of physical media (floppy disks and CD-ROM)

- network messaging

- secure electronic data interchange transmission over the Internet

- electronic document and message formats.

Guidelines issued by the project include ICH M2 E2B (M) (Electronic transmission of individual case safety reports message specification), which incorporates the ICH ICSR DTD version 2.1, in November 2000.

ICH E1 – The extent of population exposure to assess clinical safety

The E1 EWG was formed to develop a set of principles for the safety evaluation of drugs intended for long-term administration (more than 6 months) to patients with non-life-threatening diseases. The resultant guideline reached Step 4 in October 1994.
  Key principles presented within the guideline include:

- Standards for the safety evaluation of drugs should be based on previous experience with the occurrence and detection of ADRs, and statistical and practical considerations.

- AEs are most frequent in the first few months of treatment; the number of exposed subjects should be large enough to observe whether the more frequent events (0.5–5 per cent) increase or decrease over time (300–600 patients should be adequate).

- Some patients should be treated for 12 months; 100 patients exposed for at least 1 year is considered acceptable.

- The total number of individuals treated, including short-term exposure, should be approximately 1500.

There are exceptions to these general standards, e.g. where there is:

- concern from clinical studies, other similar drugs or pharmacokinetic or pharmacody-namic properties of late onset ADRs;

- an expectation of low-frequency serious ADRs;

- only a small benefit from the drug;

- concern that the drug may add to a significant background morbidity or mortality.

The European Union

At present, the EU has 15 member state authorities, each setting regulatory requirements for ADR reporting from a framework of EC legislation and guidelines. Although there has been some attempt to harmonize regulatory requirements for the conduct of pharmacovigilance within the EU, implementation of new legislation has not been a total success in this regard, as some authorities persist with divergent national practices.

Legal basis and regulatory framework for adverse drug reaction reporting

The current EU system for authorizing medicinal products came into effect on 1 January 1995, further to implementation of Council Regulation (EEC) 2309/93 and Council Directive 75/319/EEC (as amended by Council Directive 93/39/EEC). The directive has since been further amended by Commission Directive 2000/38/EC, with all requirements subsequently codified within Council Directive 2001/83/EC. In addition, Council Directive 2001/20/EC specifies requirements for the conduct of clinical trials within the EU, including ADR reporting requirements, with effect from May 2004.

Although this legislation forms the basis for the present pharmacovigilance system in the EU, as shown in Table 9.3, it has necessitated a mixture of EU legislation, national legislation and various guidelines for full implementation. As a result of this regulatory framework, the decision to notify an ADR to the EU regulatory authorities has to take into account several factors in addition to its clinical characteristics:

- product status (investigational or marketed)

- source of the ADR (e.g. clinical trial or spontaneous report)

- country of origin (EU or non-EU)

- method of market authorization (centralized, mutual recognition or national procedure).

Table 9.3 Regulatory framework governing expedited and periodic reporting requirements within the EU

Investigational products	Marketed products
Council Directive 2001/20/EC	Council Regulation (EEC) 2309/93
	Council Directive 2001/83/EC
	• Council Directive 75/319/EEC (as amended)
	• Commission Directive 2000/38/EC
	Commission Regulation 540/95
Clinical Trial Directive guidelines	Pharmacovigilance Guidelines[a]
CPMP guidelines ICH/135/95, ICH/287/95	CPMP guidelines ICH/288/95, ICH/377/95,
and ICH/377/95	CPMP/175/95 and CPMP/183/97
National legislation	National legislation

[a] PhVWP/108/99 (December 2001).

Clinical Trials Directive (Council Directive 2001/20/EC)

The 'Clinical Trials' Directive was formally adopted and published as EU legislation on 4 April 2001, the objective being to provide uniform standards for the conduct of clinical trials across the EU, primarily in the interest of protecting subjects that take part in those clinical trials. Member states had until 1 May 2003 to apply the provisions of this directive through national legislation, although this has taken longer in most instances. National legislation should come into effect no later than 1 May 2004.

The Clinical Trials Directive applies to all clinical trials conducted within the EU, throughout all phases of clinical development (including bioequivalence and bioavailability studies), but does not apply to non-interventional trials. It stipulates that all clinical trials should be conducted and reported in accordance with the principles of GCP.

The ADR reporting requirements specified within the directive are generally in accordance with standards expressed within the relevant ICH guidelines, although the directive does contain provisions for annual safety reports, a relatively novel concept at the EU level for investigational products.

A series of guidelines were issued during April 2003 under the sponsorship of the EC in support of the Clinical Trials Directive. These include two guidelines related to clinical drug safety: *Detailed guidance on the collection, verification and presentation of adverse reaction reports arising from clinical trials on medicinal products for human use* ('ADR reporting' guideline) and *Detailed guidance on the European database of suspected unexpected serious adverse reactions (Eudravigilance – Clinical Trial Module)* ('SUSAR database' guideline).

Council Regulation (EEC) 2309/93 and Council Directive 2001/83/EC

In 1993, the EC published legislation comprising Council Regulation (EEC) 2309/93 and Council Directive 75/319/EEC (as amended by Council Directive 93/39/EEC), which came into effect from 1 January 1995. Although the primary purpose of this legislation was to define the requirements for the approval and maintenance of MAAs, they also define the requirements for the conduct of pharmacovigilance by any company marketing medicinal products within the EU.

In addition to 'ethical' pharmaceutical products, the legislation applies to generic products available on prescription, over-the-counter products or those sold under licences for parallel imports. The regulation applies to all medicinal products registered under the 'centralized' process, including biotechnology products, and was immediately binding to all member states. The directive applied to all products registered under mutual recognition or national procedures, but it required endorsement through national legislation.

Commission Regulation 540/95 was implemented on 14 March 1995, as a supplement to Regulation 2309/93, specifically to clarify that pharmaceutical companies should notify all non-serious unexpected ADRs, for products authorized under the centralized procedure, in a separate section of PSURs, regardless of their country of origin.

Further amendment to Directive 75/319/EEC occurred with the issue of Commission Directive 2000/38/EC (5 June 2000). These amendments were then incorporated, through codification, into Council Directive 2001/83/EC (6 November 2001).

Almost all member state authorities have issued legislation in accordance with Council Directive 93/39/EEC. However, there has been some variation in their interpretation of ADR reporting requirements, such that ADR reports still require consideration on a country-by-country basis when reporting to member state authorities.

Recently, as part of a mandatory review of existing pharmaceutical legislation, the EC has made proposals to amend many aspects of the EU medicines regulatory regime, as set out in Regulation 2309/93 and Directive 2001/83. The proposals include the following relevant to the conduct of pharmacovigilance:

- replacement of 5-yearly product licence renewals with a system based on the submission of 3-yearly PSURs;

- an enhanced role for the EC in the coordination of EU-wide pharmacovigilance and inspection work.

Committee for Proprietary Medicinal Products guidelines

The Committee for Proprietary Medicinal Products (CPMP) has provided several guidelines relating to expedited and periodic reporting for investigational and marketed products:

- ICH/135/95: Good clinical practice (implementing ICH E6)

- ICH/287/95: Data elements for transmission of individual case safety reports (ICH E2B)

- ICH/288/95: Periodic safety update reports for marketed drugs (ICH E2C)

- ICH/377/95: Definitions and standards for expedited reporting (ICH E2A)

- CPMP/175/95: Note for guidance on the procedure for competent authorities undertaking of pharmacovigilance

- CPMP/183/97: Conduct of pharmacovigilance for centrally authorized products.

Although these guidelines lack formal legislative power, it is generally accepted that they represent the requirements of member state authorities with regard to meeting reporting requirements. Hence, companies are advised to observe these guidelines, and the provisions of the Notice to Marketing Authorisation Holders (see below), when developing ADR reporting procedures.

Pharmacovigilance Guidelines

In accordance with Article 24 of Council Regulation 2309/93 and Article 29g of Council Directive 75/319/EEC (as amended), the CPMP drafted several guidelines in order to provide MAHs with guidance on the implementation and practical procedures involved in complying with the legislation. These were originally incorporated into Chapter V of the Notice to Marketing Authorisation Holders (synonym: Notice to Applicants), effective from 1 January 1995. This was superseded by formal incorporation of the guidance into Volume 9 of 'The rules governing medicinal products in the European Union – Pharmacovigilance' (synonym: Pharmacovigilance Guidelines) in December 2001.

Volume 9 is presented in four parts:

Part I – pharmacovigilance of medicinal products for human use

Part II – pharmacovigilance of medicinal products for veterinary use

Part III – general information on EU electronic exchange of pharmacovigilance data

Part IV – general reference to administrative and legislative information relevant to human and veterinary products.

Perhaps of greatest practical relevance to meeting EU pharmacovigilance requirements, Part I contains the following chapters:

1. Notice to Marketing Authorisation Holders

    1.1 Legal basis and purpose

    1.2 Adverse reaction reporting

    1.3 Reporting requirements in special situations

    1.4 Periodic safety update reports

    1.5 Company-sponsored post-authorization studies

    1.6 Ongoing pharmacovigilance evaluation during post-authorization period

2. Guidance and procedures for competent authorities

3. Terminology

Upon issue, the foreword in Volume 9 indicated that certain chapters within Part I were expected to be revised during 2002 and legal references taking into account the 'codified' Council Directive 2001/83/EC, although this has yet to occur.

Data privacy legislation

Many EU member states have had legislation in place for several years to govern the privacy of personal data, reinforced by the issue of the Data Protection Directive (Council Directive 95/46/EEC) in October 1995 and its subsequent implementation though national legislation. The legislation has had a variable impact with regard to the management of drug safety information. In general, it should not prevent healthcare professionals from notifying ADRs to pharmaceutical companies, provided that appropriate informed consent is obtained from the patient and anonymity preserved to the extent required by local laws.

However, company pharmacovigilance departments need to be aware of the legislation so that they do not contravene national laws when managing ADR data, especially when communicating to third parties in non-EU countries. In particular, companies need to take into account the provision that personal data should not be communicated to 'third' countries that do not maintain comparable standards of privacy protection. In such circumstances, possible solutions to this issue may need to be considered:

*   utilize an exemption, provided by the directive, that allows for the transfer of data to a 'third' country for reasons of substantive public interest;

*   develop inter-affiliate contracts to ensure that data transferred from the EU are handled in accordance with European law;

- anonymize the data in accordance with EU data privacy legislation before transfer to a 'third' country.

Role of member state authorities

Council Regulation 2309/93 and Council Directive 2001/83/EC require that each member state should establish a pharmacovigilance system for the collection and evaluation of safety information relating to marketed medicinal products, and take appropriate measures to encourage doctors and other healthcare professionals to report suspected ADRs to member state authorities. Details of the requirements are specified within CPMP guideline CPMP/175/95 (revised 1998). These cover the following topics:

- Establishment of a pharmacovigilance system
- Management of pharmacovigilance data
    - spontaneous reporting systems
    - company-derived pharmacovigilance data
    - pharmacovigilance data from other sources
    - procedures for communication and evaluation of pharmacovigilance issues within the EU, including:
        - transmission of ADR reports (to MAHs)
        - transmission and management of detected signals
        - evaluation of company-sponsored post-authorization safety studies
        - evaluation of PSURs
        - special safety monitoring of medicinal products
        - electronic data transmission.

Specifically, the guideline instructs member state authorities to:

- Notify all serious ADRs occurring within their respective countries to the relevant MAHs, and the EMEA, within 15 days of receipt of information from local healthcare professionals; the data should be sufficient to allow an evaluation of each ADR, although it is not mandatory for the authority to have made a formal evaluation before notification to the MAH.

- Make information on non-serious ADR reports available in summary form to all relevant parties, including MAHs.

- Regarding ADR reports received from MAHs, each authority should ensure that:

    - reports submitted by an MAH conform to Pharmacovigilance Guidelines, and that all data included in these reports are validated and verified, as far as possible, and that these reports are followed up by the MAH, where appropriate;

- PSURs are evaluated and, if a Reference Member State, assessment reports are issued;

- the progress of post-authorization safety studies should be reviewed on a regular basis; final study reports should be evaluated and changes to the Summary of Product Characteristics (SPC) made, if appropriate.

• Ensure that they have the capability to send and receive ADR reports electronically.

European Agency for the Evaluation of Medicinal Products Council Regulation 2309/ 93 also established the EMEA, situated in London. Initially, the EMEA's primary role related to medicinal products authorized under the 'centralized' procedure. Recently, their role has seemingly broadened and will soon encompass investigational products as well as marketed products subject to mutual recognition procedures or national authorization procedures.

EudraVigilance EudraVigilance is the EU's new data-processing network and database management system, financed by the EC, for the exchange, processing and evaluation of safety data relating to marketed products, and came into operation on 5 December 2001. Further development in the system's functionality is expected to occur during 2003 and 2004, including provision for a Clinical Trial Module.

EudraVigilance has been presented as a milestone in the development of electronic exchange of pharmacovigilance data, between member state authorities and also between companies and authorities. Its main functional components are:

• EudraVigilance Gateway for the secure transmission of ICSRs;

• EudraVigilance Database Management System, including the safety and acknowledge-ment message exchange, routing and loading mechanisms, the guided ICSR creation procedure, the user management and security mechanisms;

• EudraVigilance Standard Terminology, with a focus on MedDRA and a product dictionary being developed by the EMEA.

Definitions

Although the EU legislation incorporates most of the relevant ICH definitions, there are some anomalies. However, most have minimal impact upon company working practices and are not considered further.

Guidelines supporting the Clinical Trials Directive have introduced the concept of suspected unexpected serious adverse reactions (SUSARs), with regard to expedited report-ing requirements, seemingly without definition. However, it is evident that these simply refer to ADRs that are serious *and* unexpected in nature.

Health professional

At present, companies are required to notify only those cases that have been confirmed by health professionals to EU authorities, whether for investigational or marketed products. These are defined within the Pharmacovigilance Guidelines as medically qualified doctors, dentists, pharmacists, nurses and coroners.

When a report originates from a pharmacist or nurse, the company should attempt to obtain further information about the case from a medically qualified doctor responsible for the patient.

General requirements

The Pharmacovigilance Guidelines indicate that the MAH must ensure that it has an appropriate system of pharmacovigilance in place within the company in order to assure responsibility and liability for its products on the market and to ensure that appropriate action can be taken.

In addition, since 1995, any company marketing a medicinal product within the EU should have 'permanently and continuously at its disposal' within the European Economic Area (EEA; i.e. EU plus Iceland, Liechtenstein and Norway) a 'qualified person' responsible for pharmacovigilance at the EU level. This person should have experience in all aspects of pharmacovigilance and, if not medically qualified, should report to or have access to a medically qualified person. Otherwise, the qualifications necessary for filling such a role are less well defined than those evident for the person with analogous responsibilities for manufacturing standards.

The MAH should provide the name of the qualified person to all member state authorities and, for centrally authorized products, to the EMEA.

Although it is clear that each company must have at least one qualified person resident within the EEA, the Pharmacovigilance Guidelines recognize that national regulations in some member states require a nominated individual from within that country who has specific legal obligations with regard to the conduct of pharmacovigilance at a national level (e.g. France, Germany and Spain).

The responsibilities of the qualified person are:

- Establish and maintain a system that ensures that information about all suspected ADRs reported to company staff, including medical representatives, is collected and collated so that it may be accessed at a single point within the EU.

- Prepare expedited ADR reports, PSURs and company sponsored post-authorization study reports for the EMEA and member state authorities in accordance with the respective requirements of Council Regulation 2309/93 and Council Directive 2001/83/EC.

- On-going pharmacovigilance during the post-authorization period, ensuring that any request from member state authorities, for the provision of additional information necessary for the evaluation of benefits and risks of a medicinal product, is answered fully and promptly, including provision of sales/prescription information for the product concerned.

- Provision to member state authorities of any other information relevant to the evaluation of benefits and risks of a medicinal product, including appropriate information on post-authorization safety studies.

Licensing agreements

The Pharmacovigilance Guidelines contain specific requirements relating to licensing agreements between pharmaceutical companies. Part I Section 1.1.1 requires MAHs to ensure that the arrangements for meeting pharmacovigilance obligations are specified in writing to relevant member state authorities at the time that an authorization is granted, and subsequently when any changes to the arrangements are proposed.

In addition, Part 1 Section 1.2.2 indicates that the 'clock' for expedited reporting starts as soon as any personnel of the MAH receive the minimum information. However, wherever possible, the time frame for regulatory submission should be no longer than 15 days from first receipt by the second company, and explicit procedures and detailed agreements should exist between the MAH and the second company to facilitate achievement of this objective. Although challenging, these requirements seemingly take into account the consideration that the MAH cannot have sufficient control over, or be made responsible for, the operations of the partner company and that each ADR report usually has to be processed at least twice before notification to regulatory authorities.

Review of scientific literature

The Pharmacovigilance Guidelines indicate that the MAH is expected to 'screen the relevant worldwide scientific literature' and report suspected ADRs arising from this source in accordance with expedited and periodic reporting provisions. Although the guidance is ambiguous, in that it fails to define the terms 'screen' or 'relevant', it is generally accepted that companies should review relevant journals from across the world, with relevance being determined by the nature of the medicinal product sold within the EU. The review should have two objectives:

- to discover suspected ADRs relating to identifiable patients;

- to identify new safety issues that might impact on the benefit–risk of the marketed product.

The Pharmacovigilance Guidelines (Part I Section 1.2.2) indicate that the regulatory 'clock' should start on the date that the MAH first becomes aware of the article or case report. This takes into account the consideration that there is often a time lag between the date of publication of an article and access by the MAH, as determined by the arrival of the relevant journal on site, its availability on MedLine or other recognized literature databases, or its international broadcast in publications that summarize the literature.

Reporting requirements for investigational products

Expedited reports

The Clinical Trials Directive stipulates that clinical investigators should notify serious AEs, and other safety-related information to the sponsors of clinical trials to standards that are in accordance with the ICH E6 guideline. Once notified to the sponsor, each serious AE should be assessed opposite national expedited reporting requirements and notified accordingly.

Although CPMP guideline ICH/377/95 endorsed the ICH E2A guideline, it was formally implemented in only a small number of member states. Hence, at present, expedited reporting requirements vary across member states to a considerable extent, as illustrated in Table 9.4. This situation should change with implementation of the Clinical Trials Directive, which will require that member states implement 7 and 15 day requirements in full accordance with ICH E2A.

Table 9.4   EU expedited reporting requirements – investigational products

Country	ADR type		
	Local origin	Foreign origin	Time frame (days)
Austria	Serious	Not required[a]	Not specified
Belgium	Serious[b]	Serious[b]	Not specified
Denmark	Serious[c]	Serious unexpected[a]	Not specified
Finland	Serious unexpected	Not required[a]	7/15
France	Serious[d]	Serious unexpected[e]	7/15
Germany	Serious	Serious	15
Greece	Serious	Serious unexpected[f]	15
Ireland	Serious	Serious unexpected	15
Italy	Serious unexpected	Serious unexpected	7/15
Luxembourg	Serious	Not required	Not specified
Netherlands	Serious unexpected	Serious unexpected	7/15
Portugal	Serious	Serious unexpected[g]	15
Spain	Serious unexpected	Serious unexpected	7/15
Sweden	Serious unexpected	Serious unexpected	7/15
UK	Serious unexpected	Serious unexpected	7/15

[a] Report only if having an impact upon the conduct of clinical trials in that country.
[b] Only once MAA submission has been made.
[c] To be reported by investigators; report events rather than reactions.
[d] If drug- or trial-related.
[e] All serious if from a multicentre trial involving French centres (drug- or trial-related).
[f] Only if from non-EU countries.
[g] If from a multicentre trial involving Portuguese centres.

The 'ADR reporting' guideline clarifies that expedited reporting requirements will apply to all SUSARs associated with the investigational product regardless of which trial they occur in, whether within the EU or a third country, as well as those that arise from other sources such as spontaneous reports, the published literature or those transmitted to the sponsor by another regulatory authority.

Once implemented, the Clinical Trials Directive will require sponsors to provide the same information to ethics committees as and when notified to 'concerned' member state authorities. In addition, sponsors are to keep all 'concerned' investigators informed. The 'ADR reporting' guideline provides clarification with regard to both of these requirements.

Sponsors should notify SUSARs to all ethics committees that have approved clinical trials on the related investigational product simultaneous with notification to the authorities. Notification should generally be via the issue of individual case reports to the ethics committees, although sponsors may use a periodic line listing (accompanied by a summary report) for notification to an ethics committee of SUSARs from outside of the ethics committee's home country, if they wish.

Notification to an ethics committee may also be delegated from the sponsor to the coordinating/principal investigator in some circumstances.

The sponsor should immediately inform all investigators with regard to findings that could adversely affect the safety of subjects participating in ongoing or planned clinical trials. Safety issues that impact upon the course of a clinical trial or development project should also be considered significant; these include suspension of the trial programme and safety-related amendments to trial protocols.

Otherwise, safety information may be provided to investigators as an aggregated line listing of SUSARs on a periodic basis, the periodicity being determined by the nature of the clinical development project and the volume of SUSARs generated. The line listing should be accompanied by a concise summary of the evolving safety profile of the investigational product. With regard to data from blinded clinical trials, the line listing should present data on all SUSARs, regardless of the medication administered, with the blind maintained.

In addition, the 'ADR reporting' guideline indicates the following:

- All case reports will require causality assessments; this requirement will apply equally to serious and non-serious AEs reported during the conduct of clinical trials; in addition, reports submitted to the authorities should include both the investigator *and* sponsor causality assessments when these differ.

- Treatment codes should always be broken before serious unexpected ADRs are reported to the competent authorities and ethics committees:

  - cases involving placebo do not meet the criteria for expedited reporting;

  - the 'blind' should be maintained for those persons responsible for the analysis and interpretation of results.

- Expedited reports will also be required for any finding that could affect ongoing benefit–risk assessment of the investigational product or would be sufficient to require changes to the conduct of a clinical investigation; this includes serious 'protocol-related' events.

- Annex 3 of the guideline presents details on the data elements for inclusion in expedited reports; reports should include the relevant 'Eudract' number plus the sponsor's case report reference number; reports with insufficient information may be returned to the company for completion and resubmission.

- In due course, electronic reporting will be the expected method for the notification of

SUSARs to the authorities, using the format and content as defined within the 'SUSAR database' guideline; until then, the CIOMS-I form will be accepted, although other important observations qualifying for expedited reporting should be notified by letter.

Periodic reports

At present, only a few EU member states have periodic reporting requirements for investigational products (see Table 9.5). Again, this situation will change with implementation of the Clinical Trials Directive, which requires that the sponsor should provide information to relevant member state authorities and ethics committees relating to the safety of subjects participating in clinical trials in the EU. Although the Clinical Trials Directive indicates that periodic reports should be submitted annually on a trial-by-trial basis, the 'ADR reporting' guideline indicates that companies will be allowed to prepare a single periodic report to cover each clinical development programme, to an annual schedule determined by the date of first authorization of a clinical trial by a member state authority.

Table 9.5   EU periodic reporting requirements – investigational products

Country	Periodic reporting requirement
Austria	Not required
Belgium	Not required
Denmark	Not required
Finland	Annual report (list of serious ADRs and summary of safety)
France	Not required
Germany	Not required
Greece	Not required
Ireland	Line-listing (non-serious ADRs) at end of study
Italy	Semi-annual reports (serious ADRs and summary of ongoing/completed studies)
Luxembourg	Not required
Netherlands	Not required
Portugal	ADRs to be listed in copy of study report
Spain	Annual report (list of serious ADRs and summary of safety)
Sweden	Annual reports, provided by investigators and sponsors (serious ADRs, withdrawals due to ADRs, progress of trial)
UK	Reports on completion of individual studies and at time of update/renewal of CTX (summary tabulations and comments)

Each report should include:

- A line listing of all serious ADRs that have occurred during the period under review; these should be presented trial by trial.

- Aggregate summary tabulations of serious ADR terms; to be presented trial by trial.

- A summary overview of the subjects' safety, to include:

  - a concise benefit–risk evaluation of the product under study;

–   supporting results of non-clinical studies or other experience with the investiga-
    tional product that are likely to affect the subjects' safety;

–   where appropriate, measures proposed to minimize identified risks, including a
    detailed rationale with regard to any proposals to amend trial protocols, to change
    or update the consent form, patient information leaflet and/or the investigator's
    brochure.

Annexes 4 and 5 of the 'ADR reporting' guideline provide further detail on the content of
the line listings and summary tabulations respectively.

Reporting requirements for marketed products

Although expedited and periodic reporting requirements for marketed products are defined
in Council Regulation 2309/93 and Council Directive 2001/83/EC, a single standard
currently does not exist within the EU, due to the impact of national legislation. However,
there are elements common to all member states, as presented by the guidance contained
within the Pharmacovigilance Guidelines.

Expedited reports

MAHs should submit expedited reports to relevant member state authorities (including the
EMEA) within 15 calendar days following receipt of relevant information. In principle,
ADR reports should be notified as follows:

•   ADRs originating from within the EU – report all serious ADRs to the member state
    authority where the reaction occurred and, if subject to mutual recognition or referral,
    also to the reference member state;

•   ADRs originating outside the EU – report serious unexpected ADRs to all member
    state authorities (where authorized) and the EMEA.

In practice, the above requirements hold true across all member states for products
authorized under the centralized requirements. However, requirements for products subject
to mutual recognition or national authorization procedures vary across some member states
(see Table 9.6).

The Pharmacovigilance Guidelines indicate that reporting forms acceptable to member
state authorities should be used until electronic reporting standards are established and
implemented (see below). Paper-based forms may be computer generated but should follow
an accepted content and layout.

The Pharmacovigilance Guidelines indicates that reports from post-authorization studies
should be unblinded by the sponsor prior to reporting. However, cases of serious expected
ADRs should only be reported in an expedited manner if the blind has already been broken
for some other reason. Otherwise, reporting may be deferred until the study has been
completed and the study data locked. The Pharmacovigilance Guidelines also confirm that
reports from post-authorization studies that qualify as clinical trials will be subject to the
requirements of the Clinical Trials Directive from its date of implementation.

Table 9.6 EU expedited reporting requirements – marketed products (mutual recognition or national authorization)

Country	ADR origin	
	EU	Non-EU
Austria	Serious[a]	Serious unexpected
Belgium	Serious[b]	Serious unexpected
Denmark	Serious[b]	Serious unexpected
Finland	Serious[b]	Serious unexpected
France	Serious[b]	Serious unexpected
Germany	Serious	Serious
Greece	Serious[b]	Serious unexpected
Ireland	Serious[b]	Serious unexpected
Italy	Serious[a]	Serious unexpected
Luxembourg	Serious[b]	Serious unexpected
Netherlands	Serious[b]	Serious unexpected
Portugal	Serious[a]	Serious unexpected
Spain	Serious[b]	Serious unexpected
Sweden	Serious[b]	Serious unexpected
UK	Serious[c]	Serious unexpected

[a] Local cases plus serious unexpected ADRs from other EU member states.
[b] Local cases only; reports not required for ADRs from other EU member states.
[c] Local cases plus serious ADRs from other EU member states for products covered by the UK 'Black Triangle' scheme.

Evaluation of case reports   The EU legislation does not mandate causality assessments on individual ADR case reports for marketed products. However, the Pharmacovigilance Guidelines indicate that MAHs may opt to comment whether they consider that there is a causal association between the reported suspect product(s) and reaction(s), together with the criteria used for the assessment. However, some member states retain local requirements for mandatory assessments, e.g. France ('imputability') and Germany ('scientific evaluations').

The CPMP Pharmacovigilance Working Party has recommended that regulatory authorities and companies perform causality assessments using an 'ABO' classification, as presented below:

A   'Probable' – the case report contains a good rationale and sufficient documentation to support a causal relationship in the sense of it being plausible, conceivable or likely (but not necessarily highly probable).

B   'Possible' – the case report contains sufficient information to consider a causal relationship as possible, in the sense of it being not impossible and not unlikely, although the relationship may be uncertain or doubtful; for example, because of missing data or insufficient evidence.

O   'Unclassified' – the causality of the case report cannot be assessed for one or more reasons; e.g. insufficient evidence, conflicting data or poor documentation.

In addition, the Pharmacovigilance Guidelines indicate that, 'in exceptional cases, when a reported ADR impacts significantly on the established safety profile of the product', the MAH should indicate this within the report. Examples include:

- the report is one of a series of similar or linked cases;
- there is *prima facie* evidence in favour of a causal relationship for a serious unexpected ADR;
- there is a suggested change in the nature, severity or frequency of expected ADRs;
- new risk factors are identified.

Information on the frequency of ADRs should provide the basis on which the estimate has been made, including data on the total number of ADR reports and patient exposure.

Special situations   The Pharmacovigilance Guidelines specify reporting requirements for several 'special' situations:

1. Reporting during the period between MAA submission and approval.
   ADR reporting should be in accordance with clinical trial regulations. In addition, the applicant should expedite reporting of any information that impacts upon the ongoing benefit–risk assessment, e.g.:
   - a serious unexpected ADR that has good evidence of a causal relationship;
   - multiple reports of serious unexpected ADRs where there is a possible relationship;
   - suspicion of change in frequency or severity of a known effect;
   - results from studies which impact on efficacy assessment.

2. Reporting of outcomes of use during pregnancy.
   MAHs are expected to follow up all reports of pregnancy. Abnormal outcomes are subject to post-marketing expedited and periodic reporting requirements. In addition, reports from prospective registries should be evaluated and information included in PSURs, including:
   - details of cases during report period;
   - aggregated data of overall exposure and normal/abnormal outcomes.

3. Reporting from other post-marketing initiatives.
   This section distinguishes between situations where there is a systematic process for reporting of adverse events and where no such process exists. The MAH should report only those events that are specifically reported as serious ADRs, as for expedited reports from post-authorization studies.

4. Compassionate use/named patient supplies.
   The MAH should establish a protocol for controlling the supply of a medicinal product for compassionate/named-patient use, which encourages the prescriber to report any

suspected ADRs to the company (and competent authority if required on a national basis).

5. Lack of efficacy.
Reports of lack of efficacy are not normally subject to expedited reporting within the EU but should be discussed in the relevant PSUR(s). However, expedited reports may be required if lack of efficacy occurs in certain circumstances, e.g. treatment of life-threatening disease, vaccines and contraceptives, or where lack of efficacy indicates a change in the benefit–risk balance, e.g. lower than expected efficacy or higher than expected death rate due to progressive disease in the case of anti-neoplastic agents.

6. Reporting of overdoses and abuse.
The MAH should report cases of overdose and abuse (accidental or intentional) that lead to serious (EU) or serious unexpected (non-EU) ADRs. This includes reports that indicate that the taking of the product led to suicidal intention and a subsequent overdose of the same or different medicinal product. However, it does not include reports of overdose or abuse that have no associated ADR, although follow-up is required to obtain relevant details.

7. Reporting of misuse.
The MAH should collect any available information related to misuse of its products, which may have an impact on their benefit–risk evaluations, and provide expedited reports for any cases of misuse that lead to serious (EU) or serious unexpected (non-EU) ADRs.

Periodic safety update reports

Companies operating within the EU are required to submit PSURs to member state authorities and the EMEA (for products authorized under the centralized procedure) in accordance with Council Regulation 2309/93 and Council Directive 2001/83/EC. Full details of the requirements are provided within the Pharmacovigilance Guidelines, which indicate that the content and format of the PSURs should generally be in accordance with standards expressed in the ICH E2C guideline.

Schedule for submission   PSURs should be prepared at the following intervals, unless specified otherwise as a condition of marketing authorization:

- six-monthly for the first 2 years after authorization;
- annually for the subsequent 3 years;
- at the time of first licence renewal;
- thereafter five-yearly (at the time of licence renewal).

The MAH's safety database should be frozen at the time points defined above ('data lock points'). Each report should cover the period since the last PSUR and be issued within 60 calendar days of the data lock point.

The Pharmacovigilance Guidelines indicate that the schedule for submission may be reset to 'zero' when a product receives approval for a new indication, dosage form, route of administration or patient population beyond the initial authorization for the active substance. Unfortunately, member state authorities have been inconsistent in their interpretation of this requirement, leading to some practical difficulties for MAHs.

Birth dates   The EU legislation specifies a periodicity for PSURs based upon the date of marketing authorization within the EU. Therefore, although the principle of an IBD was supported by the EC through their endorsement of the ICH E2C guideline, each product should have an EU birth date based upon procedure used for marketing authorization:

- centralized procedure – date of marketing authorization granted by the EC;

- mutual recognition – date of marketing authorization granted by the reference member state;

- national – the MAH may propose an EU birth date that can be applied to reporting requirements across member states.

In order to harmonize the international production of PSURs, the Pharmacovigilance Guidelines have allowed some flexibility in this requirement, to the extent that the IBD can be used to determine the schedule for submission of PSURs within the EU provided that the IBD is within 6 months of the EU birth date. Nevertheless, some national authorities have persisted with a requirement for submission of PSURs based upon the national approval dates. In practice, companies may circumvent this requirement by submitting selected PSURs early in order to synchronize the schedule across member states.

One further difficulty has arisen when some member state authorities have required updates to 5-year PSURs submitted in support of product licence renewals, if the time of renewal is in excess of 6 months from the time that the previous 5-year PSUR was written. Companies have been able to overcome this obstacle in many instances by submitting line listings and short summaries of regulatory actions and safety issues that cover the intervening period.

Content of reports   Member state authorities require and/or accept PSURs produced in accordance with the content and format specified within the ICH E2C guideline, as subsequently supported by guidance provided within the Pharmacovigilance Guidelines.

In addition, for products authorized under the centralized procedure, in accordance with Commission Regulation 540/95, all non-serious unexpected ADRs should be included within the relevant PSUR, regardless of their source or country of origin, usually as a separate line listing. These ADRs should also be considered as part of the overall evaluation of the ongoing safety profile of the product under review.

Variations in Summary of Product Characteristics   The Pharmacovigilance Guidelines requires that, if the PSUR indicates that the new safety information warrants an amendment to the SPC, the variation application should be submitted at the same time as the PSUR. Two factors sometimes make it difficult for companies to comply with this requirement:

- in-house processes often require lengthy consideration of proposed label changes, taking the decision point beyond 60 days from the data lock point;

- review of the data presented in the PSUR may generate new safety signals that will then require detailed evaluation, something that may take more than the 60 days allowed from the data lock point if the evaluation is to be thorough and considered.

Inconsistencies in EU requirements for periodic safety update reports   Since implementation of the current EU requirements for PSURs, it has become evident that several member states persist with specific national requirements in addition to the general requirements detailed above. These include:

- France, Germany, Portugal, Spain – national birth dates are applied, although they do allow companies to synchronize these with the EU birth date.

- France and Germany appear to have a relatively low threshold for resetting clock start.

- Italy requires PSURs per EU schedule *plus* abridged semi-annual reports.

- Germany requires PSURs per EU schedule *plus* 2-year and 5-year 'experience' reports.

- UK, Germany, Greece – line-listings to include non-serious listed ADRs (usually as an addendum to the report).

- Ireland – MAH to provide non-serious listed ADRs upon request.

- Belgium – PSUR to include scientific evaluation and benefit/risk statement in Dutch or French.

- Belgium, Denmark, Finland, Germany, Italy and Sweden often require *ad hoc* reports in support of product licence renewals.

Post-authorization safety studies

Post-authorization safety studies (PASSs) may be conducted for a variety of reasons:

- to identify previously unrecognized safety issues;
- to investigate possible safety hazards;
- to confirm the safety profile of a product under marketed conditions;
- to quantify or identify risk factors for established ADRs;
- to explore the clinical relevance of toxic effects apparent in pre-clinical studies.

Although the Notice to Applicants has specified requirements for the conduct of PASSs for a number of years, the legal basis for these provisions was provided by Commission Directive 2000/38/EC. The directive defines a PASS as 'a pharmaco-epidemiological study or a clinical trial carried out in accordance with the terms of the marketing authorization, conducted with the aim of identifying or quantifying a safety hazard relating to an authorized medicinal product'. This definition seemingly limits PASSs to:

- observational post-marketing surveillance or pharmacoepidemiological studies;

- 'Phase IV' clinical trials (i.e. clinical trials within the terms of the approved SPC), with evaluation of clinical safety as a primary objective.

However, the Pharmacovigilance Guidelines complicate matters by indicating that, in addition to the above definition, 'any study where the number of patients to be included will add significantly to the existing safety data for the product will also be considered a post-authorization safety study'. In theory, this could then include the large 'Phase IIIb' clinical trials usually conducted to evaluate new indications, formulations or methods of administration (i.e. outside the terms of an approved SPC), which would presumably be otherwise covered by the requirements of the Clinical Trials Directive. Hence, companies are advised to clarify their own understanding of the definition of a PASS, if necessary with the assistance of legal advice.

Regulatory requirements For each PASS, companies should interact with relevant member state authorities as follows:

- discuss the draft protocol at an early stage;

- submit for comment a copy of the final protocol and any proposed communications to doctors, at least 1 month prior to initiation of the study;

- inform the authorities when the study has commenced;

- provide interim reports on study progress every 6 months from the time of initiation, or as requested by the authorities;

- provide a copy of the final study report within 3–6 months of study completion.

In addition, companies are expected to comply with ongoing expedited and periodic ADR reporting requirements and submit the findings of the study for publication.

Electronic communication of safety information

Several member state authorities have been active in the development of technology for the electronic communication of safety data. In 1999, the EMEA, in collaboration with member state authorities and the European pharmaceutical industry, initiated a joint pilot for the electronic communication of ICSRs in accordance with ICH recommendations. This activity has culminated in the production version of the EudraVigilance system, which should facilitate a single standard for the electronic communication of safety data within the EU. The EMEA issued a policy paper in January 2002 (EMEA/H/5255/01) specifying the activities and schedule for rapid implementation of the electronic transmission of ICSRs within the EU. These include the following measures:

- Initiation of electronic transmission of ICSRs amongst member state authorities from 5 December 2001.

- Implementation of electronic transmission from pharmaceutical companies to member state authorities and/or EMEA utilizing EudraVigilance, with pre-coding of ICSRs using current versions of MedDRA and the EudraVigilance product dictionary; this was due to take effect on a mandatory basis from 31 January 2003, but delays have occurred due to technical issues, which should be resolved by end of 2003.

- Completion of migration of legacy data for all medicinal products sold within the EU from pharmaceutical companies to EudraVigilance; this was due to be completed by 31 January 2004, but delay will also occur due to technical issues.

In addition, the EC has issued the 'SUSAR database' guideline, in support of the Clinical Trials Directive, that indicates that the EudraVigilance database will eventually contain a 'Clinical Trials' module to accommodate SUSAR case reports from clinical trials.

Compliance concept paper

In November 2001, the CPMP issued the 'Position paper on compliance with pharmaco-vigilance regulatory obligations', effective from January 2002. This paper sets out the legal basis for pharmacovigilance obligations in the EU, how compliance should be monitored and the types of regulatory action that may be considered in the event of non-compliance.

The paper indicates that member state authorities will be required to conduct more frequent inspections of companies' pharmacovigilance capabilities, and that these inspec-tions will be random, systematic and targeted to facilitate, as well as to enforce, compliance with regulatory requirements.

The paper indicates that the following will be regarded as 'serious' non-compliance:

- failure to notify changes in benefit–risk profiles
- deliberate non-compliance
- failure to improve, in response to inspection findings and recommendations.

The actions that can be taken by member state authorities will include:

- education and facilitation, with advice on how to remedy non-compliance
- repeat inspections
- formal warnings
- 'naming and shaming' of serious/persistent non-compliant companies
- formal caution, if a non-compliant MAH admits that a criminal offence has occurred
- prosecution of serious/persistent non-compliant companies, including their directors, managers or the qualified person responsible for pharmacovigilance.

The United Kingdom

Legal and regulatory basis

The legal basis for UK regulations governing the conduct of pharmacovigilance and notification of safety information within the UK is provided by the Medicines Act 1968, which provides the power to make regulations using statutory instruments (SIs). The Medicines (Exemption from Licences) (Clinical Trials) Order 1995 (SI 1995/2808) and Medicines (Exemption from Licences and Certificates) (Clinical Trials) Order 1995 (SI 1995/2809) currently provide the basis for ADR reporting requirements associated with the conduct of investigational clinical trials within the UK although these will soon be superseded by SIs used to implement the requirements of the 'Clinical Trials Directive', at which time the Clinical Trial Certificate (CTC) and Clinical Trial Exemption (CTX) schemes will cease to function.

The Medicines for Human Use Regulations (SI 1994/3144) relate to medicinal products marketed within the UK. It cross-references relevant EC provisions and specifies reporting requirements for pharmaceutical companies relating to the notification of ADRs to the MCA, now known as the MHRA (Medicines and Healthcare products Regulatory Agency). More recently, SI 236/2002 transposed Commission Directive 2000/38/EC into UK law, thereby bringing the UK's ADR reporting requirements into full accordance with EU legislation.

SI 1994/3144 (Schedule 3) also created a series of criminal offences relating to failure to comply with the legal provisions governing pharmacovigilance and ADR reporting in the UK. Persons found guilty of such offences may be liable to large fines and/or terms of imprisonment. Although the offences apply to the 'person placing the medicinal product on the market', it is evident that some are also applicable to the UK company's qualified person and/or senior management.

The MCA/MHRA have provided guidance within various Medicines Act Leaflets (MAL) and Medicines Act Information Leaflets (MAIL). Although only guidelines, they do represent the agency's interpretation of UK and EU provisions for the conduct of pharmacovigilance. Hence, compliance with the guidance should minimize risk of indictment or conviction of any offence under Schedule 3 of SI 1994/3144.

Adverse drug reaction reporting requirements for investigational products

Expedited reports

Sponsors of clinical trials are required to notify relevant safety information to the MHRA's Licensing Division, whether as expedited or periodic reports. It is apparent that this division relies on sponsors to limit their expedited notifications to serious unexpected suspected ADRs (i.e. clinically important cases), and to provide (relatively) less important safety information in annual reports.

With effect from 1995, UK expedited reporting requirements, for medicinal products under clinical investigation within the UK, have been in full accordance with ICH E2A requirements. However, it is possible that some aspects may change with implementation of the Clinical Trials Directive in 2004.

Expedited reporting requirements apply to all serious unexpected ADRs occurring in association with an investigational product covered by a CTC or CTX, regardless of source or country of origin. The term 'investigational product' applies to all new chemical entities, as well as to marketed drugs being evaluated for new indications, formulations, etc.

Further to guidance issued in MAL 4 and MAIL 105, the general understanding is that:

- the 7- and 15-day time frames start on the date that the company is informed about any serious unexpected ADR on a worldwide basis;

- treatment codes should be broken prior to the expedited notification of serious unexpected ADRs from blinded clinical trials; the code break should occur at the time of receipt of information on a case report;

- case reports involving placebo do not require expedited notification.

All AEs that occur in a clinical trial conducted under a CTC or CTX should be subject to causality assessments – all cases qualify as suspected ADRs where the clinical investigator or sponsor considers that there is a 'reasonable possibility' of a causal relationship with the investigational product. Guidance in MAL 4 indicates that the MHRA considers that the expression 'reasonable causal relationship' is meant to convey that there is a rationale, based on facts or other evidence, to suggest that a causal relationship exists.

In addition to the minimum requirements for expedited reporting specified within ICH E2A, each submission needs to be clearly identified as an ADR report from a clinical trial and include the CTX number, protocol number and company reference number. Reports lacking such information will be returned for completion and resubmission by the company.

All clinical trials case reports, whether of UK origin or not, should be submitted on the Clinical Trials Unit's variation of the 'Yellow Form', as specified in MAL 4.

Periodic reports

Guidance contained in MAL 4, MAIL 88 and MAIL 105 indicates that companies are required to monitor and keep records of *all* AEs occurring during a clinical trial conducted under a CTC or CTX. The following should be reported in summary tabulations, either at the conclusion of the trial or at the time of updating or renewal of the CTX (if they occurred within the UK), or with the MAA (if from abroad):

- deaths

- serious expected ADRs

- non-serious ADRs

- withdrawals due to ADRs.

Comment should be included as to the relationship of the events to the pharmacological effects of treatment on the patient population receiving the trial drug. The report may also indicate any instances of significant lack of efficacy, and any new pre-clinical findings that are significant and/or have had an impact on the studies being conducted under the CTX.

Data Safety Monitoring Boards

The MHRA encourages companies to appoint a Data Safety Monitoring Board (DSMB) for any clinical trial that involves a patient population with a high mortality disease state, although this is not a mandatory requirement. The expectation is that this committee would:

- decode trialists' reports

- construct the group sequential analysis

- report ADRs directly to the MHRA using line listings, at agreed time intervals.

Reports submitted by the DSMB should discuss any clinically important difference in the rate of serious AEs between the investigational product and comparator(s), although a formal frequency analysis may not need to be performed.

In addition, serious unexpected ADRs should still be reported by the sponsor to the MHRA in accordance with the ICH E2A guideline.

Arrangements for establishing and reporting the line listings, and other safety information, should be defined within each trial protocol. The procedures for this form of reporting may be discussed with the MHRA Clinical Trials Unit in advance of the protocol being finalized, although there is no indication that this is mandatory.

Adverse drug reaction reporting requirements for marketed products

It is evident that the MHRA's strategy for ADR reporting has been based upon full and prompt implementation of relevant EU legislation and the guidance provided within the Pharmacovigilance Guidelines. In addition, the MHRA has been a leading proponent of requirements relating to post-authorization safety studies.

Expedited reports

Although the guidance provided within MAIL 87 refers only to spontaneous ADR reports and reports from post-marketing (safety) studies, the UK expedited reporting requirements for marketed products apply to ADRs that arise from any source, if related to the product's approved marketed use – this also includes relevant ADRs from Phase IV clinical trials and the published literature.

The UK's expedited reporting requirements are in full accordance with the requirements specified within Council Regulation 2309/93 and Commission Directive 2000/38/EC. However, as published in MAIL 130 (April 2002), the MHRA has requested that MAHs continue to notify all serious ADRs arising from within the EU for any medicinal product subject to the UK's 'Black Triangle' scheme, until such time that electronic reporting into the EudraVigilance system becomes fully operational.

The MAH is also expected to inform the MHRA without delay if any new information is received which may adversely affect the benefit–risk evaluation of the medicinal product In all instances, expedited reports should be submitted to the MHRA within 15 calendar days of initial receipt of information by the MAH – the MHRA have indicated (informally) that this applies once the information has been received by the UK company or by any of its overseas businesses (parent company or affiliates).

Expedited reports should be submitted to the MHRA using the 'Yellow Form'. This form should be used for the notification of ADRs from the UK and other EU member states; although the MHRA would also prefer that this form is also used to notify ADRs from non-EU sources, it will accept such reports on a CIOMS I form.

Periodic safety update reports

PSURs are required for all medicinal products sold within the UK, regardless of when they were first licensed or the authorization procedure used, with a periodicity for submission in accordance with that specified in Council Directive 2001/83/EC.

In general, the format and content of each PSUR should be consistent with that specified within the ICH E2C guideline. However, guidance provided in MAIL 101 indicates that the MHRA have some specific requirements:

- The timing of submission should be based on the date of first marketing authorization for the product, granted to *any company* in any country; after UK marketing authorization approval, the relevant PSURs should be submitted to the MHRA as and when they become available.

- The section on worldwide marketing authorization status should contain information on the dates of renewal as well as dates of marketing authorization.

- Line listings should include the following:

    - cases selected in accordance with ICH E2C criteria, plus

    - non-serious listed ADRs, as an addendum.

- Summary tabulations should be presented for serious and non-serious, listed and unlisted ADRs.

- A comment should be provided for any differences that exist between the CCDS and the UK Data Sheet/SPC, together with their consequences for the overall safety evaluation.

With regard to the addendum containing the line listing of non-serious listed ADRs, the guidance contained within MAIL 101 does not specify whether this applies to all non-serious listed ADRs (i.e. including those from clinical trials, named-patient use and other regulatory authorities), or whether it can be limited to non-serious listed ADRs from spontaneous reports and published literature. A reasonable assumption is that the latter situation should prevail, as most company post-marketing safety databases do not contain non-serious ADRs from clinical trials.

In addition, the MCA indicated in MAIL 101 that it 'would appreciate a more proactive approach from companies', with companies paying particular attention to the analysis of data presented in the PSUR. Hence, they suggested that the conclusion of each PSUR should cover the action required to investigate emerging safety signals, together with proposals for amending and updating the marketing authorization and product information in the light of the findings of the PSUR and cumulative experience.

Post-authorization safety studies

The MHRA is a strong advocate of the concept of post-authorization safety studies, as one of the five parties that contributed to the Safety Assessment of Marketed Medicine (SAMM) guidelines issued in 1993, which then formed the basis for the EU's provisions in this regard. Guidance issued in MAIL 87 and MAIL 104 indicates that they expect pharmaceutical companies to comply with these obligations – this will probably be supplemented by SIs implementing Council Directive 2001/83/EC, now that it provides a formal legal basis for provisions relating to post-authorization safety studies.

It is apparent that the requirements are not restricted to studies conducted within the UK, in that they may apply to any company-sponsored PASS conducted worldwide if it relates to a product authorized in the UK. In addition, MAIL 104 indicates that the company should actively seek information about the study objectives, design, time frame and results if it becomes aware of a relevant study planned or being performed in the UK by a third party, and inform the MHRA accordingly.

ADROIT Electronically Generated Information Service

For several years, the MHRA has been a strong advocate of electronic transmission of safety information. This includes the development of the ADROIT Electronically Generated Information Service (AEGIS).

The MHRA receives over 80 per cent of its ADR reports directly from UK healthcare professionals via the 'Yellow Card' scheme. In accordance with EU legislation, it is important that the agency is able to pass on information from this source to MAHs to augment their own understanding of the safety profile of products that they have on the UK market. Hence, AEGIS was introduced in 1993 to facilitate the electronic exchange of information between the pharmaceutical industry and the MHRA.

AEGIS provides companies with (restricted) on-line access to anonymized data on the ADROIT database. For a nominal sum, a company may be granted access to the following information on the ADROIT database:

- Drug Analysis Prints – summary prints of any drug substance marketed within the UK

- Product Analysis Prints – summary prints of the company's own medicinal products

- Anonymized Single Patient Prints (ASPPs) for any drug substance marketed by that company

- Reaction Analysis Prints (listing of drug substances associated with a particular reaction term)

- Fatal reports (cumulative analysis of the cause of death in ADR reports for a specific substance)

- *Ad hoc* query service.

AEGIS allows the MHRA to meet its obligation to supply information on serious ADRs to pharmaceutical companies. ASPPs for serious and non-serious reports are made available to AEGIS users on a weekly basis; companies with access to AEGIS then have the responsibility of accessing the database at regular intervals to obtain the information. In addition, the MHRA continues to send ASPPs as paper prints by post every 2 weeks to companies that do not have access through AEGIS (MAIL 87).

Reporting requirements for marketed products still under clinical investigation

There remains some ambiguity with regard to the reporting requirements for medicinal products that are marketed within the UK but which are still subject to clinical investigation.

The MHRA has previously indicated that new chemical entities and marketed drug substances that are subject to clinical investigation for new indications, formulations or routes of administration qualify as investigational products within the UK. Hence, ADRs that arise from clinical studies conducted within the remit of the UK Data Sheet/SPC (i.e. Phase IV clinical trials or PMS studies) should be notified to the Post-Licensing Division in accordance with the guidance specified in MAIL 87. ADRs that arise from clinical studies on investigational products should be notified to the Clinical Trials Unit in accordance with the provisions of MAIL 88.

France

Legal basis and regulatory framework

In general, the French ADR reporting requirements are consistent with those mandated by EU legislation and guidelines. It is evident that the Agence Française de Sécurité Sanitaire des produits de Santé (AFSSAPS) has adopted a pragmatic attitude to ADR reporting, thereby facilitating international harmonization of requirements. However, there are two French idiosyncrasies that require specific consideration, namely protocol-related events and imputability assessments (see below).

The French ADR reporting requirements for investigational products are defined by the Loi Huriet (22 December 1988), which concerns all forms of trials and medical experiments on living human beings in France, specifically Article (L1123-8) du Livre II bis du Code de la Sante Publique. The law is applicable to all biomedical research and aims to protect all subjects participating in clinical investigations.

Detailed requirements for the reporting of adverse events from clinical trials are currently specified in two guidelines, 'Recommendations du 12 Septembre 1994', issued by the AFSSAPS, and 'Recommendations for the reporting of serious events likely to be attributable to research', issued by Syndicat National de l'Industrie Pharmaceutique (SNIP) on 21 February 1997. Although draft legislation was issued in March 2003, amending the Loi Huriet in order to implement the Clinical Trials Directive, at the time of writing it is not known what changes, if any, will occur in response to implementation of the Clinical Trials Directive.

With regard to marketed products, the French government issued Decree No. 95-278 on 13 March 1995, modifying the Code de la Sante Publique and thereby implementing Council Directive 75/319/EEC (as amended). This is supported by a guideline from the AFSSAPS ('Notification of Adverse Reactions'), issued by SNIP on 18 October 1996.

Definitions

For marketed products, the AFSSAPS has applied definitions consistent with EU legislation and regulations. However, the definitions used for the notification of ADRs from clinical trials differ slightly from those in use for marketed products, most notably with regard to protocol-related events and the definition of a serious AE.

Protocol-related events

An adverse event is defined as any noxious and new medical condition occurring during the conduct of a clinical trial, whatever its cause; this specifically includes events that occur during diagnostic procedures and the washout phase of any study. Likewise, an adverse reaction is defined as any event due to the study conduct, i.e. it may relate to the design of a trial and need not be related to the study drug.

Hence, all AEs that occur during a clinical trial and cannot be related to a cause independent of the trial conditions are considered as protocol-related events. This is relevant, as such events may qualify for expedited notification to the AFSSAPS even if clearly not drug related.

Foreign patients are included in this requirement when the trial is multinational and involves French centres. This means that companies operating outside France need to be aware of which trials involve French centres.

Serious adverse events

Within the context of clinical trials conducted in France, an AE is considered as 'serious' if, in addition to the widely accepted (ICH) criteria, it meets one or more of the following criteria:

- is judged as serious in a clinical sense by either the investigator or sponsor
- is a clinically important laboratory abnormality
- is specified within the trial protocol as a serious AE (regardless of clinical outcome)
- is from the list of WHO critical terms.

Although these additional criteria appear unique to France, they all probably fall within the ICH concept of 'medically important' events and, hence, should have minimal impact upon working practice in those companies that utilize the ICH definition.

General requirements for pharmaceutical companies

In addition to the general requirements specified within the Pharmacovigilance Guidelines, any company marketing a medicinal product within France must inform the AFSSAPS of the name of the designated person responsible for pharmacovigilance within the company, who must be a physician or a pharmacist. Article R 5144-17 of the Code de la Sante Publique states: 'Every company or organization exploiting a medicine ... must have a pharmacovigilance department. The name of the person responsible for this department, medical doctor or pharmacist, must be communicated to the Drug Agency by the Responsible Pharmacist of this company or organization'.

Investigational products

French expedited reporting requirements for investigational products are generally consistent with ICH E2A, although it is possible that some details could change with implementation of the Clinical Trials Directive in 2004.

The AFSSAPS requires that the following be notified as expedited reports:

- fatal or life-threatening unexpected events – preliminary notification within seven calendar days of initial receipt of information by the sponsor, with a written report within a further eight calendar days (if the 7-day report is incomplete);

- all other serious events – written report within 15 calendar days from initial receipt of information by the sponsor.

The events that qualify for expedited reports also depend on their country of origin:

- French cases – all serious adverse experiences that are potentially related to the clinical research, i.e. study drug, active comparator, placebo or protocol-related;

- foreign cases – all serious adverse experiences that are potentially due to the clinical research (as above) when a multicentre trial involves French sites, plus all serious unexpected ADRs (i.e. only related to the study drug) when the trial is conducted abroad and lacks French centres.

In addition, companies are required to notify the AFSSAPS within 15 calendar days of acquiring any new information that can decrease the benefit–risk ratio for the subjects participating in a trial. This includes:

- serious unexpected ADRs from spontaneous reports, published literature, other regulatory agencies and foreign trials;

- results from interim analyses concerning safety or lack of efficacy;

- increased incidence of serious AE/ADRs in special groups;

- discontinuation of other clinical trials;

- new safety information arising from pre-clinical studies.

The AFSSAPS has not decreed that the study drug must be identified prior to expedited reporting. Companies may maintain the study 'blind' if they wish and submit reports to the AFSSAPS as 'code unbroken'. However, the AFSSAPS should then be notified of the drug's identity once the 'blind' has been broken at the end of the study.

Companies are required to use a local form (CERFA Form 65-0040) for the expedited notification of cases arising in France; foreign cases may be submitted using the same form or a modified CIOMS I form. In addition, the French law requires companies to notify relevant facts to ethics committees, although it appears that this seldom happens in practice. Periodic reports are not required for investigational products within France.

Marketed products

Expedited reports

In full accordance with EU legislation, the following have to be notified to the AFSSAPS within 15 days of receipt of information by the company worldwide:

- serious ADRs occurring in France

- serious unexpected ADRs from non-EU countries.

However, companies may also notify serious suspected ADRs that have come from other EU member states, although this is not a mandatory requirement.

If a serious ADR leads to an expedited modification of a French SPC, then the company involved should inform the AFSSAPS by telephone at the same time that the dossier supporting the amendment is sent by mail.

Companies are required to conduct a formal causality assessment of all serious ADRs that originate in France prior to notification to the AFSSAPS. The assessments are mandatory for all French cases, but are optional for foreign cases, and must use the official French imputability method as defined by Begaud et al. (1985). This combines chronological and semiological criteria, and results in the ranking of the suspect drug at one of five levels of causality.

Periodic safety update reports

The AFSSAPS has stipulated that PSURs should be produced in full accordance with the content, format and periodicity specified in the Pharmacovigilance Guidelines.

In addition, for products registered under French national procedures, companies should submit information on the French experience during the period under review, for the purpose of comparison with the international experience. The information required on French cases in this additional report includes:

- number of cases reported;

- summary table of ADRs classified by nature and imputability to drug;

- number of 'serious' case reports;

- serious ADRs classified as 'unexpected' with reference to the French SPC;

- evaluation of the number of patients treated in France;

- conclusion, including a comparison with the previous situation and implications for the French SPC.

The AFSSAPS has indicated that companies having to satisfy international periodic reporting requirements, may present PSURs made up of 6-month units, with a global evaluation of the period covered by the report. In addition, manufacturers may consult with the AFSSAPS in order to agree birth dates that would be mutually acceptable to both parties.

Germany

Legal basis and regulatory framework

The German Drug Law (AMG), most notably Sections 29(1) and 49, provides the legal basis for current German ADR reporting requirements. This covers the manufacturers' obligations relating to the conduct of pharmacovigilance, expedited and periodic reporting and the graduated plan (Stufenplanverfahren). The 3rd Promulgation (May 1996) on the Notification of Adverse Reactions, Interaction with Other Products and Drug Abuse, produced by the Federal Institute for Drugs and Medical Devices (BfArM) and the Paul-Ehrlich Institut for Sera, Vaccines and Blood Products, provides the German authorities' interpretation of the AMG.

The AMG specifics a series of offences and penalties for non-compliance with its requirements. For example, there is an administrative offence relating to non-compliance with the requirements of Section 29(1) that may incur a large personal fine for the Stufenplanbeauftragter (see below). In addition, the Stufenplanbeauftragter may also be liable to criminal prosecution for bodily injury or involuntary manslaughter.

Definitions

The BfArM has adopted most of the relevant ICH definitions and those stipulated by EU legislation. However, the 3rd Promulgation introduced some variation, providing some definitions that appear applicable only in Germany, as presented below.

Adverse reaction

In addition to the definition provided by Council Directive 2001/83/EC, the BfArM considers that an ADR should be suspected if an AE meets two other criteria:

- the event has a temporal association with administration of the product (including an allowance for the possibility of delayed effects), and

- the event has evidently not been brought about by any cause other than administration of the drug.

All events attributable to causes other than administration of the drug should be considered as unrelated to the drug. This includes symptoms due to a patient's underlying disease or concurrent disease, although deterioration of a patient's symptoms should be evaluated to determine whether this has been due to natural disease progression or caused by the drug.

Lack of efficacy

Occurrences of lack of efficacy should be treated in the same way as conventional ADRs when the lack of efficacy is considered to have damaged the patient's health. This is especially so when associated with drug interactions or insufficient efficacy of sera, vaccines, blood preparations, test allergens, test sera and test antigens.

Serious adverse event

The BfArM has clarified two aspects of the definition of a serious AE:

- the term 'unexplained death' should be used to describe the event when the cause of death cannot be determined;

- the term 'disability' applies when the patient has suffered considerable disability or permanent damage, including, in particular, the inability to work as a result of lasting damage to health.

Healthcare professionals

German regulations require that ADRs should be confirmed by healthcare professionals in order to qualify for notification to BfArM, although BfArM will accept consumer reports if they are of clinical importance and have been evaluated by the Stufenplanbeauftragter.

The 3rd Promulgation indicates that non-medical practitioners (Heilpraktiker) and psychotherapists qualify as healthcare professionals in Germany, in addition to those specified within the Pharmacovigilance Guidelines.

Commissioner for the Graduated Plan (Stufenplanbeauftragter)

Any company marketing a medicinal product in Germany must appoint a Commissioner for the Graduated Plan (Stufenplanbeauftragter). The individual must be qualified in human or veterinary medicine or pharmacy and should have an appropriate level of knowledge and reliability necessary for the collection, evaluation and notification of ADR reports, and coordination of any measures that might be required consequent to any changes to the company's product safety profile. The company is required to notify the name of this individual, and any changes in personnel thereafter, to the local German authority.

The Stufenplanbeauftragter has personal responsibility for ensuring that their company complies with the relevant parts of the AMG, and is personally liable for meeting any fines in the event of an administrative offence.

Expedited reports

German expedited reporting requirements are currently identical for investigational and marketed medicinal products, although, at the time of writing, it is not known what changes (if any) will occur with regard to investigational products as a result of implementation of the Clinical Trials Directive.

At present, unlike the rest of the EU, *all* serious ADRs qualify for expedited reporting to the BfArM, within 15 days from the date of initial receipt by the German company/affiliate, whether they originate from a clinical study or from post-marketing use, and regardless of the country of origin. The only exceptions relate to:

- ADRs associated with medicinal products authorized under the EU's centralized procedure – these require notification in accordance with the case selectivity specified by Council Regulation 2309/93;

- ADRs cited in the scientific literature – single case reports should be notified to the BfArM within 15 days if they are serious and unexpected.

German and foreign cases may be notified in German or English, either using a specific German form, the 'Bericht uber unerwunschte Arzneimittelwirkungen' ('Adverse Drug Reaction Report'), or a CIOMS I form.

Reporting requirements before marketing authorization

The requirement for the expedited notification of reports for investigational products depends upon the German registration status of the product. Reports should be submitted prior to submission of an MAA simply for the purpose of registration with the BfArM, whereas, following submission of the MAA, cases should be notified expeditiously if they are considered relevant to the ongoing evaluation of the submission.

Hence, prior to submission of the dossier, serious ADRs should only be sent as expedited reports to the BfArM if they arise from clinical trials conducted in Germany or international clinical trials that have centres in Germany. Once the submission has been filed, then serious ADRs of foreign origin should be notified, whether arising from post-marketed use or clinical trials that do not have German centres, in addition those of German origin.

Minimum criteria for expedited reports

Although case reports should contain at least the minimum information specified within the Pharmacovigilance Guidelines, the BfArM has indicated that expedited reports are still required should follow-up of serious unexpected ADRs that lack specific patient identification (e.g. 'in several patients', 'in x per cent of patients') not result in further detailed information.

Management of adverse drug reactions from 'blind' clinical trials

The 3rd Promulgation indicates that randomization codes should be broken prior to notification of ADRs that arise from 'blinded' clinical trials. However, the guidance does not explicitly state that the 'blind' must be broken at the time that the German company receives information on a serious ADR. Instead, it indicates that the period for immediate notification commences with the breaking of the blind.

In practice, it is apparent that BfArM expects companies to break the blind for serious unexpected ADRs on an immediate basis and report these accordingly. However, companies may elect to defer the code break for serious expected ADRs until completion of the trial and its database lock, with an expectation that expedited notification will occur within 15 days of the eventual code break.

Scientific evaluations

All expedited reports, regardless of their country of origin, are subject to 'scientific evaluation' prior to submission to the BfArM. Each evaluation should include:

- the case description;

- assessments of causality and expectedness, and whether the status of scientific knowledge regarding the product has changed;

- evaluation of whether measures are required with regard to the approval status of the product or reduction of the risk to other patients.

Drug abuse and misuse

The AMG places a significant emphasis on the need for companies to report drug abuse, defined as the deliberate maladministration of a drug, especially when associated with damage to human health. Companies should notify all known instances of frequent abuse or significant abuse in a single individual, if the abuse may (directly or indirectly) endanger human health.

The 3rd Promulgation specifically indicates that AE occurring in association with off-label use should be managed in the same manner as ADRs that occur during licensed use of the drug.

Periodic safety update reports

Periodic safety updates are not required for investigational products.

For products licensed in Germany, PSURs should be submitted, in English or German, in the same time frame as that used elsewhere within the EU. However, the 'clock' is often reset in any circumstance that requires renewal of the marketing authorization, most notably approval of a new indication (even for a well-established 'mature' product).

Although the BfArM has indicated that the schedule for submission should be based on the German date of marketing authorization, it allows German MAHs to submit their initial PSURs early so that the schedule can then be synchronized with that determined by the EU birth date.

Strict interpretation of Section 29 of AMG requires that a PSUR should include all ADRs notified to the company during the period under review. In practice, the BfArM accepts PSURs produced in accordance with the Pharmacovigilance Guidelines, supplemented with a line listing of non-serious expected ADRs.

In addition, PSURs submitted to the BfArM should include a section focusing on the product's ongoing safety profile with regard to marketed use in Germany. Current understanding is that this section should highlight differences between the CCDS and the German SPC, and indicate the actions that the German company/affiliate will undertake in response to new information generated within the PSUR

Experience reports

In addition to PSURs, companies are also expected to submit 'experience' reports 2 years and 5 years after initial marketing authorization, in accordance with Section 49(6) of AMG. 'Experience' reports should be structured as follows:

- Registration status.

- Details of marketing authorizations in other countries, including conditions of approval and reasons for any withdrawals or rejections.

- German sales data and foreign sales data, plus an estimate of the number of patients exposed.

- List of studies performed, together with copies of all study reports finalized during the reporting period.

- Summary of type and frequency of ADRs.

- Summary and conclusion, with an assessment of any change to the benefit–risk evaluation and justification for any unexpected ADR report that remains absent from the German SPC.

United States of America

Legal and regulatory framework

In the USA, the legal basis for drug regulation, including those governing pharmacovigilance and ADR reporting, is provided by the Kefauver–Harris Amendments ('1962 Amendments') to the Federal Food, Drugs and Cosmetics Act of 1938. The 1962 Amendments also provide the FDA with the power to revoke authorization for clinical trials at any time, if it suspects that the drug under investigation is unsafe. In addition, although the amendments do not mandate PMS, the FDA is empowered to require that a manufacturer conducts post-marketing clinical studies as a condition of approval of a New Drug Application (NDA), if it considers that further demonstration of safety is necessary once a product is on the market.

Federal regulations oblige the sponsor of an IND or the manufacturer granted an NDA to report suspected ADRs to the FDA, for all medicinal products sold or being developed in the USA. These are specified in Title 21 of the Code of Federal Regulations, as follows:

- 21 CFR 310.304: 'grandfathered' drugs (pre-1938)

- 21 CFR 312.32: IND Safety Reports

- 21 CFR 314.80: post-marketing reporting (drugs) – applicable to medicinal products granted a marketing licence, either as a full NDA or abbreviated application [ANDA]

- 21 CFR 314.98: generic products

- 21 CFR 600.80: post-marketing reporting (biologics) – applicable to licensed biological products (including vaccines).

The Expedited Safety Reporting Final Rule, published in the Federal Register on 7 October 1997 and effective from 6 April 1998, amended the above regulations in order to improve harmonization of US expedited reporting standards with other ICH regions.

In March 2003, the FDA issued a proposed rule, 'Safety Reporting Requirements for Human Drug and Biological Products', otherwise known as the 'Safety Tome', which proposes significant changes to for pre- and post-approval safety reporting requirements. At the time of writing, the proposals have been subject to extensive review and comment by interested parties, and it is likely that they will not become fully effective before the latter part of 2004.

FDA guidance on ADR reporting is provided in several documents, including:

- Guideline for Post-marketing Reporting of Adverse Drug Experiences (March 1992)

- Guideline for Adverse Experience Reporting for Licensed Biological Products (October 1993)

- Guidance for Industry Post-marketing Adverse Experience Reporting for Human Drug and Licensed Biological Products: Clarification of what to report (August 1997).

Federal regulations clearly indicate that ADR reporting requirements are not specific to the US company that holds the IND application or NDA, but also apply to any of its affiliates, these being any corporate entity relating to the applicant, including all subsidiaries, licensees or licensors.

Food and Drug Administration

The FDA is responsible for assuring the safety and efficacy of all regulated medical products developed or marketed in the USA, including biological products. Two departments within the FDA bear this responsibility:

- Center for Drug Evaluation and Research (CDER), responsible for monitoring the safety of the majority of drugs sold or developed in the USA.

- Center for Biological Evaluation and Research (CBER), responsible for monitoring the safety of licensed biological products and vaccines.

Safety information on investigational products should be notified to the relevant therapeutic division within the Office of New Drugs. The Office of Drug Safety has responsibility for post-marketing ADR reporting for non-biological products and operates the Adverse Event Reporting System (AERS) database for post-marketing pharmacovigilance purposes. The AERS database also generates compliance reports that enable the Office of Compliance to determine whether companies are submitting reports in accordance with federal regulations. A programme is currently ongoing to develop the methodology for manufacturers to download safety data electronically onto AERS in accordance with ICH standards.

Definitions

Definitions relevant to ADR reporting are provided within 21 CFR Sections 312.32(b) and 314.80(a) for IND applications and NDAs respectively. In general, these are consistent with the corresponding ICH definitions. Those specific to the USA are presented below.

Sponsor

The sponsor is the person or corporate entity that takes responsibility for, and initiates, a clinical investigation, and may be an individual or pharmaceutical company, government agency, academic institution, private or other organization. In practice, the sponsor is the individual/organization that submitted the IND application covering the clinical investigation.

Adverse drug experience

Within the USA, the term 'adverse drug experience' (ADE) tends to be used rather than the terms AE or ADR. In practice, an ADE is considered synonymous with an AE. Indeed, FDA guidance on this matter indicates that reporting an ADE does not necessarily reflect a conclusion by the company or the FDA that the event is causally related to the drug.

An ADE is defined as any AE associated with the use of a drug or biological product in humans, whether or not considered to be product related. It includes AEs occurring in the usual course of professional practice (i.e. 'spontaneous' reports), as well as those occurring in association with overdose or abuse of a product, whether accidental or intentional. An ADE also includes any *significant* failure of expected pharmacological action.

Adverse drug reaction

At present, there is no federal definition of an ADR. However, expressions are used in the IND and NDA regulations that are synonymous in their meaning.

Under the terms of an IND, sponsors are required to notify ADEs that are 'associated with the use of the drug'. This means that there is a 'reasonable possibility' that the experience may have been caused by the drug, analogous to the philosophy that has since been adopted by the ICH in its definition of a suspected ADR.

All ADEs notified on an unsolicited basis to pharmaceutical companies or direct to the FDA, by healthcare professionals or consumers, are considered as 'spontaneous reports'. In the context of federal regulations, all spontaneous reports are regarded as ADRs: the mere act of unsolicited notification implies that the reporter suspects that a causal relationship exists.

Serious adverse drug experience

As of 6 April 1998, the FDA formally adopted the ICH definition of a serious AE and applied it equally to the pre- and post-marketing situations.

The FDA has clarified that the term 'persistent or significant disability' equates with a substantial disruption in a person's ability to conduct normal life functions.

With regard to the 'important medical event' criterion, the FDA's MedWatch programme has simplified this to 'requires intervention to prevent permanent impairment or damage'. Under IND regulations, a serious ADE also includes any experience suggesting a significant risk for human subjects, including any finding of mutagenicity, teratogenicity or carcinogenicity with respect to results obtained from pre-clinical testing.

Unexpected/unlabelled adverse drug experience

The terms 'expected' and 'labelled' tend to be used interchangeably within the USA, as are 'unexpected' and 'unlabelled'. Although the IND and NDA definitions of 'unexpected' relate to different reference documentation, they are consistent in that they both refer to the specificity or severity of the event in the reference documents. However, whilst the IND definition of 'unexpected' is consistent with that provided by the ICH, under the terms of an NDA, an ADE is regarded as 'unexpected' simply if it is not listed in the current Professional Information Brochure (PIB) for the product.

Federal regulations also clarify that the term 'unexpected' refers to an ADE that has not previously been observed during the use of the product, rather than from the perspective of such an experience not being anticipated from the product's pharmacological properties. In addition, an observed event does not necessarily equate with an 'expected' event: its frequency and severity need full characterization before it can be considered as 'expected'. This is clarified by the Federal Register, which indicates that 'a sponsor would be required to report each successive case of a serious and unexpected adverse experience until the risk posed by the experience is sufficiently well understood to be described in the Investigator's Brochure or until an equally satisfactory resolution of the issue is reached (for example, a determination that the experience is not drug related)', i.e. a serious ADR that had been reported previously could still be regarded as 'unexpected'.

The 1992 guideline on post-marketing reporting indicates that class-related effects should be considered as 'unexpected' if they are not mentioned with specific regard to the product within its label. For example, a rash should be considered as unexpected even if the label refers to 'Rash may be associated with this class of antibiotics', when it lacks a specific reference to the occurrence of rash from the product itself.

Interpretation of Food and Drug Administration guidance on reporting deaths

Although there is no specific reference to death in relation to 'unexpectedness' in the IND or NDA regulations, the FDA issued guidance on this topic in its 1992 guideline on post-marketing reporting. Although issued with regard to NDA reports, it can be assumed that this guidance also applies to IND reporting.

The guideline indicates that death is 'unlabelled' (i.e. 'unexpected') when labelling does not specify that the event may be associated with a fatal outcome. The guideline indicates that the FDA expects to be notified about all ADRs that have a fatal outcome, even when the cause of death is unknown. Manufacturers and sponsors only need to determine whether notification occurs on an expedited or periodic basis, the primary consideration being the 'expectedness' of the fatal outcome.

However, the guideline oversimplifies the clinical relevance of a fatal outcome and disregards the clinical context within which that fatality occurs. Hence, companies must decide for themselves the extent to which they will act in accordance with this guidance.

Reporting requirements for investigational products

IND regulations require that the sponsor shall promptly review all information relevant to the safety of the drug obtained or otherwise received from *any* source, foreign or domestic. Sponsors are required to notify ADEs that are associated with the use of the drug and have a reasonable possibility of a causal relationship (i.e. suspected ADRs), either as expedited or as periodic reports, dependent upon the nature of the ADE.

Investigational New Drug safety reports

Consistent with ICH E2A, expedited reports ('IND safety reports') are required for the following:

- all serious unexpected ADRs associated with the use of the investigational drug product, regardless of source, including trials not covered by the IND and post-marketing use, or country of origin;

- any significant finding from pre-clinical tests, including reports of mutagenicity, teratogenicity or carcinogenicity.

The only qualification relates to the time allowed for the sponsor to notify the relevant division of CDER or CBER:

- 7 days (via telephone/fax) – fatal or life-threatening unexpected ADRs, to be followed by a written report within a further 8 days;

- 15 days (written report) – other serious unexpected ADRs and significant pre-clinical findings.

The 7-day reports need only be notified to the FDA. However, all 15-day reports should be sent simultaneously to the FDA and investigators covered by the IND.

There is no need to notify ADRs that occur in association with administration of placebo. If an active comparator is involved, then ADRs should be notified either to the FDA or manufacturer of the comparator. In the latter instance, it is the responsibility of the receiving company to assess whether the ADR is ultimately reportable to the FDA.

All relevant follow-up information relating to a previously submitted IND safety report should be notified to the FDA as soon as the relevant information becomes available. If the results of the follow-up establish that an ADE initially considered as non-reportable has become reportable under the provisions of an IND, then the sponsor is required to send an IND safety report to the FDA within 15 days of making such a determination.

Each written notification should be submitted as follows:

- domestic case – Form 3500A or in a narrative format;

- foreign case – Form 3500A or CIOMS I form, or in a narrative format;

- results from animal or epidemiological studies – narrative format.

The sponsor should identify all safety reports previously filed under the IND that concern a similar adverse experience, together with an analysis of the significance of the adverse experience in the light of previous, similar reports.

An FDA commentary issued in the Federal Register (7 October 1997) indicates that sponsors should break the 'blind' for reportable events that occur during 'blind' clinical investigations, at the level of the individual subject/patient in question. It also advises that sponsors should consult with the FDA division responsible for the product's IND if they are concerned that breaking the 'blind' would compromise their study, e.g. when a fatal or other serious outcome is the primary efficacy endpoint in the clinical trial.

Further guidance indicates the following for ADEs that occur in association with products approved for marketing within the USA:

- ADRs that occur during an IND clinical study, relating to a product with an approved NDA, are subject to both IND and NDA reporting requirements; evaluations of 'expectedness' should be based on the use of IB and PIB for respective reference purposes.

- ADRs that occur outside an IND study, relating to a product with an approved NDA, are only subject to NDA reporting requirements, even if the product has an 'open' IND.

Thus, the only time that an event should be reported to both IND and NDA would be when a serious suspected ADR occurs in an IND study, and the event is classified as 'unexpected' on the basis of both IB and PIB.

Investigational New Drug annual reports

The sponsor is required to submit a report on the progress of clinical investigations within 60 days of each IND anniversary. This annual report should include:

- Individual study information – status of each study covered by the IND in progress or completed during the year under review.
- Summary information:
  - most frequent and most serious adverse experiences;
  - all IND (15 day) safety reports submitted during the year under review;
  - list of all subjects who died, with their cause of death;
  - list of subjects withdrawn in association with adverse experiences;
  - brief description of information relevant to the understanding of the drug's actions;
  - list of pre-clinical studies completed and a summary of major findings;
  - summary of any significant manufacturing or microbiological changes.
- Other information:
  - description of the general plan of investigation for the forthcoming year;

- description of any revisions to the IB and a copy of the updated IB;

- description of any modifications made to Phase I protocols not previously reported to the IND in a protocol amendment;

- brief summary of any significant foreign regulatory or marketing developments;

- log of any outstanding business with respect to the IND for which the sponsor expects a reply, comment or meeting.

Reporting requirements for marketed products

Each company (the 'applicant') having a product cleared for marketing is required to review all ADEs obtained, or otherwise received, from all sources, whether foreign or domestic. Whether through expedited or periodic reports, the following must currently be reported:

- all spontaneous reports of ADEs occurring within the USA ('domestic' reports);

- foreign, literature and study reports involving

  - serious unexpected ADEs

  - increased frequency of serious labelled ADEs.

Study reports should only be submitted if there is 'reasonable possibility' that the drug caused the ADE, i.e. it is a suspected ADR.

Responsibility for submission of reports also applies to any person or entity whose name appears on the label of a marketed drug as its manufacturer, packer or distributor. However, the regulations do allow the 'non-applicant' to discharge responsibility by ensuring that all relevant information is communicated to the applicant within 5 days of its receipt by the non-applicant. However, the non-applicant is then obliged to maintain a record of any such action.

Expedited reports

The applicant must notify to the FDA all ADEs that are both serious and unexpected, regardless of source, within 15 calendar days of the time of initial receipt of information by the applicant. With regard to ADEs from clinical trials or post-marketing studies, the applicant should report only those cases that are serious, unexpected and considered as having a reasonable possibility that the drug caused the event, i.e. serious unexpected ADRs. Although not specifically stated in the regulations, it is apparent that the 'regulatory clock' for 15-day reports starts at the time that the applicant receives sufficient information to identify a valid case as 'serious'. For foreign cases, the 'clock' begins when the applicant or its foreign affiliate/HQ has received sufficient data to suggest that the 15-day criteria have been met.

If the initial 15-day report contains incomplete information, the applicant should file a preliminary report pending the receipt of further information. Additional follow-up information should then be sought, at least sufficient to complete a Form 3500A, and submitted to the FDA within 15 calendar days after receipt of any new information. If additional information is not obtainable, then the applicant should maintain records of the steps taken to seek additional information.

Domestic case reports should be notified using the FDA Form 3500A or, for vaccines, a

VAERS form. Foreign cases may be submitted using Form 3500A or a CIOMS I form. Reports may be submitted using a computer-generated format provided that the content is equivalent in terms of the information that would otherwise have been provided on a Form 3500A and that the format is agreed in advance with the FDA.

Data elements for a post-marketing safety report   The August 1997 CDER/CBER guideline indicates that case reports should meet minimum criteria for reporting, analogous to those specified within ICH E2A, before submission to the FDA. Case reports not meeting this standard should not be submitted to the FDA. If a report is submitted that lacks one or more of the basic data elements, then it will be returned to the reporter marked 'insufficient data for a report'.

Case reports should contain enough information to indicate that a specific patient was involved. For example, a report stating that 'an elderly woman had anaphylaxis' or 'a young man experienced anaphylaxis' is acceptable, whereas one that states 'some patients got anaphylaxis' does not meet the specified requirements.

The ADE being reported should have some specificity, e.g. one or more signs (including abnormal laboratory findings), symptoms or disease diagnosis. Reports that state, for example, 'experienced unspecified injury' or 'suffered irreparable damage' should not be submitted until more specific information about the nature of the AE can be determined.

Scientific literature   Serious unexpected ADEs reported in the scientific literature, either as case reports or as results of clinical study, must be submitted as 15-day reports on a suitable form together with a copy of the article, translated into English if published in a foreign language. A separate Form 3500A should be completed for each identifiable patient.

If the article refers to more than one drug product, then the manufacturer of the 'suspect drug' is responsible for submission of the report to the FDA; the 'suspect drug' is usually that identified by the article's author, often within the article's title.

Solicited information   The 1997 CDER/CBER guideline indicates that information concerning potential ADEs received during planned contacts and active solicitation of information from patients (e.g. patient support programmes, disease management programmes) are not considered as 'spontaneous' reports. They should be handled in the same way as case reports obtained from post-marketing studies, i.e. ADEs should only be submitted if they are serious, unexpected and there is reasonable possibility that the drug caused the event.

Overdose   Reports of overdose should be submitted only when the overdose was associated with an adverse experience; the ADE would qualify for a 15-day report if it was serious, unexpected and suspected as being drug related.

Reporting of events on another company's products

There are no regulated requirements for sponsors of clinical trials to notify ADRs that occur with active comparator agents on an expedited basis to the FDA. However, the FDA has indicated that sponsors should choose to notify serious unexpected ADRs that occur in patients given active comparators either to the relevant regulatory authorities or to the manufacturer of the product concerned.

With regard to marketed products, the 1992 guideline indicates that the recipient of reports of serious unexpected ADRs that occur in patients administered products subject to another company's NDA should notify the product's manufacturer, not the FDA.

Periodic reports

Periodic reports are due on a quarterly basis during the first 3 years after NDA approval and annually thereafter. If there is a delay between the granting of a licence and initial marketing within the USA, then quarterly reports will be required for the first 3 years after initiation of marketing. Federal regulations also allow the FDA to extend the time over which quarterly reports should be submitted, e.g. after the submission of a major supplemental NDA.

Quarterly reports must be submitted to the FDA within 30 calendar days of the last day of the reporting quarter. Annual reports must be submitted within 60 calendar days of the anniversary date of NDA approval.

Cases that qualify for inclusion in the report are summarized in Table 9.7.

Table 9.7   Case reports qualifying for inclusion in a US periodic report

Source	Type of case report
Spontaneous reports	All domestic ADEs (serious and non-serious)
	Foreign serious unexpected ADEs
Published literature	Serious unexpected ADEs
Clinical trials and PMS studies	Serious unexpected ADRs

In addition, all domestic spontaneous reports of 'lack of effect' (i.e. failure to produce the expected pharmacological effect) should be submitted in the periodic report with other domestic ADEs. However, reports of 'lack of effect' do not require notification to the FDA if from abroad and/or associated with an unapproved indication.

The FDA has specifically indicated that the following cases do *not* need to be submitted as part of a periodic report:

- domestic serious unexpected spontaneous ADEs (as they should already have been notified as 15-day reports);

- foreign marketing experience (except serious unexpected ADEs);

- ADEs from post-marketing studies, except serious unexpected ADRs;

- ADE reports within the scientific literature, except serious unexpected ADEs.

Each periodic report should contain four sections arranged in the following order:

1. Form 3500As – for each serious expected and non-serious unexpected spontaneous report.
   The 1997 CDER/CBER guideline indicates that the FDA will issue a waiver for the requirement to submit Form 3500As for non-serious expected case reports, upon specific request by the applicant.

2. Line listing of Form 3500As submitted in Section 1.

For any drug interaction listed as an ADE, the interacting drugs should be identified in this line listing.

3. Narrative summary and analysis of information in the periodic report, as well as an analysis of the 15-day reports submitted during the reporting period.
    This section should include:

    *   a listing of the 15-day reports submitted during the period under review;

    *   a listing of all ADE terms and counts of occurrences during the period under review, taken from the 15-day reports of serious unlabelled ADEs notified during the period;

    *   a summary of ADE reports in which the drug was listed as one of the suspect drugs but the report was filed to another NDA held by the applicant;

    *   a narrative discussion of the clinical significance of the 15-day reports, assessing the clinical significance and an overall evaluation of the new information received during the period under review relating to that already known about the drug.

4. Narrative discussion of action(s) taken as a result of new safety information, including any labelling changes or studies initiated since the last periodic report, a summary of important foreign actions (e.g. new warnings, limitations in indications and use of the product), any communications of new safety information (e.g. 'Dear Doctor' letters) and a copy of the current PIB.

ICH E2C periodic safety update reports   The FDA has indicated that it will accept periodic reports in accordance with ICH E2C format and content, provided that the applicant first secures a waiver from the FDA. Current experience indicates that the waiver could be subject to some or all of the following conditions:

*   PSURs are prepared in accordance with the ICH E2C guideline, as published in the Federal Register (19 May 1997).

*   PSURs are submitted in accordance with the usual periodicity and time frames for US periodic reports, i.e. quarterly reports may still be required for new products, with 30-day deadlines for submission; however, there are instances whereby the FDA will accept PSURs every 6 months for the first 2 years after approval, and annually thereafter, based upon the IBD and all with 60-day deadlines for submission.

*   All indications, dosage forms and formulations may be covered in a single PSUR, subject to the following:

    –   a copy should be submitted to each approved NDA/ANDA covered by the PSUR;

    –   information on different dosage forms, formulations and/or indications should be presented in separate sections, if needed to portray accurately the safety profile of the product, e.g. do not combine safety information from ophthalmic drop dosage forms with solid oral dosage forms.

- Appendices should be attached, as follows:

  - copies of 3500A forms as required by 21 CFR 314.80(c)(2), including consumer reports;

  - tabular listing of all consumer-reported AE terms and counts of non-serious listed ADRs, if such cases are not already included in the international PSUR;

  - a narrative that references the changes considered as appropriate in the CCDS, as well as any changes considered appropriate to the approved US labelling for the product(s) covered by the PSUR;

  - a copy of the most recently approved US labelling for the product(s) covered by the PSUR.

Record keeping

The applicant is required to keep records of all ADEs for 10 years, including raw data and any correspondence relating to ADEs. Manufacturers, packers and distributors are required to permit any authorized FDA employee to have access to, copy and verify such records.

The 'Safety Tome'

On 14 March 2003, the FDA published a 93-page proposed rule to change the requirements associated with pre- and post-approval safety reporting for drugs, biologics, and devices. Significant revisions to existing definitions and reporting requirements are proposed, with a number of new definitions and reporting requirements added, which, if implemented, will have significant practical implications for industry.

An extended period has been allowed for comments by interested parties owing to the length of the proposed rule, with final comments not due to the FDA until October 2003. The final rule will become effective 180 days after its publication in the Federal Register, likely to be in early 2004, although a full year will be allowed for compliance with the requirement for use of the MedDRA coding dictionary.

In summary, the major changes being proposed are as follows:

- New definition for a suspected ADR, to replace the term 'adverse drug experience'; to be 'a noxious and unintended response to any dose of a drug product for which a relationship between the product and the response to the product *cannot be ruled out*'.

- Definitions for 'Actual' and 'Potential' medication errors; all (actual and potential) medication error reports would require 15-day expedited reporting.

- Nineteen medical conditions, which, if reported as AEs, would always be subject to 15-day expedited reporting, regardless of seriousness, outcome, or expectedness.

- 15-day expedited safety reporting requirements will be applied to human bioavailability and bioequivalence studies, whether or not conducted under an IND; additionally, any information that leads to a consideration of change in product administration or consideration of a change in the conduct of a study would also qualify for 15-day expedited reporting.

- A healthcare professional at the company will have to speak directly to the initial reporter of an ADR or medication error to obtain the information needed for a complete data set, i.e. letters will no longer be acceptable as a method of obtaining follow-up information; all active query efforts will have to be documented in detail in the report narrative.

- In addition to the usual 15-day follow-up reports, the sponsor will also have to submit a 30-day follow-up report to document specific efforts taken to obtain new information and the reason for the inability to obtain complete information if there is no new information.

- If the sponsor is unable to determine whether the outcome of an ADR was serious or non-serious, a report will need to be submitted to FDA in 45 days from time of first awareness with a detailed description of all active query attempts.

- Completion of all fields of the MedWatch Form 3500A will be required for US cases; completion of all fields on a CIOMS report will be required for cases of non-US origin.

- Use of the MedDRA dictionary will be required for coding ADRs in individual case safety reports.

- All licensing partners and others defined as 'contractors' would have to exchange all serious and non-serious ADRs and medication errors within five calendar days.

- US-specific implementation of ICH E2C periodic reporting standards. Although the framework for periodic reports will be based upon E2C, the proposal includes unique Interim Periodic Safety Reports (IPSRs) and semi-annual submission of individual case safety reports. It is also proposed that there are various US-specific addenda as a supplement to each PSUR. The schedule for submission of reports will be amended, although it will remain different to the schedule in operation in the EU and Japan. Retention of 'traditional' US periodic reports for legacy products will be allowed for those companies that wish to retain this system for the older products.

Japan

Legal basis and regulatory framework

The Pharmaceutical Affairs Law provides the legal basis for pharmacovigilance requirements in Japan, supplemented by a variety of communications issued by the MHLW.

The management of safety information obtained during clinical trials conducted in Japan is specified in the Notification No. 227 (1995), MHLW Ordinance No. 28 – Good Clinical Practice (1997) and Notification No. 445 – Operation of GCP (1997).

In response to health scares associated with HIV contamination of blood products used by haemophiliacs in the 1980s and, more recently, unexpected side effects from various drug products, there are a series of post-marketing provisions. The most important are provided by:

- Standard for implementation of post-marketing surveillance for the re-examination application of new drugs (1991)

- Standard for the conduct of good post-marketing surveillance practice (GPMSP) (1993) and MHLW Ordinance No. 10 (GPMSP) (1997)

- Ordinance No. 29 – Enforcement of the pharmaceutical affairs law, Article 66-7 (1997)

- Notification No. 1324 – Implementation of early post-marketing phase vigilance (2001)

- Notification IYAKUAN No. 0531001 – Electronic ADR reporting (2002).

General requirements

All Japanese companies must make the following provisions for the conduct of PMS:

- establish 'PMS Management Departments' with sufficient qualified staff and independent of sales/marketing departments;

- appoint a 'Responsible Person' for PMS management;

- prepare and comply with relevant standard operating procedures.

Definitions

Japanese definitions are generally in accordance with those specified in ICH guidelines. The MHLW has utilized the ICH definition of a serious AE but without the inclusion of the 'medically important' criterion and 'disability' is defined as any disablement that is a permanent dysfunction such that it causes a disturbance in daily life; in practice, companies can operate successfully in Japan using the ICH definitions.

Investigational products

Japanese expedited reporting requirements for investigational products are generally consistent with the ICH E2A guideline. However, the requirements also specify that fatal or life-threatening *expected* ADRs qualify for 15-day reports (see Table 9.8). These requirements are regardless of the country of origin of the case report. The requirements also apply to the following:

- ADRs that relate to products marketed in Japan that are also subject to clinical investigation for new formulations or indications; such ADRs require duplicate reporting to the respective divisions within the MHLW that handle investigational and marketed products;

- any reports of infection that occur in association with the administration of a parenteral drug product.

Table 9.8 Japanese expedited reporting requirements – investigational products

Report	ADRs that qualify for reporting
7-day	Fatal or life-threatening unexpected
15-day	Serious unexpected
	Fatal or life-threatening expected

In addition, 15-day reports should be filed if results from clinical research indicate an increased frequency of ADRs, lack of efficacy or the possibility of an association with onset of cancer, important medical events, disability/incapacity, or a fatal outcome.

The MHLW has indicated that the sponsor should assess the causal relationship for all serious AEs that occur in clinical trials on products that are under clinical investigation in Japan, even if the AE occurs abroad. In addition, each report should include a formal assessment of the clinical importance of the case and relevant previous experience with the same or similar medicinal products.

There are no requirements in Japan for submission of periodic safety updates before marketing authorization is granted. However, as submissions in Japan often taken place once a product has been marketed elsewhere, it is usual for the Japanese NDA ('Gaiyo') submission to include a PSUR summarizing overseas post-marketing safety experience.

Marketed products

Post-marketing surveillance activities

Once a company secures approval to market a drug in Japan, it must evaluate the product's safety over a 4, 6 or 10 year 're-examination' period, dependent upon the nature of the drug.

The activities that must take place in the early post-marketing phase are as follows:

- early post-marketing phase vigilance (EPPV);

- Clinical Experience Investigation (CEI) studies;

- special studies and post-marketing clinical trials as instructed by the MHLW at the time of approval; these may include

  - drug utilization studies;

  - studies deemed necessary as a result of issues arising from pre-approval clinical trials, reports of ADRs, communicable diseases, etc.,

  - studies for identifying, validating or confirming information about the appropriate use of the product.

Early post-marketing phase vigilance Recent regulations require companies to conduct

EPPV during the first 6 months after launch of a new product on the Japanese market, the objectives being:

- to assure that appropriate information has been provided to prescribers;

- to encourage caution;

- to promote an understanding of appropriate use of the product in medical institutions;

- to report promptly spontaneous information on serious ADRs and infections and to implement the consequent safety measures and minimize the associated public health risk.

Clinical Experience Investigation studies   CEI studies are also a post-marketing requirement, their objectives being:

- to detect unlabelled ADRs;

- to understand ADR development during actual use of the drug;

- to define factors suspected to influence the product's safety and/or efficacy profile.

In addition, for orphan drugs and others where required, CEI studies also have the purpose of characterizing efficacy and safety in actual drug usage conditions.

The number of cases to be studied is determined according to the characteristics of the drug.

Special studies and post-marketing clinical trials   Special studies include the following:

- studies on efficacy and safety in patients with special situations, e.g. children, elderly, pregnant women, and patients with renal or hepatic disease; conducted to refine or confirm associated prescribing information relating to 'special' patients that were not adequately investigated in pre-approval clinical studies.

- studies on long-term use.

- studies for the detection or confirmation of factors likely to affect efficacy and safety, e.g. the time to onset of ADRs.

- studies concentrating on the collection of information on AEs for which causality cannot be easily determined due to the small number of cases, to confirm or refute causality to the drug in question.

Post-marketing clinical trials may include:

- studies for establishing the most appropriate use in patients with special backgrounds, e.g. patients with renal disorders.

- studies based on pharmacoepidemiological methods for verifying prolongation of life from long-term use, improvement in quality of life, etc.

- studies for verifying efficacy and safety in accordance with the guidelines for the clinical evaluation of new drugs.

- studies for verification that factors identified as likely to affect efficacy or safety do so in practice.

Expedited reports

Expedited reporting requirements for marketed products depend on several factors, including the country of origin and the seriousness, severity and 'expectedness' of the ADR, as illustrated in Table 9.9.

Table 9.9 Japanese expedited reporting requirements – marketed products

Report	Origin	ADRs that qualify for reporting
15-day	Domestic	Serious unexpected[a]
	Foreign	Serious unexpected
	Scientific literature	Serious
30-day	Domestic	Serious expected
		Severe/moderate non-serious

[a] Fatal unexpected ADR: immediate preliminary notification to be followed by full written report.

Thirty-day reports should also be filed if results from clinical research indicate that a marketed product is associated with an increased frequency of ADRs, lack of efficacy or the possibility of an association with onset of cancer, important medical events, disability/incapacity, or a fatal outcome.

Although not explicitly stated in the legislation, common understanding is that the time frame for reporting begins from the date of receipt of information by the Japanese business/affiliate. All reports should be submitted on Japanese forms and in one of the Japanese languages.

A recent Notification (IYAKUAN No. 0531001) indicates that electronic reporting will be mandatory for post-marketing expedited reports with effect from 1 October 2003, with relevant data fields coded using MedDRA.

Infections The Pharmaceutical Affairs Law requires all domestic and foreign reports of fatal/life-threatening or other serious infections, associated with possible contamination of marketed drug products, to be notified immediately to the MHLW as preliminary reports by fax, with written reports within 15 days, whether labelled or not.

Domestic cases of moderate unexpected infection must be notified within 30 days.

Measures taken abroad In addition to the requirements that apply to individual ADR reports, companies should notify the MHLW on an expedited basis about any measures taken abroad that relate to safety issues, e.g. addition of a new precautionary statement to a US product label. This applies equally to marketed products and those under clinical investigation in Japan.

Periodic reports

PSURs should be submitted to MHLW for all marketed products. These should be produced in full accordance with ICH E2C and include foreign data. Within (or attached to) each PSUR there should be a commentary on the safety information presented in the Japanese prescribing text(s) for the product.

In addition, periodic reports are required to summarize the progress of all Japanese post-marketing studies. Their content should include:

- the number of patients recruited, including the reason for any delay in the planned schedule for recruitment;

- comments on any factors derived from the statistical analysis that might influence the safety/efficacy profile of the product;

- a list of reported ADRs and/or infections, organized by body system;

- copies of ADR case reports previously sent to the MHLW;

- future measures to be taken as a result of the investigation.

Periodic safety updates (whether PSURs or post-marketing study updates) should be submitted every 6 months for 2 years following approval of the JNDA, and on an annual basis thereafter during the defined 're-examination' period. Following completion of 're-examination', the reports then revert to a 5 year periodicity.

The 'clock' may be reset to zero if the product has been approved for a new indication or formulation (depending on negotiation with the MHLW). Although the schedule for submission should be based on the date of marketing approval in Japan, the reporting period for each set of data may be determined from the IBD, in order to facilitate harmonization of Japanese PSURs with those produced elsewhere.

Acknowledgements

Wherever possible, the information provided within this chapter has been drawn from publicly available regulations and guidelines produced by CIOMS, ICH and regulatory authorities. On occasions, additional information has been included that was made available to the author through publications or symposia on ADR reporting, as well as personal communications with colleagues within AstraZeneca or other companies.

Indeed, I am indebted to my many colleagues in AstraZeneca who have provided the necessary information, and who have reviewed draft sections, for this chapter to be completed.

References

Arnold BDC (1999). Global ADR reporting requirements: 2nd Edition. Scrip Report BS 980.

Begaud B, Evreux JC, Joulard J and Lagier G (1985). Imputabilité des effets inattendus ou toxiques des médicaments. Actualisation de la méthode utilizé en France. *Thérapie* **40**: 111–118.

Bibliography

Commission Directive 2000/38/EC (2000). Amending Chapter Va (Pharmacovigilance) of Council Directive 75/319/EEC on the approximation of provisions laid down by law, regulation or administrative action relating to medicinal products. *Official Journal of the European Communities* 10 June 2000.

Commission Regulation (EC) 540/95 (1995). Laying down the arrangements for reporting suspected unexpected adverse reactions which are not serious, whether arising in the Community or in a third country, to medicinal products for human or veterinary use authorized in accordance with the provisions of Council Regulation (EEC) No. 2309/93. *Official Journal of the European Communities* 11 March 1995.

Council Directive 75/319/EEC (1975). On the approximation of provisions laid down by law, regulation or administrative action relating to proprietary medicinal products. *Official Journal of the European Communities* 24 August 1993.

Council Directive 93/39/EEC (1993). Amending Directives 65/65/EEC, 75/318/EEC and 75/319/EEC in respect of medicinal products. *Official Journal of the European Communities* 24 August 1993: 22.

Council Directive 2001/20/EC (2001). On the approximation of the laws, regulations and administrative provisions of the Member States relating to the implementation of good clinical practice in the conduct of clinical trials on medicinal products for human use. *Official Journal of the European Communities* 1 May 2001.

Council Directive 2001/83/EC (2001). Community code relating to medicinal products for human use. *Official Journal of the European Communities* 28 November 2001.

Council for International Organizations of Medical Sciences (1990). Final Report of CIOMS Working Group: International Reporting of Adverse Drug Reactions. CIOMS, Geneva, 1990.

Council for International Organizations of Medical Sciences (1992). Final Report of CIOMS Working Group II: International Reporting of Periodic Drug-Safety Update Summaries. CIOMS, Geneva, 1992.

Council for International Organizations of Medical Sciences (2001). Final Report of CIOMS Working Group V: Current Challenges in Pharmacovigilance: Pragmatic Approaches. CIOMS, Geneva, 2001.

Council Regulation 2309/93/EEC (1993). Laying down Community procedures for the authorization and supervision of medicinal products for human and veterinary use and establishing a European Agency for the Evaluation of Medicinal Products. *Official Journal of the European Communities* 24 August 1993.

European Agency for the Evaluation of Medicinal Products (1998). Notes for guidance on procedure for competent authorities on the undertaking of pharmacovigilance activities. CPMP/175/95 Rev 1.

European Agency for the Evaluation of Medicinal Products (1996). Note for guidance on good clinical practice. Step 5 Consolidated guideline CPMP/ICH/135/95.

European Agency for the Evaluation of Medicinal Products (1996). ICH Topic E2A. Clinical Safety Data Management: Definitions and Standards for Expedited Reporting. Step 4 Consensus guideline CPMP/ICH/377/95.

European Agency for the Evaluation of Medicinal Products (1996). ICH Topic E2C. Clinical Safety

Data Management: Periodic Safety Update Reports for Marketed Drugs. Step 4 Consensus guideline CPMP/ICH/288/95.

European Agency for the Evaluation of Medicinal Products (1997). Conduct of pharmacovigilance for centrally authorized products. CPMP/183/97.

European Agency for the Evaluation of Medicinal Products (2000). ICH Topic E2B(M). Clinical Safety Data Management: Data Elements for Transmission of Individual Case Safety Reports. Note for guidance CPMP/ICH/287/95 (modified).

European Agency for the Evaluation of Medicinal Products (2001). Position paper on compliance with pharmacovigilance regulatory obligations. CPMP/PhVWP/1618/01.

European Agency for the Evaluation of Medicinal Products (2002). Policy paper on the implementation of the electronic transmission of individual case safety reports for medicinal products for human use authorized in the European Union. EMEA/H/5255/01.

European Commission (2001). Volume 9 of 'The rules governing medicinal products in the European Union' – Pharmacovigilance, December 2001.

European Commission (2003). Detailed guidance on the collection, verification and presentation of adverse reaction reports arising from clinical trials on medicinal products for human use, April 2003.

European Commission (2003). Detailed guidance on the European database of suspected unexpected serious adverse reactions (Eudravigilance – Clinical Trial Module), April 2003.

European Commission Pharmacovigilance Working Party (1991). Causality classification in pharmacovigilance in the European Community. III/3445/91.

Federal Institute for Drugs and Medical Devices (BfArM) (1996). 3rd Promulgation on the notification of adverse reactions, interactions with other products and drug abuse pursuant to §29(1) sentences 2–8 of the German Drug Law. Unauthorized translation (BPI), 15 May 1996.

Food and Drug Administration (1992). Guideline for Postmarketing Reporting of Adverse Drug Experiences. March 1992.

Food and Drug Administration (1993). Guideline for adverse experience reporting for licensed biological products. 15 October 1993.

Food and Drug Administration (1997). Guideline on Clinical Safety Data Management: Periodic Safety Update Reports for Marketed Drugs; Notice, Federal Register, 19 May 1997.

Food and Drug Administration (1997). Guidance for Industry Postmarketing Adverse Experience Reporting for Human Drug and Licensed Biological Products: Clarification of What to Report'. August 1997.

Food and Drug Administration (1997). Expedited Safety Reporting Requirements for Human Drug and Biological Products; Final Rule, Federal Register, 7 October 1997.

Food and Drug Administration (2003). Safety reporting requirements for human drug and biological products; proposed rule. Federal Register, 14 March 2003.

France (1995). Code de la Sante Publique, modified by the Decree 95-278 of 13 March 1995. *Journal Officiel de la Republique Francaise* 14 March 1995.

France (1994). Article L209–12 du Live II bis du code de la Sante Publique, completed by recommendations du 12 Septembre 1994. Issued November 1994.

Germany (1994). German Drug Law (Gesetz uber den Verkehr mit Arzneimitteln: AMG). Fifth Amendment, 17 August 1994.

HMSO (1994). The Medicines for Human Use (Marketing Authorisations Etc) Regulations 1994. Statutory Instrument 1994 No. 3144.

HMSO (1995). The Medicines (Exemption from Licences) (Clinical Trials) Order 1995. Statutory Instrument 1995 No. 2808.

International Conference on Harmonization (1994). Clinical safety data management: definitions and standards for expedited reporting (ICH E2A). International Conferences on Harmonization, Geneva, 25 October 1994.

International Conference on Harmonization (1994). The extent of population exposure to assess clinical safety for drugs intended for long-term treatment of non-life-threatening conditions ICH E1). International Conferences on Harmonization, Geneva, 27 October 1994.

International Conference on Harmonization (1996). Clinical safety data management: periodic safety update reports for marketed drugs (ICH E2C). International Conferences on Harmonization, Geneva, 6 November 1996.

International Conference on Harmonization (1996). Guideline for good clinical practice (ICH E6). International Conferences on Harmonization, Geneva, 1 May 1996.

International Conference on Harmonization (2000). Clinical safety data management: data elements for transmission of individual case safety reports (ICH E2B(M)). International Conferences on Harmonization, Geneva, 10 November 2000.

International Conference on Harmonization (2000). Recommendations on electronic transmission of individual case safety reports message specification (ICH M2(M)). International Conferences on Harmonization, Geneva, 10 November 2000.

International Conference on Harmonization (2003). Addendum to E2C: periodic safety update reports for marketed drugs. International Conferences on Harmonization, Geneva, 6 February 2003.

ICH Steering Committee (1997). Statement of principles (MedDRA). 15 July 1997.

Medicines Control Agency (1995). Pharmacovigilance in the new European system. Medicines Act Information Letter 87.

Medicines Control Agency (1995). AEGIS update: new version of AEGIS includes electronic ADR reporting for industry. Medicines Act Information Letter 87.

Medicines Control Agency (1995). Clinical trials: adverse reaction reporting by companies. Medicines Act Information Letter 88.

Medicines Control Agency (1996). Guidance notes on applications for clinical trial exemptions and clinical trial certificates. Medicines Act Leaflet, MAL 4.

Medicines Control Agency (1997). New ICH guideline on periodic safety update reports. Medicines Act Information Letter 101.

Medicines Control Agency (1997). Studying the safety of marketed medicines. Medicines Act Information Letter 104.

Medicines Control Agency (1998). Handling of clinical trials adverse drug reactions. Reminders! Medicines Act Information Letter 105.

Medicines Control Agency (2002). Directive 2000/38/EC: changes to UK pharmacovigilance requirements – interim requirements for 'black triangle' products. Medicines Act Information Letter 130.

Pharmacovigilance Working Party (1991). Causality classification in pharmacovigilance in the European Community. 29 April 1991.

SNIP (1997). Notification of adverse reactions – guideline from Medicines Agency. Circular No 96-0763, 18 October 1996.

SNIP (1997). Recommendations for the reporting of serious events likely to be attributable to research. Circular No 97-0197, 2 February 1997.

USA (1995). Title 21 of the Code of Federal Regulations. 4 January 1995.

10

Legal Aspects of Pharmacovigilance

C. Bendall

Introduction

Chapter 9 has already addressed the detail of the requirements currently applying in different jurisdictions to pharmacovigilance activities and adverse reaction reporting. Specific requirements that are laid down in legislation, and/or powers that are described generally in legislation to be exercised by regulators (who add detail administratively), form the legal basis for adverse drug reaction (ADR) recording and reporting obligations and for the enforcement of those obligations by regulatory authorities. Often, legislation is broadly worded, dealing in general requirements, concepts and principles; the practical detail of how the obligations are, or may be, satisfied is left to guidelines and administrative provision made by regulators. In the UK, for example, before the revision of the Medicines Act 1968 in 1994, a marketing authorization (MA) holder (MAH) was required (by 'standard provisions' attaching to the MA) simply to report ADRs in accordance with whatever requirements were laid down by the Licensing Authority from time to time. These were set out and amended periodically in (Medicines Act Information Letters MAIL) issued every 2 months by the Medicines Control Agency. Currently, Statutory Instrument (SI) 1994 No. 1344 simply provides that the requirements of European legislation – which includes the provisions for pharmacovigilance (for national, decentralized[1] and centralized products) – are applied under UK law. In contrast, legislative provisions in the USA are relatively detailed, both for investigational new drug authorizations and new drug applications.

Any consideration of relevant legislation raises the following issues:

- Determining how to arrive at the proper interpretation of legal texts, particularly where they are broadly written.

- Determining the status of guidelines and the extent to which guidelines are themselves enforceable.

- Assessing the extent to which guidelines assist interpretation.

---

[1] Also known as 'mutual recognition' or 'MR', although the Commission now prefers to think in terms of 'decentralized'.

Stephens' Detection of New Adverse Drug Reactions Fifth Edition edited by John Talbot and Patrick Waller
© 2004 John Wiley & Sons, Ltd   ISBN: 0 470 84552 X

It is self-evident that laws are made in an effort to regularize and control activity across a range of situations. In order to achieve a high level of compliance, the rules need to be clear, coherent and comprehensive and there must be certainty about the nature and scope of the requirements. In fact, this is a goal that relatively few pieces of legislation ever fully attain. Unsurprisingly, therefore, European Community (EC) law on drug safety has given rise to a number of issues relating to its scope, interpretation and application.

The legal status of guidance depends upon whether it is incorporated into the relevant legislation. In some cases, specific cross-reference to a document or documents may be made in statute, together with a requirement for compliance that operates actually to incorporate the contents of guidelines into the legislation. In general, however, guidance is merely guidance, and, therefore, is not legally enforceable; non-compliance with such guidance may be censured by regulatory authorities but is not a breach of legal require-ments, nor is it subject to legal penalty. As a matter of law, it is the legislation that binds and is enforceable: a fact that is acknowledged in Guideline ICH/288/95 which emerged from the ICH process (International Conference of Harmonization involving EU, USA, Japan): 'Guidelines are not legally binding. Some portions of this guideline may not be reflected in existing regulations. To that extent, until the regulations are amended, MAHs must comply with existing regulations'.

However, guidelines are, at least, a strong indication of a competent regulatory authority's approach to interpreting and applying the law and, in practice, regulatory guidance will play an important part in determining the MAH's policy and practice. Moreover, adopted guidance can have marked legal significance in the context of determining 'civil' liability. In cases where negligence is alleged, guidelines (especially those written by, or with the support of, regulatory authorities), provide a benchmark against which the civil courts tend to judge the 'reasonableness' of a defendant company's systems, standards and conduct of its business activities.

Although it is not intended to revisit the detail of relevant legislation and guidelines in this chapter, the adequacy of legal requirements in terms of clarity, ease of interpretation and comprehensiveness and the role of guidance with reference to compliance and enforce-ment will be addressed. Otherwise, this chapter will focus upon legal responsibility for compliance and the legal consequences, in terms of both regulatory procedures and liability proceedings (civil and criminal), of failures in the practice of pharmacovigilance in relation to marketed products for human use. This discussion will concentrate upon the European Union (EU).

Legal responsibility for pharmacovigilance

The marketing authorization holder

Under EC law (Directive 2001/83/EEC, Regulations 2309/93 and 540/95; see Table 10.1) pharmacovigilance is one of several legal obligations imposed upon the MAH. Others include: establishment in the EU, establishment of an information service, an obligation to keep product manufacture in line with the state of the art, obligations for record keeping, appointment of qualified personnel, etc. (See: Notice to Applicants, Volume 2A, Chapter 1.)

The duty of pharmacovigilance attaches whether the MAH intends itself to perform the obligation by applying its own resources, or to invest in third-party services. The legislation does not prohibit buying in services for the purposes of achieving compliance; indeed, guidance recognizes the practice (Volume 9 of the Rules Governing Medicinal Products in the European Community ('Volume 9'), Part 1, paragraph 1.1.1[2]), but the responsibility for compliance, as a matter of law, continues to rest with the MAH. For example, in relation to marketing the guidance states:

> "such arrangements for joint pharmacovigilance data collection and analyses are acceptable to competent authorities, provided the MAH confirms in writing that it understands that legal responsibility rests with it."

Whilst current legislation generally imposes pharmacovigilance obligations upon the MAH in terms of reporting ADRs of which it is aware, with time limits running from the date of knowledge,[3] regulatory authorities in practice are rarely, if ever, impressed by excuses for regulatory reporting failures based upon the breach of a contractual obligation by some person other than the responsible MAH. Moreover, the current draft of the revised pharmaceutical legislation clearly indicates an intention that an MAH should be judged according to data 'of which he/she may reasonably be expected to be aware ...' (Article 22, Regulation 2309/93 – draft amendments dated 5/3/02). Whatever view is taken of legislation framed in this way, the point is that the MAH must take steps necessary to ensure that the system upon which it relies is properly set up, managed, reviewed and audited; the authorities, moreover, expect to be satisfied that proper arrangements are in place.

There is, therefore, a level of risk to contracting-in services that are crucial to drug safety, regulatory confidence (i.e. in the relationship with the regulatory authority) and compliance, especially where a breach may give rise to criminal or other administrative sanctions and/or civil liability. It is a commercial risk that many companies take. In some cases they may have little choice. Smaller entities simply may not possess the resources and infrastructure to set up and run a 'full service' drug safety unit. Foreign companies establishing a presence in new markets may not possess the necessary experience of the local regime to undertake the full range of pharmacovigilance activities (or other MAH obligations) without external help. A lack of experience and local resource in a new market is a common (although not the only) reason for the commercial practice of licensing out of products by smaller developer/niche companies to larger entities with well-established products, practices and procedures. Within joint ventures/partnering arrangements, it is common to see companies 'allocating' the performance of regulatory functions between them according to their respective abilities, resources and experience.

The provision of a contract and careful contractual drafting is essential in these circumstances. A high level of trust is placed by the MAH in a third party whose non-compliance with regulatory requirements, should it occur, may have significant consequences for the MAH. In the more complex commercial arrangements, it is generally more practical and therefore preferable, to set out the relevant obligations generally in the contract itself and to incorporate by cross-reference a detailed document providing standard operating procedures (SOPs). These SOPs should ideally have been developed for and been

---

[2] The Rules Governing Medicinal Products in the European Community form the fundamental collection of guidelines and reference legal texts in the EU.

[3] E.g. Article 22 of Regulation 2309/93: 'The person responsible for placing the medicinal product on the market shall ensure all suspected serious adverse reactions ... are reported ... no later than 15 days following receipt of the information'.

adapted to the particular circumstances and parties to the contractual relationship. Such a document must thereafter be regularly reviewed, updated and amended in line with changes in the legal requirements and developments in standards of good practice. This approach avoids producing a turgid, lengthy contract and facilitates subsequent amendment of the working document (SOP) as necessary to maintain currency with the changing legal and ethical environment.

Care with the accuracy and clarity of cross-referencing is important. There should be no mistake as to the documentation that is referenced which may affect the terms or even the validity of the contract. In some jurisdictions, if two commercial entities sign a contract and agree to take on certain obligations then they are bound by those terms, whether or not they have properly read the contents. In practice, the best policy is to ensure that all parties are familiar with (and fully understand the terms of) the agreement. In other jurisdictions the courts will look critically at the circumstances of inclusion (e.g. in Sweden the party agreeing to comply must have had sight of and understand the content of the referenced document at, or before, signing). Contractual safeguards, involving the detailed spelling out of the third-party's obligations, are essential, therefore, and maximize the MAH's degree of protection. Moreover, in practice, the MAH may well be asked to supply details of the 'arrangements for meeting pharmacovigilance obligations' to the regulatory authority (i.e. including a copy of the contract), and to update the authority when changes to the arrangements are 'proposed'. (Volume 9, Part 1 paragraph 1.1.1.) In theory, this suggests the possibility that the regulators will comment upon/make demands with regard to the adequacy of the contractual arrangements designed to achieve compliance.

A well-written contract cannot, however, guarantee *total* indemnity against all losses consequent upon a breach of contract, or compensate for any criminal liability that could arise where failure nonetheless occurs. These concerns apply irrespective of the jurisdiction to which the MAH is subject. The precise penalties for failure to comply with phamacovigilance obligations do, however, differ from country to country. Whether there is individual, or merely corporate, exposure to them also depends upon local law (see below).

The potential consequences of a breach of pharmacovigilance requirements are not only regulatory (e.g. action against the authorization and/or MAH and/or others by the regulatory authorities, and the imposition of penalties). They can also be civil, where they may arise in the context of claims for personal injury based upon allegations of negligence and/or the supply of a defective product causing injury. (The liability issues are discussed in more detail below.) With regard to product liability, the basic issues to which the MAH must give thought are again common to most jurisdictions, although the precise principles and approach will depend upon local provisions.[4] In such cases, the claims might be expected to be framed in terms that a failure or delay in relation to the collection, analysis, periodic review and/or reporting of ADRs has meant that a significant safety issue was not identified at all, was identified too late, or was insufficiently characterized for proper action to have been taken to place appropriate limitations upon the availability and/or use and administration of a product. This would, for example, include failure in relation to implementing labelling changes or product withdrawal where, at the time, with proper attention, one or

---

[4]In certain countries, for example, the burden of proof in claims for product-related personal injury is 'relaxed' in favour of the claimant and the courts are quick to find that the burden has been satisfied (e.g. in the Netherlands). In others, there may be special provision made for pharmaceutical product claims through insurance pools, which pay out (usually at levels less than those obtainable through court proceedings) on proof of causation alone; there are such schemes in Sweden and Finland.

other would have been the appropriate course to have taken to safeguard patient health. If the MAH relied upon a third party in the performance of pharmacovigilance obligations, it may be argued that the MAH failed to impose and monitor an adequate system to ensure compliance and the discharge of its legal duty of care.

Thus, in claims based on negligence, a plaintiff might seek to establish that:

• The MAH knew, or ought to have known through appropriate pharmacovigilance activities, of the risk posed by the product.

• The MAH should have acted, or should have acted sooner or more expansively.

• The system was (still is) generally below reasonable operational standards when compared against prevailing legal requirements and/or industry practice.

The evidence for this type of pleading often arises from the defendant company's own documents examined by claimant lawyers under court rules for disclosure of all relevant documents by one party to proceedings to the other. "Document" is widely interpreted to include all records, in whatever medium (electronic, paper, microfiche, etc.). If a claimant can then show, on the balance of probabilities (which in law means more likely than not, i.e. 51 per cent or greater chance), that the deficiency identified was 'causative' of the injury suffered, the claim will be established and damages obtained.

In strict liability cases there is no need to show fault, as there is in negligence claims. The mere fact of some inadequacy in (pharmacovigilance) practice having occurred which has led to the product being less safe than persons would generally be entitled to expect (i.e. 'defective') will be sufficient (e.g. because the labelling fails properly to present the side effects, warnings or precautions for use of the product accurately), providing that causation is established. The majority of defences made available by statute in strict liability cases are unlikely to apply. Again, the basic principles of strict liability are more or less common to the European and USA jurisdictions.

Contracting with a third party to perform a regulatory function for and on behalf of the MAH will not isolate the MAH from suit, or a finding of liability, but the MAH may be able to recover (at least part of) any damages and costs awarded against it from the service provider who defaults under the terms of the contract, who has contributed to or caused the personal injury. Clearly defined obligations and indemnities in the contract are of central importance to such recovery.

The 'qualified person responsible for pharmacovigilance'

A feature of European legislation (and practice) in the pharmaceutical sector in recent years has been its focus upon the appointment of specific individuals to take charge of core functions for the MAH. The amendment of Directive 75/319/EEC and introduction of Regulation 2309/93 as part of the development of the 'New Systems' for registration in the early 1990s established a requirement for the appointment of a person responsible for pharmacovigilance (PRP) whose obligations are outlined in the legislation. Guidelines further emphasize the importance that regulators attach to the role of the PRP and their consequent expectation that the appointee will be a more senior person of experience and appropriate qualification. Regulators in the EU also require the name of the PRP to be notified to them by the MAH. (Volume 9, Part 1, paragraph 1.1.1.) This focus upon individual personal responsibility, however, does not mean that attention is directed away from the MAH: the MAH remains responsible. The responsibility of the PRP and MAH is concurrent. For the PRP, a compliance failure *may* expose him/her to regulatory sanctions as well as the MAH when, according to local law, provision is made for individuals to be sanctioned; e.g. in the UK, under Medicines Act legislation, regulatory breaches may expose both natural and corporate 'persons' to fines and/or (in the case of natural persons) imprisonment.

A PRP also has to bear in mind (and negotiate an appropriate protective contractual term in his/her contract of employment/for services) that, in theory at least, it is possible to be sued by the MAH for damages in respect of a breach of contract and/or negligence leading to loss on the part of the MAH. In practice, however, this is unheard of, and employment contracts would normally be expected to contain clauses limiting/ruling out such claims between the parties. In practice, individuals rarely have the resources to warrant a civil claim being made against them. Realistically, were MAHs to take action against their employees, it would soon prove impossible to recruit individuals to the position of PRP.

Interpreting legal provisions

Table 10.1 lists the relevant legislative texts in which the EC has set out the pharmacovigilance requirements applicable in the EU (subject to formal implementation into local law in the case of directives). Different pieces of legislation apply depending upon the route by which a medicinal product has been authorized and the place where the adverse reaction occurs. These provisions are 'over layered' in several EU member states by additional provisions of local law. This, unfortunately, leads to a level of complexity in terms of compliance (regarding nationally authorized and decentralized or 'MR' products), which arguably could and should be further reduced without any compromise of public safety. However, until member states act to simplify the position, the tone of Volume 9 seems to indicate that the EC is prepared to accommodate local requirements that exceed EU-level requirements. It is accepted, for example, that some member states (e.g. Germany) will not be satisfied with a PRP resident in *a* member state as the law provides, but insist upon a locally based PRP.

In looking at EC law (i.e. law passed by EC institutions) the approach to interpretation is 'purposive'. This means that interpretation is not simply a matter of the wording of the provisions, but relies upon the intention underlying the legislation. It is normal practice,

Table 10.1   EC legislation relevant to pharmacovigilance

Product	Legislation
Centrally authorized medicinal products	Regulation 2309/93 (Articles 15, 18, 19–26, 51) Regulation 540/95 (non-serious ADRs). N.B.: includes definitions in Article 1 of 2001/83, and 1085/2003 (variations and urgent safety restrictions)
Decentralized (or MR) medicinal products	Directive 2001/83 (Articles 1, 101–108) incorporating 75/319/EEC (as amended by Directive 2000/38) plus local provisions
Nationally authorized medicinal products	Directive 2001/83 (Articles 101–108) incorporating 75/319/EEC (as amended by Directive 2000/38) plus local provisions

therefore, in considering EC legal provisions to look closely at the recitals (which are often set out in great detail) at the beginning of directives and regulations. The aim is to encourage interpretation in line with the objectives that the legislation was designed to achieve.

In relation to pharmaceuticals, the legislative objective is to 'safeguard public health' without hindering the development of the pharmaceutical industry or trade within the Community; Regulation 2309/93 ("the Regulation") on centrally authorized products states:

"Whereas it is also necessary to make provision for the supervision of medicinal products which have been authorized by the Community and, in particular, for the intensive monitoring of adverse reactions ... in order to ensure the rapid withdrawal from the market of any medicinal product which presents an unacceptable risk under normal conditions of use."

Directive 2001/83 ("the Directive") (on national and decentralized products) refers to the need to *'ensure the continued safety of medicinal products in use'* through modern pharmacovigilance systems. In considering risk, the EU has moved increasingly in recent years towards a precautionary approach to consumer safety (Communication on the precautionary principle, 2/2/2000): crudely, 'a better safe than sorry' style of approach which allows regulators discretion in the absence of 'proof' but on the basis of reasonable suspicion/concern.

EC legislation must also be understood in the context of certain fundamental European legal principles, including:

- Respect for natural justice (which includes the right to equal treatment in the EU, and the right to be heard).

- 'Transparency' in relation to the requirements imposed and in respect of the criteria and procedures applied.

The EC provisions for pharmacovigilance under New Systems were intended to be supported by guidance (listed in Table 10.2) issued by the CPMP and the Commission. The original legislation (Directive 93/39/EEC, which amended 75/319/EEC) referred directly to guidelines that were to be adopted by the Commission:

"The Commission in consultation with the Agency, Member States and interested parties shall draw up guidance on the collection, verification and presentation of adverse reaction reports."

That guidance (following a considerable process of evolution during the 1990s) is now contained in Volume 9. The current version 'is ... intended to update and replace pharmacovigilance guidance published in the Community prior to 30 September 2001', (some further guidelines, including CPMP Guideline 1618/01, have been issued since this date; see Table 10.2) and clearly constitutes an important source of reference for MAHs. There have been difficulties over the years with aspects of the developing guidance, both finalized and in draft. During the late 1990s there were elements of inconsistency, with differences arising between the legislation and the guidelines and also between guidelines. The amendment of the pharmacovigilance provisions by the introduction of Directive 2000/38 and the more recent work done in relation to Volume 9 and subsequent guidance, means

Table 10.2 Guidance texts on pharmacovigilance (CPMP: Committee for Proprietary Medicinal Products; ICH: International Conference on Harmonization)[a]

Description	Comment
Volume 9 of the Rules Governing Medicinal Products in the European Community	Contains a range of guidelines – Part I (1): Notice to MAH; (2) Guidance and procedures for competent authorities; (3) Terminology: Part III exchange of pharmacovigilance information; (6) periodic safety update reports (PSURs); (7) data elements for transmission of individual case safety reports
Guideline 1618/01 Concept Paper on Compliance with pharmacovigilance regulatory obligations	Provides that further guidance is needed and will be brought forward to improve the value and availability of information reported

[a] Contained in Volume 9 of The Rules Governing Medicinal Products in the European Community, updated to 30/9/2001.

that some of the early issues (e.g. the reporting of ADR data other than spontaneous ADRs by the MAH) have now been better clarified or settled, but there is still room for improvement (see below).

The relationship between European Community pharmacovigilance legislation and guidelines

Centrally authorized products

Article 24 of Regulation 2309/93 refers to the obligation of the Commission, pursuant to consultation, to draw up guidance on the collection verification and presentation of adverse reaction reports. This is a reference to Volume 9 and guidelines subsequently adopted. There is nothing, however, that is designed specifically to incorporate the provisions of that guidance into the legislation. Technically, this guidance remains guidance and is not law. However, in terms of day-to-day management this may have little practical impact, as MAHs are aware of the expectations of the European Medicines Evaluation Agency (EMEA) based upon the guidance and they generally seek to satisfy them. Occasionally, however, such as when there is a dispute with, or threatened enforcement action by, a competent authority, the distinction is important; that is the difference between, on the one hand, a breach of the law with its attendant consequences and, on the other hand, the dissatisfaction of the competent authority (although this, too, may carry significant consequences in terms of the regulatory relationship). However, the proposals for the amendment of the Regulation (dated 5/3/02), which are currently under consideration pursuant to the 2001 Review of the pharmaceutical legislation (hereafter, the Review), cross-reference Article 106(2) of Directive[5] 2001/83 and apply it 'for the purposes of' the pharmacovigilance chapter contained in the Regulation, thus applying Article 106 to centrally authorized products. If enacted, this will enhance the status of the guidelines, since, as is explained below, Article 106 seems to require certain activities to be carried out specifically 'in accordance with' the relevant guidance. Pending the introduction of these amendments, there is an apparent disparity in the legal status of the guidance between centrally authorized and other MAs which is discussed below.

[5] Article 106 refers to Volume 9 of the Rules, etc.

Nationally authorized and 'mutual recognition' products

In contrast to Regulation 2309/93, Directive 2001/83 specifically cross-refers to current guidance and requires action to be taken 'in accordance with' that guidance. Article 106 identifies the guidance as that published in Volume 9.

Thus:

1. The person responsible must establish and maintain a system within the MAH and is responsible for the preparation of 'the reports referred to in Article 104 ... in accordance with the guidance referred to in Article 106(1)'.

2. Reports should be made of 'Other suspected serious adverse reactions' (i.e. not brought to the PRP's attention by a healthcare professional) that meet the reporting criteria 'in accordance with the guidance referred to in Article 106(1) ...'.

3. The same form of reference, i.e. 'in accordance with the guidance' is applied to reporting suspected serious and unexpected ADRs from third countries.

4. Article 107 refers to the guidance in the context of the consideration by member states of the suspension, withdrawal and variation of an MA. It also states that, in relation to the definitions contained in Article 1 of the Directive ('ADR', 'serious ADR', etc.) and the principles set out in the Title IX on pharmacovigilance: 'the MAH and the competent authorities *shall* refer to the guidance ...' (emphasis added).

However, what will be considered to constitute a 'referral' to the guidance and what exactly it means for something to be done 'in accordance with the guidance' may not be entirely straightforward. 'Referral' means that reference must be made or consideration given, but this does not necessarily mean its application to the letter. Where the guidelines leave issues open, to be handled according to the particular circumstances, discretion must be exercised to determine a practical course in line with the spirit of the requirements. Where guidelines leave matters to be handled according to local rules, the regulatory authority at national level remains the arbiter (subject to determination by local courts). It is possible, therefore, to envisage differences of understanding arising between the regulators and the regulated. This is important if a failure to comply is to be judged and enforcement action taken, on the basis of reference to guidelines. This is especially problematic if the guidelines are unclear or ambiguous. There is, in any event, a real distinction to be drawn between the extent to which guidance fulfils the *legitimate* function of assisting in the understanding and interpretation of legal requirements/restrictions already set out in legislation and an attempt to legislate through guidance in an effort to supplement deficient legislation.

National implementation

As indicated above, EC directives (not regulations, which have immediate application and effect in all member states upon the date earmarked following adoption by the Community) need to be implemented by member states before they can be enforced against MAHs by those authorities. In relation to EC legislation, it is inevitable that some differences in local interpretation and, therefore, in the results of implementation, will arise during this process.

Similarly, the treatment of guidelines in the process of implementation may differ between member states, with some member states actually incorporating guidance into their national laws. Member states can be brought to book by the Commission through the European Court of Justice (ECJ) for improper implementation of, or failure to implement, EC legislation. In this connection, not all member states have yet fully implemented the amendments to Directive 75/319/EEC made by Directive 2000/38 (now found in Directive 2001/83), which should have been achieved by 5 December 2001. Such failure would mean that these provisions could not be used by the authorities against a local company who failed to comply with the revised non-implemented requirements (see: Organon Laboratories Ltd versus DHSS; 1990 2 CMLR 49).

In the UK, concern with regard to achieving proper implementation of EC law has led to a change in the approach to drafting legislation. By tradition, English law is drafted precisely, with careful use of language (the words, rather than the purpose, determining what the law is) and, until recently, efforts were made to transpose or 'translate' new European requirements to fit them into and around whatever UK legislation already existed. However, particularly in the field of medicines law, following the discovery of some legislative shortcomings in the early 1990s, the practice has developed so that the draftsmen now tend either simply to cross refer to the EU legislation or to 'lift' large sections of the text from European legislation and place it in local legislation. This may be done without any attempt to mould, interpret, or alter the language to fit that previously used in English legal texts. Such 'importation' can be problematic, as the text used has been drafted in accordance with a different legal culture and is comparatively ambiguous or vague. The alternative approach, i.e. merely to cross refer to the 'relevant Community provisions' and incorporating them as they stand in full, again imports locally any inherent problems or issues of interpretation that are part and parcel of the European text (see SI 3144 of 1994, Article 7(1): 'Every holder of an UK marketing authorization ... shall comply with all obligations which relate to him by virtue of the *relevant* Community provisions including in particular obligations relating to providing or updating information ... to pharmacovigilance ...'). Such problems may be less of an issue in other systems. For example, in German legislative practice, laws are produced together with statements of reasons for both general and more specific provisions, so allowing regulated individuals, the national authority and the courts to make use of these explanatory statements in interpreting the provisions.

In any event, it is also a requirement of EC law that local laws must be interpreted in the light of, to give effect to and consistently with, the relevant EC law and its objectives. Uncertainties as to the meaning of EC law may be 'referred' for resolution to the ECJ by national courts. In the context of pharmacovigilance, both the general and specific aims of medicines legislation must be borne in mind:

- 'The primary purpose of any rules concerning the production and distribution of medicinal products must be to safeguard public health'. (Directive 65/65/EEC now incorporated in Directive 2001/83.)

- The competent authority 'shall suspend or revoke an authorization ... where that product proves to be harmful in normal conditions of use ...'. (Directive 65/65/EEC now incorporated in Directive 2001/83.)

National competent authorities enforce local law and are also bound to enforce and give effect to Community Regulations within their jurisdictions as they would national provisions (Council Resolution 25/6/95 OJ 22.7.95 C188/1). This is spelled out, so far as pharmacovigilance is concerned, in Article 69 of Regulation 2309/93.

Uncertainties in European Community provisions

The content of EC provisions is discussed length in Chapter 9. There are certain deficiencies and uncertainties relating to them. A selection of some of these issues is discussed below. They range from problems in the drafting of the legal texts to inconsistency between the Regulations (2309/93 and 540/95) and the Directive (2001/83), inconsistency between the legislation and Volume 9 (including 1618/01) and uncertainties in Volume 9 itself.

Definitions

Directive 2001/83

Directive 2001/83 contains the definitions of a number of terms relevant to the pharmacovigilance requirements set out in Title IX. However, it is not comprehensive.

Despite the reference in Article 102 to the collection by pharmacoviligance systems of 'information on misuse and abuse' of medicinal products, only 'abuse' is defined in Article 1. What is 'misuse', therefore, and, in contrast, what is use in 'normal conditions' are not defined.

There are a number of other terms that are crucial in judging matters of compliance (and, therefore, penalty) which are also absent from the glossary in the legislation, e.g.:

- 'permanently and continuously at his disposal'

- 'healthcare professional'

- 'immediately'.

Whilst it might be said that Article 106, by providing that 'For the interpretation of the definitions referred to in Article 1 points 11 to 16 and the principles outlined in the Title' both MAH and competent authorities 'shall refer to the guidance referred to in paragraph 1' (Volume 9) fills in the legislative gaps, this is neither a neat nor satisfactory means of approaching the definition of central terms and there is no obvious rationale for including some such terms in Article 1, but not in others. Moreover, it assumes, that definitions for the absent terms are to be found in Volume 9. So far as Part 1 of Volume 9 (Terminology) is concerned, this is true only for 'healthcare professional'. For the rest, it is necessary to read through the voluminous text of the guidelines. Thus, 'immediately' cannot be a period running beyond 15 days of receipt of ADR data and, by inference from the guidelines, must be related to the point at which 'minimum information' to enable a report to be made (per the Guidelines) is available; but this link is not stated expressly. There would be merit in ensuring comprehensive coverage of all terms used in legislation and guidelines in Volume 9, and in ensuring that all of the terms actually appearing in the legislation are part of the definitions section in Article 1 of Directive 2001/83.

Regulation 2309/93

Article 19 refers to and incorporates the definitions contained in the Directive; consequently the same issues of interpretation arise.

Volume 9

The guidance contained in Volume 9 necessarily introduces a range of new terms that are introduced by the guidance, not the legislation. Additionally, there are significant phrases used, particularly in relation to discussions of non-compliance. Therefore, it is important that all such terms are clear and unambiguous. Setting aside questions of whether the 'obligations' in the guidance are consistent with obligations in the legislation, it would be helpful if greater clarity attached to the following:

- 'all' or 'any relevant information' – which the guidelines state should be shared between the MAH and competent authority;

- 'appropriate information' – on post-authorization safety studies;

- 'well in advance of' – relevant to notifying competent authorities of a voluntary product withdrawal by the MAH;

- 'expedited report' – this term is much used, but, in fact, not defined by reference to the immediate/15 day reporting requirements;

- 'misuse' – the guidance imposes a 'requirement' upon MAHs to collect data on misuse.

For practical ease of reference, if terms are to be used in the guidance and Volume 9 is intended to include a working glossary, then it would be convenient to have the terms and an explanation of what the terms mean, in that glossary. For example, it would be helpful to have what constitutes 'the literature' (see paragraph 1.4.3.6.1, Volume 9) and explanatory text in the glossary, rather than only in the body of the extensive text, which suggests that 'literature' at least *includes* 'standard, recognized medical and scientific journals'.

The guidance also seeks to add to the definitions in Article 1 of the Directive. In relation to 'Serious Adverse Reaction' it provides:

"It also includes serious adverse clinical consequences associated with use outside the terms of the SPC, overdoses or abuse."

The meaning of 'Post-authorization Safety Study' (also defined in the Directive) is expanded in the guidance, which adds that the term includes any study where the number of patients will significantly add to existing safety data for the product. The definition in the Directive is specific to studies 'conducted with the aim of identifying or quantifying a safety hazard …' and is consequently narrower in scope. This creates an inconsistency which could be cured by the amendment of the legislation or guidelines, depending upon which version is intended to apply.

The guidance introduced the concept of the reportable ADR or 'minimum information' necessary to make a valid report. This provision is arguably important enough to warrant inclusion in the legislation. It is implicit that, in the absence of minimum information, no report is expected to be made to competent authorities (see Part 1, paragraph 1.2.2). However, in practice, it is not clear that this would be consistent with the expectations of regulators, especially in cases of serious ADRs.

Volume 9 is a collation of separate guidelines. As time progresses, tightening of drafting styles and use of terminology would facilitate compliance.

Requirements

Relationship between legislation and guidelines

Pending amendment of Regulations 2309/93 and 540/95, which is expected following the Review of the pharmaceutical legislation, there are differences in the obligations imposed upon the holders of centralized and national MAs. The specific cross-reference to Volume 9 guidance that appears in Directive 2001/83/EEC is absent from Regulation 2309/93.

Who has the reporting obligation?

The Directive (because 75/319/EEC was amended by 2000/38/EEC) has included a further obligation for the *PRP*, namely paragraph (d) Article 103: 'the provision of any other information relevant to the evaluation of the benefits and risks' of an authorized product. This provision drew together the legal obligation of competent authorities to *collect* information useful in the surveillance of medicinal products and that of MAHs to report such information; MAH reporting obligations had been more narrowly drafted in 75/319/EEC.

Whilst in Article 20 the Regulation includes a general obligation of the MAH to 'ensure that all relevant information' about suspected adverse reactions is brought to the attention of the Agency, this is not yet a specific aspect of the PRP's duties. Volume 9, however, draws no such distinctions.

Source of reports

Volume 9 guidance interprets Article 22 of the Regulation as comprehending ADR data appearing in worldwide literature and states that 'receipt' of the data occurs on the date of 'awareness' of the publication by a member of the MAH's personnel for the purposes of calculating reporting time. This is not an apparent meaning of Article 22.

Volume 9 states that the reporting of ADRs occurring outside the EU is required where they are brought to the MAH's attention by a healthcare professional. Whilst Article 104.4 of the Directive is consistent with this, the Regulation does not refer to a healthcare professional in this context (see Article 22.1 paragraph 2).

The Regulation does not obviously refer to ADR reports received by MAHs from competent authorities. The Regulation is also silent on what Volume 9 calls 'reporting requirements in special situations' (i.e. overdose, pre-grant of an MA, lack of efficacy, abuse, etc. (paragraph 1.3)).

As written, the legislation requires PSURs to be furnished at the end of time periods calculated from the grant of the product MA in the EU. Guidelines have introduced the concepts of the European birth date (EBD) and the international birth date (IBD). This approach was developed to avoid a multiplicity of different reports for the same product where it is marketed in several countries. The guidelines also permit the altering of the periodicity of PSURs when new products, derived from the same active ingredient, are authorized by a competent authority. Technically, the legislation includes no such flexibility. However, member states who agree variation from the 'rule' would be estopped from taking any action against the MAH who files reports pursuant to such agreement. If the guidelines are considered to be more practical, then it might be preferable for the legislation to be amended to require submission in accordance with the guidelines, rather than to lay down provisions that are routinely modified in practice.

The guidance contains specific references to MAH obligations in relation to voluntary product withdrawal on which the legislation is currently silent. This may change pursuant to the Review.

The guidance on compliance (1618/01 – see below) requires the MAH to notify 'immediately' any change in the balance of risk and benefits. This seems to comprehend even minor or positive changes. Clarification is needed here : perhaps by the addition of the word 'significant' and an explanation of what that would mean.

It is important to clarify the relationship between the law and the guidance. If there is to be legislation setting out obligations for competent authorities and MAHs, but also guidance to which specific cross-reference (i.e. requiring tasks to be done 'in accordance with', or by reference to, such guidance) is made, then where the parameters are drawn is crucial. This is particularly so in cases where they overlap, but are not identical, and where the drafting of the guidance as a whole is much less disciplined than that of the legislation.

There would be merit in the legislation reflecting guidelines, by making express the requirement to conduct ongoing, proactive safety evaluation of an authorized product post-MA grant, what this means and the requirement/process/time for notification linking in with the PSUR obligations.

Article 22 of the Regulation and Article 104 of the Directive display drafting differences, despite the stated intention of the EU authorities to have the same requirement for all marketed products irrespective of route of authorization.

Article 104.3 of the Directive includes an obligation to record and report (on an expedited basis) 'all other serious ADRs which meet the reporting criteria in accordance with the guidance referred to in Article 106(1) of which he can reasonably be expected to have known . . .'. There is no equivalent in the Regulation. Furthermore, precisely what is meant by 'other serious ADRs which meet the reporting criteria', the 'reporting criteria' and 'reasonably be expected to have known' (except regarding literature reports, as this is mentioned in Volume 9) is an open question.

Concept Paper on Compliance with Pharmacovigilance Regulatory Obligations (1618/01)

The draft of this paper emerged in March 2001 for consideration in the Pharmacovigilance Working Party (CPMP) and was adopted in November 2001 with a view to becoming operative in January 2002. Its drafting, as is the case with Volume 9, pre-dated the introduction of the codifying Directive 2001/83/EEC. The time lag generally complicates the reading of all the guidance at present.

The document addresses compliance and therefore, what constitutes 'non-compliance' with the pharmacovigilance rules which are to be enforced through inspection or 'monitoring' by the competent authorities.

It emphasizes the importance of PSURs and states that non-compliance with obligations 'may include':

- Submission outside the correct cycle, outside correct time frames or non-restart of the cycle when necessary.

  As discussed, what is the 'correct time frame' may be a matter of discussion with competent authorities. In relation to all products, EC legislation is drafted by reference to the authorization date for the product concerned. In guidance and practice, this has been recognized as inadequate and other approaches have been adopted, from using an IBD (first authorization worldwide), to the EBD (first authorization in the EU), to a revised EBD based upon the introduction of further products to a 'family' related to the originally authorized product.

  Thus, in relation to centralized products, – technically there is no legal flexibility or option as to time frame: the date of central authorization is the start date and basis for establishing a timetable.

  What is the correct cycle at national level may well vary country to country. This is messy and confusing and does not promote ease of compliance.

  In practice, for any authorized product, the key must be what has been agreed with competent authorities and/or imposed as part of the MA.

- 'Poor quality reports'.

  This leaves the judgement of when compliance is achieved (i.e. what is acceptable 'quality') with the competent authority but seems to take no account of the potential for dialogue between the MAH and an authority, or the difficulties that the MAH can experience (through no fault) in obtaining follow-up information to complete and contextualize ADR reports received. It would no doubt be assumed that, for reasons of fairness and proper process, the judgement of non-compliance must follow prior notification of the MAH of the alleged deficiencies, followed by requests for correction, supplementation or explanation and the opportunity for the MAH to improve/remedy the situation before action is taken/sanctions set in motion. However, this is not addressed in the guideline. The idea that the authorities might judge the adequacy of the MAH's follow up by reference to the data received direct by the competent authority ignores the fact that a healthcare professional may be more cooperative and forth-coming in the reports made to regulatory authorities than to the MAHs.

- Failure to highlight differences between company core data sheets and national/EU summaries of product characteristics (SPCs) will be considered an instance of non-compliance, but the guidance fails to say which areas of these documents need to be compared, and multiple comparisons against many national SPCs is a potentially long and involved process.

- The guidance provides that competent authorities 'will' scrutinize post-authorization safety study protocols prior to initiation of the study. It is left to member states to determine the process for this. The potential outcome of this liaison or scrutiny is undefined, i.e. should there be a means by which the study is blocked, changes required to the protocol, etc?

It will be evident that there yet remains some scope for refining EC legislation and guidelines.

The potential impact of the 2001 Review of pharmaceutical legislation

The Commission's proposals for the amendment of Directive 2001/83 and Regulation 2309/93 are currently working through the legislative process. The European Parliament's first report and multiple suggested amendments were debated in October 2002. Political agreement was reached in the Council in June 2003. The formal Common Position and Second Reading in Parliament are anticipated in the Autumn of 2003.

In its current draft form (which may change), the following changes are worth noting:

1.   The Regulation

• Article 20 will specify the ability of the CPMP to determine that variation is a measure necessary to ensure safe and effective product use.

• Article 21 will include the additional obligation for the PRP (paragraph (d)) to provide 'any other information relevant to the evaluation of the risks and benefits' to regulatory authorities.

• Article 22 will be broadened to require reporting 'in accordance with guidelines' of suspected serious ADRs which meet the notification criteria 'of which the MAH may reasonably be expected to be aware …'. At face value, the latter wording would mean that if an MAH could, in the view of the authorities and bearing in mind the advice given in Volume 9 and perhaps the practices applied in industry generally or in relation to the class of/similar product, have made itself aware of certain information, then it will be a breach not to have reported that data even though in reality it did *not* actually know of that data.

• Electronic communication will become a requirement of reporting, and adherence to the guidelines in Volume 9 on that topic will become an obligation.

• The periodicity of PSURs will be altered (to take account of the removal of the requirement for renewal of MAs):

Current	Future
• Upon request	• Upon request
• Six monthly in first 2 years	• Six monthly in the first 2 years
• Annually for the next 3 years	• Annually for the next 2 years
• Thereafter, every 5 years	• Thereafter, every 3 years

• Accepted international medical terminology will have to be used by MAHs.

2.   The Directive

- Article 104 will be amended to require electronic reporting of ADRs.

- Reporting of suspected serious unexpected ADRs occurring outside the Community will not be dependent upon the reports being communicated to the MAH by a 'healthcare professional'.

- PSUR periodicity will be changed to the same timetable as in the Regulation (above).

- In the case of concertation and MR products, reports must be made additionally to the Reference Member State.

- Article 107 will introduce provisions in relation to the process of handling urgent safety measures to protect public health.

European powers and procedures in the event of a product safety issue

The interplay between national and EC authorities on pharmacovigilance matters, and in particular, the action that can be taken and procedures applicable to the processing of a safety concern, is dependent upon the nature of the product authorization.

Single national marketing authorizations

If the product concerned is authorized through the national route in only one member state, then dealing with pharmacovigilance signals indicating a product safety concern is a matter for the national authority, following national procedures, pursuant to national legislation (Table 10.3). This national legislation must implement and take account of EC provisions, in particular Articles 126 and 116 of Directive 2001/83/EEC, which define the circumstances in which revocation or suspension may occur.

In 1993 the ECJ determined in the case of Pierrel Spa versus Ministero della Sanita (C183/92) that a national authority could revoke or suspend an authorization only on the grounds provided by what was then Directive 65/65/EEC and could not add to their national provisions other bases which extended beyond the scope of the EC provisions. The case did not (as Article 21 does not), however, address the matter of the compulsory variation of national authorizations. This remains at local discretion for purely nationally authorized products. It should, however, be noted that Article 107 of Directive 2001/83 obliges (apparently without limit of situation) member states to notify the EMEA, and other member states (and the MAH) where it considers that an MAH should be suspended, withdrawn, or varied in accordance with guidance in Volume 9. In urgent cases, an authority may suspend an MA provided notice is given within one working day to the Agency Commission and other member states. The legislation does not confine itself to MR cases.

Table 10.3   Product authorized nationally in one member state: procedure

- National law and procedures apply
- Article 126 of Directive 2001/83/EEC applies: 'An authorization to market a medicinal product shall not be refused, suspended or revoked except on the grounds set out in this Directive'
- The grounds are to be found in Article 26, 2001/83/EEC

  'The marketing authorization shall be refused if:

  a) the medicinal product is harmful in the normal conditions of use

  b) its therapeutic efficacy is lacking or is insufficiently substantiated

  c) its qualitative and quantitative composition is not as declared

  ... the particulars and documents submitted in support of the application do not comply with Articles 8 and 10(1)'.

  And in Article 116:

  'The competent authorities of the Member States shall suspend or revoke an authorization to place a medicinal product on the market where that product proves to be harmful in the normal conditions of use, of where its therapeutic efficacy is lacking, or where its qualitative and quantitative composition is not as declared.

  Therapeutic efficacy is lacking when it is established that the therapeutic results cannot be obtained with the medicinal product'.

  'An authorization shall also be suspended or revoked where the particulars supporting the application ... are incorrect or have not been amended in accordance with Article 25 or where the controls referred to in Art 112 have not been carried out'.

- Article 117 further allows member states to take 'appropriate measures to ensure that the supply of the product[a] shall be prohibited and the medicinal product withdrawn' on the same grounds as appear in Article 116 and in the event of the occurrence of manufacturing defects.

[a] Or an appropriate batch.

Products marketed in more than one member state

Where the product is also authorized (by national route) in more than one member state or where it has been authorized by the decentralized/MR route in several member states, there is the potential (national products) or the requirement (MR) for a safety question to be examined by the CPMP (in future, following the Review, to be referred to as the CHMP – Committee for Human Medicinal Products).

EC provisions make arrangements for the dissemination of alerts and information between member states and between member states and the EMEA (see Article 105 of Directive 2001/83/EEC and Article 24 of Regulation 2309/93). Article 122 of Directive 2001/83/EEC states: 'Member States shall take all appropriate measures to ensure that the competent authorities concerned communicate to each other such information as is appropriate to guarantee that the requirements for the ... marketing authorizations are fulfilled'. The speed and means of transmission of the information depend upon the level of seriousness assigned to the concerns arising from the information received. The system is such that an MAH cannot expect a safety issue to remain ring-fenced within a particular member state when the product is marketed in other parts of the EU.

Where a product is authorized in more than one member state, the reference provisions in Articles 30 and 31 of Directive 2001/83/EEC (formerly Articles 11 and 12 of Directive 75/319/EEC) allow a member state (or the MAH, or the Commission) to refer certain questions (which would include a safety issue) to the CPMP, which is obliged, under Article 27.2, to examine it. When a reference is made by a member state, it must be notified, not only to the

CPMP, but also to the MAH. Both the member state and the MAH are, thereafter, obliged to supply to the CPMP all available information relating to the matter in question which is in their possession. In this way, the issue and its solution are thrown into the European arena for a 'European solution' to be adopted.

The nature of this process and CPMP obligation was, during 1996, the subject of some debate in the context of the review of oral contraceptives relating to the degree of risk of serious thromboembolic events in third-generation pills. It was unclear whether the UK had made a formal reference under what was then Article 12 of Directive 75/319/EEC (now Article 31 of 2001/83) to the CPMP and whether this was the only option that could be used by a member state – in other words, whether the matter had to be addressed through a formal process. In the event, the CPMP dealt with the matter on an informal basis. An examination of the wording of the legal obligations of the CPMP, does not suggest any CPMP discretion as to whether to accept a reference. However, there must be a 'reference' for the procedure to be set in motion, and the legislation does not spell out any particular method by which one is to be made or recognized. Volume 9 refers to a 'letter' initiating the process. The Annex to Volume 2A of the Rules also contains examples of forms of reference. In theory, therefore, a reference can be made simply by a clear, identifiable request addressed to the CPMP to examine a question that is adequately set out and described. Equally, it would seem a matter may be brought to the CPMP for consideration without the instigation of a formal reference.

The Commission and CPMP view appears to be that it is in the general interest for there to be a less formalized process available for the CPMP's scientific experts, specifically through the Pharmacovigilance Working Party, to evaluate a product safety issue without the Committee being drawn immediately into formal and time-limited procedures requiring them to reach a formal opinion that is binding in the EU (once adopted by the Commission). The discussion of matters raised by member states within the CPMP's Pharmacovigilance Working Party is not, therefore, uncommon with the working party reporting its views on an issue informally to the CPMP, a practice that is not covered specifically by legislation.

Referral to the Committee for Proprietary Medicinal Products

There are a number of possible bases for referral to the CPMP in the event of a product safety concern. These are discussed below. In practice, in the context of pharmacovigilance, it is Articles 31 and 36 that are most important.

Article 30 (formerly Article 11 75/319/EEC)

Article 30 applies where several applications have been made for authorization in the EU and member states have taken 'divergent decisions' *inter alia*, concerning the suspension or withdrawal of the product authorization.

In such a case, either the MAH, a member state(s) or the Commission may refer the matter to the CPMP. In practice, references borne out of a Pharmacovigilance issue are likely to be brought increasingly by Reference Member States re decentralized products as a result of guidance stating they should take a lead role in product monitoring and in due cause, due to amendments to 2001/83 requiring all data to be reported to and accessible by the Reference Member States.

Article 31 (formerly Article 12, 75/319/EEC)

Under the provisions of Article 31, in 'cases where the interests of the Community are involved'[6] a member state(s), the MAH or Commission 'may' refer a matter 'before reaching a decision on the suspension or withdrawal of an authorization or on any other variation to the terms of the MA which appears necessary to take account of information collected in accordance with Title IX'. (Title IX of the Directive contains the pharmaco-vigilance requirements.) The burden of demonstrating that the interests of the Community are involved rests with the referring party.

There has been debate (for example, in relation to the anorectics review begun in 1996) about the use of Article 12 (now 31), in relation to a 'class' or group of authorized products, although the guidance in Volume 9, Part 2, paragraph 2.5, states clearly that *other medicinal products containing an active substance of the same therapeutic class may also be referred'*. An Article 31 reference was made in July 2002 by France in relation to Cox-2 inhibitors as a group. The Commission appears to intend to clarify its use in these cases and obviate any further discussion or doubt though the amendment of Directive 2001/83/EEC, the draft of which specifically anticipates referrals of a 'range' of products within a therapeutic class for CPMP consideration (Article 31.2).

Article 36 (formerly Article 15a 75/319/EEC)

Article 31 makes provision for cases to be referred to the CPMP, before a member state reaches a decision with regard to any application, suspension, withdrawal or variation, 'which appears *necessary*, in particular, to take account of the information collected in accordance with Title IX' (emphasis added). The reference is, in fact, not compulsory; 'may refer'. However, under Article 36 of Directive 2001/83/EEC, a member state, *in respect of a mutual recognition or a concertation* (Directive 87/22/EEC) product, i.e. 'a marketing authorization which has been granted in accordance with the provisions of this chapter', *must* refer the matter to the CPMP in circumstances where, pursuant to pharmacovigilance data, it considers a variation of the authorization, or its suspension, or withdrawal, is 'necessary for the protection of public health'. Where a product has passed through such a harmonizing EC process of registration, the resolution at EC level of a concern that a member state considers warrants a regulatory response is compulsory. Volume 9 refers to Article 36 as the *'principal legal basis'* for referrals for MR products.

The relevant procedures for references are set out in Articles 32–34 of Directive 2001/83/EEC (see Table 10.4). The drafting of the legislation is, however, significant. Articles 30 and 31 state that the procedure applicable to references made under their provisions is set out in Article 32 (alone). Article 32 deals only with the process up to and including the issue of the CPMP opinion. Article 36 states that the relevant procedure is contained in Articles 32–34. Articles 33 and 34 deal with the process of the production of a binding Commission Decision pursuant to the CPMP opinion. Since a CPMP opinion is not binding of itself, and since Articles 33 and 34 clearly seem to follow chronologically from Article 32, it may have

---

[6]Whatever discussion there may be as to the meaning of this phrase, there has been little doubt that matters of public health and safety in the EU, fall within that description. Volume 19 Pt II 2.5 provides that this is a reference to community public health in the light of *new* data relating to safety, quality or efficacy, or new pharmacovigilance data.

Table 10.4   Products authorized in more than one member state: procedure

Day 1	Reference to CPMP
	↓ Rapporteur and experts (if appropriate) appointed
	Information sought from MAH; others
	Written or oral explanation from MAH
Day 90[a]	CPMP reasoned opinion
	↓
	Opinion to EMEA
	EMEA informs MAH 'forthwith'
	↓
	Within 15 days of receipt of opinion, MAH to give notice in writing of any intention to appeal
	↓
	Within 60 days of receipt of opinion, MAH forwards detailed grounds for appeal
	↓
	Within 60 days of receipt of grounds for appeal, CPMP to consider whether to revise opinion
	↓
	Within 30 days of adoption of final CPMP opinion, EMEA forwards it to member states, Commission and MAH with assessment report and reasons for conclusions
	[and (applicable to references under Article 36 only)
	Commission prepares decision according to usual decision-making process (Articles 33 and 34)]

[a] May be extended by 90 days where Articles 30 and 31 apply. May be shorter if Committee agrees in cases of urgency. Clock may be suspended whilst preparation of explanations is under way.

been thought that this was merely a drafting error, rather than an attempt to distinguish Articles 30 and 31 references from those under Article 36. (Volume 9 Part I refers in paragraph 1.1.2.2 to decisions on the basis of CPMP opinions pursuant to Articles 13 and 14 of 75/319/EEC now Articles 32–34 2001/83/EEC.) However, in December 2002, the Court of First Instance of the European Communities gave its judgement in a group of cases (Cases T-74/00, T-76/00, T-83/00, T-84/00, T-85/00, T-132/00, T-137/00 and T-141/00 Artegodan GMBH and others versus Commission) involving several healthcare companies interested in the supply of anorectics whose MAs had been the subject of a Commission Decision pursuant to a referral to the CPMP. A crucial finding of the Court was that there *is* a distinction in the procedures that apply in respect of referrals and in the outcome of those procedures depending upon whether the reference is made under Article 36 or Articles 30 and 31. What this means is that the Commission has no power in relation to national authorizations, unless they have been granted following the application of the MR procedure, to impose the recommendations of the CPMP. Therefore, referrals to the CPMP in respect of purely national authorizations are consultative only and cannot lead to the enforcement of a Commission Decision. Competence remains with the regulatory authority that granted the national MA.

In addition the judgement reaffirmed the rule that the revocation/suspension of an authorization must only be based upon the protection of public health, which is founded upon product risk–benefit analysis. The Court held that for the withdrawal of an MA to be justified there would need to be 'a new potential risk' or 'the lack of efficacy is substantiated by new objective, scientific and/or medical data or information'.

The implications of this decision, is that only non-binding CPMP opinions are produced by referrals except under Article 36. The current Heads of Agencies initiative for referrals under Article 30, in an attempt to harmonize the SPCs of certain products, is clearly not capable of imposing variations to national MAs. It remains to be seen whether and how the Review proposals to amend the European pharmaceutical legislation may yet be altered to provide for binding decisions in all cases in the light of this judgement, which is clearly contrary to previous Commission practice and conviction.

The provisions for appeal hearings under Article 31 state only that the MAH 'may' be asked to explain itself, orally or in writing, before the CPMP reaches an opinion. To the detriment of the MAH, this appears to contrast with the provisions relating to references under Article 30, where the provision is that the MAH has a 'right' to make oral or written explanations. Article 36 references are not mentioned specifically. However, bearing in mind the principles of 'natural justice', it is strongly argued that the difference in drafting style should not be treated as legally significant, with the MAH in any of these situations, in fact, being entitled (as a matter of proper process) to be afforded the same rights to appear before, and be heard by, the CPMP in order to defend its product(s). This approach is confirmed by the text in Volume 9 and by proposed amendments to Directive 2001/83 pursuant to the Review – which remove any distinction between Articles 30 and 31 in this regard.

The CPMP 'appeal' provisions have been a matter of some debate. The concern is that the provisions do not, in fact, constitute a true appeal, but rather a mere reconsideration by the same committee of its own prior decision. Lobbying by industry groups and others, however, failed to produce any changes to this position in the draft amendments to 2001/83/EEC. Challenges to Community Decisions (Article 36 cases) lie in the European Court of First Instance. At national level, where an authority seeks voluntarily to take regulatory action against an MA in line with a CPMP opinion, such compulsory action will invoke all the usual national appeal procedures.

In the context of a product safety concern, the outcome of the CPMP's consideration may be an opinion/recommendation that the MA, the SPC (or its equivalent) and labelling should be varied, or that the MA should be suspended or revoked, with immediate, or phased product withdrawal. In the case of Article 36 referrals, delay can arise with regard to the procedural stages that occur 'after' the CPMP has delivered its opinion. Although there are time limits applicable to the decision-making process with reference to when the EMEA must forward the CPMP opinion to the Commission and when the Commission must draft the resulting licensing decision (both 30 days), time limits are largely absent from the point in the process at which the Standing Committee becomes involved (see also: Regulation 1662/95). The time between Standing Committee consideration of the decision proposed and the Commission's finalization of the decision is not time limited and can be lengthy. This is simply the result of application of a standard procedure applicable to all decision making by the Commission, which, when applied in the pharmaceutical licensing context, is not ideal. Having said this, in the field of pharmacovigilance, where the decision may concern a serious matter, the sense of urgency may well be such that the formal decision, pursuant to the CPMP's opinion, would be made with all due haste. Member states have 30 days to comply with the final decision and also to confirm with the CPMP and the Commission that they have done so. Again, although not discussed in the legislation, member states, with due regard to their responsibility/liability to local populations, would be expected to take action locally at an early stage following a CPMP opinion in an urgent case.

However, there can be difficulties in relation to local imposition of some MAH restrictions. Regulation at local level may give rise to problems in applying decisions nationally in these areas that have been treated as matters of local control to greater or lesser degrees:

- legal status distribution channels

- pack size

- specialist or hospital use and labelling.

In any event, member states do not have to wait for the final decision before taking any protective action in an Article 36 situation. Directive 2001/83/EEC (Article 36.2) allows the suspension of 'marketing and use' at a local level in 'urgent cases' pending a final EC decision and subject to notice being given within one working day to the Commission (CPMP) and other member states of the action taken and reasons for it.

In reality, the extent to which member states may deal with what they perceive to be product safety issues *without* reference to the CPMP is questionable. In the case of an MR (or decentralized) product, this is unlikely ever to be an option; it is difficult to think of a case where compulsory action is contemplated by the member state and such action is not considered 'necessary for the protection of public health', i.e. the basis upon which the obligation to refer arises. With purely nationally authorized products there is no requirement in the legislation for a reference, but it should be noted that Article 30 makes provision for references to the CPMP to be made where member states have adopted divergent decisions in relation to MAs for essentially the same product, and the Commission has made plain its interest in minimizing the extension and persistence of differences in MAs granted in different member states for the same basic product, although, as a result of the 2002 ECJ decision, it cannot lead to forced harmonization. The system of circulating information between member states and the opportunity for discussion at the Pharmacovigilance Working Party tends to work against action taking place within only one member state without others also deciding to undertake a review.

A member state's ability to deal on a purely local basis with a safety concern may also depend upon the content of national provisions. In the UK, parts of SI 1994 No. 3144 are written in a way that rules out the unilateral initiation of national procedures applicable to taking compulsory regulatory action where the product in question is 'authorized elsewhere in the Community'. Perhaps the original intention was to reflect the aims of what was then Article 15a, Directive 75/319/EEC (now Article 36), and to deal with MR products, but that limitation was not properly classified into the local law, which would require amendment to achieve this clear result and remove the uncertainty now pertaining to local procedures in such circumstances.

In practice, in the past, where product crises have arisen since the introduction of the New Systems, as discussed above, the CPMP has not been reluctant to take an informal approach to assessing the position. Hence, on a number of occasions, the CPMP has preferred to adopt a "position statement", to issue press releases and let matters be thrashed out in the Pharmacovigilance Working Party without being subject to formal process of referral. There were/are clear advantages in such a stance, but there were/are, inevitably, also difficulties. 'Informal' consideration does not result in a binding opinion/decision. Member states are free to apply the outcome of the discussion 'if' and 'as', they see fit. With the non-formal approach, neither the authorities nor the MAH has an established process or timetable to follow. The MAH has no specific rights (e.g. to make representations to adequate time) upon which to rely. The MAH can still, however, be required to supply information requested to the authorities on statutory grounds (both the Regulation and the Directive require the PRP to supply data relevant to safety evaluation fully and promptly – Article 21c 2309/93 and Article 103c Directive 2001/83/EEC). It is obliged under Title IX to provide information relevant to an assessment of risks and benefits of a product. In such circumstances, it would clearly be arguable that it would be against natural justice, even in informal circumstances, for a body charged with responsibilities to consider, advise and/or review by the Community to fail to allow representations to be made, or to take them into account. However, the lack of set time limits, procedures and requirements does mean that there is potential for these rights to be undermined when they are afforded and exercised on an *ad hoc* basis. Informal procedures are run according to time frames that are determined by the CPMP and/or the Working Party, and the process of evaluation may last for some considerable time amidst a blaze of publicity. Even after CPMP consideration that does not result in any formal opinion or informal recommendation to limit product use or availability, a product may nevertheless be 'killed off' in the marketplace owing to resulting public speculation regarding its safety and the capitalization by competitors upon such doubts. Following the anorectics judgement, that even formal referrals under Article 30 or 31 cannot result in an opinion which can be transposed into a Commission Decision, it remains to be seen whether matters are more or less likely to be referred to the CPMP in future under Article 32 procedures.

The MAH may anticipate, and thus better manage or even avoid, compulsory regulatory action by adopting (in cooperation with competent authorities) a voluntary course. This could range from product withdrawal and yielding up the MA, to proposing variations to the MA and SPC initiating the procedure. In the case of an MR product, variation must be done (Regulation 541/95) on an EC-wide basis – so there is no prospect of any irregularity developing across the EU. (Note: the current text of the Review proposals will require voluntary withdrawals by MAHs to be referred in advance to competent authorities.)

Centrally authorized products

Where products are centrally authorized, the responsibility for arranging and coordinating the consideration of safety issues is done at European level, through the EMEA upon the advice of the CPMP (in particular with the input of the Pharmacovigilance Working Party) albeit that the alert/concern may originate from one (or more) member state(s).

Regulation 2309/93 emphasizes (Recitals) that procedures must ensure the rapid withdrawal of any product which presents an unacceptable level of risk under normal conditions of use. At present, the Regulation still cross-refers to the pharmaceutical legislation prior to consolidation in the form of 2001/83/EEC, which can make it difficult to follow. The provisions relevant to product safety issues are covered in Articles 18 and 20.

Article 18

Article 18 provides a process whereby a member state or the Commission must inform the CPMP (and Commission) when it considers that one of the measures envisaged in Chapter 4 Title IX of 2001/83/EEC (previously Chapter V and Va of Directive 75/319/EEC), i.e. (inspection) variation, suspension, revocation, should be applied to a centrally authorized product. The member state, or the Commission, must give detailed reasons and indicate what it considers to be an appropriate course of action.

Notification leads to a CPMP opinion delivered within a time frame determined on a case by case basis according to the urgency of the matter. The process does not guarantee the MAH a right to be heard:

"Wherever practicable the person responsible for placing a medicinal product on the market shall be invited to provide oral or written explanations."

However, arguably, a situation would have to be serious and urgent and there would need to be no other reasonable means of dealing with the matter so as to protect the public, without cutting across the MAH's rights, for this to be justifiable. This seems more likely to be arguable, but not certain, where a temporary measure was proposed, pending a full consideration of the issues and options available which would involve representations made by the MAH.

The wording also suggests that the MAH has to choose whether to make oral *or* written representations; but again, in context, it is probably correct to read 'or' as 'and/or' as there will be circumstances when both written submissions together with oral presentation and availability to respond to questions from the CPMP would be the best means to address the issues.

The CPMP opinion is then converted into a Commission Decision. During this process, member states are able to suspend the use of a medicinal product on their territory 'where urgent action is essential to protect human health or the environment'. Again, such action must be notified immediately (the following working day) to the Commission and other member states and is only acceptable pending the final determination of the issue at EC level (Article 18.6).

Article 20

Article 20 envisages the CPMP formulating 'opinions on the measures necessary to ensure safe and effective use' of centralized products 'if necessary' in the context of ADR information received by the EMEA. The same procedure applicable to Article 18 applies.

Controversially, neither Article 18 nor 20 provides an appeal right for the MAH – 'whenever practicable'. This is in contrast to the position relevant to procedures initiated under Regulation 542/95 (as amended by 1069/98 and which has since become 1085/2003) for compulsory variation of the MA pursuant to a provisional urgent safety restriction imposed by the Commission, where the possibility of an appeal is envisaged as a result of the cross-reference to Article 9 of Regulation 2309/93 on appeals procedures.

The drafting of the legal provisions is confusing. The process for the Commission to follow in issuing a 'provisional' urgent safety restriction is not actually specified, but rather is implicit in the Regulation. The MAH is obliged in these circumstances to apply for a variation of the MA 'taking into account the safety restrictions imposed by the Commission'. Precisely how such a measure fits in with Articles 18 and 20 is also not explicit: 'without prejudice' to Article 18, the procedure is set out in Articles 6 and 7 of Regulation 1085/2003. Consideration of the Review proposals for Article 18, however, place the adoption of necessary provisional measures between the receipt of a CPMP opinion and the adoption of a final decision, the time limit for which is 6 months. This would seem, therefore, to remain a process apart from the type of action contemplated by Regulation 1085/2003.

An MAH has an option, where a safety problem seems likely to result in compulsory action, to take voluntary action ('urgent safety restriction') under Regulation 1085/2003. By making proposals to the EMEA, to which the Agency does not object within 24 hours, the MAH is able to introduce its proposed measures and to make a corresponding application for the variation of the MA.

Failures to meet adverse drug reaction reporting requirements

Assuming no deliberate concealment of information, there may be a number of reasons why compliance failures occur. In the last 10 years, the list of reasons has changed. Shortcomings, which might have been described as common in Europe in the early 1990s, are very much less likely to be encountered in the prevailing regulatory climate, in which product safety and pharmacovigilance now occupy a central position. For example, since the advent of 'New Systems' and the legal requirement for there to be an appointed 'person responsible' (in the EU) for pharmacovigilance for each MAH, the once common occurrence of corporate groups setting up their pharmacovigilance functions with reference to the rules and regulations applicable to the non-EU jurisdiction in which their head office was based, is very much a thing of the past. The legislation forces companies to focus upon operations and accountability within the EU.

Similarly, the failure of companies to devote adequate resources to pharmacovigilance is ill- advised and increasingly unusual. The profile of the regulatory function generally within pharmaceutical companies has grown tremendously over the last 10 to 15 years with the realization that unless regulatory affairs are in order and without proper regulatory input into policy and strategy development, the core of the business of pharmaceutical companies (i.e. selling products), could be seriously undermined. The priority now given at EU level to pharmacovigilance cannot be ignored. Current proposals for the review of the pharmaceutical legislation place considerable focus upon drug safety; and include proposals for the end of five-yearly MA renewal linked directly to enhanced pharmacovigilance obligations.

Nonetheless, compliance failures can occur[7] and may include:

- *Misunderstanding the requirements.* The more complex the requirements and the greater the multiplicity of requirements imposed by different authorities, the easier it is to make errors. It is still the case that the Commission's aim[8] of consistency across the EU has still not fully been achieved, given that member states continue to insist upon adding their own national requirements to those in Directive 2001/83. A misunderstanding of terminology (e.g. 'serious', 'severe' and 'relevant') is not unusual.

---

[7] A small study in 16 countries in 2001, discussed at the Drug Industry Association Euro Meeting in Basle 5–8 March 2002, found problems in the following areas: confusion amongst personnel; difficulties in arrangements with sub-contractors and non-compliance; lack of experienced personnel; lack of interaction between staff in post marketing, clinical trial and epidemiological groups/departments; poor review of functions, poor quality control/ monitoring/auditing.

[8] 'Whereas it is the interest of the Community to ensure that the pharmacovigilance systems for centrally authorized products . . . and those authorized by other procedures are consistent.' Recital 57, Directive 2001/83/EEC.

- *Poor or incomplete SOPs*. SOPs must be written to cover all aspects of pharmacovigilance procedures. Poor drafting will mean that SOPs are not comprehensive and cannot perform the function of ensuring compliance. Moreover, failure to review and update SOPs will ultimately result in out-of-date, non-compliant procedures and results. Regular audit of pharmacovigilance clause functions is also important in order to identify areas of procedure that are not applied, do not work or are incomplete/inadequate. SOPs are an identified target for inspectors looking at a company's compliance with the legal requirements. (See Guideline 1618/01 on compliance.)

- *Poor inter-company communication*. This may lead to unnecessary delays in relevant information being reported by the MAH. Increasingly, over recent years, various regulatory authorities have shown that they are minded to try to look through the separate legal personalities of different companies within (or even without) a corporate group and to expect rapid exchange of information within those corporate groups, particularly in relation to pharmacovigilance. As a matter of law, there are established principles for respecting the individuality and separate 'personality' of companies, which, although part of a global group of companies, may well be totally separate in terms of their jurisdiction, operations and internal organization. Nonetheless, from a product liability aspect, it is in the interests of the companies and corporate headquarters to ensure efficient exchange of relevant product and market information and regulatory data between group members who have products in common. Moreover, in a legal climate where the Directive and, pursuant to the Review, the Regulation; (see Article 104.3 of 2001/83/EEC and Article 22 (proposed amendment) of Regulation 2309/93) requires reporting of ADR data of which a company should 'reasonably be aware', the MAH must put in place and be able to demonstrate that it has a system in which all reasonable steps are taken to place the MAH in a position to make such reports. Even between unrelated corporate entities engaged in a contractual arrangement, the guidelines indicate the authorities' expectation that procedures in both companies should be designed so as to ensure expedited reporting within 15 days of receipt of data by the first company to receive the data, whether or not that company is the MAH.

- *Delay*. This is usually consequential upon one of the other shortcomings above. Inefficiency in company systems, can lead to backlogs developing.

- *Failure to train representatives*. As part of the company structure, representatives in the field are often the first point of contact between the company and healthcare professionals. EC law makes it plain that company representatives have a clear role in pharmacovigilance (see Article 21, Regulation 2309/93 and Article 103, Directive 2001/83/EEC). Failure to train representatives, and failure to establish procedures that require and enable them to pass on promptly, information collected in the field from healthcare professionals, can lead to companies overshooting the 15 calendar day (from receipt by the representative) reporting period for spontaneous, serious adverse reactions.

- *Failure to provide for regular review*. Before the requirements were introduced for PSURs it was not unusual to come across MAHs who did not have adequate procedures in place for regular review of the totality of ADRs and safety data received within a given period and comparison against the previous product record. In this way, for example, increased incidence might be missed. The requirements under the legislation for PSURs should make such omission impossible. However, inadequacies in PSURs are a major focus of the compliance guideline 1618/01 and it is clear that the authorities place considerable importance upon this aspect of practice. Proposals to remove the requirement for 5-yearly MA renewals are largely dependent upon the operation of a robust periodic reporting and assessment system. (Review proposals 5/3/02 COM (2001) 404-1 and 404-2.)

*   *Poor follow up*. It is a common criticism by regulators that reports are not adequately followed up by MAHs. However, it may be that the MAH's ability to undertake follow-up is severely curtailed by the attitude and lack of cooperation from the original sources of reports or lack of knowledge, such as when corroboration is sought from a doctor when the original source is a patient or pharmacist. This highlights the general absence in much of the EU of any legal compulsion for healthcare professionals to submit reports. The European rules 'allow' (Article 101 Directive 2001/83) member states to make reporting by healthcare professionals a legal requirement. In the majority of member states, however, the professionals have not had this obligation imposed upon them (an exception is Italy, where rules affecting doctors and pharmacists have been introduced). The receipt of initial reports and of follow-up information may be affected, therefore, by the knowledge of and approach to reporting that is characteristic of the health professionals in particular member states. In some cases this may not be especially well developed. For example, even in the more sponsor-controlled environment of clinical research, it seems practice may be patchy. Bohaychuk and Ball (1999), in their book '*Conducting GCP Compliant Clinical Research*' commented that it was not uncommon for investigators to decide for themselves (irrespective of protocol) whether to record an adverse event (AE) in a case report form and for follow up to be confined only to the first stages of a clinical study.

*   *Failure to tie in licensees, distributors, joint venture and other partners*. It is still common for contracts between commercial partners to give low priority to the arrangements for liaison in relation to pharmacovigilance. It is also still common for these arrangements to be addressed only after a contract has been entered into and for there to be little or, in some cases, no provision for exchange or supply of information. Although imposing obligations does not guarantee adherence by a contractual partner, total failure to set them out clearly in the first instance is a major oversight. Addressing the issue only after a contract has been completed may give rise to delay and difficulties when the parties cannot agree the arrangements in subsequent discussion, and may have more far-reaching consequences when the structural and financial provisions are, or would have been, affected by the arrangements necessary for pharmacovigilance practice (e.g. in a large contract where the cost of IT systems is an issue). Volume 9 now makes it very clear that the regulatory authorities will expect to be informed of and, by implication, satisfied by the arrangements put in place in these circumstances. Companies should be prepared to submit copy documents to provide information and to be inspected for good pharmacovigilance practice. Whatever the legal position as to whether a company has breached actual reporting requirements, a poor showing at an

inspection is clearly undesirable for a number of reasons, including loss of credibility with regulators and exposure in product liability terms.

• Failure to learn from mistakes/experience. The consequences here are self-evident.

Consequences of failure to meet requirements

The consequences of failure to meet requirements can be roughly divided into three categories:

• regulatory

• civil

• criminal.

The consequences may apply to the MAH, to the individual who is appointed as PRP and also to other officers of the MAH. It may be thought that the appointment of a 'person responsible' would insulate all other senior company officers from any responsibility in relation to a failure of compliance, but this is a misconception. As a matter of law, and depending upon the provisions applicable in the member state dealing with the breach, it is possible for other officers of the company of sufficient level of authority and having some degree of responsibility, involvement and/or knowledge to be made subject to enforcement proceedings.

Regulatory consequences

Regulatory consequences will affect the MAH and the MA itself. A loss of credibility with regulatory authorities can be a serious commercial concern. A failure in reporting compliance may ultimately result in product safety being reviewed (see below), although it is probably actually more common for failures in reporting to come to light 'after' a product safety issue has already been identified.

It is very doubtful that a breach of pharmacovigilance requirements could ever justify revocation of an MA in the absence of a clear and immediate safety concern of a serious nature (i.e. whether the technical breach alone would be significant justification). As discussed above, Directive 2001/83 provides for suspension or revocation of authorizations where the product proves harmful in normal conditions of use, its therapeutic efficacy is lacking, or where its qualitative and quantitative composition is not as originally declared where the 'particulars' supporting the MA are incorrect or have not been amended or where quality controls have not been carried out. (N.B.: the 'particulars' include details of adverse reactions, warnings, precautions, etc.; see Article 116 and Article 117; see also Regulation 2309/93 for equivalent provisions for centralized products). Directive 2001/83/EEC refers to suspension or withdrawal taking place where it is necessary for the protection of public health. As mentioned, in the case of Pierrel SPA versus Ministero Della Sanita (C183/92, 7 December 1993), the ECJ found that the only grounds upon which revocation would be justifiable by the Italian authorities were those mentioned in the Directive (then 65/65/EEC). It is not open to competent authorities (central or national) to add to those provisions.

Therefore, it seems that any failure in pharmacovigilance compliance must be more than a technical breach: it must raise a question of safety, quality or efficacy for a revocation of the authorization to be justifiable and consistent with the terms of the Directive. In contrast, US provisions for post-marketing reporting of adverse drug experiences state, 'If an applicant fails to establish and maintain records and make reports as required under this section, FDA may withdraw approval of the application and thus prohibit continued marketing ...' (Paragraph 71, 423 S314.81). (Note: amendments proposed pursuant to the Review to these provisions do not require a product to 'prove' harmful, only for the 'view to be taken', i.e. by the competent authorities, that it may be. This is a shift in emphasis that has worked its way into the draft legislation pursuant to the Review in order to clarify that the authorities may act upon reasonable suspicion rather than upon proof, applying the precautionary principle to the protection of public health.)

There is an obvious possibility that a breach of a pharmacovigilance obligation would provoke/justify competent authority inspection (*ad hoc*, and/or increased frequency of periodic inspections). Where products are nationally authorized, local law will be applicable in respect of operations taking place within the jurisdiction. Member states' national laws may assign wide powers to the competent authority inspectorate (e.g. UK Medicines Act 1968, Section 111 *et seque*). Directive 2001/83/EEC clearly envisages 'repeated inspections' to ensure compliance with legal requirements (see Article 111). Although the inspection provisions were originally placed in the legislation in the context of the regulation of manufacturing operations, it has arguably been the basis for inspections to be undertaken by certain competent authorities in much broader circumstances and, with the modification of the legislation, is more clearly applicable.

Where a product is centrally authorized, the responsibility for following up pharmacovigilance matters rests with the EMEA. However, the EMEA has no real manpower for the conduct of inspections and EC legislation generally envisages cooperation between the Community and member states. The mechanism for an inspection in those circumstances, would be liaison between the EMEA and the member state(s) in which the MAH conducted relevant operations, where the pharmacovigilance function took place. Regulation 2309/93 envisages the Commission, in such circumstances, coordinating the 'supervisory responsibilities' of member states. The concept paper envisages the results of inspections being provided to the MAH with an opportunity for comment being afforded. As a matter of proper practice, established at national level, due process would dictate an opportunity to respond and a mechanism for responding to any enforcement action that an authority may institute. Article 17 states that the 'supervisory authorities shall have responsibility for exercising supervision over MAHs' in accordance with Chapter V of Directive 75/319/EEC (i.e. pharmacovigilance activities), now Chapter 4 Title IX of 2001/83/EEC. The Regulation actually defines 'supervisory authorities' as those who have granted a manufacturing authorization, or where batch control and release of third-country imports takes place. This may not, however, be the same country as that in which the company bases it pharmacovigilance activities. However, 'supervision' and enforcement are not necessarily synonymous, and this does not seem to rule out action by another member state with legal jurisdiction, perhaps at the supervisory authority's request. This remains speculation in the absence of any actual examples.

Article 17.2 of Regulation 2309/93 provides further for 'serious disagreements' between member states as to MAH compliance with manufacturing or pharmacovigilance requirements to be settled by the Commission requesting an inspector from the supervisory authority to undertake a further inspection accompanied, if required, by an impartial member state, and/or a Rapporteur or expert nominated by the CPMP. Member states are also obliged to refer to the CPMP concerns arising and proposals for action to be taken where they consider one of the measures covered in Chapter V or VI, Directive 75/319/EEC or 2001/83/EEC (pharmacovigilance sections) should be applied.

Civil consequences: – product liability

Although, in the context of personal injury claims, the MAH and other parties (e.g. doctors, licensing authorities) may all be the target of proceedings, it is usually the MAH pharmaceutical company, perceived as having 'deep pockets', that is the prime target for claimants. Claims for negligence based upon a failure to act with reasonable care (e.g. to obtain or act upon pharmacovigilance data) and/or the supply of a product that is 'defective' in legal terms (e.g. because its labelling was not amended, pursuant to the receipt and review of pharmacovigilance data so as to give adequate warnings and precautions) are always possible.

Tables 10.5 and 10.6 set out in very simple terms the necessary 'ingredients' for establishing product liability, either in negligence or under statute: so-called 'strict liability'.

Table 10.5 Criteria for negligence (N) – D+L+F+C=N

D: Duty of care	Owed to the claimant; easy to establish in the case of the supplier/manufacturer *vis à vis* the patent who uses the product
L: Lack of reasonable care	Evidenced by a failure (through an act or omission) to conduct operations according to accepted standards applicable at the time – i.e. a breach of regulatory requirements, or possibly failure to take account or apply (industry) guidelines
F: Foreseeable injury	Of the type likely to occur following the failure identified (e.g. side effect of the drug)
C: Causation	The lack of reasonable care must have caused/contributed to the injury; if a label would not have been read by the patient in any event, then an omission from it might not have 'caused injury'

Table 10.6 Criteria for strict liability (SL) – D+D+C=SL

D: Defect	Widely defined – product design defect, manufacturing error, or deficiency in 'presentation', i.e. product information labelling which renders the product safer than persons generally are entitled to expect
D: Damage	To person (or property) flowing from the defect
C: Causation	See Table 10.5

All of the elements of each of these legal wrongs must be present in a given situation for liability to be established. In negligence, therefore, where the claim is made against the person alleged to owe the duty of care (in the context of this chapter this will be the MAH putting the product on the market), proof of causation, without a lack of reasonable care having occurred, will not afford the claimant a remedy. However, the chief distinction between negligent liability and so-called strict liability is that, in the case of the latter, fault is not required to be shown. To establish strict liability (Directive 85/374/EEC) the claimant must establish against the 'producer' (manufacturer/supplier/first importer into the EU), that the product was 'defective' (for the purpose of the law, this could refer to shortcomings in its presentation, design or manufacture) and that it caused the injury suffered. In practice, claims in negligence have outnumbered strict liability cases. It is only in recent years that strict liability claims have started to emerge in personal injury cases.

It would not be at all unusual for claimants in personal injury actions to look for a regulatory compliance failure on the part of a company defendant. The demonstration of a regulatory breach will significantly assist the plaintiff in establishing lack of reasonable care (i.e. conduct falling below acceptable standards) for the purposes of a negligence claim. In fact, whether the alleged failure is directly relevant to the injury or not, it can be used to demonstrate a more general lack of care in the operation of corporate systems with prejudicial effect. Indeed, a breach of legal requirements may not be necessary to establish lack of care. Failure to apply accepted standards (e.g. recommendations in guidelines) may be significant in the absence of good reason on the part of the MAH. Failure to warn is a common element of many pharmaceutical product liability cases, where the pleadings (of negligence and strict liability) might be expected to assert that had the labelling accurately dealt with contraindications, precautions and/or warnings, the patient would have avoided the injury allegedly suffered, either because the product would not have been used/administered at all, or the patient would have been monitored, advised (by the treating doctor), or managed differently so as to avert injury.

In a case where pharmacovigilance omissions are identified that can be said to lead to no/or an insufficient response being adopted by the MAH (especially where the regulatory authorities have taken some form of action, or simply criticised a company), then the plaintiff is a significant way towards establishing a case for lack of reasonable care in negligence, or that the product was defective in strict liability terms, because it was not presented accurately and was, therefore, less safe than persons were entitled to expect, given the content of the labelling.

Table 10.7 sets out a hypothetical example that briefly illustrates the basic issues. In this situation, the company has received reports of serious unexpected possible ADRs. The

Table 10.7 Example

Product X MA granted in 1993
Patient A prescribed product in July 1994
Company receives several reports of serious unexpected possible ADRs early May 1994
Follow-up poor and protracted
Reports not filed for 12 weeks; company takes no further action thereafter
Mr A suffers serious reaction (same as those reported) end July 1994
Following eventual receipt of reports, regulatory authority reviews product safety profile and (a) takes it off market, or (b) strictly limits its use and amends warnings and contraindications (identifying an ascertainable group of patients in whom use is discouraged) in September 1994
Mr A sues, claiming he would not and should not have been exposed to the drug at all; he falls within the contraindicated group

product has not long been on the market and is probably under intensive monitoring. Where those professionals reporting the events clearly suspect them to be ADRs, the company should have treated them as such and notified the authorities with basic information immediately, supplying follow-up data as it was obtained and affording the authorities the opportunity to pursue their own line of enquiry. To report only after follow-up and then not to consider (aside from compulsory activity by the authorities) what would be an appropriate response would not amount to reasonable, responsible conduct, especially when the authorities subsequently take action to withdraw/amend the MA.

In such circumstances, Mr A can make a good case for saying that swifter action by the company would have resulted in earlier product withdrawal/MA or labelling amendment such that he would not have been exposed to the risk of hazard.

There are factors that might alter the legal assessment of such cases. For example, had the information received been garbled and difficult to draw any conclusions upon, or insufficient to constitute an ADR report, the delay in following up until the 'minimum' information necessary was available might not be unreasonable where action could not be taken until intelligible, assessable data were obtained. If follow-up were unsuccessful, the ability to demonstrate that all reasonable steps had been taken by the company would be crucial. (Note: in the USA, regulatory requirements require a report of 'steps taken to seek additional information and the reasons why it could not be obtained' with regard to 15-day alert reports.)

It may be that even had a label change been implemented earlier, Mr A's doctor would still have prescribed X, judging the potential risks to be outweighed by the potential benefit and that Mr A would have agreed to take it, so that the omission/defect did not actually lead to the injury and the label change would not have changed the course of events. This line of argument can be problematic where the compulsory regulatory action taken is MA suspension followed by revocation. It may well be less likely (although not impossible) that the exercise of medical discretion would have led to the prescription of a withdrawn product.

The company's failure to amend labelling or withdraw the product might still be acceptable if the company can show that it did promptly, fully and properly consider the data, but reasonably (i.e. for good, identifiable, recorded reasons) decided in all the circumstances to leave the product on the market in its current presentation. Subsequent compulsory action by the authorities, defended by the company, would not render a well-considered decision unreasonable retrospectively, although that fact is likely to test strenuously the rationale of the company's earlier decision making. In general, in any event, although certainly influential, the decision of an authority will not be determinative of whether there has been negligence or whether a product is defective.

Criminal consequences

The possibility of criminal sanctions for breach of pharmacovigilance requirements arises in a number of member states, including the UK. They may be applied to MAH companies and to individual employees, including the 'responsible persons', with the resulting prosecution, in the worst cases, leading to a fine and/or imprisonment, loss of reputation and, in the case of individuals, loss of employment. These sanctions are clearly, for individuals, potentially very serious consequences and highlight the level of responsibility imposed upon those taking on the role of 'person responsible' for pharmacovigilance. Having said this, within

Europe, individual prosecutions are relatively rare in relation to regulatory breaches generally. It is difficult to identify any publicity within the EU of any prosecution of a private individual in cases of non-compliance with MAH obligations since the requirements were introduced.

Where nationally authorized products are concerned, the relevant local provisions may be applied by the member state in respect of the MAH and possibly company officers, including a 'person responsible' whose identity is notified to the authorities. With regard to mutual recognition products, these are still locally granted authorizations and breaches could be expected to be dealt with on a local level with liaison between authorities.

The relevance of local sanctions to breaches occurring in relation to centrally authorized products, where the competent authority is the EMEA/Commission, must be examined further. The Commission has no powers of prosecution, no criminal competence in this context and the regulations and legislation do not currently contain any specific reference to types of sanction. (But note, the Review provisions foresee the Commission having powers to impose fines in certain cases of breach of the Regulation.) However, the EC does expect member states to take proportionate measures in order to enforce EC law. It is expected that member states will enforce the law with the same effectiveness and thoroughness as national law (see Council Resolution 95/C 118/01). As with regulatory supervision, the mechanism, therefore, is for authorities at EC level (EMEA/Commission) to request a member state or states to take action according to their local provisions in respect of MAHs/persons responsible, etc. operating within their jurisdiction. Article 69 of Regulation 2309/93 specifically provides that member states must determine the penalties for infringement of the Regulation. These penalties must be 'sufficient to promote compliance'. If a breach occurs in certain jurisdictions, then this might constitute an offence, but the MAH could, it would seem, be subject to different enforcement action in other member states where the locally provided penalties are less strict. Table 10.8 shows the differences between some member states in their provisions for sanctions for breaches of pharmacovigilance regulations. For example, in the UK, the Medicines Act 1968 provides for criminal sanctions for several offences and, under Section 124, for the individual 'personal' criminal responsibility of corporate officers. Under Regulation 3144 of 1994, which implements all recent EC pharmaceutical directives, enforcement powers are expressly reserved in respect of 'EU obligations', which include those relating to pharmacovigilance (see Schedules 3, 10 and 14). The legislation makes no distinction whatsoever between action taken where centrally authorized products are concerned and where products have national authorizations. However, it would be unlikely that a member state would act in respect of breaches concerning a centralized product without first reporting/referring to or receiving a request from the competent authority – EMEA/Commission/CPMP.

It is clear from EC legislation (see above) that the member states' competent authorities are expected to monitor compliance and to keep the European authorities well informed. Under UK law, criminal prosecutions against individuals are still relatively rare and, indeed, prosecutions generally are undertaken only in clear-cut cases, since the competent authority must make a significant commitment of its limited resources. However, EC policy in addressing regulatory obligations and allocating regulatory responsibility is increasingly to nominate individuals within MAHs for key responsibilities at the regulatory level with the intention, no doubt, of focusing activity and attention, and improving compliance. For this to be achieved, there must evidently be potential for sanctions to be imposed where standards are not achieved, particularly where there are marked consequences for patient health.

Table 10.8 Pharmacovigilance – member states (survey McKenna & Co., autumn 1996 and spring 1997)

Country	Legislation	Offence	Sanction
Belgium	Law on Medicinal Products 25.3.1964 (as amended), Royal Decrees 3.7.69 (as amended) 7.4.95	Breach may be punished by criminal sanction or administrative fine; depends upon seriousness	Imprisonment (8 days to 1 month) and/or fine (BEF100–1000 × 200) Administrative fine (BEF100–500 × 200)
Germany	German Drug Law 1976 (as amended), Regulation (Pharm. BetrV) Federal Health Office (BGA) 1991 (due to be replaced by announcement of Federal Institute (BfArM))	Administrative offence	Fine up to DM50 000 (criminal liability for bodily injury or involuntary manslaughter)
Italy	Presidential Decree No. 93 25.1.91, Decree of Ministry of Health 20.4.91, Circular of Ministry of Health 29.4.93, Law 24.1.96, Legislative Decree No. 44.F18-2-97	Administrative sanctions for breach of rules with regard to institution of pharmacovigilance services: fines from Itl30 million to Itl180 million (MAH and person responsible)	Penalty Itl1 million Itl10 million and imprisonment up to 6 months in cases of violation of duty to record and notify serious ADRs to the competent authorities or to file a report upon request or periodic reports
Spain	Law 25/1990, Royal Decree 767/93	Administrative infringement (serious)	Fine 500 000–2 500 000 Ptas (or five times value of product)
UK	Medicines Act 1968, Regulation 3144 of 1994	Criminal offence	Fine and/or imprisonment. Fine £5000 (summary) unlimited (indictment) and/or imprisonment (2 years on indictment)

Safety in research products

Regulatory controls

Although this chapter is concerned with marketed products, some comments should be added concerning products in development. Until Directive 2001/20/EEC on Clinical Trials, there was no European-level legislation relating specifically to the conduct of clinical research. (Directives 65/65/EEC and 75/319/EEC addressed only the technical aspects of the content of dossiers compiled for the purposes of making an MA, i.e. 'analytical, pharmacotoxic ... and clinical standards and protocols in respect of the testing of medicinal products', and imposed a generalized requirement for 'good clinical practice' in research.) Controls were purely a matter for the national authorities and local legislation. This situation will continue until implementation of the new Directive by member states during 2003–04 (and by May 2004 at the latest). Until that time (and possibly even after it) the various different methods of trial authorization and control of trial products and practices will continue to vary by member state. This necessarily includes requirements relating to reporting of adverse events/reactions.

Looking ahead, the Clinical Trials Directive will lead to a number of changes in handling and reporting safety data. The objective of the directive in the context of pharmacovigilance is to introduce harmonizing provisions for 'the monitoring of adverse reactions occurring in clinical trials using Community surveillance procedures, in order to ensure the immediate cessation of any clinical trial in which there is an unacceptable level of risk'. It can be expected that monitoring of trial sponsors' compliance with the law, in particular through 'good clinical practice' (GCP) inspections, will develop significantly after the directive is implemented. In a regulatory climate in which pharmcovigilance generally has assumed major importance, safety reporting is likely to be a significant focus of such trial inspections. As indicated, research has suggested that safety reporting in clinical studies is below standard. In 41 per cent of 378 study sites audited by Bohaychuk and Ball (1999) 'significant under-reporting of safety information' was uncovered.

The requirements (a) for reporting by the investigator to the trial sponsor and (b) by the sponsor to the competent authorities of the member states (and ethics committees) are contained in Articles 16–18 of the new directive. As in the case of marketed products, the legislation sets out fundamental requirements, but envisages (Articles 1.3 and 18) the drawing up and publishing of 'detailed guidance on the collection, verification and presentation of adverse event/reaction reports together with decoding procedures for unexpected serious adverse reactions'. In the context of this directive, the guidance generated/adopted in line with Article 18 is advisory and there is no text explicitly requiring acts to be done in accordance with the guidelines. In practice, however, the authorities are likely to expect reference to the guidelines and cogent reasons for deviating from them. Some may use the guidelines in developing the implementing local legislation.

It is also worth remembering that it is already a legal requirement and will remain so, if data are to be acceptable to competent authorities, that clinical trial data should derive from trials conducted in accordance with 'GCP' (Part 4, B Annex 1, 2001/83/EEC). The new Clinical Trials Directive includes similar wording in Article 1.4. ADR reporting is a feature of working to GCP standards.

Current law, i.e. Directive 2001/83/EEC, is not specific as to the basis of determining GCP, but, in practice, the ICH guidelines (ICH/135/95), which have been in place since January 1997, are and have been an obvious relevant set of standards for application to European trials. Paragraphs 4.11, and 5.16,17 of the ICH GCP guidelines addressed safety reporting and information as follows:

- Investigator obligations (Paragraph 4.11)

    (a) To report serious AEs, immediately to the sponsor.

    (b) To provide 'detailed' follow-up reports in writing.

    (c) To comply with applicable regulatory requirements re reporting of unexpected serious ADRs to regulatory authorities and ethics committees.

    (d) To report AEs identified in the protocol as critical to safety evaluation to the sponsor according to the protocol.

(e) To supply information relating to deaths to the sponsor and ethics committees as requested.

- Sponsor obligations

  (a) Responsibility for ongoing safety evaluation of investigational products.

  (b) To notify 'promptly' all concerned investigators, institutions and the regulatory authorities of findings that could adversely affect the safety of trial subjects, impact the conduct of the trial or alter the ethics committee's approval or favourable opinion.

  (c) To expedite the reporting to investigators, institutions, ethics committees and regulatory authorities of serious and unexpected ADRs.

  (d) To comply with 'applicable regulatory requirements' and ICH guidelines on expedited reporting.

  (e) To submit to regulatory authorities safety updates and periodic reports 'as required by applicable regulatory requirements'.

By referring throughout to 'applicable' or 'relevant' requirements, the guidelines simply advise compliance with the rules applicable in the countries in which the research is conducted (and where the results may be used in a regulatory MA submission). What is interesting about the pharmacovigilance provisions of the Clinical Trials Directive is that Article 16 of the directive draws much of its text from the ICH guidelines. However, the directive does/will impose some specific reporting obligations (e.g. as to time limits) upon trial sponsors (Article 17).

It seemed highly unlikely that any future guidelines adopted pursuant to Article 18 of the Clinical Trials Directive would be inconsistent with the ICH GCP standards. In July 2002, the Commission released a draft of guidelines on the principles of GCP in the EU of clinical trials (ENTR/6416/01). It specifically cross-referred to ICH GCP (135/95), which must be 'taken into account' in the conduct of clinical trials. At the same time, the Commission released the draft ADR reporting guidelines (Detailed Guidance on the Collection, verification and presentation of adverse reaction reports arising from clinical trials . . . ENTR/6422/01). There were marked similarities between the draft and ICH guidelines, but the latter contained recommendations that were not part of the ICH guidelines. In the consultation process in relation to the draft EU guidelines a number of issues were identified as requiring further consideration or revision. These included:

- resolving what approach should be adopted in determining whether there is an adverse event or reaction, i.e. causation. The guidelines contained advice in relation to two different tests: that a causal connection could not be ruled out and that there were reasonable grounds to consider the existence of a potential link between the event and the administration of the investigational product.

- Clarifying whether Annual Reports were to be required per protocol or per programme.

The law is drafted in a way suggesting that annual reports are required per protocol at intervals determined according to commencement of an individual study.

- Determining the practicality of reporting of individual ADRs to ethics committees and the way in which ethics committees are to handle and respond to the data.

- Clarifying when trial sponsors should break a study blind in order to report to competent authorities – when the event that may be a reaction occurs or at the end of the study?

- Clarifying who determines expectedness of an ADR – investigator or sponsor?

- Addressing the overlap of trial requirements (which can include studies after the grant of an MA) with the requirements for reporting in respect of marketed products.

ENTR/6422/01 was finalized in April 2003. Several issues thrown up by the previous draft were clarified. Paragraph 6.2.2 provides that an adverse event "judged either by the investigator or sponsor as having a reasonable suspected causal relationship" to the study drug is an adverse reaction. The Annex clarifies that there should be evidence or argument to suggest a causal relationship." Paragraph 6.3.2 confirms the need to submit "once a year throughout "the clinical trial a safety report. Where several trials are being conducted on the same product, it is also provided that the report should include a "concise global analysis of the actual safety profile" of the product. The provisions are still expressed on a per trial basis. Further guidance has been given on the submission of "SUSARs" (serious unexpected suspected adverse reactions) to ethics committees (paragraph 6.3.1.6.5) allowing for quarterly reporting. Expectedness is to be determined by the trial sponsor (paragraph 6.2.3). Some post marketing studies falling within the clinical trials Directive will feed data both into an annual safety report and into reports made pursuant to Directive 2001/83. The GCP guidelines have not been finalized and are expected to re-emerge as a new directive.

Notwithstanding the finalization of Article 18 guidelines, it would not be surprising to find member state regulatory authorities imposing additional reporting requirements locally, as has happened in relation to pharmacovigilance in respect of marketed products and taking individual approaches to interpretation.

Consent and risk

Achieving regulatory compliance in terms of adverse event/ADR recording and reporting (and thus avoiding problems with regard to trial 'authorization') is only part of the legal considerations related to the handling of safety data/information. Subject consent to trial participation is not a 'one off' event. Conducting a trial lawfully and ethically requires ongoing attention to the issue. A vital component of consent is information. In particular, it is only when adequate information has been given to the individual that he/she can assess the trial and the risks attached and make a proper decision as to participation. If the facts concerning a product change, in particular in the hazards and/or level of risk relating to the product and the change in fact may be such that a trial subject's assessment of his/her participation might be affected/informed by that information, that information should be passed on promptly to the trial subject. Failure to inform may undermine consent. If information is deficient, a subject may have a claim in negligence and/or strict liability. For example, if a subject continues in a study when he/she may otherwise have withdrawn and suffers an adverse event of which he/she did not know but ought to have known was possible through trial participation, there is the basis for a claim.

Personal data privacy

A discussion of the law concerning confidentiality and the protection of personal data privacy would be a detailed and lengthy undertaking and, accordingly, is not part of the scope of this chapter. However, it is a significant legal issue in the context of "processing" (see Data Protection Directive 95/46/EEC) pharmacovigilance data. Local implementation of the EC directive has resulted in differing approaches to the processing of sensitive, personal, health-related data, the provision of exemptions from requirements and certain data – subjects' rights (e.g. access to personal data held). The rules are relevant to all aspects of the 'processing' (everything from the collection, to the recording and circulation of data) of 'personal data' (i.e. which identify an individual or from which an individual could be identifiable) and, therefore, affect:

- the drafting of consent forms in clinical trials which consent to collection, use, and transmission of personal data to regulators and also out of the relevant jurisdiction may easily be sought

- receipt recording, storage, access, anonymization of data;

- reporting to regulatory authorities (these should be anonymized, but, in practice are not always supplied in that form).

A data privacy/protection assessment of all pharmacovigilance processes and procedures is, therefore, essential.

Reference

Bohaychuk W and Ball G (1999). *Conducting GCP Compliant Clinical Research: A Practical Guide.* Wiley.

11

Operational Aspects of the Drug Safety Function Within a Pharmaceutical Company

Janet Steiner

Introduction

This chapter focuses on the operational aspects of the drug safety function as related to the adverse event reporting process within a pharmaceutical company, placed within the context of basic functions and best practices. The discussion of the process will also include the key contributory roles of technology, quality control and training, as well as recommendations for working with external partners and sharing information with external stakeholders.

Overview of the case-handling process

A drug safety department in a pharmaceutical company performs many functions, although corporate structures in the pharmaceutical industry are extremely diverse in how the drug safety function fits within the company. Drug safety work may be performed within the regulatory function, the medical affairs function, the clinical development function, or as an independent area. The remit of drug safety may also be variously defined to include medical information activities, product complaint management, submission of regulatory documents, pharmacoepidemiology and/or safety support of clinical trials, as well as safety surveillance and other pharmacovigilance activities. However, the task most common to all safety departments is the reporting of adverse events to health authorities according to regulatory requirements. The process of collecting, processing, analysing, and reporting adverse event (AE) information will be collectively referred to here as *the case-handling process*. In addition to maintaining regulatory compliance, this process is a key component of pharmacovigilance. As discussed in Chapter 8, effective monitoring of drug safety not only requires a systematic approach to collection of information, but a means of organizing that information into a database that allows retrieval in a format amenable to screening and analysis. Much of the safety data available to a pharmaceutical company regarding its products arises from individual reports of AEs. Without effective management of this data

Stephens' Detection of New Adverse Drug Reactions Fifth Edition edited by John Talbot and Patrick Waller
© 2004 John Wiley & Sons, Ltd   ISBN: 0 470 84552 X

through the case-handling process, pharmaceutical companies would be less able to under-stand the evolving benefit-to-risk balance of their products in order to act responsibly in protecting patients (CIOMS, 1998).

Specifics of the case-handling process

Introduction

The case-handling process may be defined as the process by which single case reports of AEs (from clinical studies or from marketed use) are collected, evaluated and commu-nicated. This process forms the basis for an important part of the generation of safety signals and is a necessary prerequisite for enabling the company to comply with international regulations for reporting to regulatory authorities. Although this may vary widely between companies, certain common tasks exist. These tasks may be performed by different skill types, or they may be performed in slightly different sequences, but the steps described in this section provide the basic framework of almost any case-handling process.

The five basic steps in the case-handling process

The basic steps of the case-handling process are shown in Figure 11.1. Each of those individual steps is now discussed.

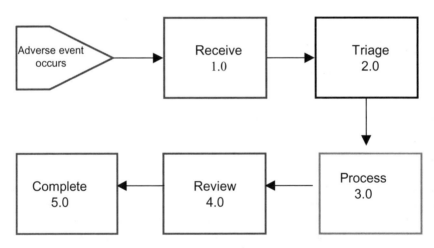

Figure 11.1   Overview of the case-handling process

Step 1: Case receipt

Companies receive AE reports from a variety of sources via a wide range of methods. Each method of case receipt has special case-handling considerations, but the one absolute requirement for all is that the date of receipt by the company or company's agent must be captured and recorded, since this becomes the clock start date for regulatory reporting (Figure 11.2).

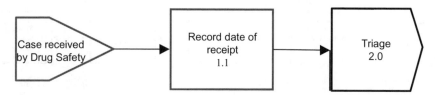

Figure 11.2   Step 1: Case receipt

- *Telephone calls.* Consumers and healthcare professionals may call the company to complain specifically about side effects they believe to be caused by medications, or they may call the company for other reasons, for instance to obtain reimbursements or medical information, and incidentally mention an AE. The company employee or agent taking the call must be sufficiently trained not only to recognize AEs, but also to know what information should be collected concerning the event. Additionally, it is essential to obtain contact information enabling further follow-up with the reporter. If the calls are received in an area outside of the safety department, then a means must exist to transmit the information quickly.

- *Facsimile transmission.* Although paper facsimiles, or 'faxes', have the advantage of providing automatic confirmation and date stamping, frequently there are legibility problems with the fax copies, and the use of faxes increases the amount of paper that must be tracked and archived. The use of 'e-fax' technology, in which faxes are automatically scanned into an electronic document that is received via electronic mail, allowing them to be viewed on-line and stored electronically, mitigates this problem.

- *Standard mail.* Since letters containing AE information may conceivably be received by anyone in the company, it is essential that all personnel are trained in recognition of AEs and understand that this information needs to be forwarded to the safety department as soon as possible. This training needs to include the highest levels of management within a company, since many times such letters are sent to the president or CEO of a company. The legal department is also a frequent recipient of such correspondence, and every effort must be made to ensure that the safety department is notified promptly.

- *Electronic media.* This category includes company electronic mail systems, company Web sites, Internet chat rooms, diskettes and compact discs, and electronic data capture systems used in clinical trials. Although the regulations do not require companies to search the Internet for AE reports, companies are required to monitor any company-sponsored Web sites for potential reports. The issues with electronic media are mainly issues of validity and verification.

Step 2: Case triage

Within the context of the case-handling process, triage is the assessment, classification and prioritization of the information received according to key regulatory, scientific and medical criteria in order to determine what route for processing the case should follow (Figure 11.3). This is the most important step in the case-handling process, when one considers the impact

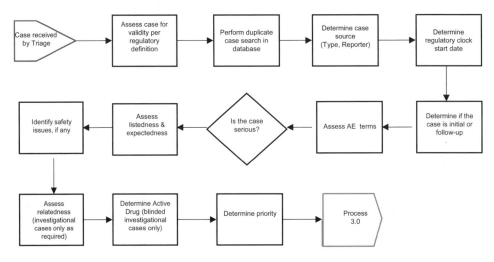

Figure 11.3   Step 2: Case triage

on the rest of the workflow as well as the consequences of triage errors, e.g. late regulatory reports, missed safety signals and/or waste of case-handling resource. Key issues for consideration in the triage process include the need for clear communication of triage decisions to subsequent participants in the workflow of the case, adequate knowledge level of those involved in triage, and the need for appropriate checks and balances to ensure that errors are caught early. Triage should be performed as early in the process as possible in order to ensure compliance with regulatory reporting timelines. Since this critical step in case handling has such a huge impact on the overall work of drug safety, experienced and qualified safety personnel should always supervise triage.

Step 3: Case processing

For the purposes of this chapter, case processing (Figure 11.4) is the creation of a case in the safety database from source information. Case processing includes the tasks of data entry

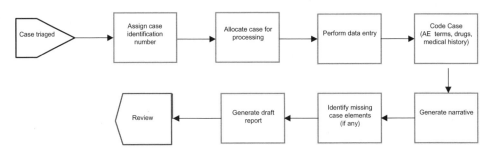

Figure 11.4   Step 3: Case processing

into the safety database from source documents, coding (AEs, medical history, concomitant conditions, concomitant medications, etc.), writing the case narrative and identifying missing information that should be pursued in follow-up.

Step 4: Case review

All cases should be reviewed after processing to ensure that regulatory, scientific and medical standards are met. Case review (Figure 11.5) may be characterized as a two-step process:

- quality review (see Figure 11.6)

- medical/scientific review (see Figure 11.7)

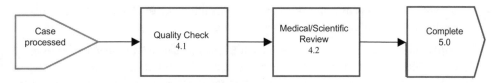

Figure 11.5   Step 4: Case review

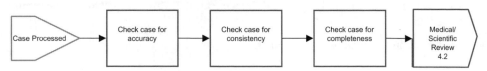

Figure 11.6   Step 4.1: Quality check

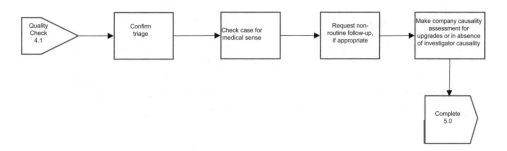

Figure 11.7   Step 4.2: Medical/scientific review

The key difference between the medical/scientific review and quality review concerns the focus of the review, rather than who does it, when it is done, or how it is done. The appropriate focus of the quality review should be:

- confirmation of the triage assessment of regulatory reportability;

- consistency of data-entry with source documents.

- consistency with established report standards (ICH, 1995).

In contrast, the appropriate focus of the medical/scientific review should be:

- Appropriateness of the AE terms selected.

- Confirmation of the seriousness classification of the AE terms.

- Agreement with the listedness/expectedness classification of AE terms.

- Agreement with outcome classification.

- Agreement with the coding of AEs, concomitant conditions, and medical history.

- Review of the narrative to ensure that it makes clinical sense and includes all important elements (the 2001 CIOMS V Working Group Report contains an excellent description of key components of AE report narratives).

- Authoring the company clinical comment, including determination of the company causality assessment, when appropriate.

- Identification of any specific additional information needed for medical assessment purposes other than routine follow-up requests required for case completion. Pursuit of follow-up on single case reports should be tailored according to the importance of the case in terms of attempts made and methods used (CIOMS, 2001).

- Consideration of 'upgrade' or 'downgrade' to the case's regulatory reportability classification.

- Identification of potential safety signals.

A rapid and clearly understood error resolution process must support case review.

Step 5: Case completion

The case is considered ready for completion when it has gone through triage, processing, review and approval. The case completion process (Figure 11.8) includes any updates to the case as required by the review cycle, incorporation of additional information requests into standard follow-up requests, generation of a final report and distribution of the final report to appropriate internal and external parties, which may include regulatory submission. Case

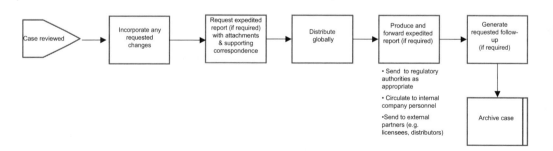

Figure 11.8   Step 5: Case completion

completion also includes archiving the report and the accompanying source documents. Strategies for document management should allow for paper as well as electronic storage.

Periodic safety updates

Introduction

In addition to the processing of individual case safety reports, drug safety departments are expected to collate, evaluate and report aggregate analyses of AE cases. Examples of these aggregate reports include the US Food and Drug Administration (FDA) periodic reports, International Conference on Harmonization (ICH) periodic safety update reports (PSUR) and European license renewals. This section will focus on PSURs, in particular on the process for the collection, review and analysis of aggregate safety data.

Re-evaluation of the benefit/risk ratio of a drug is usually not possible for each individual adverse drug reaction (ADR) case, even if serious. Therefore, PSURs present the worldwide safety experience of a medicinal product at defined times post-authorization, in order to:

- report all the relevant new information from appropriate sources;

- relate these data to patient exposure;

- summarize the market authorization status in different countries and any significant variations related to safety;

- create periodically the opportunity for an overall safety re-evaluation;

- indicate whether changes should be made to product information in order to optimize the use of the product (ICH, 1996).

Overview of the periodic safety update report document

Pharmaceutical companies are responsible for providing safe and effective drugs. To meet this responsibility, companies are expected to collect safety data on their medicinal products, perform pharmacovigilance throughout the entire life cycle of a product and provide accurate information to healthcare professionals and patients. In addition, companies are expected to keep regulatory authorities informed of the results from the ongoing safety evaluations of their drugs. A standard format for reporting safety evaluations to health authorities is the PSUR.

According to the current ICH E2C guideline (ICH, 2002), see Chapter 9, the PSUR should contain all relevant safety information collected within a specific time period along with a clinical evaluation of the data. Ideally, the data lock point or cutoff date of the PSUR is based on the date of the first market authorization for the drug, i.e. the International Birth Date. In general, authorities require a PSUR for a drug to be submitted every 6 months for the first 2 years after approval, annually for the next 3 years and every 5 years thereafter.

The PSUR consists of the following sections.

1. *Introduction.* A brief description of the purpose of the document, time period covered and reference to previous PSURs.

2. *World-wide marketing authorization status.* Tabular presentation of trade names and marketing authorization dates for all countries.

3. *Update of regulatory authority or marketing authorization holder (MAH) actions taken for safety reasons.* Details of the types of action relating to safety that were taken during the reporting period.

4. *Changes to the reference safety information.* A listing of specific changes made to the reference safety information during the reporting period.

5. *Patient exposure.* An estimate of the number of patients exposed during the reporting period along with the method used for calculation.

6. *Presentation of individual case histories.* Line listings and summary tabulations for cases received during the reporting period plus a brief description of cases considered particularly important.

7. *Studies.* A brief summary of any important safety studies and a review of published safety studies from the literature.

8. *Other information.* Explanation of any efficacy-related information collected during the reporting period. Presentation of any important late-breaking information received after the data lock point.

9. *Overall safety evaluation.* A concise analysis of the data collected during the reporting period followed by an assessment of the significance of the data from the perspective of cumulative experience. This experience includes a review of drug exposure in special populations, e.g. paediatric, elderly, organ impaired, exposure during pregnancy, overdose, drug abuse, drug misuse, drug interactions.

10. *Conclusions.* A comment on whether the data presented are in accord with the reference safety information and a description of recommended or initiated actions.

Collection and preparation of case-related data

The sections of the PSUR that deal specifically with case-related data are Sections 6 and 9. The main case-related components of the PSUR are the summary tabulation and line listing of medically confirmed serious (listed and unlisted) and non-serious unlisted ADR cases, the cumulative tabulation of medically confirmed serious unlisted ADR cases and the summary tabulation of the non-serious listed ADR cases found in Section 6. Effort should be made to ensure that the data contained in the tabulation and line listing are accurate and inclusive. This effort should focus on the following:

- Inclusion of all cases initially received or with significant follow-up received during the reporting period.

- Accuracy and completeness of the key data elements, particularly those related to the patient, adverse experience and drug exposure.

- Accuracy and consistency of the coding of the verbatim adverse experience terms against a standard medical terminology coding dictionary, e.g. MedDRA.

This initial review of the data can be facilitated by the generation of data quality reports that direct the reviewer's attention to specific data inconsistencies and omissions.

The PSUR line listing provides the reviewer with key information regarding the patient, adverse experience and drug exposure, along with a brief assessment of the case. The data in the line listing are usually sorted by the medical dictionary body system/system organ class and date of receipt of the case by the company.

Although ICH E2C requirements can be fulfilled by providing the summary tabulation and line listing of medically confirmed serious (listed and unlisted) and non-serious unlisted ADR cases, the cumulative tabulation of medically confirmed serious unlisted ADR cases and the summary tabulation of the non-serious listed ADR cases, companies should prepare listings and tabulations that are acceptable to all regulators. This is particularly important when submitting PSURs to the FDA, who require submission of consumer cases in addition to medically confirmed cases. The FDA also requires the submission of all spontaneous cases regardless of causal relationship to the drug. Companies can meet the reporting requirements of most regulators and still follow a consistent practice across all PSURs by including the additional cases in the ICH line listing or by providing the cases in an addendum or optional case listing.

The ICH line listing format is a useful standard; however, the output can quickly become overwhelming in PSURs containing a large number of cases. Therefore, it is helpful in the review process to complement the standard line listing with supplemental data reports. The reports should be in line listing and/or tabulation format for ease of review. Reports containing full case data and narratives could also be provided to allow a detailed review of selected cases. Topics of interest for supplementary review reports include serious medically confirmed unlisted cases received during the reporting period, cases with an outcome of death, cases involving drug use in special patient populations (pregnant women, elderly, paediatric, organ-impaired patients) and safety issues identified during the current review process or carried forward from previous PSURs. If appropriate, the results of the review of the topics of interest should be presented in the 'Overall safety evaluation' section.

The topics described above are common to most PSURs and can be delivered to PSUR authors as uneditable or not easily edited output. They can also be delivered in formats that allow sorting and subsetting of the data. However, the computer programs that generate the output are not usually accessible to individuals involved in writing PSURs and analysing safety data.

The complexity and inaccessibility of the underlying computer programs prevent data end-users from generating *ad hoc* data queries and reports that may be pertinent to the data in the specific PSUR. However, as computer software applications become more sophisticated and user friendly, data end-users will more accurately be able to query, subset and analyse data without the need for technical programming skills. These sophisticated software tools will provide greater data query and reporting flexibility and allow less reliance on preprogrammed data searches and rigid output.

Collection of other safety data

Certain sections of the PSUR, namely Sections 2–5 and 7, contain information relating to drug approvals and regulatory actions (Sections 2 and 3), reference safety information (Section 4), drug exposure (Section 5), studies and published literature (Section 7). In many pharmaceutical companies, the source data required to complete these sections are not readily available to individuals in drug safety departments. In these situations, it is necessary to include a 'call for information' step in the PSUR generation process. The call for information ensures that the appropriate business units are informed of the need for the information, the format required and the deadline for delivery.

The information relating to market authorizations, regulatory actions and changes to safety reference information (Sections 2–4) can generally be requested from the regulatory affairs business unit.

Patient exposure data, reported in Section 5, should be solicited from the business unit with access to worldwide sales information, such as global product information, global sales or global marketing organizations. It is important to collect this information from a consistent and reliable source. This will allow year-on-year comparisons of exposure data. Exposure data can be collected as kilograms or units sold for a specific time period and converted to patient exposure using an appropriate algorithm based on the use of the drug. The conversion method should be included in the section.

The clinical studies information contained in Section 7 should be collected from worldwide clinical project or clinical development teams. The purpose of the section is to highlight completed, ongoing or planned studies that provide important safety information that may affect product information. A detailed description and analysis may be appropriate for some studies; however, a simple listing of the study name, brief description of the study, start date, completion date, number of subjects exposed and brief description of the pertinent safety data is sufficient for most situations.

The compilation of published studies should be performed by individuals or groups experienced in search strategies within literature databases, such as library services or information management groups. Only those published studies containing safety information relating to the drug should be included.

Although the current practice within most pharmaceutical companies is to solicit non-case-related data from individual business units outside of drug safety, there is a trend in the industry to integrate data from various databases into a single 'data warehouse'. Once this is accomplished, the collection and review of these data, particularly the regulatory, clinical and exposure data, can be accomplished within the drug safety units, resulting in a more timely and efficient delivery of information.

Presentation of case histories

Section 6 of the PSUR provides an opportunity for the company to discuss cases of interest, including cases considered particularly serious, unanticipated or related to a particular safety issue. The sources of these types of cases can often be found in the pool of unlisted cases.

Individual cases selected for presentation should be described in narrative format. Groups of related cases should be summarized collectively. Use of the verbatim case narrative should be avoided. Case narratives, particularly those for expedited cases, are usually more detailed than is necessary for a PSUR. Case narratives may also contain information specific to follow-up expedited submissions that do not fit well in the PSUR context.

Overall safety evaluation

The overall safety evaluation for the PSUR is presented in Section 9. This section summarizes the results of the review of the line listings and tabulations, results of the continued analysis of ongoing safety issues and any appropriate safety signals generated through the ongoing pharmacovigilance process.

The organization of the overall safety evaluation section should be based on the types of issues discussed. PSURs with large numbers of cases, lengthy discussion or multiple issues should be based on a body system or system organ class organization, as appropriate.

The overall safety evaluation is followed by the assessment of the cumulative experience of the drug, such as effects of long-term use, effects of use during pregnancy, drug interactions, etc. The source of data for these evaluations is the supplemental data reports described above.

Managing the periodic safety update report process – scheduling and timelines for delivery

At any point in time, major pharmaceutical companies will have many drugs on the market with varying market approval periods in different regions of the world. For instance, a drug may have been in the marketplace for over 3 years within a European Union (EU) country and only recently approved in Japan. Under current regulations, the PSUR will be submitted annually in the EU countries but semi-annually in Japan. Additionally, ICH E2C (ICH, 2002) currently requires that PSURs be submitted to regulators within 60 days of the data lock point. Because of these complexities it is essential that companies devise a suitable project management and workload balance approach to the generation and delivery of PSURs. The project management approach begins with a centralized scheduling procedure for PSUR generation.

The source of information regarding worldwide market authorizations is generally the regulatory affairs business unit. Regulatory affairs would be responsible for compiling the PSUR needs for the drug, including reporting period(s), planned and actual submission dates and contact information. Drug safety units could then augment the centralized schedule with milestone dates pertinent to the generation of the PSUR, such as due dates for submission of non-case-related data, document review, approval and delivery dates.

Because the time interval between the data lock point and regulatory submission is relatively short (60 days), particularly for large reports, companies should enforce a strict set of deliverable action points for the compilation, review and delivery of the PSUR. The action points should actually start well before the data lock point to allow contributors to produce accurate and timely information. A sample timeline based on a 60-day submission and ongoing pharmacovigilance is shown below.

Day −28: initiate process

- send out call for information for non-case-related data

- meet with contributors to discuss relevant issues, known safety signals and deliverables

Day 0: data lock point

- run draft tabulations and line listings
- perform necessary data clean-up

Day 12: completion of Sections 1–5, 7 and 8

Day 21: completion of first draft of the PSUR

- send draft out for review

Day 35: close of draft review

- revise document and send out subsequent drafts if necessary

Day 45: approval, sign-off and internal delivery of final document

- send to business unit responsible for regulatory submission
- publish document using internal publishing standards
- archive document

Day 60: due to worldwide regulators.

Staffing models for the case-handling process

Definitions and standards associated with the case-handling process are covered in Chapters 1 and 9 and will not be reiterated here. The focus of this section will be on a description of common approaches to case management from both the medical/scientific and the staffing/ organizational perspectives.

There are several common staffing models used to organize a case-handling group to deal with AE reports efficiently. There are advantages and disadvantages to all. Below are some brief descriptions.

- *Division according to reporting source.* Traditionally, this sort of division refers to having one group process reports from clinical trials and another group process spontaneous reports from the post-marketing environment, i.e. post-approval, since safety regulations are similarly divided. However, there may be further subdivision by report source, e.g. one group may handle consumer reports exclusively while another group may handle reports from healthcare professionals, one group may handle reports just from Phase IV trials and another may be focused on earlier phase studies, etc. The efficiencies gained from this type of approach include: decreased training time, since the scope of work is narrowly focused; the ability for the groups to develop a deeper knowledge in their particular specialty; and the potential for developing a closer working relationship with their counterparts in key interface areas, such as clinical teams, because of the increased frequency of interaction. The disadvantage is that there is less flexibility in the ability of staff to cross-cover during absences and peak workload periods. Also, job satisfaction and retention may be adversely impacted if the employees feel that the limited variety in their work experience is boring and/or makes them less marketable.

- *Product life-cycle approach.* This structure typically divides products among persons or teams who are responsible for them through the entire product life cycle, from the earliest phase of clinical development until the product is no longer marketed. This ensures that persons processing the reports have in-depth knowledge of the product's safety profile, and can provide knowledge continuity to others outside of drug safety working with the product over time. The danger is that these knowledge experts may be lost to attrition or become impediments in the process if they do not share their expertise freely. Frequently, the product life cycle approach also utilizes therapeutic alignment, since it makes sense to group similar classes of products or those used in similar indications. This allows focused hiring of persons with backgrounds in the specialty area, which can shorten their learning curve and bring an additional knowledge resource to the group.

- *Therapeutic alignment.* This may not work well for companies with a diverse portfolio, and most companies will have a number of products that fall outside of their main therapeutic areas. If these 'orphan' products are distributed among therapeutically aligned teams, then they may suffer from neglect. If a 'miscellaneous team' handles these products, then the team may suffer from a perceived loss of status among the teams more therapeutically focused. Also, therapeutic alignment can limit flexibility in staffing coverage.

- *Pooled case approach.* In this staffing model, the cases are assigned as they are received, i.e. the first case is assigned to Person A, the second case is assigned to Person B, etc. This is based on the principles that:

  (1) over time, the workload will tend to even out so that no one person has more work than another, and

  (2) each person can be expected to process cases within similar time frames.

In reality, this is seldom true, since cases can vary widely in complexity, clusters in case types received frequently occur, compliance can be jeopardized by work overload, and productivity can vary widely from person to person. Additionally, this approach carries the risk that the least experienced person may process the most complex or medically important case. In order for this model to work, some sorting of cases must be done to align expertise with complexity, priority with availability, and case input with case output. If managed appropriately, this model ensures the greatest staffing flexibility, supports knowledge transfer, and, indirectly, employee satisfaction. That being said, it is difficult for this model to work in very large departments without robust tracking mechanisms, and, if there are a large number of products, training time will be prolonged.

Aside from staffing models at the organizational level, there are also staffing models at the role level that should be considered:

- *Data entry model.* In this model, the largest number of employees involved in case handling are devoted to data entry only, e.g. the rote transfer of information from source documents to proscribed fields in the safety database. These roles are supervised by a small number of persons with scientific, medical, and/or regulatory expertise who assess and analyse the cases, but who perform little of the hands-on case processing. The focus of such a model is primarily on regulatory compliance rather than on safety surveillance. This model is similar to the data management model used in clinical trials, although double data-entry is seldom performed. The advantage of this model is that it can handle a large number of cases very efficiently, and relatively cheaply, since it relies on a less expensive staffing pool. Additionally, it is much easier to recruit and train data-entry staff than more skilled healthcare professionals. The disadvantage is that fewer skilled persons means scrutiny of incoming cases is more cursory and less focused, so signals may be missed.

- *Case owner model.* In this model, healthcare professionals who have been trained in safety regulations perform all aspects of case handling. This ensures that all cases are subject to highly qualified scrutiny. The person who first processes the case becomes the 'owner', i.e. accountable for the quality, compliance and completion of the case through all initial and follow-up versions, and is responsible for tracking the case through the process, ensuring that required actions, such as physician review and regulatory submission, are performed as required. The disadvantage of this model is that it requires a greater number of expensive skill types, who are frequently difficult to recruit. Additionally, marketplace competition for these types of individual makes them more difficult to retain, especially as the data-entry component of the work may become tedious to these persons over time. Also, for many types of reports this level of expertise may be overkill, since simple non-serious reports of expected AEs may not merit expert scrutiny.

- *Hybrids.* Cost effectiveness and efficiency can frequently be increased by using a combination of the data entry and case owner strategies according to the types of product and report received. For example, if the bulk of incoming reports are from consumers, then it may make sense to use the data entry approach, and reserve the case owner model for serious cases from clinical trials. The available labour pool at any given time may also influence staffing; for example, during a period when local hospitals are downsizing, it may be relatively easy and cheap to recruit nurses and pharmacists to safety work.

- *Matrix model.* In this model, similar to that used by some innovative clinical teams, a cross-functional team comprised of persons with different skill sets and responsibilities work together in a defined process flow to take the 'raw material', e.g. source documents, and produce the 'end product', i.e. the completed report. This team includes persons outside of the drug safety department who may be performing functions that are traditionally considered to be drug safety roles. For example, there may be a designated safety specialist on the clinical team (or within the clinical research organization (CRO) working with the clinical team) who is the primary contact with the investigator to collect the necessary information. This person may enter the report into the safety database, and then interface with a counterpart within drug safety to ensure clarity and resolve outstanding questions. The clinical team physician and the drug safety physician partner in the assessment of the case.

Document management personnel (again either internal or external to drug safety), manage the incoming source documents, case files, and archiving. Data management and/or quality assurance personnel may perform quality checks, which enables ongoing reconciliation between the safety and clinical databases. A safety subgroup within the regulatory department may perform additional review and submission of the report. Other members of the matrix cross-functional team could include safety surveillance scientists, epidemiologists, medical information scientists, and those involved in communicating with independent ethics committees (IECs) and institutional review boards (IRBs). The key to the success of the matrix model is to avoid silo thinking, and evaluate each step of the process in terms of best fit within existing functions rather than in terms of traditional or legacy roles.

- *Out-sourcing.* Increasingly, companies are out-sourcing case-handling work to so-called 'safety CROs' – organizations that offer a menu of safety-related services ranging from taking incoming phone reports of AE to regulatory submissions of case reports (Chukwujindu *et al.*, 1999). Owing to the set-up costs of such an approach, out-sourcing is most cost effective as a means of handling peak volumes, such as the large number of spontaneous reports typically received after product launch or to handle the large number of serious AE reports expected from a large mortality/morbidity trial. If a company wishes to maintain a complete safety database on its products, a means of data transfer from the CRO must be found, either by electronic import through E2b files, or by giving the CRO access to the company safety database so that they can enter reports directly. Lessons learned from use of CROs in clinical trials would indicate that success of out-sourcing is dependent on a clear understanding of expectations among both parties, robust supporting processes, and good communication.

Other points to consider

In summary, consider the following 'good process principles', or 'GPP', when evaluating a case-handling process:

- Processes should be mapped into categories of work with defined inputs and defined outputs. This will help eliminate redundancies and duplication of effort, as well as define roles.

- Skill sets in the organization must be correctly aligned with each category of work. Efficient staffing is dependent on accurate assessment of the skills needed to perform the work. If it is difficult to find the right skill sets for a role, then one should consider redefining the role.

- To maximize efficiency in time and effort, it is absolutely essential to maintain a linear workflow and minimize hand-offs. Back-loops, which lead to re-work, duplication of effort, and redundancies, should be eliminated.

These principles should be considered when setting up a new department, merging two or more existing departments, or re-engineering an existing department for gains in efficiency.

Technology and the case-handling process

Introduction

Perhaps the most profound change to the structure and function of safety departments within pharmaceutical companies in recent years has occurred as a result of advances in technology. Leaps in the ability to collect electronically, analyse, and store data have revolutionized the case-handling process. However, the benefits of new technology have also brought new policy and process challenges for safety departments. This section will attempt to provide an overview of both sides of this blade of 'cutting-edge' technology.

Selection and implementation of a drug safety case-handling system

Although the terms are often used synonymously or interchangeably, for the purposes of this discussion, 'system' will be used to refer both to the application for case processing and to the database for storage of case reports. The choice of systems available for drug safety work continues to expand. A number of vendor packages, or 'off-the-shelf' systems, currently exist, allowing companies to purchase wholly functional safety systems ready for immediate use, complete with ancillary functions such as training and technical maintenance services. Alternatively, a host of information technology (IT) consultant firms exist that are experienced in helping pharmaceutical companies develop their own custom safety systems for collecting, reporting, tracking and storing case reports. There are pros and cons to both approaches.

Companies are frequently attracted to vendor packages because the system is immediately available, comes with a user-training program and technical support services, and negates the need to expend internal resources on a development program. However, vendor packages are restrictive in terms of flexibility to meet the company's specific data capture needs, and the vendor may be slow to make requested changes, even when new regulations would seem to require it. Additionally, the instability and volatility of the technical marketplace may result in a company being contractually tied to a totally different corporate entity from that of its initial system purchase – one that may be less customer-focused.

In contrast, custom applications ensure complete company control over system design and the timetable of subsequent upgrades, as well as integration with other company systems. However, development and maintenance are very resource-intensive, both from an IT and a user perspective. Some companies attempt to tread the middle ground by purchasing a vendor package and then modifying it with customization. Although this approach may address specific data capture needs, depending on the level of customization, it may also result in an inability to incorporate system upgrades from the vendor, leading eventually to an outdated system that is as dependent on internal maintenance as a custom system.

When assessing a vendor package for purchase, or when designing an internal system, the following factors should be considered:

- Critical features or 'must-haves'

  1. *Validation*. Any safety system must be fully validated in order to be compliant with regulations. Validation documentation is a frequent focus of health authority inspections, and auditors expect to have access to these documents even when the company was not the developing entity.

  2. *System security*. A safety system must have, at a minimum, certain features to ensure the integrity of the data. It must:

     - be compliant with regulations regarding electronic records and signatures;

     - have controlled access

     - have a robust, easily accessible audit trail to track changes to the data.

  3. *Technical compatibility*. The safety system must also be technically compatible with company technical platforms and other system interfaces. For example, duplicate data entry could be avoided if personnel in the company call centre could transmit information regarding reported AEs from their database to the safety system through a direct link. Any system that interfaces with the safety system must also be fully validated or the validated state of the safety system is, by definition, compromised.

  4. *Storage capability*. A safety system must also have adequate storage capability for long-term use. Adding additional storage at a later date may adversely impact system performance. It is unlikely that one can overestimate the volume of reports that may be received over time. As several companies have found, one well-publicized safety issue with one drug can generate an avalanche of reports for prolonged periods.

- Desirable features or 'nice-to-haves':

  1. *Easy input and easy output*. Most systems are better at one than the other, but both are essential. The importance of one over the other may be relative to internal company needs. For example, if the safety department has limited resource for data entry, then the ease of input may be valued most. On the other hand, if the safety department has to respond to a lot of queries to support other functions and has limited technical support to do this, then ease of output may be more important.

  2. *User friendly*. If data entry and data extraction are intuitive, then the learning curve of new users will be minimized, decreasing the need for long training periods and minimizing the potential for error. Systems developed solely by technical staff, without naïve user input, are notorious for being difficult to learn by persons without an IT background. This tends to be more prevalent among off-the-shelf systems rather than those developed in-house.

3. *Flexibility to support process changes*. The work of a safety department is constantly influenced by many internal and external changes: corporate priorities, product portfolio, organizational structure, regulations, staffing, customer demands, etc. Systems that cannot adapt to these changes can become a liability. A system that only supports one way of working, due to rigidity of the data entry workflow sequence, or an inability to support global as well as local case distribution, will quickly become obsolete.

4. *Detail of supporting documentation*. When evaluating a system for purchase, the quality of the on-line help, user manuals and other documents will say much about the quality of the system itself, as well as the customer focus of the vendor. Additionally, poor training materials mean hidden costs to the buyer, since additional training will have to be developed and provided by the company. When developing a system, the project plan should include ample time and resource for development of the content of these materials, which should occur in tandem with the technical development. This promotes a user–developer dialogue that ensures results meet expectations.

5. *Labour-saving features*. Automated features, such as auto-narratives, auto-encoders, auto-distribution, edit checks, etc., will not only decrease resource needed for data entry, but will also decrease the potential for error. For example, an automated narrative that pulls information from various database fields into a structured format will not only decrease the amount of time spent authoring the narrative, but will ensure that the information in the narrative (patient demographics, drug names and dosages, medical history, etc.) is consistent with the information that appears in other portions of the report form.

6. *Workflow support*. As the volume of cases and the number of staff increase, the ability to generate performance metrics from the system will greatly assist in identifying areas for process improvement, as well as provide data to justify resources to management. For example, automated date generation and tracking will allow analysis of bottlenecks in the process workflow. Automatic routing will ensure that minimal delay occurs in report hand-offs. The ability to generate various management reports to measure productivity and analyse case-load distribution is also helpful.

- Other issues for consideration

1. *Level of technical support required*. Many companies only consider the initial system development costs, without considering the continuing costs of long-term maintenance. A vendor package may be relatively cheap in development costs, but expensive in terms of annual licence fees and service fees for continued IT support. A custom system may be expensive in development costs, but may pay for itself with cheaper internal maintenance. The company must also consider availability of IT resource. A large company with an existing IT staff could support internal maintenance, whereas a new start-up company may have to outsource all IT needs.

2. *Ease and consistency of data retrieval.* As a further point to the need for easy output described above, the nature of safety data requires that query results are consistently reproducible and accurate. This is not as simple as it sounds. If the database structure is complex, or if the system query tool is difficult to use, then different people will come up with different results. Needless to say, this could have disastrous consequences for evaluating a possible safety signal or when responding to a query from a regulator.

3. *Flexibility to support different regulatory requirements as well as regulatory changes, especially in regulatory report generation.* Recent regulatory harmonization initiatives have made it much easier to meet basic international regulatory requirements. In today's business environment, all safety systems should be able to support these, at a minimum. When regulations change, a period of time is allowed for companies to make the required changes to their systems for compliance. However, depending upon the scope of the change, as well as what else is happening at the vendor or company, the time provided may be inadequate to test, validate and document adequately if the system is inherently inflexible or if system support resources are minimal.

4. *Change control process.* Over time, any system will require modifications, some to resolve errors and some to improve efficiency. Regardless of whether the system is customized or purchased, there must be a clearly defined process for technical changes, with unambiguous accountabilities for each step. Testing, validation, and documentation requirements must be just as rigorous as during system development. This is frequently a focus of internal audits and external inspections by health authorities, since change control is key to data integrity and validity.

Data migration and database conversion

Once a new system is in place, there is frequently a need to migrate legacy data from the old system or systems. Over time, with system upgrades, data in the existing database will need to be converted into a new database structure. Additionally, company mergers or licensing agreements may also require data migrations and database conversions. (Although data migrations and database conversions have slightly different meanings and technical differences, for the purposes of this discussion the term data migration will henceforth be used to refer to both.) Without due care, these transactions can result in 'dirty' data that is incomplete, inconsistent and incoherent. The following paragraphs describe some best practices than can ensure results that maximize data integrity (Steiner *et al.*, 2001).

Any successful data migration must begin with proper planning. The purpose of the plan is to accomplish the following:

*   *Define the project scope.* What is the target data for migration (e.g. how many years of data, which fields, which dates, coded or uncoded, what is the volume, what are the data similarities, what are the data differences, etc.)?

*   *Analyse costs and alternatives.* Data migration is costly and resource intensive. For relatively low volumes of data it may be more cost effective to hire temporary

data-entry resources to re-enter the data manually into the new system. It may also be cost effective to migrate only the most recent portion of data, and archive the older data in a read-only database.

- *Review business processes.* The migration team (and, in due course, the system users) must have a clear understanding of how the conventions for entering the old data differ from conventions of data entry in the new system, as well as differences in how the systems handle the data. This will require both functional and technical analyses. For example, if the old system was used to record product quality complaints as well as AEs and this will not be the case in the new system, then it may be problematic to separate the data if the old system had no nomenclature to distinguish them.

It is essential that good validation practices be built into the migration process. Not only is this essential for maintenance of data integrity, but the need to clearly describe assumptions and approaches in validation documents will assist the team in identifying potential gaps and areas of confusion sooner rather than later. Additionally, if problems arise later, comprehensive validation documents can be a key resource in identifying the root cause of the issue, as well as its resolution, especially if members of the original migration team are no longer available.

Success of the effort depends not only upon having adequate resources, but also on having the appropriate and knowledgeable resources available. This is a special challenge during merger situations, when personnel may be leaving the company or are reassigned. It may be necessary for the company to provide special incentives in order to secure the knowledge and expertise necessary for the conversion effort. Even the best legacy system documentation will not cover the historical nuances of business processes. Having access to those familiar with the old system can save much time and resource. In addition to early identification and retention of key personnel, there is also a need for a team approach and continuity throughout the project. Roles and responsibilities should be clear, and communication is key.

Flexibility should be built into the conversion schedule. Time frames should be as realistic as possible, and contingency plans should be in place to account for unforeseen problems that are almost certain to arise at the most critical moment. At least one, and preferably multiple, 'mock' migrations should be done prior to the final one. In a mock migration, a copy of a representative subset of data from the old system is migrated into a copy of the new system database. This helps to ensure that errors in the migration program are identified and corrected prior to the final effort, when the data is migrated into the 'real', i.e. production, environment.

Once the final migration is completed, it is critical to provide post-migration support to avoid continuing problems. Retaining members of the original migration team for the immediate post-conversion period is critical. If consultants are used, then their contracts should include a provision for at least a 2 to 4 week support period post-rollout. It is also important to document and track any migration issues identified by the users. Although no data migration is perfect and some problems will be expected, this will allow the maintenance team to evaluate and prioritize repairs. It is also essential that read-only access to the retired database be retained for some period of time after migration. There is frequently a need to refer to the legacy data in order to resolve errors in the migration, or to use as a resource in data queries. For example, during the initial post-migration phase, it may be useful to query both databases to ensure completeness and accuracy of surveillance search results until a reasonable comfort level is established. Finally, a 'top-down' (e.g. prioritized) and programmatic, automated approach to clean up of legacy data is recommended. Manual data clean-up of individual cases is not only labour intensive, but it can actually result in more discrepancies, with the danger of increasing inconsistencies with the original cases due to individual interpretations and lack of knowledge of legacy processes.

Quality control and the case-handling process

Introduction

In order for the AE information accumulated in the safety database via the case-handling process to be useful in pharmacovigilance, there must be an assurance of the quality and consistency of the data. As described in Chapter 8, although case-handling errors would have to be severe in order for a true safety signal to be completely missed, such random inaccuracies might lead to a delay in detection by diluting the certainty over the association between the AE and the drug. Conversely, data errors may lead to generation of a false positive, or just increase the level of 'noise' that must be filtered out to make an accurate assessment. Ongoing continuous quality control is necessary in the case-handling process in order to prevent these cumulative effects from wasting time and resource. Quality control procedures are not enough; there must be an overall quality control *system* in place to ensure that processes interface and that no gaps exist. The ultimate success measure of a company's quality control are audits, both internal and external. This section will define quality as it pertains to the case-handling process, describe the underlying principles of good quality control practices, and then provide some advice for how to prepare for an audit, how to behave during an audit, and how to respond to audit findings.

Defining quality

Before something can be measured, it must be defined. As most of today's concepts of quality were first defined in the product manufacturing area, it is useful to consider this definition of quality. Good manufacturing practice (GMP) defined product quality as the absence of defects and the fitness for use as determined by the end user. These same GMP principles were later applied to good clinical practice (GCP) and thus to the work of drug safety. One may think of case handling as the manufacturing process, and the output of that process, the AE report, as the product. The report should have an 'absence of defect' and be 'fit for use' by the end customer, e.g. the receiving regulator and others, both internal (safety surveillance staff, clinical teams, etc.) and external (data safety monitoring boards, ethics committees, etc.) With the needs of these end users in mind, quality of an AE case report can be loosely grouped into four categories, the 'four Cs' of quality:

1. *Consistent.* The information in the report should be consistent with the source documents, and the report should be processed in such a way as to be consistent with established departmental standards and applicable regulations.

2. *Correct.* The report should be medically accurate, especially in terms of any coding of terms, and the regulatory classification should be appropriate.

3. *Compliant.* The case should be processed and reported as required by company standard operating procedures (SOPs) and relevant regulations.

4. *Complete.* Completeness of the report may be thought of on two levels: enough information to make an accurate medical and regulatory assessment of the reported event(s) and/or enough information to complete the required fields of the relevant regulatory reporting form. In most instances these two should be synonymous.

Improving documentation

It is impossible to assess consistency, correctness, compliance and completeness without good documentation. The old adage 'if it isn't written down, it didn't happen' is especially true in quality control. Documentation provides the evidence that the process is defined and functioning, and may be classified into three categories:

1. Documents that specify how something should be done, such as policies, SOPs, guidelines, working practice instructions, coding manuals, data-entry manuals, etc.

2. Documents that capture information and provide evidence of the work performed, such as source documents, individual case reports, summary reports, classification work-sheets, review notes, queries, change requests, etc.

3. Documents that provide information about the results of the work performed, such as productivity reports, error reports, compliance reports, etc.

All three types play important roles in quality control of the case-handling process:

• Type 1 documents provide the standards against which the work is assessed.

• Type 2 documents provide the evidence of how the work conforms to the standards.

• Type 3 documents provide the data needed to identify problems and solutions.

The following good documentation practices should be considered. Type 1 documents should reflect the consensus and best practice experience of all involved. This means that SOPs, guidelines, manuals, and other instruction-type references should be written by those with in-depth knowledge of the processes, and be subject to wide review to identify possible gaps or exceptions and eliminate potential conflicts. Special attention should be paid to language in global documents, since certain terms may have different meanings according to the linguistic background of the reader. Additionally, it is important to ensure consistency between overlapping documents, especially in the use of terms and definitions. Subtle text variances may lead to significant differences in interpretation and implementation. Consideration should also be given to external documents, such as regulatory guidelines and software manuals, and the pool of reviewers should be chosen accordingly. Approval should only occur after a consensus is reached. Dates of implementation should be synchronized and tracked.

The biggest challenge for these types of document is ensuring that they are kept up-to-date with real-life practice. Documents that require more time for revision and approval, such as corporate policies and global SOPs, should be written at a high-enough level so as to minimize the need for frequent change. The lowest level of detail should be reserved for documents such as local guidelines and working instructions that can be updated quickly and easily to meet the changing needs of everyday work. All documents should be subject to version control and review cycles appropriate to change frequency. It is important for documents to have both a routine review cycle as well as a defined mechanism for making an *ad hoc* change quickly. Changes to more technical documents, e.g. data-entry manuals and coding manuals, should in most instances be aligned with technical changes or updates. It is also important to have strategies in place to minimize errors when changes are made, such as focused training workshops, job aids and visual reminders.

Measuring quality

Once quality has been defined and documented, the process for measuring it also needs to be defined. It is important that the focus is on key areas that have a true impact on quality, not just 'counting what's easy to count' (see Chapter 8). First, the boundaries of the process being measured should be established. For example, when measuring regulatory compliance, choices must be made when determining scope. Will global compliance be measured or will local compliance be measured as well? Will the focus be on submission compliance of expedited single reports or will it include submission of periodic summary reports? Will only external regulatory compliance be measured, or will internal compliance, e.g. compliance with company standards (SOPs, guidelines, etc.) and compliance with internal distribution timelines also be measured? If internal compliance is measured, to what level will that extend: tracking hand-offs at all levels or at a subset of levels – between individual employees, between company departments, between company divisions, such as global units and local marketing companies, between the company and licensing partners, etc? Will this be measured bidirectionally, or just unidirectionally? For example, is it important only to know the compliance of local units sending data to the global headquarters, or is it also useful to track the time frames in which headquarters sends data to the local units?

In determining both the scope and the strategy for measuring quality, the following points should also be considered:

1. *Available resources.* The scope of quality control must be consistent with the available resource; elaborate plans are useless without the means to carry them out. Resource constraints require more prioritization and focus in methodology (Burr, 1987).

2. *Management support.* Sufficient resources (time, money, people, technology) must be allocated to quality control by management. Support for this can be obtained by providing metrics documenting the need, a detailed plan that maximizes efficiency, and examples from internal or external experiences that demonstrate the costs of poor quality (Farrow, 1987).

3. *Company structure.* Quality control is not a one-size-fits-all type of process; it must be tailored to the specific organization, or otherwise risk being inefficient and inaccurate.

4. *Areas of concern.* Quality control should focus on known problem areas, although

analysis of interfaces that may be contributing factors should also be prioritized. For example, a recurring data entry error may be the result of inadequate training.

5. *Technology*. Technology should be leveraged as much as possible to improve quality control efficiency, but should be seen as an enhancement to, rather than a replacement for, human analysis.

When considering what data to collect in order to measure quality, whether manually or with the aid of technology, it is important that what is collected is:

1. *Valid and verifiable*. For example, programmed quality control reports should be validated the same as any technical query, and all findings should be supported by documentation.

2. *Clear and consistent*. Quality control should focus on objective rather than subjective data, and recognize the difference between style and substance. Persons participating in quality control should not only agree on what priorities to focus on, but should agree on common methods.

3. *Meaningful and timely*. The quality control process cannot add value if the process is so slow that results are outdated by the time the data are analysed, or if the findings are inconclusive because the right data were not collected.

Quality control does not end with data collection. It is not enough to present the number of late report submissions without providing some insight as to why the reports were submitted late. Not only must the overall findings be analysed, but the components must also be analysed. Some types of component to consider are:

- report type (e.g. post-marketing, investigational, etc.);
- report source (e.g. consumer, sales representative, clinical research organization, licensing partner, etc.);
- report origin (country, department, clinical trial, etc.).

Additionally, common contributing factors and trends should be identified:

- training issues
- communication issues
- process issues (especially identification of 'bottlenecks' in the process)
- technical issues.

Once the underlying problem is identified, quality control should assist in determining the appropriate corrective actions to be taken. Individual human error may be addressed with retraining and management counselling. Systematic process errors may be addressed with revisions and clarifications to guidelines and manuals. Agreements with outside managers may be needed to address issues with external contributors to the process (i.e. incomplete reports from clinical study monitors, late reports from sales representatives, etc). Although quality control personnel may not be involved in implementation of the corrective actions, they should be responsible for ensuring that the agreed actions are clearly documented, and should follow up at intervals to ensure that the corrective actions have occurred.

Preparing for internal audits and regulatory inspections

While the discussion below is based primarily on experience with FDA inspections, the basic principles are equally applicable to inspections by other health authorities. The term 'audit' will be used to refer to internal company audits, and 'inspection' will be used to refer to audit by a regulator. However, all audits and inspections are intended to answer the same essential questions:

- What is the system?
- Is it functioning as planned?
- If not, what is the significance of the findings?

There are three lines of evidence to be pursued in any audit or inspection:

- physical evidence
- documentation
- verbal accounts.

This is done primarily through three corresponding activities:

- physical inspection
- document review
- personnel interviews.

Internal audits are conducted so that company management knows whether company procedures are being followed, company objectives are being met, and whether regulations are being complied with by the department(s) under scrutiny. The goal of this is to prevent damage to the company, to identify areas for improvement, and to provide quality assurance, which can be defined simply as 'the activity of providing the evidence needed to establish confidence, among all concerned, that the quality function is being effectively performed' (Gryna, 1988).

Inspections by auditors from health authorities focus almost entirely on regulatory compliance. These inspections may be unannounced and do not occur on a regular basis. The inspection may be 'routine', e.g. conducted as part of the normal periodic inspection schedule to verify the accuracy and completeness of the reports submitted to the health authority, or 'for cause', e.g. prompted by evidence of non-compliance or suspicion of non-compliance with regulations (CPMP, 2001). The most common reason for a 'for cause' inspection of a safety department is late submission of expedited reports.

The best way to prepare for a regulatory inspection is to maintain a state of constant readiness. The preparations described below should not be deferred until notice of inspection is given (should one be so fortunate as to have advance notice) but should be activities that are part of the routine function of the department.

Document preparation

Special attention should be paid to ensuring all documents that are subject to inspection are accurate, complete and up-to-date, especially organizational charts, training records, job descriptions, employee CVs, SOPs, guidelines, policies, validation documentation, manuals, and any other procedural documents. All documents should show evidence of change control, including implementation dates, approval signatures, and version control. Employee resumés should include their current position and responsibilities. Regulatory inspectors may not only hold a company accountable for compliance with regulations, but they may also hold the company accountable for compliance with their own internal procedures.

Validation documentation for any application or database used by the safety department should show evidence of compliance with regulations for electronic records. This includes provision for audit trails of all changes made to electronic data and security measures to control access to the system.

Additionally, if the company was inspected in the past, then special attention should be paid to previously identified problem areas. If the company committed to corrective actions, then evidence of the implementation of these actions as well as evidence of their success in rectifying the problem should be collected.

Employee preparation

Employees should be educated about the corporate procedures for regulatory inspections. They should be aware of who should be notified, who is responsible for coordinating activities, and roles and responsibilities during the inspection. Experienced persons within the drug safety department should be identified to interact with the inspector. It is also essential that all employees are knowledgeable about the procedural documents applicable to their work, since the inspector may question them as to how they perform their daily work and compare their descriptions to what is stated in the documents. Additionally, the employees should be instructed on appropriate behaviour with an inspector. They should be instructed only to answer the questions asked, and not to volunteer additional information, as well as to admit openly when they do not know the answer to the question rather than trying to pretend otherwise. They should avoid defensive or antagonistic responses or body language, and should maintain a professional demeanour at all times.

During the inspection

A representative from the department responsible for managing activities during a regulatory inspection (in most companies, the quality assurance department) should accompany the inspector at all times. A room should be set aside to serve as the place where the inspector will interact with staff, review documents and request information. The inspector may ask to tour the department under inspection or other related areas, but is not allowed to interfere with the daily work of the company or to conduct the inspection outside of normal business hours.

Frequently, the inspector first asks for a presentation of the organizational structure of the company and the department. This is typically followed by requests for relevant SOPs, which are then reviewed for appropriateness and adequacy. The inspector often focuses on a subset of products in the beginning, although this list may expand. The selection of products is most commonly focused on drugs most likely to have serious unexpected ADRs, drugs that could cause serious medical problems if there is a failure of expected action, drugs approved within the last 3 years, new molecular entities, or those with known or suspected bioavailability or bioequivalence problems. The inspector may arrive with copies of submitted reports that he investigates further. He may also ask for line listings and randomly or selectively choose reports from the list for further analysis. He may ask for individual case reports, source documents, file notes, proof of regulatory submission, follow-up correspondence, customer complaint files, equipment service reports and periodic summary reports. Only documents specifically requested should be provided, and all documents should be reviewed and organized before giving them to the inspector. The inspector is only allowed to keep copies of documents, and these should be clearly marked 'copy' and 'confidential'. Additionally, a list of all documents provided should be maintained.

During the inspection, a plan should be in place to ensure availability of staff for support. Inspectors not only judge a company on its ability to provide the information requested, but also judge them on the speed of response, since this is a key indicator of organizational competence. Technical support should be on hand to run queries, and representatives from other departments that interface with drug safety, such as regulatory and product quality, should be available to provide information or answer questions. If it is apparent that the inspector is focusing on particular products or processes, then the most knowledgeable persons about these areas of interest should be on hand to provide expertise as needed. Additionally, arrangements may need to be made to ensure availability of staff at other company locations, which may be problematic due to time zone differences.

During the inspection, communication strategy is key in avoiding chaos and confusion. Typically, there is a designated 'inspection room' where the inspector(s) performs review, questions personnel and requests information. All requests from the inspector should be written and confirmed with him at the time of the request. One or more persons should be available at all times to receive requests from those interacting with the inspector in the designated inspection room. There should be a single point of contact at each location and in each department involved, and all requests should go through that designated person. To avoid delay, designated phone lines and fax lines should be dedicated and monitored at all times. When the request is relayed to others, all verbal communication should be followed with a copy of the written request to avoid misinterpretation.

After the inspection is complete, the inspector typically presents his findings verbally to the company inspection team and relevant management, and indicates what recommendations for regulatory action (if any) he will make. This is an opportunity to discuss the observations and seek clarification from the inspector, but should not be used as a forum for debate. The most common regulatory citations of safety departments include:

- failure to submit expedited reports for serious, unexpected ADRs;

- expedited reports not submitted on time;

- expedited reports that are inaccurate and/or not complete;
- repeated or deliberate failure to submit periodic summary reports;
- failure to conduct prompt and adequate follow-up investigation of case reports;
- failure to maintain adequate AE records for products;
- failure to have adequate written procedures.

The inspector will issue a formal written report, and the company should respond to the report in writing (usually within a specified time frame). The company response should address each item, clarifying any perceived discrepancies and specifying what corrective action the company will take, as well as what steps the company will take to avoid recurrence of the problem in the future. The health authority may accept the company's response or may require additional actions by the company if it feels the voluntary plan is inadequate. Once the action plan is agreed the company will be held accountable for implementation, and this is likely to be audited during the next inspection.

Finally, an internal summary of the inspection should be written and circulated to management. The account should be factual and avoid negative language, presenting a balanced description of what went well during the inspection and what did not. Recommendations for improvement in the preparation for, or conduct during, the inspection should be highlighted.

In the event of non-compliance, regulatory actions that may follow an inspection include (CPMP, 2001):

- required education and facilitation;
- additional inspections;
- formal warning;
- public disclosure (publication of names of companies/MAH found to be seriously or persistently non-compliant);
- formal caution (if criminal offense is admitted);
- criminal prosecution;
- suspension of marketing authorization.

Training and the case-handling process

Introduction

The cornerstone of any successful case-handling process is the training program that supports it. Drug safety departments are held accountable by regulators to ensure that persons involved in safety work are adequately qualified and trained to perform the work required. Training records are a primary focus of both internal audits and regulatory inspections. This section will discuss some best practice approaches to training as it relates to AE reporting (both inside and outside of the drug safety department), as well as provide a high-level overview of some of the new training tools available.

The importance of training records

Training records must be maintained for all personnel in a drug safety department, and are subject to audit and regulatory inspection. In order to ensure that new personnel complete all training requirements, it is helpful to develop a time-based curriculum plan for each role – a detailed, content-focused training schedule with clearly defined objectives and milestones with an accompanying checklist. Along with the traditional employee induction or orientation program, this will not only provide structure to the new-hire training program and prevent gaps in completion of requirements, but will also provide a timeline that helps the employee understand training expectations and provide an objective measurement of the employee's progress. The curriculum plan ensures that requirements are tailored to what is appropriate for each job description. The checklist can be designed with spaces for dates and signatures so that it provides verification and documentation when each task is completed.

It is also important to establish standards for maintenance of training for existing employees. Personal development plans agreed between employee and manager can be used to customize training to address individual skill gaps, as well as to accommodate pursuit of personal career interests. Annual 'refresher courses' for required SOPs and guidelines, as well as retraining when document revisions are issued, should be standard procedure. There should also be an established process for determining the appropriate level of training required when new SOPs and guidelines are issued, e.g. whether attendance at a live course presentation is required, or whether it is sufficient to read the document and sign a statement verifying comprehension. This, too, should be role specific. For example, attendance at a presentation on a new SOP for developing study protocols may not be necessary for a role focused on data entry of case reports, but it would be relevant for a drug safety physician who may assist with authoring a protocol.

Maintenance of training records has traditionally been paper based, but new electronic training tools are easing the burden of keeping these records current. Some of the functions now available include management reports to identify employee training gaps, electronic reminders when retraining is due, on-line calendars of available courses, electronic scheduling and course enrollment, and attendance tracking. Systems that are compliant with electronic records/electronic signature regulations can even serve as the sole repository of training documentation.

Suggested approaches for different audiences

When planning a training program, it is useful to understand the underlying principles of adult learning. Information presented via lectures, reading materials, or audiovisual presentations has been shown to have a retention rate of only 20 per cent or less (Brookfield, 1986). When trainees see a skill demonstrated the retention rate increases to 30 per cent, but if they actually practice a skill, then it jumps to 75 per cent. The highest retention rate, 90 per cent, is obtained when the trainees must teach someone else or immediately use what is learned. Adults learn best when they are allowed to be autonomous and self-directed, and when there are opportunities for practice and feedback (Lieb, 1998). Current research indicates that the most effective training is 'blended', e.g. provides a mixture of instructor-led and technology-based methodologies (Herron, 2002).

Internal drug safety staff

Drug safety personnel involved in case handling first and foremost need a basic understanding of the applicable regulations, since this has a direct impact on their daily work. The tight time frames of regulatory reporting are the primary drivers for process flow and task prioritization. Additionally, personnel need to have an understanding of the company interpretation of these regulations, as described in SOPs and other documents. Therefore, it is more efficient to link the two together, not only in the classroom environment but also in reading materials. Comprehension of this material can be enhanced with practical examples. A self-paced learning approach will help each student to absorb these at a rate comfortable for them. Students should be exposed gradually over time to increasing levels of complexity. For example, persons learning data entry should start with simple cases that are not under tight time frames for completion, such as reports of non-serious expected AEs, and gradually advance to more complex cases.

In addition to content, case-handling staff need technical training on the system used to process reports. Robust on-line help, detailed data-entry manuals, and other reference materials are essential. Live data-entry demonstrations and hands-on practice with sample cases in a training database environment are key to preventing new user errors in the validated production environment of the 'real' database.

Other members of drug development

Drug safety departments are frequently responsible for providing training to personnel in other areas of drug development, such as clinical study management, clinical research and experimental medicine, who are also involved in collecting and reporting AEs. The best approach for these audiences is to tailor the training materials to focus on the content that is most applicable to their daily work. For example, a clinical trial monitor has no need to learn the regulations for spontaneous AE reporting but does need in-depth knowledge of the requirements surrounding clinical studies. Cutting out the extraneous materials will allow additional time to discuss specifics pertinent to the work of the audience, e.g. requirements for informing investigators, IRBs and ethics committees. Since AE reporting for these roles may be an occasional task, rather than a daily activity, distributing simple step-by-step job aids is helpful in reinforcing the initial training. Whenever possible, the use of standard report templates to collect information will serve as reminders of what information is needed. Identifying an expert resource to be available to answer questions, and making a 'frequently asked questions' reference available will also be helpful.

Other company employees outside of the drug development area

All employees of pharmaceutical companies are required to report any AE associated with company products that they become aware of during performance of their work. The most likely other departments where this may occur are in sales, medical information and legal. All need to have sufficient knowledge to identify an AE, understand their responsibility to report these to the drug safety department, and know how to do so and in what time frame. It is important that clear and simple processes are put in place to enable this. However, especially with the sales force, the biggest challenge is to motivate these employees to report, since AE reporting is frequently seen as something that will have negative impact on their ability to sell the product. Training, therefore, needs to focus on the positive business value of AE reporting:

- *'Forewarned is forearmed'*. It is always best for the company to know about problems with its products before they become known by the press, competitors and regulators, and the sales force can serve as an 'early warning system'.

- *Increase credibility with customers.* Prescribers will be impressed with a company concerned with protection of patients, and their comfort level with use of the product will be increased when they see evidence of good pharmacovigilance practices. Providing feedback to them on the results of the company investigation and analysis of the reported AE will also give the sales representative another opportunity for interaction.

- *Improve accuracy of product labelling.* Accurate labelling protects the company and the patients. Additionally, as patient exposure increases, collecting information on AEs may actually provide data that will have a positive impact on the label. For example, percentages of expected AEs predicted by clinical trials may be found to be inaccurately high, evidence may be gained that leads to removal of warnings and precautions, and important information regarding the effects of the product in overdose situations and pregnancy exposures will be gained. There is also the potential that beneficial drug effects may be identified, e.g. minoxidil and hair growth.

Providing real-life examples of the consequences of failure to report AEs can enhance the effectiveness of training. It is fairly easy to find recent instances in the press where a company suffered a significant financial loss because of safety issues. Audiences should also be made aware of potential penalties that may be imposed on individuals as well as companies, such as fines, debarment, and imprisonment. For example, debarment may legally prohibit an individual from future employment by any pharmaceutical company or any organization associated with a pharmaceutical company, which would seriously impair the individual's ability to earn a livelihood.

Strategies for maximizing efficiency of the training process

One of the most commonly used methods for minimizing the resources required for training is the 'train the trainer' approach. When resources do not allow direct training of the target audience (e.g. a geographically disseminated group, such as the sales force), the training team can focus on training a subset of representatives who will then return to their respective locations and provide the training to their local groups. For this approach to be successful it is important that the training given to the 'trainers' is very focused and intensive, and that training materials provide a greater depth of detail than normal, since the new trainers must be comfortable with the content and be able to answer questions accurately. The drawback to this approach is that the new trainers will not have the background and experience of a true knowledge expert, which may lead to errors in interpretation and decreased knowledge retention over time.

Another frequently used strategy is mentoring, which is based on establishing trainer-level competence in specific areas among a small number of senior staff who can then share the burden of providing and, even more importantly, reinforcing training among those that they work with on a daily basis. This also provides an additional knowledge expert who is readily available to answer questions that may arise. For new employees, who have completed a basic training curriculum and are ready to begin work, it is frequently helpful to assign them to a mentor or preceptor on the same team who can provide individualized attention to them over an extended period of time. Among the disadvantages of this approach are decreased productivity of the experienced personnel who are mentoring, decreased or delayed effectiveness of training due to personality conflicts between the mentor and trainee, potential mentor burn-out, and the fact that there must be a limit on the number of new staff assigned for mentoring if the team is still to get the work done.

Overview of training tools available

Technology can also enhance the efficiency of the training process, especially if it is used in such a way as to support the principles of adult learning previously described (Kruse and Keil, 2000). Additionally, today's technology supports distance learning, which means huge cost savings can be realized because employees do not have to travel to receive training. Below are brief descriptions of some of the technical tools available, along with references that provide additional detail.

Computer-based training modules

Computer-based training (CBT) modules can be used wherever a computer is available, and can be distributed as a file by e-mail or loaded onto the computer by diskette or CD. CBT modules are self-paced, provide specific and immediate feedback, and can be hyper-linked with other resource documents. Additionally, CBT modules can be designed so that they are self-scoring, and so that they provide documentation of proficiency through a file that verifies a passing score was achieved on the tests incorporated into the material. Once loaded onto a computer, they can be revisited as needed to reinforce the initial training. CBT modules can be easily updated and reissued as needed. In the pharmaceutical industry, this methodology is frequently used to teach product information to the sales force, but it has also been applied to drug safety (Benson *et al.* 1999). However, CBT modules are not truly interactive, since additional support must be provided for the user to be able to ask questions or seek clarification.

The 'virtual' classroom

Since teleconferences do not allow discussion of visual material and CBT courses are not interactive, many are now leveraging video-conferencing capabilities to support distance learning. New tools allow instructors to control presentations using synchronized multi-media, share applications with the audience, provide electronic 'hand-raising' for questions, and acquire a screen capture of any student's desktop via a 'glimpse' feature. These tools are expensive, and without high-speed connectivity they can be cumbersome and slow during use, even more so when a large number of users are participating. This is especially problematic with international audiences, even if dedicated lines are available between sites (Anonymous, 2001).

Web-based learning

This approach attempts to bypass many of the limitations of video-conferencing by utilizing the Internet as the mode of transmission. The same methods may also be applied to internal company 'intranets'. Using a Web site for distance learning eliminates many of the technical limitations of video-conferencing while still providing interactivity, and, perhaps most importantly, allows for simulations to teach complex performance skills (Driscoll, 1998). Well-designed Web sites can result in very efficient training programs that, in some situations, have achieved results comparable to instructor-led training in 40 to 60 per cent less time. However, such success is dependent on a computer-literate audience and internal systems that enable delivery of robust programmes. And, whereas instructor-led sessions remove participants from their daily work so that they can focus on learning, there is no such protection in this environment (Zenger and Uehlein, 2001).

External partners in the case-handling process

Introduction

Pharmaceutical companies routinely hire CROs to perform all or portions of work formerly done by internal company personnel. Although companies have traditionally hired CROs to monitor clinical trials, CROs are now expanding their capabilities. There are now some CROs who can perform almost any function, including, but not limited to, data management, statistical analysis, medical writing, publishing, etc. Additionally, some CROs now offer a full menu of services normally performed by a safety department, from collection of reports (through call centres as well as other avenues), entering reports into a database, medical review, and even submitting reports to regulators. This menu of safety services is not even limited to case handling; CROs are now offering safety surveillance services as well (Doan, 2000).

There are certainly pros and cons to utilizing a CRO rather than internal company personnel for any portion of work. However, discussion of these is outside the remit of this chapter. What this section will attempt to provide are some basic principles for partnering successfully with a CRO when at least a portion of the safety work has been out-sourced to them. Additionally, the end of the section will discuss other types of external partner that may be used for safety work.

Clinical research organizations

It is to the company's advantage for the CRO to be able to perform as efficiently as possible. One key way to encourage this is to minimize the deviations the CRO is required to make from its own internal SOPs and guidelines. Part of the routine CRO selection process should include a review of all relevant SOPs and guidelines used by the CRO. Company reviewers can then not only ascertain what candidate CROs have the closest fit with the company, but the quality of these documents will provide insight as to the quality of the CRO itself.

Once the selection is made, a further in-depth analysis of differences between company and CRO SOPs should be made to identify potential areas of conflict, clarify marginal areas and agree on what deviations should be made. In many instances, subtle differences may have little impact to the work. It is best if this detailed review is performed together by knowledgeable content experts from both sides, preferably persons who will be directly involved in the out-sourced work. For example, if the out-sourced work involves safety reporting in a clinical trial, then members from the CRO safety group and the company clinical trial safety group should establish contact as early as possible to agree upon the case-handling flow for the trial. Monitors and other clinical team members should be involved in this discussion as well. Company representatives should be open to suggestions from the CRO, since they may have valuable insight about best practices from their experiences in working with other companies.

In addition to workflow, the roles and responsibilities should be clearly defined. The CRO should provide documentation to the company that their personnel are qualified to perform the services delegated to them. For example, if the CRO is providing medical review of case reports, then they should provide proof that the reviewing CRO physician meets the same standards set for internal company physicians who perform this work. Additionally, it is often helpful to have a person appointed as primary point of contact both within the CRO and within the company safety department. This ensures efficiency in communication and issue resolution. Since CROs frequently have a high rate of staff turnover, it is also reasonable for the company to require that the CRO is accountable for the transition of legacy knowledge and training replacement personnel.

In a clinical trial situation, it is also helpful for the CRO to generate a safety-reporting plan for the study, reiterating agreements on definitions, roles, accountabilities, and to include a diagram of the agreed workflow. Such a safety reporting plan will not only uncover possible misunderstandings before the trial begins, but it will also serve as a resource for new team members (for the CRO as well as the company), and may be used as a reference point in resolving future confusion. It is critical that any changes to the original plan are incorporated into the document, and that revisions are reviewed by all involved.

One key component of the safety reporting plan for a clinical study is an efficient process for tracking queries and query resolution. This should be agreed in conjunction with data management and other relevant members of the clinical team who participate in these efforts, and roles and accountabilities should be clearly defined. Plans should include a method of continuous and ongoing data comparison and corrections between the safety and clinical databases, in order to minimize the time at the end of the study needed to declare clean file for the study and lock the trial database. Furthermore, reconciliation between the safety and clinical databases should be limited to key fields, as 100 per cent agreement between the two can never be achieved, due to the fact that the safety data reflects a point in time (i.e. the time around the occurrence of the serious AE) and the clinical data reflects a continuum of visit-based data that changes over the course of the trial.

It is also important that areas of the company, such as the safety department, who are working with the CRO are able to provide feedback to the 'owner' of the contract on CRO performance. This feedback should be as real-time as possible, so that issues can be addressed quickly. For example, the safety department should notify a clinical team who is utilizing a CRO for monitoring a study if the CRO is not adhering to reporting timelines, if the quality of the reports provided is poor, and if queries are not answered in a timely manner. It is much easier to deal with poor performance with a CRO if expectations and requirements are outlined clearly in the contract itself – otherwise it may be very difficult to hold the CRO accountable. Owing to the critical nature of safety reporting, it may be useful to have an addendum to the contract or a portion of the contract itself that outlines specific safety requirements. Some companies go so far as to include automatic monetary penalties if these requirements are not met.

Other external partners

Other than CROs, there are a variety of external partners that may also be utilized by safety departments. Examples of these are temporary data-entry personnel, technical consultants and vendors contracted for document management. Regardless of function, it should be remembered that regulatory requirements for these company agents are the same as for a company employee. The same components (SOPs, training records, etc.) are subject to audit, and regulatory authorities expect that proper controls be in place to ensure system security and data integrity. Documentation is key, preferably within a contract that specifies the work to be performed.

Case distribution to external parties other than regulatory authorities

Introduction

In addition to regulatory authorities, companies frequently need to communicate safety information to parties other than regulators (in some situations, this dissemination of information may be requested or even mandated by regulators). The key to any effective safety communication is to ensure that the right message is sent to the right audience in the right way at the right time. This section will describe the methods used with three important audiences:

- data monitoring committees (DMCs)
- investigators
- health care professionals.

Data monitoring committees

As defined in the ICH E9 guideline, (ICH, 1998), a study sponsor may establish a DMC, to assess critical efficacy and safety data variables at intervals during the course of a clinical study in order to recommend to the sponsor whether to continue, modify or terminate the study. A DMC may either be a group of experts independent from the sponsor and from the investigators of a clinical trial, or may consist of internal experts from the sponsor organization. Because of the risk of compromising study integrity, it is highly desirable to have individuals who are not members of the clinical team conducting the study to monitor the incoming data.

Use of a DMC should be considered when the primary outcome of the study is a serious AE other than death, if there is a potential for short- and long-term risks to the subjects (especially if trial procedures are themselves risky or inconvenient for the subject), or when there is an alternative treatment available for the condition under study. DMCs are particularly helpful in Phase III trials that are large, multi-centre, long duration, randomized, and double-blinded, that have death as an endpoint, or are conducted in patients with a high intrinsic mortality risk. DMCs may also be useful in an earlier phase trial when the subjects are unable to give informed consent or when a new chemical entity is likely to cause serious AEs.

When study endpoints are also serious AEs, a regulatory authority waiver releasing the sponsor from expedited reporting of these endpoints is highly desirable to protect study integrity, since, unless prior arrangements are made, authorities expect expedited reports to be unblinded prior to submission. Most authorities will grant such waivers if a DMC is in place to monitor the safety of study subjects. The DMC evaluates safety in an ongoing trial through an overview of relevant points in the data flow. Responsibilities of the DMC regarding safety include:

- ensuring the safety of subjects participating in the study;

- reviewing interim reports for evidence of adverse treatment effects;

- recommending changes in the protocol to improve subject safety;

- providing advice on operational procedures affecting subject safety.

The DMC may also be charged with recommending early termination of the study for safety reasons. According to ICH E9 (ICH, 1998), the goal of any interim analysis should be to stop the study early if unacceptable adverse effects are apparent. Stopping rules must be clearly defined and understood by the DMC and the sponsor. Typically, stopping early for safety reasons does not require the same level of proof as stopping for efficacy, as it is not necessary to *prove* harm.

Most DMCs review, at a minimum, serious AE reports from the study, both at a single case level and/or in a summary fashion. The DMC charter should specify the format and frequency of safety reports sent to the DMC, as well as who will provide it (e.g. the safety department or clinical team) and the source of the data (e.g. the safety database or the clinical database). In a large company, there may be multiple large DMC-monitored trials in progress at once, so the workload of providing safety data at frequent intervals can be significant. In order to minimize the resource required for this, it may be helpful for the safety department to program a detailed individual case report suitable for distribution to an external group (e.g. with the patient identifiers encrypted to maintain confidentiality), as well as a standard DMC summary report that contains all of the key fields needed.

Investigators

The US FDA requires that a company conducting clinical trials under a US Investigational New Drug Application (IND) must submit expedited written IND safety reports to FDA and all participating investigators any time it receives information on adverse experiences associated with the use of the drug that are serious, unexpected, and possibly related to the drug under study (see Chapter 9). The regulations specifically require that these IND safety reports:

- contain the same content, whether sent to the FDA or investigators

- be sent to both the FDA and all investigators within 15 calendar days from the time that the company becomes aware of the event

- identify all safety reports previously submitted to the IND concerning a similar adverse experience

- analyze the significance of the adverse experience in light of previous, similar reports

IND safety reports sent to investigators are commonly known as 'investigator safety letters' (ISLs). The GCP guideline (ICH, 1997) requires investigators to communicate ISL information to their IRB or IEC according to the time frame specified by the IRB or IEC, and maintain evidence of this communication as well as copies of all ISLs received in their study file. These documents are subject to audit, both by company monitors and by regulatory inspectors.

Benchmarking data collected from major pharmaceutical companies regarding their ISL practices indicate that methods vary widely in terms of format: some simply send the investigators a copy of the MedWatch or CIOMS regulatory report sent to the FDA, others send a narrative summary description, with or without an attached line listing, and others send a custom report that incorporates single case as well as summary data. Although sending a copy of the regulatory report form is the easiest and quickest way to ensure that investigators receive the same information as the FDA, investigators frequently complain that the formats are not user friendly or concise, are difficult to interpret, and result in additional paper to manage. Narrative summaries, while better received by the investigators, tend to drift easily into subjective interpretation and may omit key information present in the more rigorous format of a structured report. Line listings end up being a data dump without the analysis and synthesis needed to make the information meaningful to the recipient.

The most successful solution appears to be a customized report that contains all of the same information contained in the regulatory report, but in a more user-friendly, concise format. However, since this approach has become an industry trend, investigators are now faced with interpreting a different type of report from each company (some companies even use different reports for different therapeutic areas), each attempting to provide the same basic information. Adoption of an industry standard would improve the quality of this important risk communication. It is expected that a recommendation for a standard will be made by the CIOMS VI working group.

It is a common misconception that ISLs can be considered as updates to the Investigator's Brochure (IB). The FDA has clarified that although the investigator letter may be attached to the IB as an informational update, additional cases of the same event(s) should still be regarded as unexpected (and submitted as expedited IND safety reports and ISLs) until the new ADR is added to the core safety information section of the IB. Once it is added, the revised, updated IB can be sent to all investigators as an official modification.

Studies not conducted under a US IND are subject to ICH guidelines that require study sponsors to keep investigators and IRBs/IECs informed of new safety information during the course of a clinical study. The method, format, and time frame for this are currently not specified. Guidances supporting the new EU Clinical Trial Directives are expected to provide more structure around this activity (see Chapter 9).

Dear Doctor (Healthcare Professional) letters

Although the term 'Dear Doctor' letter is often used interchangeably with the letters sent to investigators during a clinical trial (referred to above as ISLs), the two are not synonymous. 'Dear Doctor' letters, now known as 'Dear Healthcare Professional' (HCP) letters to indicate the broader target audience of pharmacists, nurses and others involved in patient care, are used to communicate important safety information in the post-marketing environment rather than solely within the confines of a clinical study. This mechanism is used as an expeditious way to highlight important safety information to those who prescribe and/or dispense and/or administer medications while other measures, such as revision of drug labels and packaging, are under way. The company may take this action voluntarily or be required to do so by a regulator. Regulators have also issued these letters independent of the company. It is to the company's advantage to participate in generating the letter in order to have some influence on the language it contains. There is also a public relations advantage to being perceived as proactive in risk communication. Chapter 8 provides a model for the essential elements that should be contained in this written communication.

Typically, the HCP recipients of these letters are generated from customer lists held by sales and marketing, professional society membership rosters, hospital employment databases, licensure registries, and even telephone directories. Companies may also pay for full-page displays of the letter in journals and other publications that target HCP audiences. These letters are also posted on company and professional Web sites, as well as the Web sites of the FDA and other regulators. When issuing a letter, it is very important to ensure simultaneous notification to regulators in all countries where the drug is marketed. Regulators monitor each other's Web sites closely, and are not pleased when companies do not inform them directly of safety issues known to other agencies.

The type of information contained in Dear HCP Letters may be categorized broadly into three types:

- *New ADRs.* When a company strongly suspects or confirms that a drug causes an ADR that is currently not described in the prescribing information, the company has a legal 'duty to warn' about this discovery quickly.

- *Notification of increased severity of ADRs.* The most severe types of ADR are usually not seen until population exposure has exceeded many thousands of patients. This includes more severe forms of known ADRs. One common example of this is drug-induced hepatotoxicity, which may have only been seen as 'elevated liver enzymes' in clinical trials, but which after market approval may result in drug-induced hepatitis, or hepatic necrosis, resulting either in the need for a liver transplant or in death.

- *Reiteration of contraindications, warnings, etc.* The company may learn that a drug is being prescribed or used in a way that increases risk to patients. Examples include co-prescribing with potentially interacting drugs, exceeding safe dosages or durations, and use in sensitive or prohibited populations (pregnant women, diabetics, etc.). Even if this information is contained in the current prescribing information, the company has an ethical obligation to re-emphasize the dangers to the public, and the Dear HCP letter may be used as one avenue of doing so.

Since the type of information described above can be complex, it was thought that communicating this type of information only to HCPs would minimize public alarm while ensuring patient safety, consistent with the concept of the intervention of 'the learned intermediary'. Today, with the technical savvy of consumer advocacy and watchdog groups, as well as lawyers and the media, publication of a Dear HCP letter frequently makes headlines in both television and the newspapers. Proponents of this wider dissemination point out that increased awareness will increase the potential for protecting patients. However, the increased publicity may also lead to unintended adverse consequences due to misinterpretation of the information, such as needless patient anxiety and potentially dangerous patient actions, such as abrupt discontinuation prior to physician consultation.

Conclusion: Vision for the future

The CIOMS 1A Working Group (CIOMS, 1994) put forth a vision (recently reiterated by the CIOMS V Working Group in its 2001 report (CIOMS, 2001)) that the interest of public health could best be served by having a single database with worldwide access, where AE cases would be entered only once, regardless of source. Until this vision is realized, even with the advent of electronic ADR submissions to regulators, safety reporting will continue to result in duplication of effort, with the danger of double counting and misinterpretation. Additionally, although considerable progress has been made over the past decade in achieving harmonization for many aspects of drug safety surveillance and reporting, much remains to be done in order to eliminate unnecessary regulatory differences and inefficiencies that consume resources and time but add little real value to pharmacovigilance.

Removal of such technical and regulatory obstacles would have a profound impact on the functional aspects of drug safety departments in pharmaceutical companies, not only in terms of organization and processes, but also in terms of the types of skill needed and work done. The majority of resources in drug safety departments could be shifted away from administrative activities, allowing increased focus on scientific analysis and medical evaluation, thus leading to enhanced public health protection through better assurance of the safety of medicinal products.

Acknowledgement

I would like to thank Mark K. Blake, Director, Drug Safety Systems, AstraZeneca Pharmaceuticals, USA, for his contribution of the excellent section on periodic safety updates to this chapter.

References

Anonymous, (2001). Managing the virtual classroom. *Training* (Jan): 14–19.

Benson L, Steiner J, Ward H and Haff L (1999). New methodologies in computer-based training for adverse event reporting. *Drug Info J* **33**(3): 899–906.

Brookfield SD (1986). *Understanding and Facilitating Adult Learning: A Comprehensive Analysis of Principles and Effective Practice*. Open University Press: Honolulu, HI.

Burr J (1987). Overcoming resistance to audits. *Qual Prog* (January): 15–18.

Chukwujindu JI, Holman C and Sanderson P (1999). Pharmacovigilance: the role of a CRO. *Int J Pharm Med* **13**: 137–141.

CIOMS (1994). CIOMS 1A Working Group, Harmonization of data fields for individual ADR reports (unpublished). CIOMS: Geneva.

CIOMS (1998). CIOMS IV Working Group, *Benefit–Risk Balance for Marketed Drugs: Evaluating Safety Signals*. CIOMS: Geneva.

CIOMS (2001). CIOMS V Working Group, *Current Challenges in Pharmacovigilance: Pragmatic Approaches*. CIOMS: Geneva.

CPMP (2001). Committee for Proprietary Medicinal Products, Position paper on compliance with pharmacovigilance regulatory obligations, November, (CPMP/PhVWP/1618/01).

Doan TVT (2000). Establishing a MedDRA safety surveillance unit. *Drug Inf J.* **34**(1): 245–250.

Driscoll M (1998). *Web-based Training: Using Technology to Design Adult Learning Experiences*. Jossey Bass: San Francisco.

Farrow J (1987). Quality audits: an invitation to management. *Qual Prog* (January): 11–13.

Gryna F (1988). Quality assurance. In *Juran's Quality Control Handbook*, 4th edn, Juran JM (ed.) McGraw-Hill: New York.

Herron M (2002). Training alone is not enough. *Training* **39**(2): 72–74.

ICH (1995). ICH Guideline E2A, Clinical safety data management: definitions and standards for expedited reporting, March.

ICH (1996). ICH Harmonized Tripartite Guideline, Clinical safety data management: periodic safety update reports for marketed drugs, November.

ICH (1997). ICH Guideline E6 Good clinical practice: consolidated guidance, May.

ICH (1998). ICH Guideline E9, Statistical principles for clinical trials, September.

ICH (2002). ICH E2C Clinical safety data management: periodic safety update reports for marketed drugs (draft consensus guideline), September.

Kruse K and Keil J (2000). *Technology-based Training: The Art and Science of Design, Development, and Delivery*. Jossey Bass: San Francisco.

Lieb S (1998). Principles of adult learning. http://www.hcc.hawaii.edu/hccinfo/facdev/AdultLearning.html [19 May 1988].

Steiner J, Cauterucci C, Shon Y and Muirhead A (2001). Planning for a successful safety data conversion. *Drug Inf J* **35**(1): 61–69.

Zenger J and Uehlein C (2001). Why blended will win. *Training Dev* (August): 54–60.

Further reading

CIOMS Working Group III and V (1999). *Guidelines for Preparing Core Clinical-Safety Information on Drugs*, 2nd edn. CIOMS: Geneva.

Galagan P (2001). Fourteen things CEOs should know about e-learning. *Training Dev* (November): 69–72.

Hamrell MR (2000). The clinical audit in pharmaceutical development. In *Drugs and the Pharmaceutical Sciences*, vol. 104. Marcel Dekker: New York.

International Conference on Developing Effective Communications in Pharmacovigilance, The 'Erice Report' (1998). *Effective Communications in Pharmacovigilance*. Uppsala Monitoring Center, Sweden.

12

Dictionaries and Coding in Pharmacovigilance

E. G. Brown

Introduction

For some reason, many professionals working in the field of drug safety do not find the topic of dictionaries exciting. Most would admit, however, that they are of critical importance. The purpose of the dictionary is to bring order to seeming chaos. They are intended to bring some discipline to the vast number of descriptive terms that health professionals and patients use for medical conditions, and to the enormous array of medicines that the former inflict on the latter. By abbreviating the original descriptions and reducing them to some form of code or standard terms, it is possible to record the data effectively and concisely on a computer database, to search for similar medical conditions associated with unique medicinal products and to present the information in summarized format or numerical tables.

The characteristics of the dictionary exert a profound effect on the data. If there are too few terms in the dictionary, then compromises have to be made when coding the data. Details that have been reported may be lost, e.g. staphylococcal bronchopneumonia and acute exacerbation of chronic bronchitis might both just become 'respiratory infection'. If the relationships within the dictionary are not completely valid, then a case reported as 'psychological problems' might be transformed into 'psychotic' in the database – which is enough to drive anyone mad.

At the other end of the scale, it could be that the dictionary accurately reflects the facts, but does not group conditions appropriately. If grouping is not effective, then it might be difficult to find items in the database. For example, if pneumonitis is classed together with some similar conditions as a respiratory disorder, but pneumonias are grouped separately under the heading of infections, then this could result in failure to identify all cases relevant to a particular safety concern about the adverse effects of a drug on the lung.

Another way in which the choice of dictionary could affect one's view of the world is, paradoxically, by being too specific. If a dictionary included 25 different types of headache, then it might be difficult to answer the simple question of whether there were there more reports of headache with the beta-blocker ololol in patients receiving active drug or placebo in a comparative trial with 100 patients in each treatment arm. The answer might be that

Stephens' Detection of New Adverse Drug Reactions Fifth Edition edited by John Talbot and Patrick Waller
© 2004 John Wiley & Sons, Ltd   ISBN: 0 470 84552 X

there were: two reports of tension headache, two reports of throbbing headache, four of unspecified headache and three of sinus headache with ololol; and one of tension headache, two unspecified headache, one vascular headache and one headache with flashing lights in patients receiving placebo. If there is no group term for 'headache', then real differences between treatments might be missed. Such 'splitting' might similarly reduce one's ability to detect signals of new adverse reactions in a post-marketing safety database.

Thus, whilst dictionaries may not be held to be universally fascinating, it is worth learning about them if serious mistakes are to be avoided in pharmacovigilance.

Scope of this chapter

This chapter describes some of the medical and drug dictionaries that are used in the safety surveillance of medicines, pre- and post-registration. I have regarded the term 'dictionary' as being synonymous with 'terminology'. The 1994 Collins Shorter English Dictionary gives one definition of 'dictionary' as: 'a reference book listing words or terms and giving information about a particular subject or activity'. A definition for 'terminology' from the same source is: 'the body of specialised words relating to a particular subject'. However, a better term might be 'thesaurus', defined in the Collins Dictionary as 'a book containing systematised lists of synonyms and related words; a dictionary of selected words or topics'.

There are a great many dictionaries currently in use in the pharmacovigilance/regulatory affairs environment. I have only considered those most relevant and widely used for general purposes in drug safety. Thus, specialist dictionaries covering specific disease areas, such as oncology or pathology, are not included; neither are those used for animals (e.g. VEDDRA). I have also ignored the many (sometimes excellent) dictionaries that have been developed in-house (e.g. the Medicine Control Agency's ADROIT dictionary, or Glaxo Smith Kline's MIDAS dictionary), as well as dictionaries used sometimes in medical practice outside the pharmaceutical environment (e.g. Read codes).

In addition to dictionaries, some issues relating to definitions of terms used for adverse reactions are also considered. It may seem strange that the existing dictionaries do not actually define the medical terms that are included – unlike dictionaries used for languages. However, there has been an initiative by the Council for International Organizations of Medical Sciences (CIOMS; Bankowski et al., 1999), to provide some definitions, and this topic is also included.

Drug dictionaries

The huge plethora of available medicines provides a challenge for those wishing to store accurate information on databases. When considering all the different formulations, dosage forms, routes of administration, therapeutic and pharmacological classes, manufacturers, approved and proprietary names for each of these, the task becomes daunting indeed. A number of standard classifications have been produced, of which the two most widely applicable are considered below.

Anatomical–therapeutic–chemical classification

The anatomical–therapeutic–chemical (ATC) classification is a system for the classification of drugs according to their site of therapeutic effect, therapeutic indication and pharmacological nature. It is widely accepted as a useful method of categorizing and recording individual drugs. The main ATC groups are shown in Table 12.1 (Anonymous, 2000).

Table 12.1   The main ATC groups

A	Alimentary tract and metabolism
B	Blood and blood-forming organs
C	Cardiovascular system
D	Dermatologicals
G	Genitourinary system and sex hormones
H	Systemic hormonal preparations excluding sex hormones
J	General anti-infectives for systemic use
L	Antineoplastic and immunomodulating agents
M	Musculoskeletal system
N	Nervous system
P	Antiparasitic products, insecticides and repellents
R	Respiratory system
S	Sensory organs
V	Various

Within each main group, there is arrangement of classes of drug as sub-groups, according to broad therapeutic area or site of action. Thus, for the Respiratory system there are the following sub-groups: R01 Nasal preparations; R02 Throat preparations; R03 Anti-asthmatics; R05 Cough and cold preparations; R06 Antihistamines for systemic use; and R07 Other respiratory products.

Additional breakdown by pharmacological category is effected under the sub-groups: e.g. under R03, Anti-asthmatics, we have: R03A Adrenergics, inhalants; R03B Other anti-asthmatics, inhalants; R03C Adrenergics for systemic use; R03D Other anti-asthmatics for systemic use.

Further specificity is then provided with additional codes under each category according to pharmacology or chemical structure. Thus: R03CA Alpha- and beta-adrenoceptor agonists; R03CB Non-selective beta-adrenergic agonists; R03CC Selective Beta-2-adrenoceptor agonists; R03CK Adrenergics and other anti-asthmatics. An extract from the Cardiovascular system group is shown in Table 12.2, to further illustrate the logic behind the classification.

The World Health Organization Drug Dictionary

This contains of the order of 45 000 proprietary drug names, with about 2600 being added annually (Uppsala Monitoring Centre, 2002). It is an international classification, giving the names used in different countries, together with all active ingredients with unique reference numbers. Drugs are classified according to ATC code. The dictionary was started in 1968 and includes all drugs mentioned on adverse reaction reports submitted under the World

Table 12.2   Example of ATC codes

C	Cardiovascular system		
	C01	Cardiac therapy	
		C01A	Cardiac glycosides
			C01AA	Digitalis glycosides
			C01AB	Scilla glycosides
			C01AC	Strophantus glycosides
			C01AX	Other cardiac glycosides
		C01B	Antiarrhythmics, class I and III
			C01BB	Antiarrhythmics, class IB
			C01BC	Antiarrhythmics, class IC
			C01BD	antiarrhythmics, class III
			C01BG	Other class I antiarrhythmics
		C01C	Cardiac stimulants excl. cardiac glycosides
			C01CA	Adrenergic and dopaminergic agents
			C01CE	Phosphodiesterase inhibitors
			C01CX	Other cardiac stimulants
	C02	Antihypertensives	
		C02A	Antiadrenergic agents, centrally acting
			C02AA	Rauwolfia alkaloids
			C02AB	Methyldopa
			C02AC	Imidazoline receptor agonists
		C02B	Antiadrenergic agents, ganglion-blocking
			C02BA	Sulfonium derivatives
			C02BB	Secondary and tertiary amines
			C02BC	Bisquaternary ammonium compounds
			C02C	Antiadrenergic agents, peripherally acting

Health Organization (WHO) Programme on International Drug Monitoring. Drugs from almost 70 countries are represented, and updates are issued quarterly.

Drugs containing the same active ingredient(s) are referred to by *Preferred name* – the international non-proprietary name (INN) in English for single ingredient drugs (or other approved name, if there is no INN). For multiple ingredient drugs, the *Preferred name* is the first reported drug name of a given combination. Drugs are given various designations, as shown in Table 12.3.

Table 12.3   WHO drug dictionary: designation of drug type

N	Single ingredient drug non-proprietary name
T	Single ingredient drug proprietary name
K	Single ingredient drug chemical name
R	Single ingredient drug code number
M	Multiple ingredient drug proprietary name
X	Multiple ingredient drug non-proprietary name
U	Non-specific name, from ATC texts (such as NSAID or benzodiazepine)

The dictionary includes a manufacturer for the drug, although this may in fact be a distributor in a particular country. The manufacturer name is abbreviated to a three- to five-letter code. Drugs are given consecutive record numbers and also two *sequence numbers*, SEQ1 and SEQ2. The first *sequence number* is used for single constituent drugs to distinguish between salts or esters of a substance and the second *sequence number* distinguishes between trade names with the same ingredients. The *Preferred name* has a SEQ2 of 001. An example showing the record number system is given in Table 12.4.

Table 12.4 Example showing the record-number system in the drug dictionary (reproduced by permission of the Uppsala Monitoring Centre)

Drug name	Des	DRECNO	SEQ1	SEQ2
Single ingredient drugs				
1. Ampicillin	N	000005	01	001
2. Ampicillin sodium	N	000005	02	001
3. Binotal for injection	T	000005	02	002
3. Polycillin-N for injection	T	000005	02	003
2. Ampicillin trihydrate	N	000005	03	001
3. Polycillin	T	000005	03	002
3. Austrapen	T	000005	03	003
Multiple ingredient drugs				
1. Ampiclox	M	001903	01	001
Ampicillin				
Cloxacillin				
3. Sinteclox	M	001903	01	002

The drug dictionary is available in paper or electronic versions and software is available for browsing the dictionary, which is held as a relational database. This comprises several files, including the drug dictionary itself, the ATC classification, substance names, ingredients, manufacturers, ATC text, sources of drug names and country codes.

Other drug dictionaries

At the time of writing, a new drug dictionary is being developed by the European Agency for the Evaluation of Medicinal Products, based on ATC codes.

Adverse drug reaction dictionaries

World Health Organization Adverse Reaction Terminology: WHO-ART

This dictionary is used by the WHO Uppsala Monitoring Centre for recording suspected adverse reactions on their worldwide database, as well as by many regulatory authorities for their pharmacovigilance activities. WHO-ART (Uppsala Monitoring Centre, 2000) has been extensively used in the past by pharmaceutical companies, but has often been modified by the addition of many new terms within individual organizations, so that these in-house versions are effectively separate terminologies. With regard to the 'standard' dictionary, this is updated at intervals by the addition of new terms and with the release of new versions. Translations are available in several languages, and there are both paper and electronic versions.

WHO-ART has a hierarchical and multiaxial structure. Of the order of 2000 *Preferred terms* are used for data input and represent separate medical concepts. *Included terms* are synonyms to the *Preferred terms* and are used for finding the most appropriate *Preferred term* for coding purposes. However, *Included terms* may also be used for data entry. *High level terms* are used to group qualitatively similar *Preferred terms*, but many *Preferred terms* have no corresponding *High level term*. At the top end of the terminology, there are 32 *System-organ classes*, which provide groupings for the *High level terms* and *Preferred terms*. A *Preferred term* may be assigned to up to three different *System-organ classes*.

Preferred and *Included* terms in WHO-ART are assigned numerical codes that provide information about the level of the term and the *System-organ class(es)* to which it is allocated. Thus, in addition to a unique record number, each *Preferred term* is assigned the number 0100.

The *System-organ classes* are shown in Table 12.5. Each *System-organ class* is associated with a four-digit code, for example 0600 for *Gastro-intestinal system disorders*, 1210 for *Red blood cell disorders*, 1820 for *Application site disorders*. Table 12.6 shows an extract from the *Autonomic nervous system disorders System-organ class.*

Coding Symbols for a Thesaurus of Adverse Reaction Terms (COSTART)

This terminology was distributed by the US Food and Drugs Administration (FDA) and has been widely used by companies for coding adverse events in clinical trials and post-marketing surveillance. However, its small size has resulted in many organizations producing their own customized versions, by the addition of new terms. At the top of the COSTART (Food and Drugs Administration, 1989) hierarchy, there are 12 *body systems*, as shown in Table 12.7.

At the next lowest level in COSTART, there is a *mid-level classification* for retrieval purposes based on pathophysiology. A classification for the *Cardiovascular System* is shown in Table 12.8. The subordinate *Coding symbols* for *Coronary Vessel Disorders* are shown in Table 12.9. As may be seen, these comprise abbreviated text. *Coding symbols* are associated with one or more *Glossary terms*, which are used to assist in selection of the *Coding symbol* when coding. For example, for the *Coding symbol ANGINA PECTORIS*, we have *Glossary terms* including *Angina at rest Prinzmetal's*; *Angina attack*; *Angina of effort*; *Angina pectoris*; *Angina pectoris aggravated*; *Anginal pain*; *Anginal syndrome*; *Effort angina*; etc.

The status of COSTART is tenuous, in view of the adoption of MedDRA® by the FDA (see below). In time it is likely that it will be completely superseded by MedDRA®.

Disease classifications

In this section, some of the classifications that are used in the drug safety environment are reviewed. Although International Classification of Diseases 10 (ICD10) is the current version, many organizations still use its predecessor, ICD9. Hence, both these classifications are considered.

The classification of diseases is defined in ICD10 as 'a system of categories to which

Table 12.5 WHO-ART System-organ classes

Skin and appendage disorders
Musculo-sleletal system disorders
Collagen disorders
Central & peripheral nervous system disorders
Autonomic nervous system disorders
Vision disorders
Hearing and vestibular disorders
Special senses other disorders
Psychiatric disorders
Gastro-intestinal system disorders
Liver and biliary system disorders
Metabolic and nutritional disorders
Endocrine disorders
Cardiovascular disorders, general
Myo-, endo-, peri-cardial & valve disorders
Heart rate and rhythm disorders
Vascular (extracardiac) disorders
Respiratory system disorders
Red blood cell disorders
White blood cell and RES disorders
Platelet, bleeding & clotting disorders
Urinary system disorders
Reproductive disorders, male
Reproductive disorders, female
Foetal disorders
Neonatal and infancy disorders
Neoplasms
Body as a whole – general disorders
Application site disorders
Resistance mechanism disorders
Secondary terms – events
Poison specific terms

---

morbid entities are assigned according to established criteria' (World Health Organization, 1992). The International Classifications have widespread application, and are accepted as worldwide standards. In the pharmaceutical environment, as elsewhere, they are used for epidemiological purposes. They have also been used for coding baseline medical history and diagnoses in clinical trials and for recording adverse events. However, they were not really designed for this purpose, and the description of conditions and their groupings is not ideal for this function. They are available in printed format as books and can generally be found in medical libraries in academic institutions and hospitals.

ICD9

In ICD9, there are 17 *chapters* plus two *supplementary classifications*: *External causes of injury and poisoning* and *Factors influencing health status and contact with health services* (World Health Organization, 1977). The chapter headings are similar to *System-organ*

Table 12.6   Extract from the WHO-ART autonomic nervous system disorders System-organ class

High level term	Record no.	Preferred term	Included term	System organ no. 2	System organ no. 3
Vasodilatation	0207	Flushing	Skin hyperaemia	1040	
Vasodilatation	0207	Flushing	Skin vasodilatation	1040	
Vasodilatation	0207	Flushing	Skin warm	1040	
Vasodilatation	0207	Flushing	Skin flushed	1040	
Vasodilatation	0207	Flushing	Blood flow sensation	1040	
Vasodilatation	0207	Flushing	Flushing aggravated	1040	
Vasodilatation	0225	Vasodilatation	Hyperaemia	1040	
Vasodilatation	0225	Vasodilatation	Vasodilation	1040	
	0202	Accommodation abnormal	Accommodation disturbance	0431	
	0202	Accommodation abnormal	Accommodation disorder	0431	
	0202	Accommodation abnormal	Distance accommodation disorder	0431	
	0202	Accommodation abnormal	Accommodation paralysis	0431	
	0202	Accommodation abnormal	Accommodation spasm	0431	
	0780	Anticholinergic syndrome		0410	
	0208	Bradycardia	Sinus bradycardia	1030	
	0208	Bradycardia	Pulse rate decreased marked	1030	
	0208	Bradycardia	Sinus arrest	1030	
	0203	Cholinergic syndrome	Parasympathomimetic syndrome	0410	
	0211	Hypertension pulmonary	Hypertension pulmonary aggravated	1010	1100

Table 12.7.   COSTART body systems

Body as a Whole
Cardiovascular System
Digestive System
Endocrine System
Hemic and Lymphatic System
Metabolic and Nutritional Disorders
Musculo-skeletal System
Nervous System
Respiratory System
Skin and Appendages
Special Senses
Urogenital System

Table 12.8   COSTART mid-level classification

Cardiovascular System
    Cardiac disorders
    Arrhythmias
    Conduction abnormalities
    Coronary vessel disorders
    Endocardial disorders
    General, functional and NEC*
    Myocardial disorders
    Pericardial disorders
    General and NEC*
    Vascular disorders
    Arterial and arteriolar disorders
    Blood pressure disorders
    Capillary disorders

---

* Not elsewhere classified.

Table 12.9   COSTART coding symbols under Coronary vessel disorders

---

Coronary vessel disorders
    ANGINA PECTORIS
    CORONARY ART DIS
    EMB CORONARY
    OCCLUS CORONARY
    THROM CORONARY

Classes, for example '*II Neoplasms*', '*VIII Diseases of the Respiratory System*', '*XIV Congenital anomalies*', etc. Each *chapter* is divided up into sub-groups represented by discrete three-digit codes, each code delimiting a more specific group of medical conditions. Thus, *Neoplasms* are covered by the codes 140 to 239 and *Respiratory disorders* by codes 460 to 519.

Within the *chapters*, diseases are grouped and classified with these three-digit codes. For example, in the *chapter Diseases of the Respiratory system*, we see six sub-headings: *Acute respiratory infections; Other diseases of upper respiratory tract; Pneumonia and influenza; Chronic obstructive pulmonary disease and allied conditions; Pneumoconioses and other lung diseases due to external agents; and Other diseases of respiratory system.*

Grouped under the sub-heading *Pneumonia and influenza* 480–487, we see the three-digit individual medical conditions, as shown in Table 12.10. Additional digits are use to represent more specific diseases. The four digit codes ending .8 refer to '*other*' related conditions; the four-digit codes ending in .9 refer to conditions that are '*unspecified*'.

Table 12.10   Example of three- and four-digit terms in ICD9

PNEUMONIA AND INFLUENZA (480–487)	
480	Viral pneumonia
481	Pneumococcal pneumonia
482	Other bacterial pneumonia
483	Pneumonia due to other specified organism
484	Pneumonia in infectious diseases classified elsewhere
	484.0* Measles (055.1†)
	484.1* Cytomegalic inclusion disease (078.5†)
	484.2* Ornithosis (073†)
	484.3* Whooping cough (033†)
	484.4* Tularaemia (021†)
	484.5* Anthrax (022.1†)
	484.6* Aspergillosis (117.3†)
	484.7* Pneumonia in other systemic mycoses
	484.8* Pneumonia in other infectious diseases
485	Bronchopneumonia, organism unspecified
486	Pneumonia, organism unspecified
487	Influenza

The use of the *asterix* and *dagger* system is demonstrated in Table 12.10. The † symbol is attached to the code showing the underlying disease, whilst the * is attached to the code in the organ system where the disease is manifested. For example, if we consider *Measles* 055, its four-digit codes include: 055.0† *Postmeasles encephalitis*; 055.1† *Postmeasles pneumonia*; 055.2† *Postmeasles otitis*, etc.

ICD9 clinical modification (ICD9-CM)

ICD9-CM provides additional specificity by having five-digit codes, so that, for example, *Mastoiditis* and related conditions are coded as 383, *Acute mastoiditis* is 383.0, *Acute mastoiditis without complications* is 383.00, whereas *Subperiosteal abcess of mastoid* is 383.01 (see Table 12.11) (Anonymous, 1994). This modification of ICD9 tends to be used more in the USA than in Europe.

ICD10

Published in 1992 (World Health Organization, 1992), this version of the International Classification has gained widespread acceptance, especially for the recording of national morbidity and mortality data and of health service resource utilization.

Table 12.11   Structure of ICD9-CM

320–389 Diseases of the nervous system and sense organs

  330–337   Hereditary and degenerative diseases of the central nervous system

  335   Anterior horn cell disease

    335.2   Motor neurone disease

      335.2 0   Amyotrophic lateral sclerosis

      335.2 1   Progressive muscular atrophy

      335.2 2   Progressive bulbar palsy

etc.

The main innovation was the use of an alphanumeric coding scheme of one letter followed by three numbers. At the end of some chapters, there is a category for post-procedural disorders. Additional three-digit codes are available to capture dual sites for aetiology and manifestation.

The classification is again divided into *chapters*. Thus, *Chapter I – Certain infectious and parasitic diseases*; *Chapter II – Neoplasms*; *Chapter III – Diseases of the blood and blood-forming organs and certain disorders involving the immune mechanism*; *Chapter IV – Endocrine, nutritional and metabolic diseases*; *Chapter XXI – Factors influencing health status and contact with health services*, etc.

Each *chapter* in the classification is prefaced with a rubric describing the inclusion and exclusion criteria for that chapter. For example, *Chapter IX, Diseases of the circulatory system*, excludes '*certain conditions originating in the perinatal period* (P00–P96); *certain infectious and parasitic diseases* (A00–B99); *complications of pregnancy, childbirth and the puerperium* (O00–O99); *congenital malformations, deformations and chromosomal abnormalities* (Q00–Q99) . . .' etc.

Within each chapter, there are sub-headings or '*blocks*'. For example, *Chapter IX* includes *blocks* for *Acute rheumatic fever, Chronic rheumatic heart diseases, Hypertensive diseases*, etc., as shown in Table 12.12. Within each *block* there are grouped related conditions, distinguished by three-character codes. In this way, for example, I20 *Angina pectoris* is distinguished from I21 *Acute myocardial infarction* within the *Ischaemic heart diseases block*, as shown in Table 12.13.

Again, the *blocks* may provide inclusion and exclusion criteria. Thus, the *block Ischaemic heart diseases* (I20–25) may include mention of *hypertension*, which may be represented by

Table 12.12   Blocks included in ICD10, Chapter IX, Diseases of the Circulatory System

---

Acute rheumatic fever

Chronic rheumatic heart diseases

Hypertensive diseases

Ischaemic heart diseases

Pulmonary heart disease and diseases of pulmonary circulation

Other forms of heart disease

Cerebrovascular diseases

Diseases of arteries, arterioles and capillaries

Diseases of veins, lymphatic vessels and lymph nodes, not elsewhere classified

Other and unspecified disorders of the circulatory system

Table 12.13   Three-character conditions classifying Ischaemic heart diseases in ICD10

Ischaemic heart diseases (I20–I25)

I20	Angina pectoris
I21	Acute myocardial infarction
I22	Subsequent myocardial infarction
I23	Certain current complications following acute myocardial infarction
I24	Other acute ischaemic heart diseases
I25	Chronic ischaemic heart disease

an additional code, if desired. There are notes provided on the way that terms are used – so, in this instance, it is stated that, for morbidity, duration refers to the interval elapsing between onset of ischaemic episode and admission to care, whereas for mortality, duration refers to the interval between onset and death.

Under the three-character *blocks* are presented four-character terms that add specificity to the disease descriptions. For example, under I20, *Angina pectoris*, I20.0 *Unstable angina* is distinguished from I20.1 *Angina pectoris with documented spasm*: see Table 12.14.

Individual chapters include refinements of the coding system. For example, in *Chapter XX, External causes of morbidity and mortality*, there are subdivisions by fourth character to indicate the place of occurrence of the external cause: .0 for the home; .1 for residential institution; .2 for school, other institution and public administrative area; .3 for sports and athletics area, etc. Each of these is provided with options for describing the detailed

Table 12.14   Four-character conditions specifying type of angina in ICD10

I20.0	Unstable angina
	Angina:
	• Crescendo
	• *De novo* effort
	• Worsening effort
	Intermediate coronary syndrome
	Preinfarction syndrome
I20.1	Angina pectoris with documented spasm
	Angina:
	• Angiospastic
	• Prinzmetal
	• Spasm-induced
	• Variant
I20.8	Other forms of angina
	Angina of effort
	Stenocardia
I20.9	Angina pectoris, unspecified
	Angina
	• NOS
	• Cardiac
	Anginal syndrome
	Ischaemic chest pain

location, such as baseball field, basketball court, cricket ground, etc. Other subclassifications in this chapter cover the activity during which the injury was sustained, such as sports activity, leisure activity, again with optional detailed descriptions.

Multiaxiality is accommodated within individual blocks in each chapter, with the site indicated by an asterisk. For example, I32* *Pericarditis in diseases classified elsewhere* includes I32.0 *Pericarditis in bacterial diseases classified elsewhere*, which covers four causal types of infection. The causal organisms are indicated by a dagger (†). These are shown under *Pericarditis in diseases classified elsewhere* as: *Gonococcal pericarditis* (A54.8†); *Meningococcal pericarditis* (A39.5†); *Syphilitic pericarditis* (A52.0†); and *tuberculous pericarditis* (A18.8†). In turn, if one refers to A18.8†, this is the block *Tuberculosis of other specified organs*, covering *tuberculosis of endocardium* (I39.8*), *myocardium* (I41.0*), *oesophagus* (K23.0*), *pericardium* (I32.0*), *thyroid gland* (E35.0*) and *tuberculous cerebral arteritis* (I68.1*).

Combination terminology

Medical Dictionary for Regulatory Activities, MedDRA®

Background and development

MedDRA® is a structured thesaurus of medical terms that has been adopted as an international standard by the International Conference on Harmonization (ICH), for use together with other standards (E2B, M2) in the electronic exchange of data between regulatory authorities and between companies and regulators (Wood, 1994; Brown *et al.*, 1999). MedDRA® was first made available for general use in March 1999.

MedDRA® scope

The dictionary includes terms that are relevant to all phases involving man in the development and post-authorization safety surveillance of medicines and to the health effects of medical devices (Maintenance and Support Services Organization, 2002a). The terms in MedDRA® cover medical diagnoses, symptoms and signs, adverse reactions, therapeutic indications, the names and qualitative findings from laboratory, radiological and other investigations, surgical and medical procedures, and social circumstances.

MedDRA® does not include a drug or device nomenclature, nor does it include terms covering study design, pharmacokinetics or patient demographics. It does not allow for adjectives such as those describing disease severity or frequency, although qualifiers such as acute, chronic, recurrent are included in terms when clinically relevant. There is a restricted range of terms for describing aggravation or exacerbation of medical conditions.

In the pre-registration phases of a product's life cycle, MedDRA® may be used, for example, for recording adverse events and baseline medical history in clinical trials, in the analysis and tabulations of data from these and in the expedited submission of adverse event data to government regulatory authorities. It may be used in constructing standard product information, such as summaries of product characteristics (SPCs) or product labelling (Brown and Clark, 1996; White, 1998), and in registration files in support of applications for marketing authorization/new drug applications. After licensing, MedDRA® is used in pharmacovigilance for the continuing evaluation of drug safety, for both expedited and periodic safety reporting.

The structure of MedDRA®

The structure of MedDRA® may be represented diagrammatically as having a five-level hierarchy, as shown in Table 12.15. As will be explained below, MedDRA® is multiaxial as well as being hierarchical, so that *Preferred Terms* (PTs), with their associated *Lowest Level Terms* (LLTs), may be represented under more than one of the 26 *System Organ Classes* (SOCs). Table 12.16 shows the MedDRA® SOCs.

Table 12.15   MedDRA® hierarchy

MedDRA® hierarchy	Number of terms	Example (primary location)	Code
System Organ Class (SOC)	26	Skin and subcutaneous tissue disorders	10040785
High Level Group Term (HLGT)	332	Skin vascular abnormalities	10047065
High Level Term (HLT)	1683	Purpura and related conditions	10037555
Preferred Term (PT)	15 709	Purpura NOS	10037559
Lowest Level Term (LLT)	55 638	Purpuric rash	10037566

Table 12.16   MedDRA® System Organ Classes (SOCs)

Blood and lymphatic system disorders
Cardiac disorders
Congenital, familial and genetic disorders
Ear and labyrinth disorders
Endocrine disorders
Eye disorders
Gastrointestinal disorders
General disorders and administration site conditions
Hepatobiliary disorders
Immune system disorders
Infections and infestations
Injury, poisoning and procedural complications
Investigations
Metabolism and nutrition disorders
Musculoskeletal and connective tissue disorders
Neoplasms benign, malignant and unspecified (incl cysts and polyps)
Nervous system disorders
Pregnancy, puerperium and perinatal conditions
Psychiatric disorders
Renal and urinary disorders
Reproductive system and breast disorders
Respiratory, thoracic and mediastinal disorders
Skin and subcutaneous tissue disorders
Social circumstances
Surgical and medical procedures
Vascular disorders

Each PT is intended to represent a unique medical concept: it is the term preferred for use in the regulatory environment and is formatted according to MedDRA® conventions. Eponymous terms may be used if recognized internationally. A PT may describe a single syndrome, even though a syndrome represents a collection of signs and symptoms. Each PT is duplicated as an LLT and may have subordinate to it one or more other LLTs that are synonyms, lexical variants or alternative spellings of the PT. In addition, some LLTs describe conditions that are more precise or specific than the PT to which they are linked; whilst not synonymous, they are considered not to warrant PT status from a pharmacovigilance perspective.

For example, the PT *Alveolitis allergic* has LLTs *Pneumonitis allergic* and *Pneumonitis hypersensitivity* which are synonyms; *Allergic pneumonitis* and *Pneumonitis allergic*, which are lexical variants; the LLTs *Bagassosis* and *Baggasosis* demonstrate differences in spelling; and the LLTs *Malt Worker's lung* and *Bird fancier's lung* are different conditions that do not warrant a separate PT from a regulatory perspective, although they may be distinct medical conditions. An example of a PT and some of its LLTs is shown in Table 12.17. Tables 12.18 to 12.20 show the hierarchical structure of MedDRA® expanded to demonstrate the nature of the terms at various levels.

Table 12.17 Hierarchy and secondary linkages for the MedDRA® PT *Purpura NOS*

	Primary SOC	Secondary SOC	Secondary SOC
SOC	Skin and subcutaneous tissue disorders	Blood and lymphatic system disorders	Vascular disorders
HLGT	Skin vascular abnormalities	Bleeding tendencies and purpuras (excl thrombocytopenic)	Vascular haemorrhagic disorders
HLT	Purpura and related conditions	Purpuras (excl thrombocytopenic)	Bruising, ecchymosis and purpura
PT	Purpura NOS	Purpura NOS	Purpura NOS
LLT	Dermatitis haemorrhagic	Dermatitis haemorrhagic	Dermatitis haemorrhagic
LLT	Dermatitis hemorrhagic	Dermatitis hemorrhagic	Dermatitis hemorrhagic
LLT	Haemorrhage purpuric	Haemorrhage purpuric	Haemorrhage purpuric
LLT	Idiopathic purpura	Idiopathic purpura	Idiopathic purpura
LLT	Purpura	Purpura	Purpura
LLT	Purpura NOS	Purpura NOS	Purpura NOS
LLT	Rash purpuric	Rash purpuric	Rash purpuric
LLT	Hemorrhage purpuric	Hemorrhage purpuric	Hemorrhage purpuric
LLT	Purpuric rash	Purpuric rash	Purpuric rash
LLT	Rash hemorrhagic	Rash hemorrhagic	Rash hemorrhagic
LLT	Rash haemorrhagic	Rash haemorrhagic	Rash haemorrhagic
LLT	Purpura symptomatica	Purpura symptomatica	Purpura symptomatica

Each PT is represented only once under a particular SOC, to which it is connected vertically via a single *High Level Term* (HLT), which in turn is fixed in location and represented only once in that SOC under one *High Level Group Term* (HLGT). It is a rule that there is only one route from LLT to PT to HLT to HLGT within the SOC. Thus, for example, the PT *Alveolitis allergic* includes LLTs *Farmer's lung* and *Malt worker's lung*. The PT is located under the HLT *Lower respiratory tract inflammatory and immunologic conditions*. It might

Table 12.18   Structure of a MedDRA® HLGT, showing its HLTs

HLGT	HLT
Skin vascular abnormalities	Capillary conditions Purpura and related conditions Skin haemorrhages Skin ischaemic conditions Skin vascular conditions NEC Skin vasculitides etc.

Table 12.19   Structure of a MedDRA® HLT, showing its PTs

HLT	PT (primary location)	PT (secondary location)
Purpura and related conditions	Ecchymosis Henoch–Schonlein purpura Increased tendency to bruise Majocchi's purpura Purpura neonatal Purpura NOS etc.	Idiopathic thrombocytopenic purpura Application site bruising Injection site bruising Petechiae Thrombotic thrombocytopenic purpura etc.

Table 12.20   Structure of a MedDRA® SOC, showing its HLGTs

SOC	HLGT
Skin and subcutaneous tissue disorders	Angioedema and urticaria Cornification and dystrophic skin disorders Cutaneous neoplasms benign Epidermal and dermal conditions Pigmentation disorders Skin and subcutaneous tissue disorders NEC Skin and subcutaneous tissue infections and infestations etc.

equally well be located under the HLT *Occupational parenchymal lung disorders*, also present in the *Respiratory* SOC. However, that would require two HLTs for a single PT within the one SOC, which is not permitted.

Every PT has a fixed location in one SOC, which is referred to as the 'primary' location. However, the parallel vertical SOC axes are not mutually exclusive; hence, a PT may also be found in so-called 'secondary' locations in one or more additional SOCs, in which it is again placed under a specified HLT and HLGT, whilst retaining all its associated LLTs. Having multiple locations for a PT within the terminology, known as 'multiaxiality', has the advantage that the term may be found when searches are carried out on any of the relevant

SOCs. The principle is similar to that seen above for WHO-ART and to the asterix and dagger system in ICD. The multiaxial linkages for a MedDRA® PT are shown in Table 12.17.

Thus, for example, to look in a database for cases that might be relevant to a new safety signal of heart failure, one would search in the *Cardiac* SOC for all the associated terms (probably PTs) that will lead to identification of the required cases. However, the PT *Paroxysmal nocturnal dyspnoea* is (appropriately) grouped with other types of dyspnoea under the *Respiratory* SOC as its primary location. This symptom of acute left ventricular failure is clearly relevant to the search, and it has a secondary location under the *Cardiac* SOC. Hence, if the search encompassed both primary and secondary locations, it would find cases with paroxysmal nocturnal dyspnoea even if the search was restricted to the *Cardiac* SOC.

The detailed MedDRA® user guide (Maintenance and Support Services Organization, 2002a) explains the development of the terminology and defines hierarchical levels and the rationale and conventions for their use. It is distributed on the MedDRA® CD-ROM, and updates are provided with new versions of MedDRA®.

A noteworthy convention applies to investigations. These are represented only in the *Investigations* SOC; there are no secondary linkages. However, terms describing clinical conditions, e.g. hypoglycaemia, hyperkalaemia, are present only in other SOCs such as *Disorders of Metabolism and Nutrition*. This has important implications for search strategies (see below). In the *Investigations* SOC, there are commonly PTs to describe a high value, normal value and a low value (e.g. *Serum sodium increased, Serum sodium decreased, Serum sodium normal*. In addition, there are terms for the names of tests themselves (e.g. *Serum sodium*). These are intended to give standard names to fields in databases.

HLGTs and HLTs are designed for data analysis, retrieval and presentation. They provide clinically relevant groupings of terms for drug regulatory purposes. However, the attempts to make the 'contents' of an HLT or HLGT transparent have resulted in some of the names becoming cumbersome; for example, the HLT *Musculoskeletal and connective tissue disorders of trunk congenital (excl spine)* or the HLGT *Miscellaneous and site unspecified neoplasms malignant and unspecified*.

MedDRA® includes data-entry terms from several sources: many of the *Preferred terms* and *Included terms* from the WHO-ART dictionary and its Japanese adaptation, J-ART; COSTART expanded *Symbols* and *Glossary Terms*; Hoechst Adverse Reaction Terminology (HARTS) terms; ICD9 three- and four-digit code terms and ICD9-CM three-, four- and five-digit code terms; there are also terms from the DSM IV psychiatric classification and other standard classifications. These terms are included as LLTs in MedDRA®: some are also PTs.

Vague, obsolete, misspelt or hybrid terms that have been 'inherited' from other terminologies are flagged as *non-current*. These are retained in MedDRA® as LLTs and can be used to preserve historical information, but will not be used for new data entry. Examples of *non-current* terms are given in Table 12.21. These terms, often derived from other terminologies, have been included in order to facilitate the migration of legacy data at the time of transfer to using MedDRA®. However, companies implementing MedDRA® have adopted different approaches to their existing data. Some transfer the previously coded data directly into MedDRA®, as exact matches with the MedDRA® LLTs. Others have recoded the verbatim (original reported) terms from their databases into MedDRA® *de novo*. It should be noted that the location of terms within MedDRA® does not reflect their position in source

Table 12.21 Examples of MedDRA® Non-current terms

Unspecified allergic alveolitis and pneumonitis
EMS
Angioneurotic edema not elsewhere classified
Traumatic amputation of foot (complete) (partial), unilateral, without mention of complication
Malignant hyperthemia
Flatulence, eructation and gas pain
Menopausal or female climacteric states

hierarchies – identical data will appear different when tabulated using MedDRA®, compared with its appearance in tables constructed from the original dictionary used in coding (Brown *et al.*, 1997).

Each MedDRA® term has an associated unique numerical eight-digit code but there is no hierarchical sequence or logic to these. These codes are not used for data entry by the coder, but they are intended for electronic transmission of the data.

Regulatory aspects

MedDRA® is being used in the new European Union (EU) safety database, Eudravigilance. From January 2003, MedDRA® has been mandatory in the EU for exchange of post-authorization safety data between marketing authorization holders and regulatory authorities (European Commission, 2001). This includes its use for expedited reports and also for periodic safety update reports. With regard to expedited reports, the Individual Case Safety Reports, the intention is that electronic transmission of data is required, using MedDRA® for adverse reaction terms, but also for other fields described in the ICH E2B guidelines, such as therapeutic indication for suspect drug, patient medical and surgical history, cause of death, etc.

In the USA, the FDA has been using MedDRA® in its Adverse Event Reporting System (AERS) database for some years. They issued an Advanced Notice of Proposed Rule Making in November 1998, stating that the use of MedDRA® would be made mandatory for expedited reporting. A reminder to this effect was published in draft post-marketing surveillance guidelines in March 2001 (Food and Drugs Administration, 2001). However, at the time of writing, there is no knowledge of when a regulation may come into force.

In Japan, the Ministry of Labour, Health and Welfare has requested companies to use MedDRA® for expedited ADR reporting and for periodic reports (Maintenance and Support Services Organization, 2002b). However, the use of J-ART (Japanese WHO-ART) is still permitted and the regulatory authority then recodes submitted data into MedDRA®.

As yet, regulatory intentions concerning pre-registration data and the use of MedDRA® in registration dossiers have not been made known. For the rest of the world, and in respect of post-marketing safety, there seems to be commitment to the use of MedDRA® on the part of the Canadian regulatory authority, and South Africa, Australia and the eastern European countries may adopt it. However, the Uppsala Monitoring Centre still uses WHO-ART, as do the majority of the WHO Collaborating centres. Indeed, the Uppsala Monitoring Centre has indicated that it is developing its own 'standard' international terminology, based on WHO-ART and ICD10 (Anonymous, 2002a).

The Maintenance and Support Services Organization

MedDRA® is owned by the International Federation of Pharmaceutical Manufacturers Associations (IFPMA – the umbrella organization for pharmaceutical industries worldwide). Licences for the distribution and maintenance of MedDRA® were issued in 1999 to the Maintenance and Support Services Organization (MSSO) for worldwide activities, and to the Japanese Maintenance Organization (JMO) for Japan. Copies of MedDRA® and licences for its use are only available from the MSSO or JMO. A maintenance framework has been developed to ensure that MedDRA® will be available at a reasonable cost, that it is updated at a frequency appropriate to the needs of users, and that there is evolution in response to advances in medical and scientific knowledge, and to changes in the regulatory environment. The MSSO and JMO are accountable to users and report to a management board.

MedDRA® is provided free of charge to regulatory authorities. Other organizations pay for an annual subscription. The main type of subscription – 'core subscription' – is charged on a sliding scale according to the financial turnover of the subscribing organization. Core subscribers receive a new version of MedDRA® as ASCII files on a CD-ROM every 6 months. Each version of MedDRA® may incorporate up to 9000 changes. Up to this annual maximum for all changes from all users, each subscribing organization may request up to 100 changes to MedDRA® each month.

Changes may include addition of new terms, moving terms, changing their multiaxial linkages, or making them non-current. When a request for a change to MedDRA® is received by the MSSO or JMO, it is considered by a medical review panel. If accepted, the change will be incorporated in the next version of MedDRA® at the time of the 6-monthly update. Notice of acceptance of the term (referred to as a 'transitional term' until it is included in the update) is posted on the MSSO Website, generally within 72 hours of the request being made.

Translations

MedDRA® is available in British English, with American English also present as LLTs, and in Japanese, using Kanji characters. Medically validated translations in French and German down to PT level, and Spanish to LLT level, will be available shortly. Work has commenced on other translations (Dutch and Portuguese – and Greek is under discussion). More translations, including LLTs for French and German, may follow.

Using MedDRA® for data entry

Because of the large size of MedDRA®, the selection of terms for data entry will generally require the use of a software program, referred to as a 'browser' for searching the terminology. Several commercial browsers are available. So too are a number of programs called 'auto-encoders' for automatic selection of MedDRA® LLTs that match the reported or verbatim terms. It is intended that data should be entered at the MedDRA® LLT level in order to capture the specificity of the information on the source document. When an LLT is selected for data entry, there is automatic assignment of PT, HLT, HLGT, and location in primary SOC, together with secondary SOC linkages. It was originally intended that data-entry staff do not select the location and linkages of the chosen LLT, although some companies have chosen to do this.

Although the large number of LLTs in MedDRA® make the chances of an exact match with the verbatim term likely, there will still be many instances where this is not the case. Under these circumstances, two approaches might be taken. Firstly, one would carry out a 'bottom-up' search for words or parts of words in MedDRA® that are similar to the verbatim term. If this does not produce an acceptable match, then it is possible to search likely locations in the terminology based on suitable HLTs or HLGTs for an appropriate PT and LLT, a so-called 'top-down' search. For example, if we are looking for a term that is equivalent to the verbatim term 'removal of part of the stomach', it would be logical to look in the MedDRA® *Surgical and medical procedures* SOC and, on an intuitive basis, to see what PTs exist under the HLGT *Gastrointestinal therapeutic procedures*, then the *HLT Gastric therapeutic procedures*, and then to choose the 'best fit' LLT, *Partial gastrectomy*, which is under the PT *Gastrectomy partial*.

If a suitable LLT does not exist, then the MSSO may be requested to allocate a new term. However, strict guidance has been provided to the MSSO to prevent the uncontrolled proliferation at this lowest level, and justification for the addition must be provided. Thus, for example, new terms including anatomical location may not be permitted unless there are particular attributes relating to the body site that are important. The objective is to provide a reasonable representation of medical concepts.

Guidance on coding and term selection (Anonymous, 2002b) has been published by a working group, which includes representation from various companies, regulatory authorities and the MSSO. The guidelines are endorsed by the ICH, although they are not formal ICH guidelines. They actually encompass far more than just coding with MedDRA® and have quite major implications for safety databases.

Data retrieval with MedDRA®

One may wish to retrieve data from a safety database for a variety of purposes (Brown and Douglas, 2000):

- to identify the number of reports of similar or associated conditions which constitute a signal of a new adverse reaction and to review the individual case reports;

- to respond to an enquiry from a regulatory authority, or health professional, about numbers of a particular adverse reaction to a product;

- when writing about a new safety issue in the body of a periodic safety update report.

Although no rules or guidelines have been issued, it seems that PTs will be commonly used for identifying cases in a database, each PT being linked through the respective LLTs to individual cases, which may thus be identified.

Display of all the data in a pre-formatted table may produce the required answer for a single drug. Thus, a table might show all the PTs in the database assembled according to SOC, with the numbers of reports of each. Compiling a list of the relevant PTs in the database provides the search criteria for identifying the desired cases.

A disadvantage of this so-called 'data dump' approach is that, for large databases, there may be many (possibly thousands) of MedDRA® PTs to review, in order to identify those relevant to the query in hand. There are some possible alternative approaches to data retrieval using MedDRA®, depending upon the way that the safety database has been constructed.

If all the levels in the MedDRA® hierarchy are represented in the database, then it may be appropriate to construct a search based on terms at different levels. By reviewing the HLGTs that have cases associated with the subordinate PTs, instead of reviewing all the PTs, the task might be simplified. For example, to identify all reports relevant to a signal that a drug may be causing or exacerbating cardiac failure, instead of searching through large numbers of irrelevant PTs, one could look at what is present in the database as HLGTs. The search would be built on all PTs present under the HLGT *Heart failure*, perhaps adding some PTs occurring under the HLGT *Cardiac disorder signs and symptoms*. It might be helpful to drill down in this HLGT, which is rather broad, and look at the HLTs. The *HLTs Cardiac disorders NEC* (not elsewhere classified) and *Cardiac signs and symptoms NEC* might contain PTs relevant to heart failure, but the HLTs *Cardiac infections and inflammations NEC* and *Cardiac neoplasms* might be ignored. It would be important also to look in the *Investigations* SOC, under the HLGT *Cardiac and vascular investigations (excl enzyme tests)*, as there could be cases represented solely by PTs for abnormalities in cardiac function, which might otherwise be missed.

If the database incorporates the full data model for MedDRA®, then it should be possible to search individual SOCs for terms that are present both in primary locations in that SOC and those that are there in their secondary locations. In other words, a multiaxial search could be performed. In the example of searching for heart failure based on the *Cardiac* SOC, this search would then also identify cases with *Paroxysmal nocturnal dyspnoea* as a symptom of acute left ventricular failure, this PT being present in its primary location in the *Respiratory* SOC, but with a secondary location in the *Cardiac* SOC.

If looking for cases with cardiac failure is likely to be a search that would have to be performed repeatedly on different databases, then one might perform a search of the whole of MedDRA® for relevant terms, and then save a list of all the PTs we have identified, to facilitate future retrieval (Fescharek *et al.*, 1996; Brown and Douglas, 2000). Unlike the previous search, the parameters for this search – a *Special Search Category* – is independent of the specific data set in question, and can be applied to any database. MedDRA® does include a small number of *Special Search Categories* (SSCs), e.g. for *Anaphylaxis*, *Cardiac ischaemia*, *Haemorrhage* and *Hypersensitivity reactions*. Searching the database for terms included in *Special Search Categories* provides automatic identification of relevant cases. However, the existing SSCs in MedDRA® are of variable quality and specificity, and it is likely that users will construct their own portfolios of searches. An extract from the PTs included in the *Haemorrhage SSC* is shown in Table 12.22.

At the time of writing, a working group of CIOMS had just been established in order to create additional standard searches along the lines of SSCs, which should be of value for pharmacovigilance purposes.

Other aspects of using MedDRA®

Little has been published on the use of MedDRA® for pharmacovigilance purposes. It is not certain at the time of writing what the effect of the high specificity of MedDRA® LLTs and PTs will be on signal detection, for example. WHO-ART has only about 2000 PTs;

Table 12.22   Preferred Terms in the MedDRA®
Haemorrhage Special Search Category (partial
list)

Abdominal aortic aneurysm haemorrhage
Abdominal haematoma
Adrenal haemorrhage
Anal haemorrhage
Anastomotic haemorrhage
Anastomotic ulcer haemorrhage
Aneurysm ruptured
Antepartum haemorrhage
Aortic aneurysm rupture
Application site bleeding
Application site bruising
Argentine haemorrhagic fever
Arterial haemorrhage NOS
Arteriovenous fistula site haemorrhage
Arteriovenous graft site haemorrhage
Auricular haematoma
Bleeding peripartum
Bleeding tendency
Bleeding time prolonged
Bleeding varicose vein
Blood blister
etc.

MedDRA®, on the other hand, has over 15 000 (Table 12.15). Therefore, MedDRA® PTs may dilute out any signals if many different terms are used to represent associated conditions (Brown, 2002). For example, there are 37 MedDRA® PTs in the *Cardiac* SOC that are grouped under the HLGT *Heart failure*, as well as numerous PTs in the *Investigations* SOC that are relevant to heart failure. If PTs are used in an attempt to identify an excess number of cases over some predetermined threshold in a safety database, or to compare incidences between two treatment arms in a study, then one may fail to show that any one PT qualifies as being greater than the threshold or greater in one arm of the study than the other, despite there being an overall difference present.

It has been suggested that HLTs may be more appropriate for detecting signals and for use in presenting data from clinical trials (Brown, 2002). However, there are some features of HLTs that may make this problematic. Some HLTs contain opposing concepts. For example, the HLT *Platelet analyses* includes the PT *Platelet count increased* as well as the PTs *Platelet count decreased* and *Platelet count normal*. Some HLTs are heterogeneous in respect of the seriousness of the conditions they include. For example, the HLT *Ventricular arrhythmias and cardiac arrest* lumps together the PTs for the serious conditions *Ventricular fibrillation* and *Ventricular asystole* with the usually benign *Ventricular extrasystoles* PT. Hence, if HLTs are to be used for purposes of data presentation, then it will also be necessary to show the subordinate PTs included in the database. For signal detection, some modifications to the existing hierarchy may be beneficial.

MedDRA® overview

MedDRA® is a new international standard, but it is not being implemented by all potential users. The manner of its implementation and use varies between users, and there is a dearth of suitable guidance from regulatory authorities and from the maintenance organization. The result is that there is still much uncertainty about how to use MedDRA® to best advantage.

It is apparent that the large number of LLTs provides specificity, which is something that was lacking in some previous dictionaries. Hence, it will be possible to better capture the actual medical condition as experienced by the patient than was previously the case. However, this very feature may lead to difficulties for finding cases within a database, for detecting patterns of reports that might constitute signals of new adverse reactions, and for presenting comparative safety data in clinical trials.

Further work on standardization of database searches is appropriate, and it is important that further guidance on its use in pharmacovigilance becomes available, so that there will be some consistency of approach. Use of MedDRA® is now required, at least for individual case safety reporting in the EU, but it is apparent that much work still needs to be done to ensure that it can be used effectively for all its intended purposes.

Definition of adverse reaction terms

A CIOMS working group published a series of papers giving definitions of terms used in adverse reaction reporting: these were subsequently collected into a book 'Reporting Adverse Reactions: definition of terms and criteria for their use' (Bankowski *et al.*, 1999). The terms defined cover 21 WHO-ART System-organ classes. The entries for each adverse reaction are generally quite concise, of the order of 200 to 300 words, and comprise a preamble, giving the context, synonyms, the definition itself and the conditions that should be applied for the use of the term.

As an example, the entry for melaena states as a preamble that this usually indicates bleeding in the upper gastrointestinal tract, but may also be due to bleeding in the middle or distal small bowel or proximal colon. The definition is given as 'Melaena is the passage of black stools'. The basic requirements for use of the term state that it should be used according to the definition, but that other causes of black stool, such as oral iron or bismuth medication, or dietary causes, such as liquorice or dark beers, should be excluded. To give an impression of the scope of the definitions, the cutaneous adverse reaction terms covered by the definitions are listed in Table 12.23.

The definitions may be of help when reviewing individual cases, allowing a comment to be added as to whether or not the standard definition has been satisfied by the available information. They are also likely to be of use when exploring a possible adverse drug reaction signal, in facilitating the selection of a sub-group of cases that satisfy standard criteria. However, care needs to be exercised in the way that the definitions are used. Thus, it would not be reasonable to exclude cases from a safety database or from regulatory reporting, simply because the criteria are not satisfied. If a health professional has reported the case as a particular suspected adverse reaction, then this is what should be recorded, whether or not the criteria are met.

Table 12.23 Range of term definitions for Skin and appendage disorders SOC (Bankowski *et al.*, 1999)

Dermatitis (eczema)
Dermatitis exfoliative
Fixed drug eruption
Lichenoid drug eruption
Pustular eruption
Urticaria/Angioedema
Erythema multiforme
Stevens–Johnson syndrome
Toxic epidermal necrolysis
Photosensitivity reaction
Phototoxic reaction
Photoallergic reaction

Conclusion

In this chapter, some of the available dictionaries for drug names, diseases and adverse reaction terms have been considered, as well as the application of definitions to the latter. The complexity of some of the dictionaries is notable, as is the way that safety data can be profoundly affected according to the dictionary used and the manner of its employment.

This is a continually evolving area, and we are just beginning the process of standardization in the pharmacovigilance field. If true standardization of dictionaries and their mode of use is ever achieved, then it will greatly facilitate the sharing of safety data and should improve the effectiveness of the pharmacovigilance process.

Acknowledgements

I thank David Pallett, of Software Technics Ltd, for assistance with MedDRA® tables and for free use of Medicoder software. Malin Nord, of the Uppsala Monitoring Centre, is also thanked for assistance with the WHO Drug Dictionary.

References

Anonymous (1994). *International Classification of Diseases. 9th Revision. Clinical Modification.* Medicode Publications: Utah.

Anonymous (2000). ATC system. In: A guide to the quarterly output for signal detection from the WHO database. Uppsala Monitoring Centre, Uppsala.

Anonymous (2002a). Drug dictionary developments. Uppsala reports (19) 16. Uppsala Monitoring Centre, Uppsala.

Anonymous (2002b). MedDRA Maintenance and Support Services Organization Website: http://www.meddramsso.com [1 November 2002]. MedDRA® Term Selection: Points to Consider, version 3.

Bankowski Z, Bruppracher R, Crusius I, *et al.* (1999). *Reporting Adverse Reactions: Definition of Terms and Criteria for their Use.* CIOMS: Geneva.

Brown DR, Brown EG and Moulvad TB (1997). A comparison of two medical terminologies in coding and analysing clinical trial safety data. *Int J Pharm Med* **11**: 85–89.

Brown EG (2002). Effects of coding dictionary on signal generation: a consideration of use of MedDRA compared with WHO-ART. *Drug Saf* **25**(6): 445–452.

Brown EG and Clark E (1996). Evaluation of MEDDRA® in representing medicinal product data sheet information. *Pharm Med* **10**: 1–8.

Brown EG and Douglas S (2000). Tabulation and analysis of pharmacovigilance data using the Medical Dictionary for Regulatory Activities. *Pharmacoepidemiol Drug Saf* **9**: 479–489.

Brown EG, Wood L and Wood S (1999). The Medical Dictionary for Regulatory Activities (MedDRA®). Leading article. *Drug Saf* **20**(2): 109–117.

European Commission (2001). *The Rules Governing Medicinal Products in the European Union*, Volume 9. European Commission: Brussels.

Fescharek R, Dechert G, Reichert D, Dass H (1996). Overall analysis of spontaneously reported adverse events: a worthwhile exercise or flogging a dead horse? *Pharm Med* **10**: 71–86.

Food and Drugs Administration (1989). Coding Symbols for a Thesaurus of Adverse Reaction Terms, 3rd edition. Food and Drugs Administration: Rockville.

Food and Drugs Administration (2001). Guidance for industry postmarketing safety reporting for human drug and biological products including vaccines. Notice of proposed rulemaking. *United States Federal Register.*

Maintenance and Support Services Organization (2002a). *Medical Dictionary for Regulatory Activities (MedDRA®) Introductory Guide (End User Manual).*

Maintenance and Support Services Organization (2002b). MedDRA Maintenance and Support Services Organization Website: http://www.meddramsso.com [July 2002].

Uppsala Monitoring Centre (2000). *WHO Adverse Reaction Terminology.* Uppsala Monitoring Centre: Uppsala.

Uppsala Monitoring Centre (2002). Website http://www.who-umc.org/umc [November, 2002].

White C (1998). A preliminary assessment of the impact of MEDDRA® on adverse event reports and product labelling. *Drug Inf J* **32**: 347–362.

Wood KL (1994). The Medical Dictionary for Drug Regulatory Affairs (MEDDRA®) Project. *Pharmacoepidemiol Drug Saf* **3**: 7–13.

World Health Organization (1977). *International Classification of Diseases*, 9th Revision. World Health Organization: Geneva.

World Health Organization (1992). *International Classification of Diseases and Related Health Problems*, 10th Revision. World Health Organization: Geneva.

13

Safety of Biotechnology Products

B. Brown and M. Westland

Introduction

Medicines based on the application of recombinant technology are relatively new to the therapeutics industry. This chapter will focus specifically on purified and recombinant proteins, collectively termed protein therapeutic agents (Gallupi *et al.*, 2001), used in the treatment of disease that are able to affect the growth or metabolism of cells *in vivo*. This rather broad definition includes proteins derived from a variety of different sources, including the purification of proteins from various sources (e.g. serum and urine), and proteins created using recombinant DNA technology in either bacterial or mammalian cells, including hormones, enzymes and antibodies. This is in contrast to the traditional method of developing medicines by the application of organic chemistry; medicines developed in this manner are usually referred to as 'small molecules'. It should be noted that other molecules, such as steroids and vaccines, as well as gene therapy techniques and various diagnostic tests, might also be considered biologics. However, for the purposes of this discussion, these molecules will be excluded from this chapter; vaccines will be discussed in the Chapter 14.

Protein therapeutic agents have had an enormous impact on the treatment of many diseases that previously did not have adequate therapies. For example:

- Prior to the widespread availability of therapeutic human growth hormone, children with growth hormone deficiency had no viable treatment options, and uniformly developed short stature as adults (Mehta and Hindmarsh, 2002).

- Prior to the development of recombinant granulocyte-colony-stimulating factor (G-CSF), patients with severe chronic neutropenia had no protection against bacterial infections and usually succumbed to the disease at a young age. With the advent of G-CSF, these patients are now able to lead much more normal lives (Cottle *et al.*, 2002).

These conditions, along with many others, are now successfully treated with protein therapeutic agents. Now that the human genome has been successfully mapped (International Human Genome Sequencing Consortium, 2001; Venter *et al.*, 2001), newer, perhaps more complex recombinant proteins will be developed to treat diseases that are currently untreatable. However, with the development of new therapeutics comes a need to increase

Stephens' Detection of New Adverse Drug Reactions Fifth Edition edited by John Talbot and Patrick Waller
© 2004 John Wiley & Sons, Ltd   ISBN: 0 470 84552 X

our understanding of the differences in safety profiles seen with these molecules from those seen with traditional small-molecule therapeutics. Clinicians in particular need to be aware of a few classes of adverse reactions seen most commonly with biological products.

Properties of proteins

To be able to understand adequately and anticipate the types of adverse reactions that are likely to be observed for new protein therapeutic agents, it is necessary to have a fundamental understanding of the general properties of proteins. There are several important differences between small molecules and proteins created from the application of biotechnology. As many companies are now using biotechnology to develop new medicines, it is imperative that these properties, as contrasted with those of small molecules, are understood by research and development personnel, as well as healthcare providers, so that patient safety is optimal.

Proteins, which are composed of specific sequences of amino acids, are the building blocks of all life. In general, protein therapeutic agents are large molecules composed of many amino acids. However, the size of currently available biotechnology-based medicines ranges from a few amino acids for small oligopeptides, such as sermorelin, which is a 29 amino acid amino terminal segment of naturally occurring growth-hormone-releasing hormone (GHRH), to large proteins with hundreds of amino acids. For example, the α and β chains of recombinant follicle-stimulating hormone (FSH) have 92 and 111 amino acids respectively. The amino acid backbone of these molecules means that they are highly degradable by the various proteases released by the stomach and small intestine during digestion, effectively decreasing the bioavailability of orally administered proteins to zero. Therefore, proteins must be given by injection, generally by the intravenous, subcutaneous, or intramuscular routes. Because of the routes of administration necessary to administer these molecules, patients must be closely monitored for the onset of hypersensitivity reactions (discussed in more detail below).

Proteins produced by the human body, as well as those created in mammalian cells using recombinant DNA technology, may contain carbohydrate modifications to the amino acid backbone (Lehninger et al., 1993). The process of adding carbohydrate moieties to the protein structure, called post-translational modification, begins in the endoplasmic reticulum and is completed in the Golgi complex. These are cellular organelles found only in cells of eukaryotic organisms (i.e. those that contain a nucleus). Therefore, recombinant versions of naturally occurring proteins produced in prokaryotic cells, such as bacteria, lack these carbohydrate additions. Some molecules, such as recombinant human growth hormone, have been successfully and safely developed using both bacterial and mammalian cells.

Another property of proteins is that they are often somewhat unstable and are prone to denature, which means that they lose their structural conformation and, therefore, efficacy, under specific known physical conditions. For example, this can occur if the storage temperature is not maintained within a tight range and the molecule becomes too warm. Many of these products require refrigeration to ensure that they do not denature.

Categories of protein therapeutic agent

Protein therapeutic agents can be classified in several ways. The most obvious way is to organize the molecules by function. Currently approved protein therapeutic agents include:

- hormones and cytokines (or smaller sequences of amino acids that retain the properties of the naturally occurring hormone);

- enzymes; and

- antibodies, both monoclonal and polyclonal.

However, for the purposes of safety monitoring, proteins can also be organized by manufacturing method. Currently, proteins are either purified from various sources, such as serum and urine, or are created in bioreactors using recombinant DNA technology.

Grouping by function

The most familiar proteins used in a therapeutic setting are recombinant versions of naturally occurring hormones. Hormones are molecules released from various glands in the body that act on target organs or cells. Examples include insulin and human growth hormone. Recombinant versions of both of these hormones were developed in the 1970s, early in the biotechnology era. Since that time, recombinant versions of other naturally occurring hormones have been developed, including recombinant erythropoietin and recombinant FSH. These recombinant molecules have very specific actions *in vivo* and normally have well-characterized safety profiles.

More recently, recombinant versions of naturally occurring cytokines have been developed using recombinant DNA technology, such as various interferons and growth factors. Examples include recombinant G-CSF and various types of recombinant interferon. Similarly, molecules have been developed to block the actions of naturally occurring cytokines, such as recombinant IL-1 receptor antagonist (Breshnihan, 2001) and etanercept, which is a hybrid molecule (used to treat active rheumatoid arthritis) that contains the extracellular ligand binding portion of the tumour necrosis factor receptor bound to the Fc portion of human IgG1 (Alldred, 2001).

Enzymes are proteins that catalyse chemical reactions in the body. Several recombinant versions of enzymes have been developed or are being developed to treat rare genetically inherited disorders, such as alpha galactosidase A for the treatment of Fabry disease and iduronate-2-sulfatase in Hunter syndrome.

Antibodies are glycoproteins that are created by B cells against foreign antigens. Therapeutic antibodies are of two types: monoclonal and polyclonal. Monoclonal antibodies arise from a single clone of cells and are specific for a single antigen. Rituximab is a monoclonal antibody directed specifically against the CD20 antigen found on normal and malignant B cells and is used to treat non-Hodgkin's lymphoma. Polyclonal antibodies arise from multiple clones and interact with many antigens. For instance, intravenous immune globulin can be used to provide passive immunity to infectious agents, such as hepatitis A (Stapleton, 1992).

Organization by manufacturing method

The earliest proteins to be used in a therapeutic setting came from the purification of proteins from various sources, including serum, urine, and even organs. Immune globulin (pooled immunoglobin from donor serum) has been available since the 1950s. Similarly, for many years, urine-derived FSH was used to treat female infertility. Pituitary-derived human growth hormone, which was derived from pooling growth hormone from the pituitary glands of cadavers, was for years the only source of human growth hormone. Depending on the level of purity achieved, the possibility exists for contamination, including by proteins and infectious organisms. Most products that were originally derived from purification are now manufactured using recombinant technology.

The biotechnology era truly began in the late 1970s, when recombinant insulin was first produced in 1978, followed by recombinant human growth hormone in 1979. Whereas prior to this time, any protein that was used for therapeutic purposes was derived from purifying it from a biological source (see previous section), now the technology became available to insert the gene for a protein into prokaryotic (i.e. bacteria) host cells. Next, technology was developed that enabled eukaryotic cells, such as Chinese hamster ovary cells, to be used as host cells. Since that time, many different proteins have had their genes sequenced and expressed. The use of recombinant DNA technology during the past two decades has revolutionized the practice of medicine.

The earliest host cells were bacteria, as the generally much smaller genomes of prokaryotic organisms were much easier to manipulate. However, because they are simple one-celled organisms that lack a nucleus, as well as cellular organelles such as the endoplasmic reticulum and Golgi complex, they also lack the capacity to post-translationally modify proteins. This means that protein therapeutic agents produced by bacteria will not contain the carbohydrate modifications found on recombinant proteins produced by eukaryotic organisms. Also, as the protein must then be purified from the bacteria, the finished product could theoretically contain bacterial breakdown products, such as bacterial cell walls, that can result in toxic side effects (Lauta, 2000).

Today, many of the more recent protein therapeutic agents have been developed using eukaryotic cells, such as Chinese hamster ovary cells. As previously discussed, eukaryotic cells contain nuclei and cellular organelles that are able to post-translationally modify proteins. Post-translational modification allows the glycosylated recombinant protein to resemble the naturally occurring protein more closely.

Safety monitoring for protein therapeutic agents

Owing to the above properties of protein therapeutic agents, and the differences cited between them and small molecules, some general observations can be made regarding the safety profiles of proteins as a class. By grouping together various types of protein therapeutic agent, including hormones, cytokines, enzymes and antibodies, and looking at their common characteristics, it is possible to recognize certain categories of adverse reactions that are common to all groups. Whereas individual molecules will obviously have unique overall safety profiles, these categories of adverse reactions must be carefully monitored to ensure the safety of patients. These categories, which are discussed in detail below, include the following:

- allergic and hypersensitivity reactions;

- infectious disease transmission;

- decreased efficacy secondary to neutralizing antibody development; and

- adverse reactions related to the efficacy of the molecule itself.

It should be noted that, practically speaking, there is no difference in the regulations that govern safety monitoring of protein therapeutic agents or small molecules. Some biologics, such as vaccines, and methods of treatment, such as gene therapy, require specific pharmacovigilance efforts as defined by regulatory agencies, and certain events, such as the development of neutralizing antibodies, require specific assays to confirm a diagnosis. However, the therapeutics described below are managed in the same way, from a regulatory perspective, as small molecules, and the monitoring procedures are essentially the same between the two.

Allergic and hypersensitivity reactions

As previously discussed, proteins are generally much larger than traditional small molecules and are easily digestible by the gut. Therefore, they must be administered by injection. While this decreases the potential of direct irritation of the gastrointestinal tract when compared with orally administered products, adverse reactions associated with the injections themselves are relatively common. These reactions can range from local oedema, erythema and pain at the injection site to injection site necrosis, severe rashes, including erythema multiforme and Stevens–Johnson syndrome, and anaphylactic shock, possibly leading to death. The mechanisms of these reactions vary from local tissue irritation and release of inflammatory mediators at the injection site to systemic reactions that involve antibody production.

The types of hypersensitivity seen with protein therapeutic agents that involve antibodies are:

- type I (immediate) hypersensitivity, and
- type III, or immune-complex hypersensitivity.

Type I, or IgE-mediated, hypersensitivity usually occurs after re-exposure to the protein and occurs within minutes of injection, when the antigen binds to IgE on the surface of mast cells, causing release of inflammatory mediators such as histamine. The signs and symptoms of type I hypersensitivity can range from urticaria and asthma to systemic anaphylaxis, which is characterized by laryngeal oedema, bronchoconstriction and hypotension, and can be fatal. Whereas reports of type I hypersensitivity are rare for most products, owing to the serious nature of these reactions, patients must be closely monitored for any evidence of anaphylaxis and appropriate treatments should be readily available.

Immune-complex hypersensitivity occurs when antibody binds to antigen and subsequently precipitates out of solution and is deposited in tissues, causing an inflammatory response. Antithymocyte globulin (ATGAM) is a collection of equine-derived polyclonal antibodies against human thymocytes. These antibodies are produced by repeatedly inoculating horses with human thymocytes, which causes the horse to produce antibodies against the thymocytes. These antibodies are then purified from the horse serum. Antithymocyte globulin is used primarily to treat acute renal allograft rejection. As these antibodies are not of human origin, hypersensitivity reactions are of particular concern, including serum sickness. When given to humans, the patient may develop 'serum sickness', which is a form of type III hypersensitivity characterized by fever, urticaria, joint pain, lymphadenopathy and splenomegaly. The symptoms usually develop between 1 and 2 weeks after administration of ATGAM. As the immune complexes are cleared from the tissues, the symptoms begin to resolve (Lawley *et al.*, 1984, 1985).

Even though recombinant versions of naturally occurring proteins are chemically very similar to the native proteins, allergic reactions can occur when these recombinant proteins are administered. Although these products are made using sophisticated recombinant technology, there still exists the possibility that the process of extracting the protein from the cellular reactors leaves some impurities in place. It is also possible that the excipients present in the formulation are able to elicit an allergic reaction.

Infectious disease transmission

Because several protein therapeutic agents, especially older products, are derived from purifying the target protein from a biological source, infectious disease transmission must be monitored very carefully. Monitoring of these types of reaction is complicated, because many of the infectious diseases contracted from the administration of tainted product, such as human immunodeficiency virus (HIV) and hepatitis C, may not manifest themselves for months, even years, after exposure. Also, these diseases are often difficult or impossible to treat effectively once they are diagnosed. Therefore, safety monitoring is crucial.

Perhaps the most well-documented example is the transmission of HIV to haemophiliacs through contaminated blood products. Patients with haemophilia A, the most common type, have extremely low circulating levels of factor VIII, causing them to be unable to develop clots effectively. Prior to the development of recombinant DNA technology, factor VIII was obtained by pooling sera from multiple donors, as it is normally present in small quantities in the blood. The availability of factor VIII concentrate had a profound impact on these patients' lives. Unfortunately, in the early 1980s, a majority of patients with severe haemophilia A were infected with HIV, and ultimately died of AIDS, as there were no effective treatments of the disease at that time (Koerper, 1989). Since then, techniques have been developed to reduce or, in the case of recombinant factor VIII, eliminate the transmission of all infectious diseases, including HIV (Horowitz and Ben-Hur, 2000).

Another prominent example is pituitary-derived growth hormone and the transmission of Creutzfeldt–Jakob disease, which is classified as a transmissible spongiform encephalopathy (TSE). Prior to the 1980s and the advent of recombinant DNA technology, human growth hormone for therapeutic use was only available via pooling and purifying the pituitary glands of cadavers. Unfortunately, in 1985, the Food and Drugs Administration and the National Institutes of Health received the first three reports of patients that had developed Creutzfeldt–Jakob disease, which is a uniformly fatal neurological disease that has been associated with a prion infection of the brain (Fradkin *et al.*, 1991; Preece, 1993). In these cases, it was discovered that the disease was transmitted through contaminated human growth hormone extract from the cadaver pituitary glands. These patients, who were adults at the time of diagnosis, had been treated with pituitary-derived growth hormone as young children, and had not developed symptoms of the disease for years after exposure. Human growth hormone is no longer available as a pituitary gland extract, and is now manufactured using recombinant DNA technology.

TSEs may also be transmitted from animal sources. Products containing bovine gelatin, tallow derivatives and serum are of particular concern. There has been increasing interest in this area due to recent reports of the development of bovine spongiform encephalopathy (BSE), or mad cow disease, in parts of Europe after ingesting infected beef. To date, there have been no reports of patients developing a TSE after exposure to a biologic that contains animal by-product. However, because it is currently thought that all reports of BSE received to date have been transmitted orally, and it has been estimated that intravenous and subcutaneous inoculation of a particular pathogen responsible for a TSE is up to 100–1000-fold more potent than an oral inoculation, there is cause for concern (Rohwer, 1996). As the TSE agents are extremely difficult to detect and remove from animal tissue, it is of the utmost importance that all steps are taken to ensure that no infected animals are used in the manufacturing process (Asher, 1999). In spite of the fact that no reports have been seen, it is prudent to monitor both proteins and small molecules that contain animal-derived excipients for events suggesting possible prion transmission.

For immune globulin there is also an increased risk of transmitting blood-borne infectious diseases, such as hepatitis C. For instance, one preparation of IVIG resulted in 137 reported cases of hepatitis C infection (Bresee *et al.*, 1996), prompting the manufacturer to recall the product. The manufacturer replaced the original preparation with one containing a solvent and detergent, which is effective in ridding the immune globulin of infectious agents. Immune globulin preparations are now considered to be safe with respect to known viruses, but companies and healthcare professionals must remain vigilant in monitoring for reports of infectious disease transmission.

Development of neutralizing antibodies

Another major safety concern for all injectable proteins, especially for recombinant versions of naturally occurring human proteins, is the development of neutralizing antibodies against the protein. This can occur because the body recognizes the injected protein as foreign and develops antibodies against it. In the case of naturally occurring substances, such as hormones and cytokines, the antibodies may cross-react with the native protein. These antibodies have the potential to neutralize the actions of the native protein by binding to the active site of the protein. This can lead to profound medical conditions, such as aplasias of blood cell lines.

Patients with chronic renal failure are unable to produce adequate endogenous erythropoietin to maintain normal haemoglobin levels (Eckhardt, 2000). As a result, these patients develop anaemia, causing them to feel fatigued and short of breath. The introduction of recombinant erythropoietin to treat anaemia has helped patients maintain adequate haemoglobin levels and reduce their need for transfusions. Beginning in 1999, however, there has been a significant increase in the number of cases of pure red cell aplasia (PRCA) in patients receiving epoetin alfa in Europe, Australia, and Canada (Casadevall *et al.*, 2002; Gershon *et al.*, 2002). PRCA is a condition in which there is an absence of erythroid precursors in the bone marrow, causing patients to develop profound anaemia requiring red cell transfusions to maintain haemoglobin levels. An increased incidence of PRCA has not been observed with erythropoietic agents or in other geographic areas. The majority of these patients have developed neutralizing antibodies to this treatment, which cross-react with the patient's endogenous erythropoietin, as well as with other erythropoietic agents. At this time, the reason for this outbreak of cases is not known. Although data on the treatment and outcome of these patients is limited at this time, some of these patients remain transfusion dependent for years after diagnosis.

The availability of factor VIII has made living with haemophilia far more tolerable. However, 25 to 50 per cent of patients with severe haemophilia A that require treatment with factor VIII concentrate develop antibodies (called 'inhibitor') against factor VIII (Lusher, 2000). These antibodies may neutralize the action of the factor VIII therapy and can greatly complicate treatment. Patients may require enormous doses of factor VIII during the treatment of haemorrhagic episodes, and some of these patients might not respond to at all. Once other potential aetiologies for non-response have been excluded, neutralizing antibodies should be considered.

Adverse reactions related to efficacy of the protein

Patients can experience adverse reactions as a direct result of the mechanism(s) of action of the recombinant version of a naturally occurring protein. In effect, these patients develop adverse reactions that result from the efficacy of the molecule itself, sometimes resulting in syndromes similar to genetic or malignant processes. For example, recombinant proteins have been developed to treat rheumatoid arthritis by blocking the effects of inflammatory mediators, such as tumour necrosis factor. Although these products are efficacious in relieving the pain and inflammation associated with rheumatoid arthritis, they also can increase the incidence of serious infections in these patients by blocking these inflammatory mediators and thereby decreasing their ability to develop an appropriate immunologic response against infection (Keane *et al.*, 2001). Patients are at increased risk of developing serious infections, possibly requiring hospitalization. Some patients have also developed opportunistic infections normally seen only in severely immunocompromised patients (i.e. patients with HIV).

Infertility is routinely treated with injections of FSH and luteinizing hormone to stimulate the ovaries to develop multiple follicles, in preparation for *in vitro* fertilization. During the process of *in vitro* fertilization, high doses of FSH are given to the patient daily during the early part of her menstrual cycle. Because of the high doses, a common, treatable, but extremely serious associated condition is the ovarian hyperstimulation syndrome (Whelan and Vlahos, 2000). The mechanism for this syndrome is unknown, but the patient develops increased vascular permeability, which manifests itself in pleural and pericardial effusions, ascites and extreme hypovolaemia, predisposing the patient to intravascular thrombosis. Patients are hospitalized and treated with fluids; infertility injections are stopped. Once the patient's FSH levels begin to decrease, the patient usually fully recovers. However, it is imperative that the condition be diagnosed and treated early by a physician experienced in this field.

Off-label use

The use of therapeutic agents for indications other than those that have been approved by the appropriate regulatory agencies is a significant safety issue for all pharmaceutical products, not just proteins. Once an agent has been approved for one use, a treating physician is free to prescribe the drug for any indication that he or she chooses, with few restrictions. However, these drugs are also often obtained and distributed illegally. In the case of some biologics, often the aim is to give supraphysiologic doses to people to increase one's physical strength or endurance. In other cases, the use is based on a perceived benefit to the patient that has little or no scientific data to support its use. In either case, this is a major area of concern in safety monitoring for biologics, and is likely to continue to increase in frequency.

Enhanced athletic performance

One of the most commonly misused biologic classes is anabolic steroids, which are commonly used illegally to increase strength in athletes (VanHelder *et al.*, 1991; Silver, 2001). Though technically not proteins, these molecules help illustrate the types of safety monitoring that must be done when there is the potential for off-label abuse. Anabolic steroid use has been banned from most major sports worldwide since the mid-1980s, when use was considered to be rampant among professional and Olympic athletes. However, every year, several players receive mandatory suspensions for testing positive for steroid use. It is also becoming increasingly popular among adolescent athletes (Bahrke *et al.*, 1998). The side effects of anabolic steroid abuse can be devastating, especially to younger athletes who are still growing. The side effects range from skin disorders, such as acne or increased rate of hair loss, to testicular atrophy, hypertension, amenorrhea, cardiac disease, and even mental disturbances, such as 'roid rage', characterized by aggressive behaviour and uncontrollable temper. Although some of these side effects can be reversible, many, such as cardiac disease, are not, and may result in an increased risk of early death (Lamb, 1984; Strauss and Yesalis, 1991).

Athletes looking for increased muscle mass and decreased body fat have also misused recombinant human growth hormone (Bidlingmaier *et al.*, 2001). However, the long-term adverse event profile of supraphysiologic doses of human growth hormone is not well defined. In patients with AIDS wasting, a syndrome characterized by loss of muscle mass and total body weight in patients with advance HIV infection, high-dose daily injections of recombinant human growth hormone can help reverse some of these effects (Mulligan *et al.*, 1999). In these patients, however, new-onset hyperglycaemia, to the point of diabetes mellitus, has been reported. Also, these patients tend to develop increased tissue turgor from fluid retention, sometimes precipitating carpal tunnel syndrome (Van Loon, 1998).

In contrast to athletes looking to increase strength, endurance athletes have been known to use recombinant erythropoietins to increase their haemoglobin concentrations to supraphysiologic levels, increasing oxygen carrying capacity and giving the athlete an edge in distance competition. Use of these drugs in distance cyclists and other endurance athletes, such as cross-country skiers, is well documented (Simon, 1994; Gareau *et al.*, 1996). The side effects associated with increased haemoglobin levels are similar to those seen in patients with polycythaemia, including an increased risk of hypertension, myocardial infarction, stroke and sudden death (Sawka *et al.*, 1996).

Other off-label use

In contrast to athletes using biologics for a performance advantage, use of some biologics is becoming more common for conditions that have very little scientific data to back them up. For instance, in the USA, some physicians are prescribing human growth hormone injections for middle-aged patients, citing the 'anti-aging' benefits of growth hormone, including its ability to increase muscle mass and decrease body fat (Cuttica *et al.*, 1997). Although human growth hormone does in fact have these physiologic actions, there is little evidence to suggest that these properties in any way retard the aging process. There have also been reports of patients being given growth hormone injections before and after surgery to help 'increase healing' (Carli *et al.*, 1997). Also, it is unclear what benefit, if any, these patients derive at the doses given, considering that the patients usually have normal growth hormone levels for their age. At the same time, these patients are exposing themselves to all of the potential risks of taking protein therapeutic agents, including those cited throughout this chapter.

Conclusion

Protein therapeutic agents are still relatively new compared with their small-molecule counterparts. Whereas small molecules extracted naturally from plants have been used to treat all sorts of maladies for centuries, proteins have only begun being used therapeutically beginning in the 20th century, with recombinant technology only becoming available within the last 25 years. However, with the human genome recently being sequenced, it is anticipated that many new therapeutics, including both proteins and small molecules, will be developed with specific targets over the coming decade. Knowledge of the specific properties and safety profiles of proteins as a class will become increasingly more important for all therapeutics companies, as many traditional pharmaceutical companies develop their own in-house biotechnology divisions – or merge with companies that already have the expertise. Although each individual molecule will obviously have a unique side effect profile, having a working knowledge of the types of adverse reactions to be expected from proteins as a therapeutic class will ultimately benefit patients and companies alike.

References

Alldred A (2001). Etanercept in rheumatoid arthritis. *Expert Opin Pharmacother* 2: 1137–1148.
Asher D (1999). The transmissible spongiform encephalopathy agents: concern and responses of United States regulatory agencies in maintaining the safety of biologics. *Dev Biol Stand* 100: 103–118.
Bahrke M, Yesalis C and Brower K (1998). Anabolic–androgenic steroid abuse and performance enhancing drugs among adolescents. *Child Adolesc Psychiatr Clin N Am* 7: 821–838.
Bidlingmaier M, Wu Z and Strasburger CJ (2001). Doping with growth hormone. *J Pediatr Endocrinol* 14: 1077–1083.
Bresee J, Mast E, Coleman P, Baron M, *et al.* (1996). Hepatitis C virus infection associated with administration of intravenous immune globulin: a cohort study. *J Am Med Assoc* 276: 1563–1567.
Breshnihan B (2001). The prospect of treating rheumatoid arthritis with recombinant human interleukin-1 receptor antagonist. *Biodrugs* 15: 87–97.
Carli F, Webster J and Halliday D (1997). A nitrogen-free hypocaloric diet and recombinant human growth hormone stimulate postoperative protein synthesis: fasted and fed leucine kinetics in the surgical patient. *Metab Clin Exp* 46: 796–800.
Casadevall N, Nataf J, Viron B, Kolta A, *et al.* (2002). Pure red-cell aplasia and anti-erythropoietin antibodies in patients treated with recombinant erythropoietin. *New Engl J Med* 346: 469–475.
Cottle T, Fier C, Donadieu J, Kinsey S (2002). Risk and benefit of treatment of severe chronic neutropenia with granulocyte colony-stimulating factor. *Semin Hematol* 39: 134–140.
Cuttica C, Castoldi L, Gorrini G, Peluffo F, *et al.* (1997). Effects of six month administration of recombinant human growth hormone to healthy elderly subjects. *Aging (Milano)* 9: 193–197.
Eckhardt K (2000). Pathophysiology of renal anaemia. *Clin Nephrol* 53: 2–8.

Fradkin J, Schonberger L, Mills J, Gunn W, *et al.* (1991). Creutzfeldt–Jakob disease in pituitary growth hormone recipients in the United States. *J Am Med Assoc* **265**: 880–884.

Galuppi G, Rogge M, Roskos L, Lesko L, *et al.* (2001). Integration of pharmacokinetic and pharmacodynamic studies in the discovery, development, and review of protein therapeutic agents: a conference report. *Clin Pharmacol Ther* **69**: 387–399.

Gareau R, Audran M and Baynes R (1996). Erythropoietin abuse in athletes. *Nature* **380**: 113.

Gershon SK, Luksenburg H, Cote TR and Braun MM (2002). Pure red cell aplasia and recombinant erythropoietin. *New Engl J Med* **346**: 469–475.

Horowitz B and Ben-Hur E (2000). Efforts in minimizing risk of viral transmission through viral inactivation. *Ann Med* **32**: 475–484.

International Human Genome Sequencing Consortium (2001). Initial sequencing and analysis of the human genome. *Nature* **409**: 860–921.

Keane J, Gershon S, Wise R, Mirabile-Levens E, *et al.* (2001). Tuberculosis associated with infliximab, a tumour necrosis factor alpha-neutralizing agent. *New Engl J Med* **345**: 1098–1104.

Koerper M (1989). AIDS and hemophilia. *Immunol Ser* **44**: 79–95.

Lamb D (1984). Anabolic steroids in athletics: how well do they work and how dangerous are they? *Am J Sports Med* **12**: 31–38.

Lauta VM (2000). Pharmacological elements in clinical application of synthetic peptides. *Fundam Clin Pharmacol* **14**: 425–442.

Lawley TJ, Bielory L, Gascon P, Yancey K, *et al.* (1984). A prospective clinical and immunological analysis of patients with serum sickness. *New Engl J Med* **311**: 1407–1413.

Lawley TJ, Bielory L, Gascon P, Yancey K, *et al.* (1985). A study of human serum sickness. *J Invest Dermatol* **85**: 129–32.

Lehninger A, Nelson D and Cox M (1993). Protein metabolism. In *Principles of Biochemistry.* Worth Publishers: New York; 925–927.

Lusher JM (2000). Inhibitor antibodies against factor VIII and factor IX: management. *Semin Thromb Hemost* **26**: 179–188.

Mehta A and Hindmarsh PC (2002). The use of somatropin (recombinant growth hormone) in children of short stature. *Paediatr Drugs* **4**: 37–47.

Mulligan K, Tai V and Schambelan M (1999). Use of growth hormone and other anabolic agents in AIDS wasting. *J Parenter Enter Nutr* **23**: S202–S209.

Preece M (1993). Human pituitary growth hormone and Creutzfeldt–Jakob disease. *Hormone Res* **39**: 95–98.

Rohwer R (1996). Analysis of risk to biomedical products developed from animal sources (with special emphasis on the spongiform encephalopathy agents, scrapie and BSE). *Dev Biol Stand* **88**: 247–256.

Sawka M, Joyner M, Miles D, Robertson R, *et al.* (1996). American College of Sports Medicine position stand. The use of blood doping as an ergogenic aid. *Med Sci Sports Exer* **28**: i–viii.

Silver MD (2001). Use of ergogenic aids by athletes. *J Am Acad Orthop Surg* **9**: 61–70.

Simon TL (1994). Induced erythrocythemia and athletic performance. *Semin Hematol* **31**: 128–133.

Stapleton JT (1992). Passive immunization against hepatitis A. *Vaccine* **10**: 545–547.

Strauss R and Yesalis C (1991). Anabolic steroids in the athlete. *Ann Rev Med* **42**: 449–457.

Van Loon K (1998). Safety of high doses of recombinant human growth hormone. *Hormone Res* **49**: 78–81.

VanHelder W, Kofman E and Tremblay M (1991). Anabolic steroids in sport. *Can J Sport Sci* **16**: 248–257.

Venter J, Adams M, Myers E, Li PW, *et al.* (2001). The sequence of the human genome. *Science* **291**: 1304–1351.

Whelan J and Vlahos N (2000). The ovarian hyperstimulation syndrome. *Fertil Steril* **73**: 883–896.

14

Vaccine Safety Surveillance

E. Miller

What is special about vaccine safety compared with other drugs?

Though many of the concepts relating to evaluation of drug safety are common to vaccines, there are a number of important differences that generate challenging methodological issues for those charged with vaccine safety surveillance.

First, unlike drugs that are given therapeutically to patients with disease, vaccines are given prophylactically to healthy individuals, often young children. As a consequence, expectations about vaccine safety are much higher than for therapeutic drugs. For example, a patient receiving chemotherapy for cancer will accept a high incidence of drug-induced morbidity, whereas the patient accepting a vaccine for disease prevention expects it to be 'safe'. Although the definition of 'safe' is clearly subjective, in the context of vaccines, serious side effects occurring at around 1 in 10 000 are usually considered unacceptable. Detection of rare adverse events is, therefore, of paramount importance for vaccine safety surveillance.

Second, the high population exposure to vaccines, together with their administration to children around the time when unrelated developmental conditions may be naturally evolving, means that temporal associations between vaccination and serious disabling conditions will inevitably occur. When such conditions are of unknown aetiology and occur in a previously normal child, there can be a strong parental perception that a temporal association is necessarily evidence of a causal association. This is particularly so when the timing of the onset of the condition relies on parental recall, as for example in autism (Andrews *et al.*, 2002). The ability to mount analytic studies of rare adverse events that can distinguish coincidental from causal associations is, therefore, an additional requirement for vaccine safety evaluation.

Third, vaccines have the potential to affect the unvaccinated through the indirect protection generated by herd immunity. This can profoundly change the risk–benefit balance for the prospective vaccinee. Providing that herd immunity is maintained by vaccination of the majority, then the optimum strategy for the individual is not to be vaccinated, thereby avoiding any risk from the vaccine while relying on the benefit of the protection afforded by herd immunity (Fine and Clarkson, 1986). Continued acceptance of vaccination in the face of a greatly reduced risk of disease requires an understanding of disease epidemiology and how this is affected by vaccine coverage. Ideally, it not only involves a risk assessment at the

Stephens' Detection of New Adverse Drug Reactions Fifth Edition edited by John Talbot and Patrick Waller
© 2004 John Wiley & Sons, Ltd   ISBN: 0 470 84552 X

individual level, but also an acceptance of the concept of the public health good and the responsibility of the individual to contribute towards this. The risk–benefit for vaccines is, therefore, considerably more complicated than for therapeutic drugs, since it depends on the behaviour of the population as a whole, not just the individual.

Finally, the emergence in many countries of a vocal anti-vaccine lobby that can rapidly promote unsubstantiated claims of vaccine harm through the Internet poses a real threat to the population acceptance of vaccination. Sustaining public confidence in immunization, therefore, requires an increasingly proactive approach by those charged with managing and delivering the national vaccination programme. Unless public concerns about a vaccine's safety can be addressed, the programme may collapse with the consequent rapid resurgence of disease, as happened with whole cell pertussis vaccination programmes in a number of countries in the 1970s (Gangarosa *et al.*, 1998). Approaches that have been adopted to help sustain high compliance include making vaccination a requirement for eligibility for some other benefit, e.g. schooling, and ensuring that national vaccine compensation schemes are available for those who have been damaged as a result of immunization without requiring recourse to litigation. The provision of readily accessible, authoritative and evidence-based information on the risks of the disease and of the vaccine underpins these approaches.

All these factors make it essential that the systems responsible for safety surveillance are as robust as possible and are accompanied by equally robust systems for surveillance of vaccine-preventable infections.

Pathogenesis of vaccine reactions

Direct effects

As with any pharmaceutical product, adverse events from a vaccine may arise as a result of a toxic or other direct effect of one of its components. With inactivated bacterial vaccines, the inclusion of endo- or exo-toxins can result in a local inflammatory reaction at the injection site or a systemic effect such as fever. A typical example of an endotoxin-mediated adverse effect is that seen with whole pertussis vaccines (Baraff *et al.*, 1989). Exotoxin-mediated effects are exemplified by anthrax vaccine, which consists of a cell-free filtrate of *Bacillus anthracis,* containing various amounts of exotoxins such as oedema and lethal factor (Brachman and Freidlander, 1999). Such toxin-mediated effects, usually occur within 24 h of immunization and resolve within a day or two. The effect of subsequent doses is difficult to predict; for example, endotoxin-mediated adverse effects are often age dependent, with an increase in reactogenicity with age. On the other hand, generation of antibody responses to vaccine toxins may result in a decrease in reactogenicity with subsequent doses.

With live vaccines, adverse events can result from the replication of the attenuated vaccine strain, the clinical picture resembling, albeit in a milder form, that seen with the wild infection. For example, attenuated measles vaccine produces a mild fever in about a quarter of children around 7–12 days after vaccination caused by the viraemia that occurs when vaccine virus replicates in the body (Peltola and Heinonen, 1986). As expected, such effects decrease with subsequent doses, as the induction of immunity prevents viral replication. On rare occasions the direct pathological effect of a live viral vaccine may be severe, as with the aseptic meningitis seen with some mumps vaccine strains; identification of vaccine virus in the cerebrospinal fluid (CSF; Forsey *et al.*, 1992) together with a statistically significant increased risk of aseptic meningitis in the immediate post-vaccination period (Miller E *et al.*, 1993) have confirmed the causal relationship with vaccination. Other examples of serious reactions that are directly attributable to the pathogenic effects of the live organisms in a vaccine are acute flaccid paralysis from oral poliomyelitis vaccine (OPV) and the disseminated infection seen in immunocompromised individuals given bacille Calmette–Guerin (BCG) vaccine.

Immune-mediated effects

Vaccines are designed to produce beneficial effects by the induction of immune responses to protective antigens in the vaccine and may also contain adjuvants such as aluminium-containing compounds that are designed to stimulate the immune system in order to enhance these immune responses. Immune-mediated adverse effects are, therefore, to be expected. There are four main types of immune-mediated vaccine reaction (Stratton *et al.*, 1994). These are as discussed below.

Type 1 reactions: anaphylaxis and other immediate hypersensitivity reactions

Anaphylactic reactions are rare but potentially fatal and can occur with any inhaled, ingested or injected pharmaceutical agent. They are caused when antigen binds to IgE antibodies on mast cells and basophils, causing release of mediators such as histamine. Sensitization by prior exposure to the antigen is required for the formation of IgE antibodies and is an idiosyncratic reaction. The characteristic symptoms/signs of hypotension, pallor, tachycardia, subcutaneous oedema, facial swelling, laryngeal spasm and wheezing are caused by smooth muscle relaxation in blood vessels with constriction elsewhere. Fluid leaks from capillaries, causing hypotension and hypovolaemic shock. Symptoms generally occur within a few minutes of exposure to the allergen, although they may be delayed for a few hours (Stratton *et al.*, 1994). Anaphylactic reactions can occur as a result of sensitization to vaccine excipients such as thiomersal (van't Veen, 2001) and gelatine (Sakaguchi and Inouye, 2000; Patja *et al.*, 2001), as well as to the intended antigenic components of the vaccine, e.g. diphtheria toxoid (Skov *et al.*, 1997).

In practice, anaphylactic reactions to vaccines are extremely rare. In the UK, no fatal cases have been reported after any of the paediatric vaccines over the last decade, despite the vaccination of around a third of a million infants each year with three doses of combined diphtheria–tetanus–pertussis/*Haemophilus influenzae* type b (DTP/Hib) vaccine, and a similar number of toddlers and pre-school children with respectively measles–mumps–rubella (MMR) and a diptheria–tetanus booster. Nevertheless, all healthcare staff giving vaccinations are required to undergo anaphylaxis training and to have adrenaline and an airway to hand.

Milder forms of immediate hypersensitivity reactions, such as urticaria, facial swelling or wheezing but without circulatory collapse, are reported more commonly than full anaphylactic reactions. For example urticaria and facial swelling were the most common serious adverse events reported after a mass immunization programme with meningococcal serogroup AC polysaccharide vaccine in Quebec, yet even then the risk was only 9.2 per 100 000 doses (Yergeau *et al.*, 1996).

When any symptom/sign of immediate hypersensitivity occurs after a vaccine, then further doses are usually contraindicated. For combined vaccines, such as DTP/Hib, where the antigen responsible for the hypersensitivity reaction is not known, rather than leave the child unprotected against all the diseases, vaccination in hospital with close observation may be undertaken. Use of skin tests to try and identify the responsible allergen may be unreliable and are not normally undertaken for vaccines. Desensitization to induce IgG rather than IgE antibodies has been done for some vaccines, for example tetanus (Carey and Meltzer, 1992).

Type II reactions: interaction of antibody with normal tissue antigens

These could theoretically occur if an antigen or other vaccine component shares a common epitope with a host tissue antigen such that the antibodies induced by the vaccine react with that tissue. Such autoantibodies may be the basis of the acute thrombcytopenic purpura reported after MMR vaccines for example (Nieminen *et al.*, 1993) but, overall, there is little hard evidence of a role of vaccine-induced autoantibodies as a cause of disease (Shoenfeld and Aron-Maor, 2000). One of the claims that MMR can cause autism is based on the postulated induction of autoantibodies to myelin basic protein (MBP) by the vaccine (Singh *et al.*, 1998), which uses embyonated chicken eggs in the manufacturing process. However, there is no evidence of MBP residues in MMR vaccines (Afzal *et al.*, 2000).

Type III: Arthus reaction

This is the most common cause of immune-mediated vaccine reactions and occurs when antigen combines with IgG antibody leading to deposition of antigen–antibody complexes on the walls of blood vessels and a local inflammatory reaction. Typically it is the mechanism whereby a vaccine, such as tetanus, produces increasing erythema and swelling at the injection site with each dose. As IgG antibody levels increase with subsequent doses, revaccination in the presence of excess antibody predisposes towards the formation of antigen–antibody complexes. Symptoms generally occur within a few hours of vaccination, peaking 1–2 days after. Although large local reactions often cause concern, they are self-limiting and usually resolve within a few days.

Systemic formation of antigen–antibody complexes gives rise to a generalized Arthus reaction (serum sickness) characterized by deposition in joints, skin and kidney, giving rise to arthritis, rashes and renal damage. This generalized type of type III reaction is extremely rare after vaccination, it being typically associated with administration of immunoglobulins raised in other species, e.g. the horse.

Type IV reactions: cell-mediated/delayed-type hypersensitivity

This occurs when antigen-specific T lymphocytes are activated by the vaccine, causing the lymphokine release and macrophage stimulation typically associated with a cell-mediated response. In a naïve individual responding for the first time to the vaccine antigen, the onset of the reaction will be delayed, peaking at about 3 weeks, whereas on revaccination the onset is more rapid, within 48 h. The classic example of a delayed-type hypersensitivity reaction to a vaccine is that seen with BCG. This is a live bacterial vaccine that replicates at the site of injection causing an ulcer that takes some weeks to heal, leaving a scar. The use of the term hypersensitivity is perhaps misleading in this context, as the BCG reaction represents a normal cell-mediated response to a replicating pathogen. However, serious adverse events may be caused by this mechanism if a cell mediated response is induced by a vaccine antigen that cross-reacts with a tissue antigen. The occurrence of demyelination after early rabies vaccines that were produced in animal brains and contaminated with nervous tissue was likely to be due to this type of immune-mediated effect. Guillain–Barré syndrome (GBS), after influenza vaccine, may also represent a delayed-type hypersensitivity reaction although the nature of the putative cross-reacting antigens is not known.

Criteria for establishing causality for vaccine adverse events

The main planks of evidence that have been used for establishing causal associations for adverse vaccine events are summarized in Table 14.1. Although there are well-established criteria for causality assessment of adverse events for pharmaceutical products, some of these cannot be applied to vaccines. For example, unlike therapeutic drugs, vaccines offer little opportunity to study dose response, since the quantity of antigen and excipients in the product is fixed. In addition, absence of a response to rechallenge does not preclude a causal association, because of the development of immunity to the vaccine antigens. Furthermore, the application of precautionary recommendations that contraindicate further doses after a suspected serious adverse event has occurred limits the opportunity for observing the effect of rechallenge. As discussed in Chapter 7, dose response and rechallenge form one of the planks of evidence for establishing causality for drug adverse events.

Table 14.1 Main criteria for establishing causality for a vaccine adverse event

Is it biologically plausible? – e.g.
- Fever after an endotoxin containing vaccine
- Acute flaccid paralysis after oral polio vaccine

Is there laboratory evidence of vaccine involvement? – e.g.
- Urabe mumps vaccine in CSF of a patient with meningitis symptoms
- Disseminated BCG in an immunocompromised patient

Is there evidence of an increased risk after vaccination? – e.g.
- Clustering in a post vaccination period
- Higher risk in vaccinated compared to unvaccinated

Is the evidence consistent across studies? – e.g.
- Consistent increased risk of aseptic meningitis within 15–35 days of a Urabe mumps vaccine
- Consistent inability to find evidence of an association between MMR vaccination and incidence or timing of onset of autism

However, other criteria, such as biological plausibility and laboratory evidence of vaccine involvement, may assume greater importance for vaccines than for non-biological agents. For example, it is biologically plausible that a live attenuated vaccine could produce reactions similar to those seen with infection due to the wild organism, although at a much lower rate. A typical example is the occurrence of acute flaccid paralysis within a few weeks of OPV. Although this could be due to unrelated conditions, such as GBS, a causal association with OPV is considered probable if the clinical syndrome is typical of poliomyelitis, the temporal relationship with vaccination is compatible with vaccine-associated paralytic poliomyelitis and alternative aetiologies have been excluded. Isolation from the case of vaccine viruses that have mutated towards virulence provides powerful laboratory confirmatory evidence.

The ability to obtain laboratory evidence to support a causal association between a vaccine and an adverse event has, so far, been restricted to live vaccines where either the vaccine strain can be shown to be involved in the pathogenic process, e.g. BCG in the lesions of patients with disseminated mycobacterial infection (Grange, 1998) or, in the case of OPV, the excretion by the vaccinee of a mutated vaccine strain. By itself, evidence of recent seroconversion to the vaccine does not confirm a causal association, since this will be present in any recently vaccinated individual. For example, the detection of mumps-specific IgM in a child with aseptic meningitis following Urabe mumps-containing MMR vaccine cannot be used to establish a causal association since it merely confirms that the child has recently been vaccinated. Laboratory evidence supportive of a causal association would be demonstration of mumps vaccine virus in the CSF (a normally sterile fluid) with a cellular reaction characteristic of a viral meningitis (a lymphocytic CSF; Forsey et al., 1992).

If laboratory evidence is used to support a causal relationship with vaccination then it must be technically robust. Unfortunately, because of the intense media interest in vaccine scare stories, unpublished reports using unvalidated laboratory methods may be given prominence that the quality of the science does not merit. For example, a recent conference abstract reporting that measles vaccine virus had been found in gut biopsies of autistic children was given wide media publicity in the UK although it was based on an assay that could readily be shown to be incapable of distinguishing wild from vaccine virus (http://www.hpa.org.uk/infections/topics_az/vaccination/response.htm).

Even when vaccine virus or other vaccine material has been shown to be present in a lesion it does not necessarily imply a causal relationship with a clinical condition. For example, it has been shown that inactivated vaccines containing the adjuvant aluminium hydroxide can produce a local histological condition called macrophagic myofasciitis (MMF) in which macrophages containing aluminium are identified at the injection site. The detection of MMF lesions in patients undergoing muscle biopsies for myopathic symptoms has led to the suggestion that MMF causes systemic disease (Gherardi et al., 2001). However, while MMF lesions are probably a consequence of vaccination, they may nevertheless be a chance histological finding in vaccinated patients who have a muscle biopsy for unrelated symptoms and could perhaps be found with equal frequency in asymptomatic vaccinated individuals were they to have muscle biopsies performed. If this is the case, then MMF lesions are simply a 'vaccine tattoo' and of no clinical consequence. Indeed, the demonstration in animals of MMF-type lesions without systemic effects following injection of vaccines containing aluminium hydroxide suggests that this is probably the case (WHO, 2002).

Finally, even when there is convincing laboratory evidence of presence of a vaccine constituent in individuals with a putative vaccine reaction but not in normal controls it may simply be the consequence rather than the cause of the disease process. In the case of wild measles infection, for example, the raised IgG titres to measles and the traces of measles virus genome reported in patients with chronic active hepatitis are not thought to be the cause of the disease but rather a consequence of the underlying immunological abnormality that is the origin of the condition (Triger et al., 1972; Black, 1988). The involvement of measles virus is, therefore, a bystander effect or epi-phenomenon.

If laboratory evidence of vaccine involvement is to be used to establish a causal association between a disease and vaccination then it is important that Koch-type postulates, employed in microbiology to establish a causal association between the presence of a pathogen and a disease, are applied to such evidence. Koch's first postulate (evidence of the presence of the organism in cases but not in healthy individuals) is not by itself sufficient and requires additional criteria for establishing a pathogenic role for the organism, e.g. the ability to culture the organism from the diseased individual and the ability to transmit the infection by inoculation of the cultured organism. In the case of adverse vaccine events, the first of these additional criteria has been met for BCG-associated disseminated mycobacterial infection, OPV-associated acute flaccid paralysis and Urabe-associated aseptic meningitis, where replicating vaccine organisms, associated with a clinico-pathological response characteristic of the wild infection, have been shown. In the case of OPV-associated acute flaccid paralysis the second additional criterion has also been satisfied, since transmission of vaccine virus to contacts can result in the same condition. In contrast, the reported detection of fragments of measles virus genome in the intestinal tract of autistic patients with ileal lymphoid nodular hyperplasia more frequently than in children without this condition (Uhlmann *et al.*, 2002) does not establish a causal role of measles virus in autism, since its presence, if confirmed, may simply be a consequence of a local inflammatory response in the gut of autistic children with bowel problems (Morris and Aldulaimi, 2002), as with the fragments of measles virus genome found in chronic active hepatitis (Black, 1988).

In practice, the opportunity to use laboratory evidence to support a causal association with vaccination is limited, and arguments based on biological plausibility, while supportive, are neither necessary nor sufficient. The main plank of evidence that been used to establish, or refute, a causal association between a vaccine and a subsequent clinical condition is epidemiological. The gold standard epidemiological method is the randomized controlled trial (RCT), which allows an unbiased comparison of the frequency of adverse events in vaccinated and unvaccinated groups. One classic vaccine example is the double-blind placebo-controlled crossover study in 686 twins that was specifically designed to document the true attributable risk of common symptoms after MMR vaccine (Peltola and Heinonen, 1986). This study established that the majority of the symptoms reported in the 3 weeks after MMR are not vaccine related and that the vaccine may even have a mild protective effect against respiratory infections in the post-vaccination period. However, a much larger study would be required to assess the attributable risk of more rare adverse events, such as febrile convulsions. Even when a vaccine RCT is powered for establishing efficacy it may still be of insufficient size to evaluate the risk of rare adverse events. Alternative methods that can be used post-licensure have, therefore, been devised to assess whether the risk of a particular clinical condition is greater in the unvaccinated than the vaccinated individual, or in a particular post-vaccination risk period. These methods will be discussed in the following sections. Though such methods may lack the rigour of an RCT, converging and consistent epidemiological evidence from different studies can provide powerful confirmatory evidence of causality, or lack of it.

Pre-licensure evaluation of vaccine safety

The main safety objective during the pre-licensure vaccine evaluation phase is to document the nature and frequency of the more common side effects and to ensure that any serious or unusual adverse events in the trial cohort are detected. This involves the active follow up of every vaccinee, at least for the occurrence of serious events. These are defined as any event resulting in death, life-threatening illness, hospitalization or permanent sequelae (see Chapter 1) even where a causal association with vaccination can reasonably be excluded, e.g. an accident. Inevitably, however the size of pre-licensure vaccine trials limits the ability to detect rare vaccine adverse events or, if they are detected, to have a statistically robust comparison of the incidence in vaccinated and placebo groups. This was situation in the efficacy trials of the live attenuated rotavirus vaccine in which intussusception occurred in 5 in 10 054 vaccinees compared with 1 in 4633 in the placebo group. Although this difference was not statistically significant, enhanced post-licensure surveillance was established which showed that this pre-licensure 'signal' was indeed evidence of a true causal association (Murphy *et al.*, 2001). Similarly, occurrence of one case of aseptic meningitis in a pre-licensure study of 10 000 children given a Urabe-containing MMR vaccine in the UK (Miller *et al.*, 1989) prompted enhanced post-licensure surveillance. This confirmed that the true risk was around 1 in 10 000 doses and not of the order of 1 in 100 000 as previously thought (Miller E *et al.*, 1993).

When differences in rare adverse events are found between vaccinated and placebo groups in an RCT, further studies will usually be required before licensure. This was the case in an efficacy study of acellular pertussis vaccines in Sweden, where an excess of invasive bacterial infection was seen in the vaccinated group (Storsaeter *et al.*, 1988). Although subsequently shown to be due to chance (Griffin *et al.*, 1992), the concern raised by this finding contributed to the delay in licensure of these vaccines. In order to maximize power for measuring vaccine efficacy the Swedish trial had been designed with a smaller placebo than vaccinated group, which unfortunately reduced power for comparing adverse events.

Other factors that can limit the ability to detect serious adverse events at the pre-licensure stage are the application of stringent exclusion criteria to potential recruits that may militate against the detection of idiosyncratic vaccine–host interactions. Interactions between vaccines, or between vaccines and other drugs, may also not come to light in pre-licensure trials, where receipt of pharmaceutical products shortly before or after the study vaccine usually constitutes an exclusion criterion. For example, administration of intramuscular injections such as antibiotics shortly after OPV has been shown to increase the risk of vaccine-associated paralysis (Strebel, *et al.*, 1995).

In light of the increasing profile given to vaccine safety issues, and the importance of sustaining public confidence in immunization programmes, it is likely that some additional requirements will be made at the pre-licensure stage of vaccine evaluation. For example, to address frequently expressed concerns about late vaccine effects, there is now a move towards extending the period of follow-up in vaccine trials to at least 6 months after the last dose. In practice, the follow up period in an efficacy trial is usually much longer in order to allow sufficient cases to accrue in the study cohorts to demonstrate protection. However, when new vaccines are licensed without efficacy trials, as for example with combination products, extension of the usual 4–6 week follow-up period to assess immunogenicity and immediate reactogenicity would seem reasonable. Furthermore, in the wake of the rotavirus and intussusception experience, is it likely that the Food and Drug Administration (FDA) in the US will require a much larger safety database to underpin a license application for a new rotavirus vaccine, and possibly other new vaccines, in the future (Black, 2001). However, a balance needs to be struck between the amount of vaccine safety data that is required for licensure and the reliance that is put on post-licensure safety evaluation in order not to prohibit the development and evaluation of new vaccines. Comprehensive guidelines on the pre-licensure evaluation of new vaccines have recently been drawn up by the World Health Organization (WHO, in press) to help ensure that appropriate but reasonable requirements for evaluation of vaccine safety and efficacy are put in place by national regulatory agencies (NRAs), particularly those in developing countries where new NRAs are being established.

Objectives of an ideal post-licensure vaccine safety surveillance system

Ideally, a post-licensure vaccine safety surveillance system should be able to detect novel or rare adverse events not identified at the pre-licensure stage, to measure both the absolute and attributable risks of such events and to identify risk factors so that sound evidence-based contraindications to vaccination can be developed. When signals of a putative causal association have come from pre-licensure studies or there are other grounds for focusing on certain adverse events, such as intussusception with a new rotavirus vaccine or aseptic meningitis with a new mumps vaccine, then there should be an ability to establish post-licensure surveillance of these events and to mount analytic epidemiological studies to address causality.

Although these ideal objectives may appear somewhat challenging, there are now many examples where they have been achieved. Moreover, there is an increasing use of sophisticated technical and statistical tools that have been specifically developed for the post-licensure investigation of vaccine safety.

Passive post-licensure surveillance systems

Most NRAs have established pharmacovigilance systems that include vaccines. However, because vaccines can be considered a special case, as outlined earlier in this chapter, institutions with relevant epidemiological expertise may also be involved in running the passive vaccine reporting system. For example, in the USA, the Vaccine Adverse Event Reporting System (VAERS) is run jointly by the Center for Disease Control in Atlanta and the FDA. In the UK, the Medicines Control Agency, collects and analyses vaccine adverse event reports as part of its general pharmacovigilance reporting system (the so-called 'Yellow Card' scheme) but will approach the Immunization Division of the Communicable Disease Surveillance Centre, or other institutions with relevant expertise, if analytic epidemiological studies of specific vaccines are indicated.

To assist countries with less well-developed pharmacovigilance systems the WHO has produced a field guide on how to establish an adverse vaccine event reporting system (WHO, 1999). As a minimum such a system should be able to detect temporal or spatial clusters of novel or serious adverse events and to investigate their aetiology, e.g. whether this is due to a problem with a particular batch or manufacturer's vaccine, or whether there has been a programmatic error such as wrong product given or wrong route of administration. Some recent examples of the ability of routine passive surveillance systems to detect such clusters are cases of an unusual oculo-respiratory syndrome occurring within a few hours of giving a new influenza vaccine in Canada (Boulianne et al., 2001), the increased reactogenicity that occurred when a manufacturer of a tick-borne encephalitis vaccine in Austria changed production methods to remove albumen (Marth and Kleinhappl, 2001) and a cluster of infant deaths in the Yemen caused by injection of insulin instead of DTP vaccine

(WHO, 1999). In each case, an epidemiological investigation of the cluster identified the causal factor.

In addition to identifying programmatic errors or problems with particular batches or makes of vaccine, passive reports should be able to identify subgroups who may have an increased likelihood of an adverse outcome by showing an overrepresentation of individuals with a particular risk factor compared with the general population. In practice there have been few examples of this: the identification of asymptomatic vertically transmitted HIV infection as a risk factor for disseminated BCG is one example (Scheifele *et al.*, 1998) and the demonstration that a personal history of convulsion is risk factor for a DTP-associated convulsion is another (Rosenthal and Chen, 1995).

Despite such successes, simple passive reporting systems have obvious limitations. First, reporting is inevitably incomplete even if there is a mandatory requirement to report suspected reactions, as in the USA with the National Childhood Vaccine Injury Act of, 1986. To try and improve the quality and completeness of adverse vaccine event reporting in the USA, the VAERS system was established in 1990. Under this system, reports are accepted from parents as well as healthcare professionals, a special form is provided that solicits descriptive information on the event and its treatment and outcome, a 24 h toll-free telephone line is provided and there is a list of conditions that are mandated for reporting. All fatal adverse events and other selected serious events are followed up. Information on the VAERS system is made widely available to parents, and healthcare professionals are regularly reminded to report (Rosenthal and Chen, 1995). Even with these attempts to stimulate passive reporting to VAERS, the reporting efficiency for known adverse events is still poor. For example, it has been estimated that only one in three convulsions after MMR vaccine are reported and about 1 in 25 episodes of ITP (Rosenthal and Chen, 1995). Surprisingly, the sensitivity of the UK Yellow Card system for MMR-associated idiopathic thrombocytopenic purpura episodes appears to be higher with about one in five reported (Farrington *et al.*, 1995).

A second limitation of a passive adverse event reporting system is the inability to use the data for testing causal associations, its value being largely limited to hypothesis generation. Analysis of the distribution of onsets after vaccination to identify periods in which there may be an excess of reports can be useful in defining *a priori* risk periods for subsequent analytic studies, as for example with aseptic meningitis after MMR vaccines (Miller E *et al.*, 1993). Finding an excess of passive reports in a particular post-vaccination period may suggest a causal association but could simply reflect reporter bias, based on expectations of when a vaccine-attributable effect should occur. For example, an analysis of claims submitted to the National Vaccine Injury Compensation Board in the USA involving acute encephalopathy after measles-containing vaccines found a statistically significant excess of cases with onset 8 or 9 days after vaccination. This clustering was used to argue for a causal association (Weibel *et al.*, 1998); but, given the well-known temporal sequence between measles vaccination and onset of side effects, such as febrile convulsions associated with the vaccine-induced viraemia, preferential reporting of cases with onset in the known risk period is likely. The authors also argued biological plausibility in support of a causal association, quoting as a model the post-infectious encephalitis that occurs in about 1 in 1000 acute measles cases about a week after onset of rash. However, this is not associated with the viraemic phase of the illness, but is thought to involve a later auto-immune demyelination process. Based on the wild model, if there was post-vaccination encephalitis then this should not occur at 8–9 days but about a week after the rash, which in vaccine recipients typically occurs 10–12 days after immunization (Miller *et al.*, 1989). While absence of a biological explanation for an adverse event does not preclude a casual association, independent confirmation by a controlled epidemiological investigation is required to show convincingly that there is an increased risk of encephalopathy 8–9 days after a measles-containing vaccine. The only controlled study of acute encephalopathy after measles vaccine failed to find an excess after removal of cases of febrile convulsions (Miller *et al.*, 1997).

Active surveillance of adverse vaccine events

Because of incomplete and potentially biased reporting with passive surveillance systems, various attempts have been made to overcome these deficiencies by establishing active systems for ascertaining adverse events after vaccination. If the active surveillance system has near-complete ascertainment of adverse events then reliable estimates of absolute risk can be derived. However, without information on the risk of such events in unvaccinated age-matched groups, causality assessment can be difficult and no estimates of attributable risk can be made.

One such active surveillance system was established in the UK to monitor the propensity of different measles vaccines to produce reactions, in particular febrile convulsions (Miller, 1982). Active ascertainment was established by ensuring that in a sentinel district all measles vaccinees were followed up by a study nurse who completed a simple questionnaire documenting significant medical events in the 3 weeks after vaccination. This surveillance was largely directed at comparison of the rates of known reactions with different vaccine strains rather than the detection of novel adverse events. Between 1970 and 1980, symptoms were documented in over 10 000 children after 62 different batches of vaccine randomly selected by the National Institute for Biological Standards and Control. No evidence of a batch or strain effect was found, and the febrile convulsion rate of 1 per 1000 in the 6–11 day post-vaccination period found in the MRC Measles Vaccine trials prior to licensure (Measles Vaccination Committee, 1966) was confirmed under conditions of routine use.

An alternative approach to active adverse event surveillance was established in Canada in 1992 with the objective of identifying all serious vaccine events that resulted in hospital admission. Specially trained nurses were installed at 11 sentinel paediatric centres with the task of reviewing the hospital notes of children admitted with possible vaccine reactions (Anon., 1993). Admissions for vaccine-preventable infections were also identified in order to provide risk assessments for the disease as well as the vaccine. The Canadian Immunization Monitoring Programme Active (IMPACT) system is labour intensive but provides a reliable measure of the absolute risk of defined adverse events of sufficient severity to warrant hospital admission and allows this risk to be compared with the morbidity attributable to the disease. However, assessment of causality is difficult and requires a judgement to be made on each case based on criteria of biological plausibility, exclusion of other causes and, where possible, laboratory evidence of vaccine involvement. In most instances, however, the biological and laboratory features of the case do not allow the adverse event to be confidentially ascribed to the vaccine or excluded as being vaccine attributable. Under these circumstances, evidence of an increased risk of the event in a defined post-vaccination period must be sought, and this requires information on the incidence of events outside the post-vaccination risk period.

Controlled epidemiological studies of vaccine safety

There are a number of methods for conducting controlled epidemiological studies to assess the relationship between vaccination and clinical conditions suspected of being causally associated. All have the same requirement, namely that ascertainment of the conditions studied should be unbiased with respect to vaccination history. The methods can either provide estimates of the incidence of events in defined post-vaccination periods relative to the age-adjusted background rate, or the risk in vaccinated compared with unvaccinated individuals. When vaccine uptake rates are high, it may not be possible to make unbiased comparisons between vaccinated and unvaccinated cohorts, since those that remain unvaccinated are likely to be an atypical subset of the population. Alternative, ecological approaches (see below) may be necessary under such circumstances.

The classic post-licensure epidemiological methods for investigating causal associations are the cohort and case-control methods. Cohort studies must be very large in order to have sufficient power to detect rare vaccine adverse events and may, therefore, be impractical as a prospective undertaking. Retrospective cohort studies using data sets already assembled for other purposes can be used instead (Ray and Griffen, 1989), although the ability to account for the effect of important confounding variables may be limited by the available data. Furthermore, when using retrospective cohorts a clear distinction must be made between an exploratory study undertaken as a hypothesis-generating exercise and a study undertaken to test an explicit *a priori* hypothesis. Ideally, exploratory analyses should be undertaken with a view to conducting a formal hypothesis-testing study if evidence of a significantly increased risk is found in a particular post-vaccination period. If sufficiently large, the data set could be split into two, with half used to conduct an exploratory analysis and the other half used to test any hypotheses so generated. Although this approach should allow the identification of statistically significant effects that have arisen by chance (a type I error), it cannot overcome the effect of bias that may be inherent in the way the data set has been collected and that results in confounding of vaccination status and the adverse event.

The large linked databases from the Health Maintenance Organizations (HMOs) in the USA have recently been used to conduct a number of cohort studies to test hypotheses about the risk of vaccine adverse events in defined post-vaccination periods, e.g. febrile seizures after whole-cell pertussis or MMR vaccines (Barlow *et al.*, 2001), or asthma exacerbations after influenza vaccine (Kramarz *et al.*, 2000). Where possible, potential confounding factors were adjusted for in the analyses, as for example in the asthma study where the unadjusted analysis showed evidence of a significantly increased risk of an exacerbation within 2 weeks of vaccination but this disappeared after controlling for asthma severity (Kramarz *et al.*, 2000). An example of using the HMO data sets for exploratory analyses is the investigation of the temporal relationship between OPV and intussusception. This was undertaken following confirmation of an increased risk of intussusception in the week after rotavirus vaccine to investigate whether this might be a generic problem with live oral virus vaccines (Andrews *et al.*, 2001). Another example of an exploratory analysis with the HMO data set is the investigation of the relationship between cumulative thiomersal exposure in the first year of life and developmental delay (http://www.cdc.gov/nip/vacsafe/concerns/thimerosal/joint_statement_00.htm). In both cases, marginally significant results in one of many analyses generated hypotheses that required formal testing in independent data sets. In each case the hypothesis generated by the exploratory analysis was not confirmed (Andrews 2001; Miller, 2002).

Case-control studies require smaller numbers than cohort studies but are subject to the same confounding with respect to acceptance/avoidance of vaccination and the putative adverse event. In addition, they may be subject to additional biases introduced by the selection of controls. For studies involving paediatric vaccines, close matching on date of birth is essential, as they are given within tight age ranges in the first and second years of life. For a fixed number of cases the power of a case-control study only approaches that of a cohort study with multiple controls per case. However, selection and matching of controls can be time consuming and, although an increase from one to two controls gives a fairly large increase in power, there are diminishing returns for more than three controls per case. In one of the most well-known case-control studies of adverse vaccine events, the National Childhood Encephalopathy Study of DTP vaccines, only two controls were selected for each case, with date of birth matched within 1 month of that of the case (Miller D *et al.*, 1993).

A case-case control study nested within a cohort study is sometimes undertaken if relevant confounders have not been measured for the entire cohort or if information on vaccination status has not been collected. Identification of subjects from a cohort should minimize selection bias between cases and controls. A recent example of a nested case-control study was the study of the risk of multiple sclerosis after exposure to hepatitis B vaccine in two large cohorts of nurses in the USA who had been followed up for a number of years as part of a nurses' health study (Ascherio *et al.*, 2001). The combined size of the cohorts was nearly a quarter of a million among whom 192 women with multiple sclerosis were identified. Five healthy controls and one ill control with breast cancer were randomly selected from the cohorts after matching on year of birth and study cohort and, for the cancer patients, date of diagnosis. Information on covariates that could be confounders for risk of multiple sclerosis, such as latitude of birth, was obtained, as well as covariates that could affect likelihood of hepatitis B vaccination, such as type of nursing job. No evidence of an increase in the risk of multiple sclerosis after hepatitis B vaccination was found.

Because of the logistic problems associated with large cohort studies, and the difficulties of ensuring adequate control of confounding factors in both cohort and case-control studies, alternative epidemiological methods have been employed for investigating vaccine safety issues (Farrington, in press). These require data collection only on cases of the putative adverse event and are not only less labour intensive but can avoid some of the potential biases in cohort and case-control studies. As with the cohort and case-control methods, case ascertainment must be independent of vaccination history. Two 'cases only' methods have been used that can provide relative risk/incidence measures, namely the case-crossover and self-controlled case series methods.

The case-crossover method was developed to investigate the effect of transient exposures on the risk of acute events (Maclure, 1991) and has frequently been used for studying the impact of potential triggers on the risk of myocardial infarction (Maclure and Mittleman, 2000). It can, under certain circumstances, also be used for investigating vaccination risks (Farrington, in press). In a case-crossover vaccine study, vaccinations for each individual are ascertained in a defined time period immediately prior to the adverse event and in one or more earlier control periods of the same duration. This produces, for each case, a matched set of exposure variables corresponding to the event and control periods, which may be analysed as in a case-control study. A case-crossover design was recently used to investigate the effect of hepatitis B on the risk of relapse in multiple sclerosis in the subsequent 2 months (Confavreux *et al.*, 2001). Four 2 month periods prior to the risk period were used as control periods. Each period was classified as 'exposed' if vaccination occurred within it, and 'unexposed' otherwise. This gave an odds ratio of 0.67 (95 per cent confidence intervals 0.20, 2.17) for relapses 2 months after hepatitis B vaccination. The authors concluded that there was no evidence that vaccination increased the short-term risk of relapse.

The strength of the case-crossover method is that it does not require separate controls and that, by matching time periods within individuals, all individual-level confounders such as social class, geographic location, underlying state of health, etc. are automatically controlled for. However, the method has limited application for investigating the risk of adverse events after paediatric vaccines, since it requires the underlying probability of vaccination to be the same in the prior control and subsequent risk intervals. This is unlikely for vaccines such as DTP and MMR that are given within narrow age ranges in the first and second years of life, and where the adverse events likely to be temporally associated with these vaccines are also highly age dependent, e.g. febrile convulsions or onset of autism. The case-crossover design is also not suitable for use with seasonally administered vaccines (Farrington, in press).

The self-controlled case series (SCCS) method overcomes these limitation and was specifically developed in the early 1990s to allow rapid, unbiased estimation of the incidence of events in putative risk periods after various paediatric vaccines relative to the age-adjusted background incidence (Farrington et al., 1996, in press; Andrews, 2001). The the SCCS method uses cases as their own controls, but, unlike the case-crossover method, derives from cohort rather than case-control logic. In particular, ages at vaccination are regarded as fixed, and the random variable of interest is the age at adverse event, conditionally on its occurrence within a predetermined observation period (Farrington, in press). In the SCCS method, like the case-crossover method, individual-level confounders are corrected for because individuals are matched to themselves, thereby eliminating one of the sources of bias in cohort and case-control approaches. As with the cohort method, age effects must be strictly controlled for in the statistical model. The power of the SCCS method is nearly as good as that of a cohort study when vaccine uptake is high and risk intervals are short, and it is superior to that of a case-control study (Farrington et al., 1996).

The comparative features of the cohort, case-control and SCCS methods are summarized in Table 14.2. Because the experience of an entire population is captured in a cohort study it provides both relative and absolute incidence estimates, whereas the case-control and SCCS methods provide relative incidence measures only.[1] However, if other data are available to derive the incidence of the event in the population and if the proportion of all cases in the population that have been captured in the case-control or SCCS study can be estimated, and the vaccination coverage in the study population is known, then absolute and attributable risk estimates can be derived (Andrews, 2001). For example, in a study of hospital-admitted febrile convulsions after MMR vaccine given in the second year of life, a relative incidence of 3.04 (95 per cent confidence intervals 2.27–4.07) for convulsions in the 6–11 day post-vaccination period was found using the SCCS method (Farrington et al., 1995). The attributable fraction (67 per cent) was converted into absolute and attributable risks (1 per 2000 and 1 per 3000 respectively) based on estimates of the number of doses of MMR vaccine given in the second year of life in the population from which the study cases arose and on assumptions about the completeness of ascertainment of the cases of febrile convulsion in the study population (Farrington et al., 1995). These SCCS risk estimates were later confirmed by a cohort study using a large linked database in the USA (Barlow et al., 2001).

---

[1] In a case-control study the odds ratio approximates to the relative risk for rare events.

Table 14.2 Comparison of case-control, cohort and self-controlled case-series studies for assessment of adverse events

Feature	Case-control studies	Cohort studies	Self-controlled case-series studies
Cost	Intermediate	High	Low
Typical time taken to perform study	Intermediate	Slow	Fast
Power	Low, unless >2 controls per case	High	High
Control for individual level bias	Only if information on confounders is included, prone to control selection bias	Only if information on confounders is included	Full
Direct estimates of risk	No, also requires information on the incidence of the event	Yes	No, also requires information on the incidence of the event
Type of analysis	Logistic or Conditional Logistic regression	Poisson regression	Conditional Poisson regression

The SCCS method has now been employed in a number of vaccine safety studies (Farrington *et al.*, 1995. 2001; Taylor *et al.*, 1999; Andrews *et al.*, 2001; Miller *et al.*, 2001, 2003; Sardinas *et al.*, 2001). In some, the results have been directly compared with those generated by the cohort or case-control method (Kramarz *et al.*, 2000; Murphy *et al.*, 2001). The study that investigated whether influenza vaccine given to asthmatic children caused asthma exacerbations in the 2 weeks following vaccination did not show an elevated relative incidence using the SCCS method, whereas the cohort analysis without adjustment for asthma severity did (Kramarz *et al.*, 2000). This illustrates the ability of the SCCS method to control for individual confounding variables without explicitly measuring them (Andrews, 2001). In a study of the risk of intussusception after rotavirus vaccines, the relative incidence estimates from an SCCS analysis were higher than from the case-control analysis study, indicating that the latter had probably underestimated the vaccine-attributable risk due to incomplete adjustment for confounding variables (Andrews, 2001; Murphy *et al.*, 2001).

However, as stated above, the cohort, case-control and SCCS analysis methods all have a common limitation, namely that when vaccination coverage is high and hypotheses about 'ever vaccinated' as opposed to 'vaccinated within a critical period prior to onset of putative adverse event' require testing, none of the analytic methods can adequately control for the bias that is likely to arise from confounding of acceptance/avoidance of vaccination and the putative adverse events. Under these circumstances, recourse to ecological approaches may be necessary.

Ecological studies of vaccine safety

A vaccine safety study can be described as ecological if it compares the incidence of adverse events in populations with different vaccine exposures without obtaining information on vaccination at the individual level. Groups in the analysis are typically geographically or temporally defined and, if valid comparisons are to be made between them, convincing arguments should be advanced that such geographical/temporal differences are unlikely to have affected the comparison of adverse event rates.

Vaccination campaigns conducted within a short period of time in one population offer a unique opportunity for powerful ecological studies of vaccine safety. For example, da Silveira *et al.* (1997) used the acute flaccid paralysis surveillance established for the poliomyelitis eradication programme to investigate the hypothesis that measles vaccine causes GBS within 42 days of vaccination. The interval of 42 days was based on that observed with GBS and swine flu vaccine for which a causal association had been established. Data on cases of acute flaccid paralysis that met the clinical and laboratory criteria for GBS were obtained for the period 1990–94 from four South American countries where mass measles immunization campaigns were conducted for a single month in 1992–93. The number of GBS cases in the risk period (1 month plus 42 days, counting from the day the campaign started) was compared with that in the non-risk periods between 1990 and 1994. No excess was found, the observed number being 97, compared with 92 expected in any 72 day period. The authors concluded that there was no evidence of a causal link between measles vaccination and GBS and that the negative evidence was sufficiently strong to allow removal from the measles vaccine product insert of any mention of an association with GBS.

A similar ecological study was carried out with MMR vaccine (Dourado *et al.*, 2000) to confirm the association reported elsewhere (Miller *et al.*, 1993) that the Urabe mumps vaccine strain causes aseptic meningitis. The study took advantage of a 2 week mass immunization campaign in children aged 1–11 years with a Urabe-containing MMR vaccine that began in mid August 1997. Cases of aseptic meningitis were ascertained using standardized criteria from referrals to specialist hospitals for infectious diseases for the period March to October 1997. The weekly frequency of cases demonstrated a marked peak in incidence following the start of the vaccination campaign, confirming the causal association reported elsewhere and providing similar risk estimates.

As can be seen, ecological studies in which a brief pulse of vaccination is applied to a population can provide compelling evidence for or against a causal association. Other ecological approaches involving comparisons of secular trends in vaccine uptake and the incidence of the putative adverse events provide much weaker evidence, since a correlation cannot establish causality. If a correlation is found in an ecological analysis, then this may generate hypotheses that can be tested in more robust epidemiological studies. Although an ecological correlation cannot establish a causal relationship, lack of a correlation may provide compelling evidence against it. For example, the hypothesis that certain vaccines given after the age of 2 months increase the risk of insulin-dependent diabetes (IDDM; Classen and Classen, 1997) has been tested in a number of ecological studies by comparing trends in the incidence of IDDM in paediatric populations before and after the addition of new vaccines; no correlations have been found (The Institute for Vaccine Safety Diabetes Workshop Panel, 1999). Another example is the hypothesized causal relationship between MMR and autism, which, it was argued, was responsible for the substantial increase in prevalence of diagnosed autism both in the USA and the UK in the past two decades (Wakefield, 1999). However, if MMR is responsible, then there should be a close temporal correspondence between autism prevalence and MMR uptake by birth cohort. None of the ecological studies conducted to date has shown such a correlation (Gillberg and Heijbel, 1998; Dales *et al.*, 2001; Kaye *et al.*, 2001; Sardinas *et al.*, 2001).

Conclusions

Sustaining public confidence in vaccination programmes has emerged as a major challenge in recent years, with a number of allegations about vaccine safety hitting the headlines in different countries. Whatever the inherent biological plausibility of a new claim about a vaccine side effect, it is essential that it is investigated rapidly and thoroughly. New statistical methods, combined with the availability of large linked databases, has greatly facilitated this process. However, detection and investigation of effects that may occur decades after vaccination remains problematic, particularly when vaccine coverage is high. Under these circumstances, ecological analyses may provide a useful methodological tool. If laboratory evidence is used to support an argument for causality then stringent criteria must be applied to such evidence. Finally, when vaccine-attributable adverse effects have been identified, it is important that the risk from the vaccine is placed in the context of the risk from the disease so that an informed decision can be made by the individual and those charged with deciding national vaccination policy.

References

Afzal MA, Pipkin PA and Minor PD (2000). Absence of chicken myelin basic protein residues in commercial formulations of MMR vaccine. *Vaccine* **19**: 442–446.

Andrews N, Miller E, Waight P, Farrington P, *et al.* (2001). Does oral polio vaccine cause intussusception in infants? Evidence from a sequence of three self-controlled case series studies in the United Kingdom. *Eur J Epidemiol* **17**: 701–706.

Andrews N, Miller E, Taylor B, Lingam L, *et al.* (2002). Recall bias, MMR and autism. *Arch Dis Child* **87**: 493–494.

Andrews NJ (2001). Statistical assessment of the association between vaccination and rare adverse events post-licensure. *Vaccine* **20**: S49–S53.

Anon. (1993). IMPACT monitoring network: a better mouse trap. *Can J Infect Dis* **4**: 194–195.

Ascherio A, Zhang SM, Hernan MA, Olek MJ *et al.* (2001). Hepatitis B vaccination and the risk of multiple sclerosis. *N Engl J Med* **344**: 327–332.

Baraff LJ, Manclarke CR, Cherry JD, Christenson P *et al.* (1989). Analyses of adverse reactions to diphtheria and tetanus toxoids and pertussis vaccine by vaccine lot, endotoxin content, pertussis vaccine potency and mouse weight gain. *Pediatr Infect Dis J* **8**: 502–507.

Barlow WE, Davis RL, Glasser JW, Rhodes PH, *et al.* (2001). The risk of seizures after receipt of whole-cell pertussis or measles, mumps and rubella vaccine. *N Engl J Med* **345**: 656–662.

Black FL (1988). Persistent measles virus genome in autoimmune chronic active hepatitis: cause or coincidence? *Hepatol Elsewhere* **8**(1): 86–87.

Black S (2001). Perspectives on the design and analysis of prelicensure trials: bridging the gap to post licensure studies. *Clin Infect Dis* **33**(Suppl 4): S323–S326.

Boulianne N, De Serres G, Duval B, Shadami R, *et al.* (2001). Clinical manifestations and incidence of oculo-respiratory syndrome following influenza vaccination – Quebec 2000. *Can Commun Dis Rep* **27**(10): 85–90.

Brachman PS and Freidlander AM (1999). Anthrax. In *Vaccines*, third edition, Plotkin SA and Orenstein WA (eds). WB Saunders Company: 629–637.

Carey AB and Meltzer EO (1992). Diagnosis and 'desensitization' in tetanus vaccine hypersensitivity. *Ann Allergy* **69**: 336–338.

Classen DC and Classen JB (1997). The timing of paediatric immunisation and the risk of insulin-dependent diabetes mellitus. *Infect Dis Clin Pract* **6**: 449.

Confavreux C, Suissa S, Saddier P, Bourdes V, *et al.* (2001). Vaccinations and the risk of relapse of multiple sclerosis. *N Engl J Med* **344**: 319–326.

Dales L, Hammer SJ and Smith NJ (2001). Time trends in autism and in MMR immunisation coverage in California. *J Am Med Assoc* **285**(9): 1183–1185.

Da Silveira CM, Salisbury BM and de Quadros CA (1997). Measles vaccination and Guillain–Barré syndrome. *Lancet* **349**: 14–16.

Dourado I, Cunha S, da Gloria Teixera M, Farrington CP, *et al.* (2000). Outbreak of aseptic meningitis associated with mass vaccination with a Urabe-containing measles-mumps-rubella vaccine. *Am J Epidem* **151**: 524–530.

Farrington CP (in press). Control without separate controls: evaluation of vaccine safety using case-only methods. *Vaccine.*

Farrington P, Pugh S, Colville A, Flower A, *et al.* (1995). A new method for active surveillance of adverse events from diphtheria/tetanus/pertussis and measles/mumps/rubella vaccines. *Lancet* **345**: 567–569.

Farrington CP, Nash J and Miller E (1996). Case series analysis of adverse reactions to vaccines: a comparative evaluation. *Am J Epidemiol* **143**: 1165–1173.

Farrington CP, Miller E and Taylor B (2001). MMR and autism: further evidence against a causal association. *Vaccine* **19**: 3632–3635.

Fine PE and Clarkson JA (1986). Individual versus public priorities in the determination of optimal vaccination policies. *Am J Epidemiol* **124**: 1012–1020.

Forsey T, Bentley ML, Minor PD and Begg N (1992). Mumps vaccines and meningitis. *Lancet* **340**: 980.

Gangarosa EJ, Galazka AM, Wolfe CR, Phillips LM, *et al.* (1998). Impact of anti-vaccine movements on pertussis control: the untold story. *Lancet* **351**: 356–361.

Gherardi RK, Coquet M, Cherin P, Belec L, *et al*, (2001). Macrophagic myofasciitis lesions assess long-term persistence of vaccine-derived aluminium hydroxide in muscle. *Brain* **124**: 1821–1831.

Gillberg C and Heijbel H (1998). MMR and autism. *Autism* **2**: 423–424.

Grange JM (1998). Complications of bacille Calmette–Guerin (BCG) vaccination and immunotherapy and their management. *Commun Dis Public Health* **1**: 84–88.

Griffin MR, Taylor JA, Daugherty JR and Ray WA (1992). No increased risk for invasive bacterial infection found following diphtheria–tetanus–pertussis immunisation. *Pediatrics* **89**: 640–642.

Kaye JA, Melero-Montes M and Jick H (2001). Mumps, measles and rubella vaccine and the incidence of autism recorded by general practitioners: a time trend analysis. *Br Med J* **322**: 460–463.

Kramarz P, DeStefanio F, Garguillo P, Davis R, *et al.* (2000). Does influenza vaccination exacerbate asthma? *Arch Fam Med* **9**: 617–623.

Maclure M (1991). The case-crossover design: a method for studying transient effects on the risk of acute events. *Am J Epidem* **133**: 144–153.

Maclure M and Mittleman MA (2000). Should we use a case-crossover design? *Annu Rev Public Health* **21**: 193–221.

Marth E and Kleinhappl B (2001). Albumin is a necessary stabilizer of TBE-vaccine to avoid fever in children after vaccination. *Vaccine* **20**: 532–537.

Measles Vaccination Committee (1966). Vaccination against measles: a clinical trial of live measles vaccine given alone and live measles vaccine preceded by killed vaccine. *Br Med J* **I**: 441–446.

Miller C, Miller E, Rowe K, Bowie C, *et al.* (1989). Surveillance of symptoms following MMR vaccine in children. *Practitioner* **233**: 69–75.

Miller CL (1982). Surveillance after measles vaccination in children. *Practitioner* **226**: 535–537.

Miller D, Madge N, Diamond J, Wadsworth J, *et al.* (1993). Pertussis immunisation and serious acute neurological illness in children. *Br Med J* **307**: 1171–1176.

Miller D, Wadsworth J, Diamond J and Ross E (1997). Measles vaccination and neurological events. *Lancet* **349**: 730–731.

Miller E (2002). Studies of exposure to thiomersal (thimerosal) containing vaccines in UK children and developmental outcome. Testimony submitted to the House Committee on Government Reform Hearing on the Status of Research in Vaccine Safety and Autism, 16 June 2002.

Miller E, Goldacre M, Pugh S, Colville A, *et al*. (1993). Risk of aseptic meningitis after measles, mumps and rubella vaccine in UK children. *Lancet* **341**: 979–982.

Miller E, Waight P, Farrington P, Andrews N, *et al*. (2001). Idiopathic thrombocytopenic purpura and MMR vaccine (short report). *Arch Dis Child* **84**: 227–229.

Miller E, Andrews N, Waight P and Taylor B (2003). Bacterial infections, immune overload and MMR vaccination. *Arch Dis Child* **88**: 222–223.

Morris A and Aldulaimi D (2002). New evidence for a vital pathogenic mechanism for a new variant inflammatory bowel disease and development disorder? *J Clin Pathol: Mol Pathol* **55**: 83.

Murphy TV, Gargiullo PN, Massoudi MS, Nelson DB, *et al*. (2001). Intussusception among infants given an oral rotavirus vaccine. *N Eng J Med* **344**: 564–572.

Nieminen U, Peltola H, Syrjälä MT, Mäkipernaa A, *et al*. (1993). Acute thrombocytopenic purpura following measles, mumps and rubella (MMR) vaccination. A report from 23 patients. *Acta Paediatr* **82**: 267–270.

Patja A, Makinen-Kiljunen S, Davidkin I, Paunio M, *et al*. (2001). Allergic reactions to measles–mumps–rubella vaccination. *Pediatrics* **107**: E27

Peltola H and Heinonen OP (1986). Frequency of true adverse reactions to measles–mumps–rubella vaccine. A double-blind placebo-controlled trial in twins. *Lancet* **i**: 939–942.

Ray WA and Griffen MR (1989). Use of Medicaid data for pharmaco-epidemiology. *Am J Epidemiol* **129**: 837–849.

Rosenthal S and Chen R (1995). The reporting sensitivities of two passive surveillance systems for vaccine adverse events. *Am J Public Health* **85**: 1706–1709.

Sakaguchi M and Inouye S (2000). IgE sensitisation to gelatin: the probable role of gelatin-containing diphtheria–tetanus–acellular pertussis (DTaP) vaccines. *Vaccine* **18**: 2055–2058.

Sardinas MA, Cardenas AZ, Marie GC, Pena MS, *et al*. (2001). Lack of association between intussusception and oral polio vaccine in Cuban children. *Eur J Epidemiol* **17**: 783–787.

Scheifele D, Law B, Jadavji T, Halperin S, *et al*. (1998). Disseminated bacille Calmette–Guerin infection; three recent Canadian cases. *Can Commun Dis Rep* **124**: 69–72.

Shoenfeld Y and Aron-Maor A (2000). Vaccination and autoimmunity-'vaccinosis': a dangerous liaison? *J Autoimmun* **14**: 1–10.

Singh VK, Lin SX and Yang VC (1998). Serological association of measles virus and human herpes virus-6 with brain autoantiboodies in autistic children. *Clin Immunol Immunopathol* **89**: 105–108.

Skov PS, Pelck I, Ebbesen F and Poulsen LK (1997). Hypersensitivity to the diphtheria component in the Di–Te–Pol vaccine. A type I allergic reaction demonstrated by basophil histamine release. *Pediatr Allergy Immunol* **8**: 156–158.

Storsaeter J, Olin P, Renemar B, Lagergard T, *et al*. (1988). Mortality and morbidity from invasive bacterial infections during a clinical trial of acellular pertussis vaccines in Sweden. *Pediatr Infect Dis J* **7**: 637–645.

Stratton KR, Howe CJ and Johnston Jr RB (eds) (1994). Immunologic reactions. In *Adverse Events Associated with Childhood Vaccines. Evidence Bearing on Causality*. Vaccine Safety Committee, Division of Health Promotion and Disease Prevention, Institute of Medicine. National Academy Press: Washington, DC: 59–66.

Strebel PM, Ion-Nedelcu N, Baughman AL, Sutter RW, *et al*. (1995). Intramuscular injections within 30 days of immunisation with oral poliovirus vaccine – a risk factor for vaccine-associated paralytic poliomyelitis. *New Eng J Med* **332**(8): 500–506.

Taylor B, Miller E, Farrington P, Petropoulos MC, *et al*. (1999). Autism and measles, mumps, and rubella vaccine: no epidemiological evidence for a causal association. *Lancet* **353**: 2026–2029.

The Institute for Vaccine Safety Diabetes Workshop Panel (1999). Childhood immunisations and type 1 diabetes: summary of an Institute of Medicine Workshop. *Pediatr Infect Dis J* **18**: 217–222.

Triger DR, Kurtz JB, MacCallum FO and Wright W (1972). Raised antibody titres to measles and rubella in chronic active hepatitis. *Lancet* **i**: 665–667.

Uhlmann V, Martin CM, Shiels O, Pilkington L, *et al.* (2002). Potential viral pathogenic mechanism for new variant inflammatory bowel disease. *J Clin Pathol: Mol Pathol* **55**: 84–90.

Van't Veen AJ (2001). Vaccines without thiomersal: why so necessary, why so long coming? *Drugs* **61**(5): 565–572.

Wakefield AJ (1999). MMR vaccination and autism. *Lancet* **354**: 949–950.

Weibel RE, Casertya V, Benor DE and Evans G (1998). Acute encephalopathy associated with further attenuated measles vaccines: a review of claims submitted to the National Vaccine Injury Compensation program. *Pediatrics* **101**: 383–387.

WHO (1999). WHO Immunisation safety surveillance. Guidelines for managers of immunisation programmes on reporting and investigating adverse events following immunisation. World Health Organisation, Regional Office for the Western Pacific, Manila, 1999. WPRO/EPI/99.01. WHO field guide for NRAs.

WHO (2002). Global Advisory Committee on Vaccine Safety 20–21 June 2002. Specific section on aluminium-containing vaccines and macrophagic myofasciitis (MMF). *Weekly Epidemiological Record*, 22 November.

WHO (in press). *WHO guidelines on Clinical Evaluation of Vaccines: Regulatory Expectations. Annex 1*. WHO Technical Report Series.

Yergeau A, Alain L, Pless R and Robert Y (1996). Adverse events temporally associated with meningococcal vaccines. *Can Med Assoc J* **154**: 503–507.

15

Ethical Issues in Drug Safety

M. D. B. Stephens

Introduction

This chapter has two sections: the first on ethics in clinical trials and the second on ethics within the pharmaceutical industry.

Ethics in clinical trials

There are two competing approaches to ethics in clinical trials:

- *Individual ethics.* What is best for the present patient? This is the approach of the practising clinician and is represented by the Bayesian methodology (Palmer, 1993). It must always prevail when dealing with serious type B suspected adverse drug reactions (ADRs).

- *Collective ethics.* What is best for the population of patients or society? This is the approach of most statisticians and epidemiologists and is represented by standard statistical methods. This is at its strongest when applied to common mild, reversible type A ADRs.

It has been suggested that individual ethics should dominate the early clinical trials, i.e. phases I and II, whereas collective ethics should dominate phases III and IV (Palmer, 1993). Those working in pharmacovigilance with clinical trials need to be familiar with the associated ethical problems and their implications.

400 BC   Hippocratic Oath

1846   American Medical Association Code of Ethics.

The Nazi experiments on humans were so deplorable that the medical world took action in:

Stephens' Detection of New Adverse Drug Reactions Fifth Edition edited by John Talbot and Patrick Waller
© 2004 John Wiley & Sons, Ltd   ISBN: 0 470 84552 X

1947   Nuremberg Code

1948   Declaration of Geneva

1964   'Declaration of Helsinki' to control clinical research and from time to time these
        have been up-dated. The last up-date was in October 2000 and one of the most
        debated points was on the use of placebo.

Arguments for and against placebo-controlled trials

Pre 52nd World Medical Association General Assembly, Edinburgh, October 2000

In the Declaration of Helsinki (South Africa 1996 amendments), it said 'In any medical
study, every patient – including those of a control group, if any – should be assured of the
best proven diagnostic and therapeutic methods'. Does the last sentence mean that a placebo
control group is not ethical unless there is no proven treatment for a disease?

- One clinical pharmacologist has said 'the blanket Helsinki recommendations which
  undermine the use of placebos generally, need revision' (Collier, 1995) and he goes on
  to say 'Incidentally, it seems to preclude study of "active" experimental drugs since
  proof of their efficacy cannot come until the trial is completed'.

- Dr Lasagna adds weight to this argument by stressing the scientific advantages of
  placebo studies (Lasagna, 1995).

- This has been countered 'But if blind assessment can be achieved in a comparative trial
  of two active treatments is there any point to using a placebo group'? And later 'If we
  adhere to these ethical guidelines, placebo controlled trials should become infrequent as
  medical knowledge accumulates. Then the scientific method of comparing active
  treatments against one another will be essential to understand' (Rothman, 1996).

- In reply to Rothman, three letters in the BMJ stress the scientific need for placebo
  studies (Georgiou, 1996; McQuay and Moore, 1996; Double, 1996).

- In an article entitled 'Comparing Treatments' there is a subtitle 'Comparison should be
  against active treatments rather than placebos'. The authors give the reasons for the
  early use of placebos, 'In the United States the Food and Drug Administration [FDA],
  historically, has required evidence from two placebo controlled trials before licensing a
  new compound, although some recent approvals have been based on a single trial'
  (Henry and Hill, 1995).

- The use of placebo in a fluticasone study of allergic rhinitis was said to be of little
  relevance to clinicians compared with the use of an active control (Gallant, 1995;
  Weinberg 1995).

What are the objections to accepting an active control group instead of a placebo group?
If the new drug seems indistinguishable from the active control 'You don't really know what

you've got' according to Dr Robert Temple of the FDA. 'The control may be a poor drug, or the trial may have been incapable of detecting true differences between the drugs. Regulators may therefore license an inferior product' (Henry and Hill, 1995).

Early trials using a surrogate endpoint, such as blood pressure, may only need a few patients when comparing a new drug with placebo to show that it works; but, if equivalence with another active drug is required then the trial numbers escalate, as will the cost and time to completion. In order to establish superiority over another active drug the number of patients required will depend on the difference demanded (see Chapter 1). Is it possible to defend the use of placebo as a control for the second drug of a new class or performing a second study after a placebo-controlled study has shown that the first drug of a new class is efficacious?

- Glaxo staff have done so in regard to peptic ulcer disease in the past. Their conclusion was that although placebo-controlled trials in appropriate patient populations place additional ethical concerns on investigators, institutional review boards and sponsors, the benefits derived from the conduct of scientifically sound clinical trials that result in the approval of new drug therapies far outweigh the risks of a placebo control group (Cocoa *et al.* 1996).

- Again, Glaxo, replying to criticism concerning placebo use in a three-arm study (placebo, lamotrigine, or lithium) for prevention of relapse of mania or depression for 1 year, says 'The use of placebo in these studies is a regulatory requirement for proof of efficacy: it also means that studies can be smaller and shorter. This exposes fewer patients to an unproven intervention and gives an answer about efficacy more quickly. If that answer is positive patients should be able to benefit early. It is difficult to see how there was 'therapeutic equipoise' between placebo, lamotrigine and lithium.

- If it is negative, fewer patients will be exposed to ineffective treatment' (Armstrong, 1998; Dollop, 1998).

'The argument that all placebo-controlled clinical trials are unethical if an effective or partly effective treatment is known has occasionally been advanced, but has not gained general acceptance. An interpretation of the ethical guidelines that has been accepted more generally is that use of placebo controls, in conditions for which there is an effective treatment, is ethical – provided that the use of placebo for the duration of the study does not place the patient at increased risk of irreversible harm or cause unacceptable discomfort' (Stein and Pinks, 1999).

- A discussion on the use of placebo, in ondansetron trials for post-operative nausea and vomiting, supports this latter view emphasizing that the ethics of recruiting patients into trials that cannot yield sensible results is dubious (Tamer *et al.*, 1998).

- The ethics of using a placebo in controlled trials with ondansetron in post-chemo-therapy vomiting have been questioned and the American Medical Association's Council on Ethics and Judicial Affairs quoted 'It is fundamental social policy that the advancement of scientific knowledge must always be secondary to primary concern for the individual' (Citron, 1993).

There are different views as to the justification of the use of placebo:

1. For a placebo-controlled trial four questions must be answered:

   - Was there any therapeutic intervention available that could be reasonably assumed to be less harmful than the placebo control?

   - Did the placebo control pose more than a minimal risk to those patients?

   - Was the study designed in every way possible to minimize potential harm to the patients receiving placebo?

   - Were the patients fully and accurately informed of the additional risk of being in the placebo group (Citron, 1993)?

2. For a placebo-controlled clinical trial to be morally justified the following conditions should appertain:

   - There must be an uncertainty as to whether the drug is any more likely to be better than a placebo, i.e. equipoise – meaning that the expectation of competing therapeutic alternatives must be equal in terms of balancing both benefit and harm. A review of therapeutic studies in multiple myeloma indicated that commercially funded studies showed violation of equipoise (Djulbegovic et al., 2000). It must be very rare that the expectations with a new drug do not outweigh the known benefits of placebo.

   - In most cases there must be no agreed alternative treatment better than placebo. Exceptions to this could arise if the statistical advantage of using a 'coarse' comparator like placebo enable a much smaller trial to be conducted as a result, though such trials give a poor picture of the rival merits of the active drugs themselves and, as such, may be of doubtful value.

   - There must be a significant need for the knowledge to be obtained by the placebo-controlled trial (it must be an important question whether the proposed treatment is better than placebo).

   - There must be a reasonable possibility that the new drug can indeed turn out to be better than placebo (see above).

   - The illness under treatment must not be so serious that any delay in receiving an active drug would be clinically harmful or dangerous.

Placebo-controlled studies should be the exception and not the norm, and it should take exceptional circumstances to justify them (Evans and Evans, 1996). These conditions have been taken from a book by the authors that is well worth reading, since it has been written for members of ethical committees.

The exception mentioned in the second condition above needs amplification, since all placebo-controlled studies require fewer patients than those with an active control.

- In the Glaxo paper, in order to show a 40 per cent difference between placebo (presumed to heal 35 per cent of ulcers) and the new drug there needs to be 28 patients in each group, or if the allocation is 2:1 then 21 patients in the placebo group to 42 in the active group. To show equivalence between two active drugs would require 408 patients under the same circumstances. Although it is possible to reduce the risk run by those in the placebo group by excluding those with predisposing factors, it is extremely unlikely to make the risks equal to those taking an active control. Can one equate the increased risk of 28 patients taking placebo with the lesser risk of the 408 taking an active control?

- The Glaxo authors also put the point that the placebo control has fewer patients at risk from the ADRs of the new study drug. The chances of discovering ADRs with a new drug increase with the number of patients treated, so this is only relevant if the drug is scrapped and no further studies are undertaken with it. Would the FDA accept an NDA with only 28 patients in each group of a placebo-controlled study? If so, then there was a large amount of overkill in the placebo studies with new drugs for peptic ulcer disease. The problem is debated further in a discussion paper (Collier, 1995).

In a leading article in the *Lancet* on the defence of the FDA, 'the acceptance of placebo-controlled evidence in preference to comparator drug trial data is a serious flaw in the regulator process (Anon., 1995). Ethics committees have been criticized for endorsing proposals for new placebo-controlled research when existing evidence shows that an active form of treatment is better than placebo (Savulescu *et al.*, 1996). In phase I studies the sponsor should consider 'Would I volunteer to take part in this study?' Ten out of 12 companies had special ethics committees for phase I studies (Baber, 1994; Gill and Baber, 1995). Unfortunately, there have been circumstances where scientists have submitted themselves as volunteers to risks that no ethics committee would ever sanction, so this question does not solve the problem. Perhaps it should be 'Would I allow any of my children to volunteer?'

Placebo run-in

Many clinical trials organized by the industry have placebo run-in periods and the reasons given are:

- weeds out non-compliers (Hulley and Cummings, 1988; Spilker, 1991);

- eliminates placebo responders (Spilker, 1991);

- ensures the patients are stable (Pocock, 1983);

- washes out previous treatment;

- provides a period for baseline measurement.

This has been said to be incompatible with informed consent (Senn, 1997). However, it would be justified if:

- the use of placebo has negligible risk and acceptable discomfort;

- it enhances the science or interpretation of the study;

- the 'deception' is covered adequately in the information provided to patients;

- agreement by an independent ethics committee that these conditions hold (Ramsay, 1997).

During the World Medical Association (WMA) Edinburgh (2000) meeting, but prior to the publication of the agreement, Rothman and Michels suggested that the declaration should be strengthened despite opposition from the FDA whilst Baum was against this (Rothman *et al.*, 2000). These are the arguments used before and after the 1996 amendment of the Declaration of Helsinki (South Africa) but prior to the 2000 amendments (Edinburgh). How do the latter modify these requirements?

Declaration of Helsinki (Edinburgh 2000 amendments)

The most important document regarding ethics in clinical trials is the Declaration of Helsinki, 1964, amended October 2000 (*Pharmaceutical Physician* **12**(1): 22–24 or **14**(5): 279–281), which should be attached to all trial protocols. The amendments of the 48th WMA General Assembly in South Africa dated 1996 have been further amended by the 52nd WMA General Assembly (Edinburgh) in October 2000. The second and third paragraphs of the introduction are:

- 'It is the duty of the physician to promote and safeguard the health of the people. The physician's knowledge and conscience are dedicated to the fulfilment of this duty' (*Collective approach*).

- The Declaration of Geneva of the WMA binds the physician with the words 'The health of my patient will be my first consideration' and the International Code of Medical Ethics declares that 'A physician shall act only in the patient's interest when providing medical care which may have the effect of weakening the physical and mental condition of the patient' (*Individual approach*).

Paragraph 16 in the section entitled 'Basic principles for all medical research' states:

Every medical research project involving human subjects should be preceded by careful assessment of predictable risks and burdens in comparison with foreseeable benefits to the subject or to others. This does not preclude the participation of healthy volunteers in medical research.

The design of all studies should be publicly available.

The sentence in the previous amendment, 'Concern for the interest of the subject must always prevail over the interest of science and society', has been removed and is now in paragraph 5 as 'In medical research on human subjects, considerations related to the well-being of the human subject should take precedence over the interests of science and society' (i.e. *individual ethic must always be put before the collective ethic*).

Paragraph 7 of the same section states:

Physicians should abstain from engaging in research projects involving human subjects unless they are confident that the risks involved have been adequately assessed and can be satisfactorily managed. Physicians should cease any investigations if the risks are found to outweigh the potential benefits or if there is conclusive proof of positive and beneficial results.

Paragraph 29 of the section entitled 'Additional principles for medical research combined with medical care' reads:

The benefits, risks, burdens and effectiveness of a new method should be tested against those of the best current prophylactic, diagnostic, and therapeutic methods. This does not exclude the use of placebo, or no treatment, in studies where no proven prophylactic, diagnostic or therapeutic method exists.

Post 52nd World Medical Association Assembly, Edinburgh, October 2000

This has implications for research in developing countries, where the testing of new drugs against the best current treatment would have massively increased the cost of research. Subsequent to the Edinburgh amendments a pharmaceutical company disallowed or postponed eight new studies because of the new guidelines (Human *et al.*, 2001). A further WMA meeting in France 'clarified' its rules on placebo. 'The association agreed that the use of placebo in research trials might be ethically acceptable in certain circumstances:

- Where for compelling and scientifically sound methodological reasons its use was necessary to determine the efficacy or safety of a prophylactic, diagnostic or therapeutic method: or

- Where a prophylactic, diagnostic or therapeutic method was being investigated for a minor condition and the patients who receive placebo would not be subject to any additional risk of serious or irreversible harm'.

The responses to these changes were:

- Professor Darbyshire, director of the Medical Research Council (MRC) clinical trials unit in London, said 'It is still not very clear, but at least it does clarify that using a trial with a no treatment group, who are taking a placebo, is no longer completely unacceptable'.

- Professor Whitworth of the MRC said that it might prevent some ethical and necessary research from going ahead (Ferriman, 2001).

- This clarification has been called a retreat from the WMA's previous position (Bland, 2002).

- The most recent version of the Declaration of Helsinki is imprecise and ambiguous (Forster *et al.*, 2001).

- Some members of the Committee on Proprietary Medicinal Products (CPMP) have said 'The section (paragraph 29) makes no exception for trials done in the specific population of patients who would subsequently benefit from a successful outcome of the research, even when there is adequate patient consent and careful avoidance of any irreversible harm or other ethically unacceptable consequences, such as long-term severe pain.' They finish by saying, 'Provided that the safety and interests of individual patients are carefully protected, the conduct of placebo controlled trials in these situations remains vital if correct regulatory decisions are to be made on the basis of reliable research. This outcome is clearly in the best interest of patients' (Lewis *et al.*, 2002).

Unfortunately, 'adequate patient consent' is problematic and 'careful avoidance of any irreversible harm or any other ethically unacceptable consequences' cannot be guaranteed. The WMA clarification has so muddied the waters that individuals will interpret the declaration differently and for their own purpose. A checklist has been designed to help Institutional Review Boards (IRBs) evaluate protocols for placebo use (available from www.centerwatch.com/irbchecklist) (Cavazos *et al.*, 2002). This leaves the ethical committees or IRBs to arbitrate, and many of those involved in clinical trial ethical committees are non-financial stakeholders.

Stopping studies

The 2000 version of the Declaration of Helsinki says 'Physicians should cease any investigations if the risks are found to outweigh the potential benefits or if there is conclusive proof of positive and beneficial results' (provision 17).

There are cases where ethically approved studies have become unethical either due to one drug having established superiority before all the patients have been recruited or that the adverse effects of one drug have outweighed any benefit and, therefore, need to be stopped. The time when a difference becomes statistically significant may not coincide with the time when the study becomes unethical.

- The basic ethical conflict in monitoring trial results is to balance the interests of patients within the trial – that is, the individual ethics of randomizing the next patient and the longer term interest of obtaining reliable conclusions on sufficient data – that is, the collective ethics of making appropriate treatment policies for future patients (Pocock, 1992). The Declaration of Helsinki says, 'Considerations related to the well-being of the human subjects should take precedence over the interests of science and society'. Professor Pocock's conclusions were, 'The ethical dilemma faced by data monitoring committees has no easy solution but it is important to note that premature stopping based on limited evidence can have severe consequences either by introducing exaggerated claims so that inadequate treatments enter clinical practice or by failing to collect sufficient evidence on effective treatments in order to convince rightly sceptical clinicians of their true merits'.

- In a paper entitled 'Premature discontinuation of clinical trials for reasons not related to efficacy, safety or feasibility' there is the phrase 'Sometimes, however, trials are scuttled by their sponsors'. They go on to cite an example. The authors finish by saying 'The usual clause according to which the sponsor "reserves the right to discontinue any study for administrative reasons at any time" should no longer be present in the protocol of a study of morbidity and mortality' (Lièvre *et al.*, 2001).

- A further comment on this study was that 'lack of commercial pay off is not a legitimate reason for stopping a trial' (Evans and Pocock, 2001).

Ethics committees

These include the IRB (USA), Research Ethics Review Boards (Canada), Local Research Ethics Committees (LRECs) and Multicentre Research Ethics Committees (MRECs, UK) and Comités Consultative pour la Protection des Personnes dans les Recherches Biomédicales (CCPPRBs, France).

'All research involving direct contact with patients or healthy people is to be submitted for independent ethical review and for the individual subject's prior consent' (Diamond *et al.*, 1994). A project which is not scientifically valid cannot be ethical (McLean, 1995).

The duties and composition of Independent Ethics Committees (IECs) are laid down in the Guideline for Good Clinical Practice, 1996 (ICH E6 CPMP/ICH/135/95 Para. 3); but, as guidelines they do not have legal status. Their main function is to safeguard the rights, safety and well-being of all trial subjects. The IEC should consist of a reasonable number of members, who collectively have the qualifications and experience to review and evaluate the science, medical aspects and ethics of the proposed trial. It is recommended that there be at least five members, of whom one member whose primary area of interest is in a non-scientific area and one member who is independent of the institution/trial site.

- *United States of America.* The US equivalent of the Ethics Committee is the IRB (Levine, 1997). The US Department of Health and Human Services (DHHS) require in an IRB consisting at least five members, of which one is a non-scientist (e.g. lawyer, ethicist, member of the clergy) and at least one member who is not otherwise affiliated with the institution. All ethical committees and IRBs exclude those having conflicting interests (21CFR 56.107).

- *United Kingdom.* LRECs and MRECs in the National Health Service (NHS) are advisory committees established under the auspices of the Department of Health. Owing to problems in seeking ethical committee approval with large multicentre studies, special committees, the MRECs, have been set up to deal with them (NHS guidance note HSG (97) 23, April 1997). These require that out of the 15 to 18 members, three to four should be non-professional lay persons and that there should be one statistician and one 'qualitative research expert', e.g. social scientist. In all, at least, one-third (but no more than six in total) will be lay (Ethics Committee Review of Multi-

centre Research, 1997). It was argued afterwards that the central problems of inefficiency and ineffectiveness . . . remained largely untouched (Evans, 1997).

- *Europe*. The Ethics Working Party of the European Forum for Good Clinical Practice
  (EFGCP) guidelines recommend the following minimum membership for ethics
  committees: two physicians sharing between them experience in biomedical research
  conducted according to GCP and independence from the institution where the research
  is carried out; one lay person, one lawyer and one paramedical (nurse, paramedic or
  pharmacist). Conflict of interest is not defined. The EFGCP board is dominated by
  members from the industry (EFGCP, 1997). For studies which are multi-national there
  is a European Ethical Review Committee (EERC) that reviews specifically multinational trials (Bennett 1995, 1997; Cordier, 1997; Foster 1997).
     In the USA, France and Scandinavia the ethical committees are an integrated part of
  drug trial regulation (Hvidberg, 1994).

- *Developing countries*. The problem of research in under-developed areas has been
  tackled by The Nuffield Council on Bioethics with *Ethics of research related to
  healthcare in developing countries*. It is important that the lack of regulation in these
  countries does not cause their exploitation (National Council of Bioethics, 2002;
  Zumula and Costello, 2002).

The ethical committee has a responsibility to monitor a study and to intervene where
necessary. This could be done either by a mid-term interim report or by receiving an interim
report every 6 months (Evans and Evans, 1996). It has been suggested that the independent
ethical committee (IEC)/IRB should be informed of adverse events as they occur (Sniderman, 1996). The Guideline for Good Clinical Practice, 1996 (ICH E6 CPMP/ICH/135/95)
states that the investigator must report to the IRB/IEC promptly all ADRs that are both
serious and unexpected and new information that may affect adversely the safety of the
subjects or the conduct of the trial. Also, changes increasing the risk to subjects and/or
affecting significantly the conduct of the trial and deviations from, or changes of, the
protocol to eliminate immediate hazards to the trial subjects must be reported (see paras:
3.3.8; 3.3.9 and 5.17).

An Independent Data-Monitoring Committee (IDMC), separate from any ethics committee, may be established by the sponsor to assess, at intervals, the progress of a clinical trial,
the safety data, and the critical efficacy endpoints and to recommend to the sponsor whether
to continue, modify, or stop a trial (ICH Guideline on GCP, 1996, section 5.5.2). In some
large phase III studies there may be an IDMC and an IRB/IEC both monitoring and possibly
stopping a study. The company pharmacovigilance staff will need to make sure that any
serious, unexpected adverse event (AE) is notified to the regulatory authority, the IDMC and
the IRB/IEC.

The guidelines on the practice of ethics committees say, referring to the situation where
society rather than the individual may benefit, 'In such situations, however large the benefit,
to expose a participant to anything more the minimal risk needs very careful consideration
and would rarely be ethical'. Minimal risk in everyday life could include travelling on public
transport or private car but not by pedal or motor cycle. In medicine they would be no more
likely and not greater than the risk attached to routine medical or psychological examina-

tion. (Tripp, 1996; CIOMS 2002). 'However, there is substantial disagreement about what constitutes minimal risk, and the concept is applied quite variously' (Woodward, 1999).

Comments:

- There is currently widespread frustration in the research community, in the regulatory authorities and in the pharmaceutical industry with the efficiency of such committees. At the same time there are doubts about the effectiveness of these independent committees in protecting patients (Ashcroft and Pfeffer, 2001).

- 'The committee is not – perhaps never could be – truly independent of those whose proposals it is scrutinizing, and this lack of independence may have an impact on the kinds of questions that researchers ask themselves' (McLean, 1995).

- There is large variation in the mode of operation of individual LRECs, and costs vary by greater than 400 per cent (Dunn *et al.*, 2000).

- Some high-profile scandals in the ethics of research in the UK and USA have caused concern, and it has been suggested that there should be less secrecy surrounding ethical committees (Ashcroft and Pfeffer, 2001). In the deaths (in the USA) of Ellen Roche (hexamethonium) and Jesse Gelsinger (gene therapy) errors of the ethics committees may have been factors (Savulescu, 2002).

- The chairman of SmithKline Beecham said, 'The processes of ethical and research committees are slow and confused' (Smith, 2000).

- There have been problems because there is no comprehensive system for compiling information regarding harm due to misjudgements or misstatements of risk, and many IRBs are overwhelmed with AE reports and do not have the capability to review them carefully (Woodward, 1999).

- 'Ethics committees are simply not set up or resourced to adequately protect the interests of participants in research' (Savulescu, 2002).

A survey of 321 GCP audits (GP surgeries or hospital departments) from 31 companies showed:

- Approval was not obtained from local ethics committee/IRB in 24 per cent of studies.

There was no evidence that the following items were reviewed and/or approved (if necessary) by an ethics committee:

- current investigators brochure – non-compliance 65 per cent;

- primary care physician to be informed of study participants – non-compliance 54 per cent;

- plans to review data collected to ensure safety – non-compliance 28 per cent;

- risks to study subjects – non-compliance 14 per cent.

- Final protocol (approved by sponsor/CRO and investigators) – non-compliance 43 percent

- Reports of serious/unexpected ADRs – non-compliance 92 per cent

- Summary of serious AE (from the current study and other studies) – non-compliance 85 per cent (Bohaychuk and Ball, 1998).

The extent to which an IRB can evaluate accurately the information in AE reports is questionable because:

1. They receive individual AEs, typically, without explanation of how the event relates to any other events previously observed.

2. In international studies, the difference in standards of care and language may make the clinical significance of reports more difficult to interpret.

3. In blinded studies they will not have the treatment code or information on efficacy.

4. Each IRB may only have access to data from trials over which it has authority.

5. It is likely that many do not have the expertise or access to appropriate information to allow them to evaluate properly the issues of safety and benefits.

6. IRBs have become inundated with AEs (Morse *et al.*, 2001).

- If an IRB expresses concerns about inclusion or exclusion criteria the sponsor may claim that the other IRBs did not question the criteria and that it cannot modify the criteria on the basis of one IRB's concerns.

- If the FDA consider an agreement about the design of a protocol 'binding on the review division' an IRB may have difficulty in effecting any change (Mann, 2002).

Conflict (competing) of interest

Definition: a set of conditions in which professional judgement concerning a primary interest (such as patients welfare or the validity of research) tends to be unduly influenced by a secondary interest (such as financial gain).

The 2000 version of the Declaration of Helsinki says 'The researcher should also submit to the committee, for review, information regarding funding, sponsors, institutional affiliations, and other potential conflicts of interest' (provision 13). 'Each potential subject must be adequately informed of ... sources of funding ... potential risks of the study and the discomfort it may entail' (provision 22). 'Sources of funding, institutional affiliations and any possible conflicts of interest should be declared in the publication' (provision 27).

In several areas of medicine, doctors are asked to declare any conflict of interest. In some cases they, themselves, decide what constitutes conflict of interest and in others they are defined for them.

The FDA (1999) criteria for investigators:

- Significant shareholdings of more than US$50 000.

- Any financial arrangement between the sponsor and the investigator whereby the value of the compensation could be influenced by the outcome.

- Compensation other than that associated with conducting the study (e.g. grant to fund ongoing research, equipment grants, or honoraria).

- Proprietary interest in the product tested held by the investigator (e.g. patents, trade-marks, etc.).

The National Institutes of Health give a level for disclosure as 'income of more than US$10 000 per year from a company that might be affected by the research involved or ownership of equity worth more than US$10 000 or representing more than 5 per cent ownership of such a company (Washington Fax, 2001).

Most major US universities have policies on conflict of interest but lack specificity about the kinds of relationship that are permitted or prohibited (Cho et al., 2000)

The Australian Drug Evaluation Committee (ADEC) competing interest guidelines give:

- A member who has at anytime been involved with a pharmaceutical product under consideration by the committee and has personally received payment for that involve-ment in any manner, including via an intermediary agent for the pharmaceutical industry.

- A member who has a current pecuniary interest in the pharmaceutical company concerned.

- A member who has a current pecuniary interest relating to a product that is a competitor to the product under consideration.

- A member who has a particular involvement in the development of pharmaceutical products (e.g. sitting on an advisory board or as principal investigator involved in the design of clinical trial protocols.

- Involvement in pharmaceutical industry sponsored trials of a product under consideration or a competitive product by the provision of patients for inclusion in a multicentre trial or participation in investigators meetings where the member does not have an involvement in trial design, monitoring or preparation of the trial report (Tattersall and Olver, 1999).

The CPMP define them as:

- Employment in the pharmaceutical industry.

- Financial interests in the capital of a pharmaceutical company, e.g. shares.

- Work currently or previously conducted by the member in return for payment, on behalf of the pharmaceutical industry.

- Other interests that the member considers the European Medicines Evaluation Agency (EMEA) ought to know about (Abraham and Lewis, 2000).

'Others, however, point with concern to the numerical dominance on most IRBs by scientists and health professionals; one presumes that such persons value things differently than the majority of the population. Almost certainly, for example, health professionals and scientists typically place a higher value on the pursuit of knowledge for its own sake than do persons outside the health professions or academia' (Levine, 1997).

'In recruiting expert members, the ADEC increasingly finds that senior specialists have been the recipients of funding from the pharmaceutical industry (McEwan, 1998).

Several American universities include any immediate family interests. Inevitably there are occasions concerning a married/unmarried couple where one works for a pharmaceutical company and the other spouse for a regulatory authority. All these refer to financial interests but there are others: the *BMJ* says to potential authors 'You might want to disclose another sort of competing interest that would embarrass you if it became generally known after publication. The following list gives some examples:

- A close relationship with, or a strong antipathy to, a person whose interests may be affected by publication of your paper.

- An academic link or rivalry with somebody whose interests may be affected by publication of your paper.

- Membership of a political party or special interest group whose interests may be affected by publication of your paper.

- A deep personal or religious conviction that may have affected what you wrote and that readers should be aware of when reading your paper.'

Is self-declared interest a sufficient safeguard? The editor of the *BMJ* has said 'Our impression, supported by the two recent papers, is that many authors are willing to sign that they don't have a conflict of interest when by our definition they do. We have two hypotheses to explain this. Firstly, authors think that an admission of a conflict implies wickedness. We don't think so. Secondly, authors are confident that they have not been influenced by a conflict of interest and so don't tell us they have one. Our response is that bias works in subtle ways and that none of us is blessed with knowledge of our own motivations and mental mechanisms' (Smith, 1998). 'Although many organisations have adopted disclosure as necessary to management of conflicts of interest, there is no evidence that disclosure alone is either sufficient or effective in protection of research integrity and prevention of harm to participants' (Forster *et al.*, 2001). Morse and his colleagues suggest that 'potential conflicts of interest should prevent any sponsor from being the sole monitor for a trial . . . . In definitive phase III trials, we recommend that the sponsor allocate responsibility for safety evaluation to an independent Data Monitoring Committee to minimize conflicts of interest among those making the necessary judgements during a trial' (Morse *et al.*, 2001).

'The impact of institutional conflicts of interest as well as non-financial conflicts of interest at all levels of the research enterprise have not been explored sufficiently and are issues that, like the development of professional norms for individual conflicts of interest, should be rigorously pursued by federal agencies and appropriate interest groups' (Federmann *et al.*, 2003)

Informed consent

Defined in the CPMP guidelines as 'The voluntary confirmation of a subject's willingness to participate in a particular trial, and the documentation thereof. This confirmation should only be sought after information has been given about the trial including an explanation of its objectives, potential benefits and risks and inconveniences, and of the subject's rights and responsibilities in accordance with the current revision of the Declaration of Helsinki'.

Section 1.28 of ICH E6 defines it as 'a process by which a subject voluntarily confirms his or her willingness to participate in a clinical trial, after having been informed of *all aspects* of the trial that are relevant to the subject's decision to participate'.

- 'The guidelines do not specify the extent of the disclosure required in terms of the detail of possible risks' (Hodges, 1991).

- It is difficult to believe that all the information available on a new drug (investigator's brochure, which is only a summary of the data produced by the company) and the standard treatment for a disease is seen, read and understood by every investigator who asks patients for informed consent. It is likely that they are selective in the information they read and again selective in the information they give to each patient. The patient is unlikely to be able to weigh the pros and cons of consent without considering their obligation towards their physician requesting consent, who is in a privileged position.

- The information to be given to the patient may, according to United States law, be of:

  1. Ordinary prudent person standard – What the average patient in the same or similar circumstances wants to know? This propagates the legal myth of the 'ordinary prudent person'

  2. Reasonable physician standard – What risks do individual investigators consider important? This paternalistic approach negates the whole logic of autonomy.

  3. Subjective standard – What risk does this particular subject consider important (Belmont Report, 1979; Klincewicz, *et al.* 2001)? This is the only valid standard .

- 'Informed consent should be an ongoing process that focuses not on a written form or a static disclosure event, but rather on a series of dynamic conversations between the participant and the research staff that should begin before enrolment and be reinforced during each encounter or intervention' (Federmann *et al.*, 2003).

A GCP audit survey of 321 protocols showed:

- Informed consent was obtained from study subjects after the start of the study or after the start of any study procedures (37 per cent).

- The consent documents submitted to the ethics committee/IRB differed from the documents actually used at the study site' (26 per cent).

There was no evidence that the following items were reviewed and/or approved (if necessary) by an ethics committee/IRB:

- consent procedures – non-compliance 12 per cent;

- contents of consent forms/information sheets – non-compliance 10 per cent (Bohaychuk and Ball, 1998).

Comments:

- 'We know how easily patients can give informed consent and we know the patients best protection is not the informed consent but rather the conscientious physician himself' (Cleophas, 1999).

- A review of clinical trial ethics concluded 'For many, informed consent seemed little more than a ritual' (Edwards et al., 1998).

- A questionnaire, 'The Quality of Informed Consent Questionnaire', has been devised and used in 207 cancer patients; 90 per cent were satisfied with process, but 70 per cent did not recognize that the treatment being researched was not proven to be the best for their cancer and only 29 per cent appreciated that they might not receive direct medical benefit from participation (Tattersall, 2001).

- In Japan there is another approach to informed consent, and at Nara Medical University, when they mandated written informed consent in all clinical trials, the rate of refusal soared from about 5 per cent to about 70 per cent (Fukuhara et al., 1997). In a survey of 1217 physicians involved in clinical trials at major medical institutes throughout Japan, 34 per cent said that they thought it was impossible to obtain written informed consent (Ueda, 1996; Fukuhara et al., 1999).

How valuable is informed consent?

- The review by Edwards et al. (1998) referred to three old studies: in one multinational study 47 per cent of responding doctors thought that few patients knew they were taking part in a controlled experiment, even though they had given written consent (Taylor and Kelner, 1987), and in two other studies three-quarters of responding doctors thought their patients rarely understood all the information given to them (Spaight et al., 1984; Blum et al., 1987).

- Four studies show that: immediately after receiving information 34 per cent of patients recall the study's purpose, 25 per cent recall the drug name, and 15 per cent recall side-effects. Ten hours after receiving information 85 per cent of patients recalled benefits and 35 per cent recalled risks. Six days after receiving information, 25 per cent of patients recall the information (DIA Program Notes, 2001).

- After an acute myocardial infarction trial, 31 per cent of patients said that they had full comprehension of the trial, 50 per cent partial understanding and 19 per cent no understanding at all (Yuval *et al.*, 2000).

- In northern Italy, patients had a poor knowledge of the principles and meaning of informed consent so that only 58 per cent recognized the true definition and 80 per cent would not enter a clinical trial involved in research on a new drug (Dazzi *et al.*, 2001).

- In multicentre cancer studies only 58 per cent of clinicians gave full information on all aspects of the trial (Willims and Zwitter, 1994).

- Re birth defects: 'Informed consents are of limited legal utility. They cannot prevent a suit from being filed' (Austrian, 1996).

- Only a third of 167 principal investigators applying to US Midwestern review boards gave a detailed description of the purpose and procedure of the proposed study, and a meaningful discussion of all other areas, such as risks, benefits and alternatives was virtually non-existent (Titus and Keane, 1996).

- Reuters Health Information quote that CenterWatch reported on a survey of 1600 volunteers that took place in January and February 2002 and that 10 per cent of volunteers admitted that they did not review the informed consent form before signing it, 30 per cent didn't understand that the study could carry additional risk, 70 per cent didn't know what to ask at the outset of a trial, 18 per cent consented to the trial without getting input from their personal physician, nurse, family member or another trusted individual. (http://www.medscape.com/viewarticle/433975).

- US government inspectors reviewed 22 clinical trials Web sites – none described the risks (http://www.medscape.com/viewarticle/434296?srcmp=phar-05). Informed consent may be invalidated by not informing the patient of any changes to their perceived state of health, i.e. 'Any information becoming available during the trial which may be of relevance for the trial subjects must be made known to them by the investigator' (CPMP Guidelines para 1.15).

- Conclusion: in my view, informed consent is a misnomer. The patient cannot be adequately informed. The question is whether, in any particular study, it is ethical for the investigator to ask for informed consent.

Patient protection in clinical studies

There are six layers of potential protection:

1. Declaration of Helsinki – depends on interpretation.

2. Sponsor's protocol – not to be relied upon.

3. Ethical committee (IRB) – lay persons in a minority and dependent on sponsor for information.

4. Investigator – will depend on any conflicts of interest.

5. Journal editor – only ICMJE members can be relied upon.

6. The patient – vulnerable.

No layer is watertight and the patient remains vulnerable.

Ethics and the pharmaceutical industry

The industry donates money to many individuals and institutions. If it is only to help the recipients accomplish their aims then there would be no ethical problem, but if the intention is to influence the recipients' decisions then many poeple would consider this to be unethical.

Recipients of money from the pharmaceutical industry

Several industries whose products may adversely affect the health of the world have been criticized for putting profits before the well-being of people, e.g. tobacco, salt, breast milk substitutes and processed foods (Anand, 1996; Godlee, 1996; Wise, 1996; Taylor, 1998). Some of these industries target the Third World. It is important, therefore, to examine the pharmaceutical industry and its behaviour.

In the past, many have criticized the honesty of the pharmaceutical industry. In recent years, regulations and guidelines have restricted the possibility of dishonesty and another generation has entered the industry. Comments will, therefore, with two exceptions, be made only on publications since 1990.

'He who pays the piper calls the tune' and 'There is no such thing as a free lunch' (www.nofreelunch.org). These two sayings reflect the general public's belief that the recipient of money or a gift is under an obligation to the donor even if, ostensibly, there are no strings attached. 'Academic medical institutions are themselves growing increasingly beholden to industry', according to Angell (2000).

In addition to looking at donations, it is necessary to examine situations where the payments are excessive compared with non-industry payment for similar work.

The following list of recipients of pharmaceutical money include those where there is an assumption that the intention is to influence the recipients' decisions, e.g. a donation or a remuneration over and above reasonable compensation for extra work and loss of income, as well as recipients where no influence is likely, e.g. where there is a set fee and no competition, and those who fall between these two extremes.

Many of these associations/societies/colleges listed below are aware of the problems and have said that if it was considered that an attempt was being made to influence policy then any offer would be refused. The fact pharmaceutical money pervades the whole of the medical system must not be taken to imply that where there is temptation all or many succumb. Some will resolutely avoid bias towards the industry, more will be affected subconsciously, others will seek to justify their failings, and some will have put money above all other considerations; but all recipients of industry money need close scrutiny if injustice is to be prevented. However, we must not forget 'Without industry funding, important advances in disease prevention and treatment would not have occurred' (Boden-heimer, 2000).

Politicians and political parties

- *USA*. A report released by Public citizen, the US consumer group, has found that the industry spent more than US$262 million to buy political influence during the 1999–2000 campaign period (http://citizen.org/congress/drugs/pharmadrugwar.html). President Bush '... received contributions of $456,000 from the pharmaceutical industry during his 2000 election campaign' (Washburn, 2001). From 1997 through 1999, the pharmaceutical/health-products industry and its employees spent more than US$14.8 million on federal campaigns through unlimited 'soft' money donations to national political parties and contributions to candidates (http://citizen.org/congress/reform/drug_industry/contrib).

- *UK*. Since November 2000 the Electoral Commission monitors political donations over £5000 (http://www.electoralcommission.gov.uk). 'Most companies now refuse to make political donations because of the controversy they attract and neither do they want to fall foul of both the Companies Act and the legislation brought in last year that says donations have to be declared' (Trefgarne, 2002). The Electoral Commission mention only one donation to the Conservative party from a pharmaceutical company for £1 000 000. The Labour party has not accepted any donations from the industry; but a director of Powderjet, Paul Drayson, gave £50 000 to the party and Isaac Kaye, chairman of Norton Healthcare, gave £10 000 to the Labour minister Frank Dobson (Guardian, 2000; Electoral Commission, 2002).

Regulatory authorities

- *USA*. 'Almost 40 per cent of the total amount the FDA spent on processing human drug applications came from user fees' (http://www.govexec.com/gpp/0299fda.htm, 1999). In total the FDA will receive US$162 million (€165 million, £104 million) from industry in 2002 (Moynihan, 2002). A survey by the Public Health Research Group among FDA regulators found that 84 per cent of Medical Officers at the FDA opposed such mutual recognition (foreign approvals) because they believed safety would be compromised (Scrip 1681/82, 5 January, 1992).

- *Europe:* Financial support for EMEA comes from two sources: a European Community grant, and the fees EMEA charges industry for the assessment of dossiers and other services (Garattini and Bertele, 2001).

- The UK National Audit Office quotes the percentage of the regulators costs funded by the industry: Sweden (Medical Products Agency) 95 per cent, Canada (Therapeutic Products Directive) 66 per cent, USA (Center for Drug Evaluation and Research) 52 per cent, Netherlands (Medicines Evaluation Board Agency) 100 per cent, France (Agence

Français de Sécurité Sanitaire des Produits de Santé) 50 per cent; the state must pay 25 per cent of funding, UK (Medicines Control Agency (MCA)) 100 per cent (NAO, 2003).

- *UK*. Medicine regulators and their expert advisors are closely identified with the interests of the pharmaceutical industry in Britain (Abraham *et al.*, 1999). The (MCA) income from the pharmaceutical industry is about £13.4 million derived from fees paid by the pharmaceutical industry (Scrip 2254, 1 August, 4, 1997) It is completely dependent on the industry's fees for its funding (Brown, 1990).

Those with financial interests in industry do not take part in matters where their interests clash. Of 23 members of the Committee on the Safety of Medicines (CSM) with financial interests in 1996, three had interests in at least 20 companies, seven in at least 10 companies and 20 in at least five companies (MCA, 1997). The CPMP figures are: of the 30 members, one was employed in the industry, one had shares, four received payment for various work, and four declared other interests (managing research institutes or coordinating clinical trials funded by the industry; see Table 15.1 (Abraham and Lewis, 2000).

Table 15.1 Industrial interests of expert advisers on medicines regulation in 1996 (Abraham and Lewis, 2000), *Regulating Medicines in Europe*). Reproduced by permission of Thompson Publishing Services

Regulatory body	No. of advisers	Personal interests	Non-personal interests	No. of interests
Medicines Commission	19	11	7	6
CSM	29	18	22	6
Total	48	29	29	12

- *Sweden*. Medicines regulation was already almost entirely funded by licensing fees from industry (Scrip 1356, 28 October, 1, 1988).

- *Germany*. The BfArM retained a government subsidy for 60 per cent of its total budget, needing to derive only 40 per cent from industry fees (Hildebrandt, 1995).

Ethics committees/Institutional Review Boards

- *UK*. Professor Stacey, Director of COREC (Central Office for Research Ethics Committees), has informed me that the LRECs and MRECs in the NHS are Advisory Committees established under the auspices of the Department of Health (DH). As such they are basically supported by public funds. Applicants from organizations which also depend on public funds (e.g. Research Councils, universities, the NHS itself) and applicants from organizations with which the DH has a 'partnership' arrangement, such as the Medical Charities, receive the advice on the ethical standards of their research free of charge. The possibility exists that other applicants may be charged and it is common practice for this to occur. MRECs charge a standard fee, currently £1000, to defray expenses. The members may be aware of this, but do not see the cash. LRECs do not (yet) have standard fees – but they may in the future.

- *USA*. 'For independent IRBs the dependence on revenue from industry sponsors exerts similar possibilities for conflict'. Some are owned by CROs (Brown 1998).

University departments and university research staff

- According to a survey undertaken by Massachusetts General Hospital Institute for Health Policy, director David Blumenthal said 'about 25 per cent of medical school faculties have research support from industry and about 8 per cent have equity in companies related to research' (NIH Catalyst, 2000). *Conjoint projects*: many universities have conjoint projects with industry to their mutual benefit e.g. Massachusetts Institute of Technology–Merck and company; Dana-Farber Cancer Institute–Novartis. Some academic institutions have entered into partnerships with drug companies to set up research centres and teaching programmes.

- The Centre for Addiction and Mental Health at Toronto University cancelled the appointment of Dr David Healey and it has been alleged that this was connected with the receipt by the centre of US$1.5 million from Eli Lilly in recent years (Boseley, 2001). In the final settlement this was denied.

- In a US survey (1994–5) 43 per cent of respondents had received a research-related gift in the last 3 years independent of grant or contract from the industry (Campbell *et al.*, 1998).

- A study of disclosures from 225 principal investigators at the University of California found that 34 per cent involved paid speaking arrangements, with 33 per cent relating to consultancy agreements between researchers and sponsors and equity ownership in another 14 per cent; 12 per cent of declarations related to two or more such relationships (Boyd and Bero, 2000).

- When the medical residency program at McMaster University adopted formal guidelines for interactions with the pharmaceutical industry and polled 24 companies, 18 responded and half of these found the guidelines unacceptable and stated that funding for the program would decrease as a result (Guyatt, 1994).

- Yale University owns the patent on Stavudine and had earned at least US$261 million since 1994. This is, of course, not a donation (Demenet 2002).

Investigators

- 'The per-patient reimbursement offered to the investigator generally exceeds the per-patient costs incurred by the investigator. This excess represents a windfall that can be used to pay for travel, equipment or supplies, or to fund research for which the investigator cannot obtain funding through peer-reviewed granting channels' (Shimm and Spece, 1991).

- Bayer paid investigators US$1200 for enrolling each patient with vaginitis; SmithKline-

Beecham US$4410 for a diabetic and Merck US$2955 for a hypertensive patient (Eichenwald and Kolata, 1999).

- 'Payments, often overtly on a per capita basis, have reached levels that are of serious concern to research ethic committees' (Rao and Sant Cassia, 2002).

- In the field of AEs the investigator's attitude can vary from bewildered ignorance to deliberate dishonesty, some fail to document and report what they should clearly recognize as an AE.

- Some are so 'invested' in the study drug and believe so strongly in its safety that their enthusiasm overshadows sound scientific and regulatory standards.

- Some chose not to report AEs, either because it requires too much effort or they were deliberately attempting to defraud.

- Some are confused over what constitutes an AE (Mackintosh and Zepp 1996).

A list of scientists with ties to industry can be found at www.cspinet.org/integrity/.

Numerous incidences of investigator fraud have been proven. In the UK, in the last 10 years, 21 cases have been referred to the General Medical Council (GMC). Of the doctors found guilty of serious professional misconduct, 12 were struck off and five were suspended from the medical register (Boardman, 2002).

Pharmacoepidemiology

Many, if not all, of the epidemiological databases will be partly financed by industry, and this is to be expected by their nature:

- Prescription Event Monitoring (PEM): Dr Saad Shakir, Director of the Drug Safety Research Unit (DSRU), has informed me that, with regard to funding of the DSRU, the unit receives funds from the pharmaceutical industry for PEM as donations to the unit in an unconditional way, i.e. PEM studies are not sponsored, the company supports the DSRU and do not sponsor individual studies. The DSRU receives other sources of funding, principally from research grants from grant-offering bodies. The DSRU has recently received a large grant from the British Heart Foundation to set up a registry for cardiovascular events associated with non-cardiovascular medications. Lastly, sometimes the DSRU undertakes studies which are defined as sponsored, *i.e.* the unit conducted a large community-based *case*-controlled study on the relationship between contraceptives and myocardial infarction, which was sponsored by Organon.

- MEdicines Monitoring Unit (MEMO): according to Dr J Parkinson, MEMO is funded by NHS (Scotland) research grants (15–20 per cent), Wellcome, Medical Research Council (MRC) and charities (15–20 per cent), pharmaceutical industry (50–60 per cent), others such as FDA (5–10 per cent) and consultancy to other healthcare databases (5 per cent). All studies are only conducted against an agreed protocol and on the understanding that the results will be published in a peer-reviewed journal.

- Boston Collaborative Drug Surveillance Program: Professor Hershel Jick of the Boston Collaborative Drug Surveillance Program says that about half of their studies are supported by industry.

- International Society for Pharmacoepidemiology: Angela Charles, of the International Society of Pharmacoepidemiology, tells me that the information is not readily available; but seven companies are benefactors.

- International Society of Pharmacovigilance: according to Dr Ana Corrêa Nunes of the International Society of Pharmacovigilance, the society does not receive any industry donations. However, its 2002 conference is sponsored by pharmaceutical companies.

- 'Many pharmaceutical companies are also increasing their investment in external pharmacoepidemiology resources' (Strom, 2000).

- 'The role of the university scientist should reflect the unique role and function of the university: the provision of disinterested inquiry and critique. This role becomes a more difficult one to fulfil as university scientists become more and more dependent on funding from sources that have vested interest in obtaining particular outcomes from the studies they fund ... Pharmacoepidemiologists are particularly at risk of becoming the targets of attempts to influence their research results, because the outcome of their studies can often affect the sales or even the licensing of drugs and medical devices' (Stolley and Laporte, 2000).

Medical journals

- Quality scores of randomized controlled clinical trials published in medical journals range from 4.2 per cent to 87.5 per cent with an average score of 37.2 per cent. Similar scores for supplement journals, 33.6 per cent, are lower than in parent journals, 38.5 per cent (Rochon *et al.*, 1994).

- Pharmaceutical advertising is placing the medical organizations in jeopardy of losing their objectivity' (Gottlieb, 1999).

- The primary clinical journals of several leading organizations had an estimated revenue from pharmaceutical advertising ranging from US$715 000 (£450 000) to $18 million (£11.4 million) – a total that they said could place the organizations in a position of dependency. Five organizations raised more than 10 per cent of their gross income from a single journal's pharmaceutical advertising (Glassman *et al.*, 1999).

- A survey of American medical journals showed that 46 per cent did not have written policies for authors concerning conflict of interest (Glass and Schneiderman, 1997).

Authors of medical articles

- Overwhelming evidence exists that single-source sponsorship is associated with outcomes favourable to the sponsor's product (Bero, 1999).

- The editor of *New England Journal of Medicine* has been criticised by the FDA for over praising a new asthma drug made by a company that he had advised as a paid consultant (Gottlieb, 2000a).

- Although 15 per cent of authors had financial ties relevant to one of their publications, no voluntary disclosures were published (Krimsky *et al.*, 1996).

- 'Although many authors of biomedical journal articles have financial competing interests, they often fail to disclose them'. A survey of five leading journals showed that only 1.4 per cent of articles declared authors' competing interests (Hussain and Smith, 2001).

- 'Author (in the *BMJ*) conclusions were significantly more positive towards the experimental intervention in trials funded by for-profit organisations alone compared with trials without competing interests ..., trials funded by both profit and non-profit organisations ..., and trials with other competing interests' (Kjaergard and Als-Nielsen, 2002).

Authors of guidelines on clinical practice

A survey of nearly 200 authors of 44 clinical guidelines showed that 87 per cent of responders admitted financial links with the industry. Only one of the guidelines carried a declaration of the competing interests of the authors. Most (93 per cent) said their relationship did not affect their judgement. There was only a 52 per cent response despite a second mailing (Choudhry *et al.*, 2002; Lenzer, 2002; Tonks, 2002a).

Hospital departments

'Requests by physicians that drugs be added to a hospital formulary were strongly and specifically associated with the physicians' interactions with the companies manufacturing the drugs' (Chren and Landefeld, 1994).

Medical colleges, associations and societies

- The Royal College of Paediatrics and Child Health. 'Sponsorship from companies which market pharmaceutical products, medical equipment, or mineral water is deemed acceptable provided that the drug company does not attempt to influence our policies. The College has accepted £7500 for the publication of a bulletin but would refuse future funding if an attempt to influence our policies was made. In addition, guidance to its individual members on commercial sponsorship recommends that great care needs to be taken so that individual paediatricians are not unduly influenced'.

- The Royal College of General Practitioners receives a small amount of support from pharma companies. Sponsorship that is directly 'product' related is not permitted and conferences or educational events are limited to an acknowledgement 'Supported by an educational grant from ...'. Subject to strict sponsorship guidelines (Jane Austen, RCGP, personal communication, 2002).

- The Association for Black Cardiologists was largely funded by industry in 1996–97 (www.integrityinscience.org). American Academy of Pediatrics, American Heart Association but not the British Heart Foundation, American Medical Writers Association.

- The Royal College of Obstetricians and Gynaecologists accepts donations towards travel scholarships and for its new conference centre (Paul Barnett, College Secretary, RCOG).

- Paul Summerfield has informed me that the Royal Society of Medicine probably receives less than 1 per cent of its income from pharmaceutical companies. A small number of conferences and section meetings are sponsored by companies and they are hoping for donations towards their redevelopment appeal.

- The Royal College of Physicians does accept donations and sponsorship from the industry, the latter, generally, for conferences, teach-ins and publications and the former for general purposes. It does not accept sponsorship which might damage the College's public standing or reputation for independence. It does not endorse a particular product.

Disease associations

American Cancer Society, Cancer BACUP, Cancer Research UK, American Diabetes Association, Diabetes UK, American Liver Foundation, American Obesity Association, American Thyroid Association, Arthritis Foundation, Arthritis Care (UK), Kidney Cancer Association, Children and Adults with Attention Deficit/hyperactivity Disorder/CHADD, Alzheimer's Society (UK). The Stroke Association (UK), Parkinson's Disease Society, The American Heart Association, has accepted US$11 million (£7.8 million, €12.6 per cent) from Genentech over the past decade (Lenzer, 2002). The International Fund for Functional Gastrointestinal Disorders (Moynihan, 2002). National Osteoporosis Society (UK) 10.5 per cent of total income.

Academic medical symposia

- At the European Society of Cardiology annual meeting in 1999, 16 per cent of the sessions were commercially sponsored satellites (Horton, 2000).

- 'Approach symposium issues, that are sponsored by a single pharmaceutical company, with scepticism' (Bero et al., 1992).

- Eminent cardiologists have admitted that, at a symposium organized by a pharmaceutical company, they were prepared to advise other doctors to prescribe the company's drug, though they had little or no experience of using it. Concerns about the safety of the drug resulted in its withdrawal weeks later. Eminent British cardiologists were paid £3000–£5000 (depending on audience size, plus travelling expenses for a 1 hour talk) to lecture to other doctors to promote the company's drugs (Wilmhurst, 2000).

Prescribers

- It has been estimated that $8000 to $13000 is spent on each physician ... the present physician–industry interactions appears to affect prescribing and professional behavior. (Wazana, 2000).

- 'Half of general practitioners' post-graduate education is sponsored by the pharmaceutical industry' (Tiner, 1999).

- Doctors were paid excessive amounts when they prescribed a TAP Pharmaceuticals drug, Lupron. The firm was fined $875 million (Peterson, 2001).

- Spanish pharmaceutical company (Kendall Institute, Barcelona) employees bribed doctors to prescribe their drugs. They and the GPs were sent to prison (Bosch, 1999).

- 'GPs in dispensing practice have told me that they have not followed my recommendations for treatment of cardiac patients because discounting by competing companies resulted in financial advantage to prescribe alternative drugs' (Wilmhurst, 2000).

- Gifts to 1600 German hospital doctors worth up to €25 000 (US$21 900, £15 400) are under investigation. In 1994, approximately 2000 German doctors were investigated and 30 found guilty of receiving bribes (Williamson, 2002).

- Well organized British general practice can earn (from the industry) an extra £15 000 annually for 3 hours work a week (Rao and Cassia, 2002), i.e. £96 per hour. This would seem to be a very reasonable payment; the BMA suggested figure is £158 per hour.

Patient associations

- National Alliance for Mental Illness (NAMI; Silverstein, 1999) received $11.72 million from 18 Pharma companies between 1996 and mid-1999 [Eli Lilly and 17 other manufacturers provided $11.72 million (£8.3 million, €13.4 million)] (Lenzer, 2002).

- International Association of Patients' Organisations was founded and funded by an industry consortium 'Center for Science in the Public Interest'.

- Citizens for Better Medicare; Alliance for Better Medicine (Gerth and Stolberg, 2000);

- Action for Access funded by Biogen (Boseley, 1999).

- The Patients Association accepted a large donation from Pharmacia and Upjohn (www.socialaudit.org.uk).

- 60 plus Association; United Seniors Association; Seniors Coalition; Centre for Addiction and Mental Health (University of Toronto) (Boseley, 2001).

- National Patient Safety Foundation (www.npsf.org).

Ethics in pharmaceutical medicine

The Ethical Issues Working Group (1998) from the Faculty of Pharmaceutical Medicine, under section 2.5 'Benefit–risk assessment'. Says:

2.5.1. If a pharmaceutical physician is not certain about all aspects of the status of a clinical research programme, even in the light of acceptable efficacy or safety, it is appropriate to delay making a decision on its future progress until any doubts have been resolved. Making an inappropriate decision before such doubts are resolved is unethical. Thus, both when assessing the outcome of a clinical trial programme before licensing and when reviewing the safety profile after marketing, pharmaceutical physicians must actively fulfil their scientific and ethical responsibilities. They must make forthright decisions where, for example, the relative evidence of efficacy is less that acceptable or where there is an unexpectedly high incidence of adverse reactions, recognising their responsibility as doctors to put the interests of patients as their top priority.

2.5.2. The management of new information suggesting the possibility of an adverse safety profile for a product can be fraught with ethical difficulty. It is essential that adequate systems are in place to ensure the timely capture and analysis of relevant data upon which a decision to withdraw a product might be based. There are situations where the potential benefit to a large number of patients has to be balanced against the possible harm to a small number. The working group recognises the ethical difficulties which these situations can create, particularly in the face of regulatory action. Pharmaceutical physicians involved in the withdrawal of a product must ensure that as much relevant information as possible is made available to enable the clinical care of patients who are affected by the withdrawal to continue with the minimum of disturbance.

This report should be read by all pharmaceutical physicians.

The accompanying editorial (Anon., 1998a) referring to the duty to safeguard the integrity of information says, referring to presenting data:

In that process there may be a temptation to 'trim' data, cutting out those that look suspiciously odd. Dealing with 'outlying' figures should be strictly defined in the statistical specification. The moment of highest risk for such 'trimming' is a tabulation in a published paper or in promotional copy. Most times any corruption of results is a typographical or unwitting error, but not always. 'Selective reporting' of only the findings that suit the researchers or the sponsors is an ever-present temptation. Such deliberate misdeeds have occurred and will happen again. The report gives no direction on 'whistle-blowing' inside a pharmaceutical company and yet information to regulatory authorities, to prescribers and to financial analysts may be incomplete or presented in a way that is favourable but fundamentally wrong.

Junior staff may be starved of information about sensitive areas and only given information 'on a need to know' basis, so it is usually senior staff who are involved in decisions where honesty is vital.

Concealing information

- A task force appointed by the US FDA has concluded that Upjohn may have obscured information material regarding the safety of Halcion (triazolam), and has recommended that the Department of Justice investigate (Barnett, 1996a). I can find no trace of any result from the Department of Justice; so, if it did investigate there were no sequelae.

- Nippon Shoji began marketing sorivudine, a shingles treatment sold as Usevir, September 1996, but had to withdraw it within weeks when it was found to be fatal when combined with cancer drugs. Evidence of the dangers began emerging in 1986, but Nippon Shoji concealed information from the government about two of the deaths during clinical trials (Gurdon, 1994).

- Pfizer received a letter from the US FDA in 1996 warning that it had failed to report adverse drug experiences on eight drugs. In reviewing Pfizer's reporting since 1983, the FDA found 'that the same or similar problems continue to recur, even though you have made promises to correct them' (Barnett, 1996b).

Publication of clinical studies sponsored by the industry

- In 1995 there was controversy concerning the safety of calcium channel blockers (CCBs). Of those physicians and researchers who were supportive of CCBs, 96 per cent had financial ties with the drug manufacturers; this compares with 60 per cent of those who were neutral and 37 per cent of those who were critical towards the drugs. Only two of the 70 articles revealed the authors' potential conflict of interest. All the supportive authors had financial relationships with the pharmaceutical industry, regardless of the product; this compares with 67 per cent and 43 per cent of those who wrote neutral and critical articles respectively (Stelfox et al., 1998). Of the 23 critical papers, 15 came from three authors all of whom were epidemiologists and, therefore, had analysed data produced by others (Meltzer, 1998). Many of the publications in support of CCB appear to be letters to the editor (Strandgaard, 1998). The authors did not refute these problems (Detsky and Stelfox, 1998).

- The Celecoxib Long-term Arthritis Safety Study (CLASS; Silverstein et al., 2000), which was funded by celecoxib's manufacturer Pharmacia, concluded that compared with the traditional non-steroidal anti-inflammatory drug (NSAID), celecoxib 'was associated with a lower incidence of symptomatic ulcers and ulcer complications combined'. It was later said that complete information available to the FDA contradicted these conclusions. The CLASS study referred to the combined analysis of the results of the first 6 months of two studies, whereas analysis according to a pre-specified protocol showed similar numbers of ulcer-related complications in the comparison group. Almost all the ulcer complications that had occurred during the second half of trials were in the users of celecoxib (Anon., 2002; Jüni et al., 2002; Skelly and Hawkey, 2002).

- Ghost-writing, where part/all of a report on a clinical trial is written by a writer employed by the sponsor who is not an author of the report, is widespread and there have been incidents where the true authors have not seen the raw data (Boseley, 2002).

• Trials with company support were much more likely to report in favour of the experimental therapy: 98 per cent to 79 per cent (Cho and Bero, 1996).

• A review of pharmacoeconomic studies of cancer drugs reported that 5 per cent of industry-sponsored studies reached unfavourable conclusions about the company's products, compared with 38 per cent of studies with non-profit funding that reached similar conclusions (Friedberg *et al.*, 1999) but differences in study reporting may have accounted for this finding (Knox *et al.*, 2000).

• Trials that are supported by pharmaceutical companies are significantly more likely to report favourable outcomes associated with use of the sponsored drug, compared with non-sponsored trials. A review of 29 randomized studies of clozapine versus 'typical' antipsychotic drugs ($N = 2490$) showed that in the 13 sponsored trials the odds of relapsing were significantly in favour of clozapine, with odds ratio 0.5 (confidence interval (CI) 0.3–0.7), and in the 10 non-sponsored studies the findings were equivocal, with odds ratio 0.4 (CI 0.1–1.4). The sponsored studies were more positive than trials not clearly supported by industry (Wahlbeck and Adams, 1999).

• A possible reason for this 'is that they (the pharmaceutical industry) are more careful about how they design their research projects and more scrupulous about how they collect their data' (Boardman, 1999).

The International Committee of Medical Journal Editors (ICMJE) are revising the uniform requirements for manuscripts submitted to biomedical journals and changing editorial practices to counter the problem of declared authors not having ultimate control over whether their studies are published (Smith, 2001):

Sponsorship, Authorship, and Accountability. As editors of general medical journals, we recognize that the publication of clinical-research findings in respected peer-reviewed journals is the ultimate basis for most treatment decisions. Public discourse about this published evidence of efficacy and safety rests on the assumption that clinical-trials data have been gathered and are presented in an objective and dispassionate manner. This discourse is vital to the scientific practice of medicine because it shapes treatment decisions made by physicians and drives public and private health care policy. We are concerned that the current intellectual environment in which some clinical research is conceived, study participants are recruited, and the data analyzed and reported (or not reported) may threaten this precious objectivity.

Clinical trials are powerful tools; like all powerful tools, they must be used with care. They allow investigators to test biologic hypotheses in living patients, and they have the potential to change the standards of care. The secondary economic impact of such changes can be substantial. Well-done trials, published in high-profile journals, may be used to market drugs and medical devices, potentially resulting in substantial financial gain for the sponsor; but powerful tools must be used carefully. Patients participate in clinical trials largely for altruistic reasons – that is, to advance the standard of care. In the light of that truth, the use of clinical trials primarily for marketing, in our view, makes a mockery of clinical investigation and is a misuse of a powerful tool.

Until recently, academic, independent clinical investigators were key players in design, patient recruitment, and data interpretation in clinical trials. The intellectual and working home of these investigators, the academic medical centre, has been at the hub of this enterprise, and many institutions have developed complex infrastructures devoted to the design and conduct of clinical trials. The academic enterprise has been a critical part of the process that led to the introduction of many new treatments into medical practice and contributed to the quality, intellectual rigor, and impact of such clinical trials. But, as economic pressures mount, this may be a thing of the past.

Many clinical trials are performed to facilitate regulatory approval of a device or drug rather than to test a specific novel scientific hypothesis. As trials have become more sophisticated and the margin of untreated disease harder to reach, there has been a great increase in the size of the trials and consequently the costs of developing new drugs.

It is estimated that the average cost of bringing a new drug to market in the United States is between $300–600 million and takes 14.9 years to come to the market (Parexel, 1998). The pharmaceutical industry has recognized the need to control costs and has discovered that private non-academic research groups – that is, contract research organizations (CROs) – can do the job for less money and with fewer hassles than academic investigators. Over the past few years, CROs have received the lion's share of clinical trial revenues. For example, in 2000 in the United States, CROs received 60 per cent of the research grants from pharmaceutical companies, as compared with only 40 per cent for academic trialists (Henderson, 2000). As CROs and academic medical centres compete head to head for the opportunity to enrol patients in clinical trials, corporate sponsors have been able to dictate the terms of participation in the trial, terms that are not always in the best interests of academic investigators, the study participants, or the advancement of science generally (Rennie, 1997).

Investigators may have little or no input into trial design, no access to the raw data, and limited participation in data interpretation. These terms are draconian for self-respecting scientists, but many have accepted them because they know that if they do not, the sponsor will find someone else who will. And, unfortunately, even when an investigator has had substantial input into trial design and data interpretation, the results of the finished trial may be buried rather than published if they are unfavourable to the sponsor's product. Such issues are not theoretical. There have been a number of recent public examples of such problems, and we suspect that many more go unreported (Blumenthal *et al.*, 1997).

The ICMJE have said:

As editors, we strongly oppose contractual agreements that deny investigators the right to examine the data independently or to submit a manuscript for publication without first obtaining the consent of the sponsor. Such arrangements not only erode the fabric of intellectual inquiry that has fostered so much high-quality clinical research but also make medical journals party to potential misrepresentation, since the published manu-script may not reveal the extent to which the authors were powerless to control the conduct of a study that bears their names. Because of our concern, we have recently

revised and strengthened the section on publication ethics in the 'Uniform Requirements for Manuscripts Submitted to Biomedical Journals: Writing and Editing for
Biomedical Publication,' a document developed by the International Committee of
Medical Journal Editors (ICMJE) and widely used by individual journals as the basis
for editorial policy. The revised section follows this editorial. (The entire 'Uniform
Requirements' document is undergoing revision; the revised version should be available
at the beginning of 2002.) As part of the reporting requirements, we will routinely
require authors to disclose details of their own and the sponsor's role in the study. Many
of us will ask the responsible author to sign a statement indicating that he or she
accepts full responsibility for the conduct of the trial, had access to the data, and
controlled the decision to publish.

We believe that a sponsor should have the right to review a manuscript for a defined
period (for example, 30 to 60 days) before publication to allow for the filing of
additional patent protection, if required. When the sponsor employs some of the
authors, these authors' contributions and perspective should be reflected in the final
paper, as are those of the other authors, but the sponsor must impose no impediment,
direct or indirect, on the publication of the study's full results, including data perceived
to be detrimental to the product. Although we most commonly associate this behaviour
with pharmaceutical sponsors, research sponsored by government or other agencies
may also fall victim to this form of censorship, especially if the results of such studies
appear to contradict current policy.

Authorship means both accountability and independence. A submitted manuscript is
the intellectual property of its authors, not the study sponsor.

We will not review or publish articles based on studies that are conducted under
conditions that allow the sponsor to have sole control of the data or to withhold
publication. We encourage investigators to use the revised ICMJE requirements on
publication ethics to guide the negotiation of research contracts. Those contracts should
give the researchers a substantial say in trial design, access to the raw data, responsibility for data analysis and interpretation, and the right to publish – the hallmarks of
scholarly independence and, ultimately, academic freedom. By enforcing adherence to
these revised requirements, we can as editors assure our readers that the authors of an
article have had a meaningful and truly independent role in the study that bears their
names. The authors can then stand behind the published results, and so can we
(www.icmje.org/sponsor.htm).

This was said by the UK Institute of Clinical Research to be 'misleading, counter-
productive and inaccurate' (Press release, September 21 2001, Institute of Clinical Research,
Maidenhead, UK) and in an editorial of the *International Journal of Pharmaceutical
Medicine* (Snell, 2001) and also in *Scrip Magazine*, December 2001 by Dr M Bowden.

- 'The Massachusetts General Hospital estimates that 30 to 50 percent of contracts
  submitted by companies have unacceptable publication clauses that must be negotiated'
  (Bodenheimer, 2000). 'Six investigators interviewed for this report cited cases of
  articles whose publication was stopped or whose content was altered by the funding
  company' (Bodenheimer, 2000).

- An objective analysis of studies, funded directly by a specific pharmaceutical company when comparing its product with that of a direct competitor, showed significant bias in favour of the product of the sponsoring company ($p < 0.001$). This persisted if studies funded by company A or company B were individually compared with those not funded by either company: $p = 0.02$ for company A and $p = 0.0002$ for company B (Thomas *et al.*, 2002).

- A survey, as to whether information on sources of funding, financial conflicts of interest of the authors and specific descriptions of the type and degree of involvement of the supporting agency were met in 268 randomized controlled trials, published by the *Annals of Internal Medicine, British Medical Journal, Journal of the American Medical Association,* the *Lancet* and the *New England Journal of Medicine* found that just over a third were supported wholly or in part by industry, and only 9 per cent failed to give the source of funding. In the trials supported by industry, a third did not provide any information on the authors' relations with industry (Gupta, 2001).

- Three studies showed an increase in venous thromboembolism (VTE) with third-generation oral contraceptives (OC) compared with second-generation OCs and their publication led to an increase in the number of abortions – over 800 (Bloemenkamp *et al.*, 1995, Jick *et al.*, 1995, WHO, 1995). Six out of ten patients on OCs in the UK stopped taking them (McPherson, 1996; Wilson, 1996a); in Norway, abortions rose by 8.2 per cent compared with the same period the previous year (Andrew *et al.*, 1996) and in the UK abortions rose by 6.7 per cent compared with the first quarter of 1995, which was 2688 more than the first quarter of the year 1996 (Feger, 1996; Wilson, 1996b). This figure was later amended to 14.5 per cent (Hall, 1996). It has been suggested that the increase was due to over-recruitment of patients with high baseline risk for VTE (Herings *et al.*, 1996; Michaels *et al.*, 1996). The original finding, that there was a doubling of the rate of thromboembolism, has been disputed (Heinemann and Lewis, 1996; Lewis *et al.*, 1996a,b, 1998; Spitzer *et al.*, 1996; Farmer *et al.*, 1997; Suissa *et al.*, 1997; Szarewski 1997). A meta-analysis of 12 studies showed a summary relative risk of 1.7 (CI 1.4–2.0). Industry studies showed an odds ratio 1.3 (CI 1.0–1.7) and 2.3 for other studies (CI 1.7–3.2) (Kemmeren *et al.*, 2001) but was sensitive to unmeasured confounding so there was no unequivocal answer (Hennessy *et al.*, 2001). Four industry-funded studies indicated no increased risk (relative risk (RR) 0.8–1.5, summary RR 1.1), whilst nine non-sponsored studies indicated an overall 2.4-fold increased risk (1.5–4.0 summary RR 2.4) (Vandenbroucke *et al.*, 2000). The industry's view on bias and confounding was not supported by the WHO's scientific committee of leading epidemiologists who were not involved in the controversy (WHO, 1998). A Dutch radio programme claimed that Wyeth suppressed research on the pill (Van Heteren, 2001).The drug firms now face a claim for £10 million by patients under the Consumer Protection Act 1987 (Dyer, 2002a,c,d; Tait and Firn, 2002). A legal action, in July 2002, taken against the manufacturers by seven lead claims was dismissed. The judge (Mr Justice Mackay) said, 'The most likely figure to represent the relative risk is around 1.7' (Section K: Conclusions on the first issue, Para 343, www.courtservice.gov.uk/judgementsfiles/j1298). The ability for the legal system to adjudicate on pharmacoepidemiological evidence has since been questioned (McPherson, 2002).

- The problems Dr Andrew Millar had with British Biotech would have been avoided had there been an independent data monitoring and safety committee, and this highlighted the need for all studies to have such a committee. Dr Millar was sued by British Biotech after he had told shareholders that the clinical trials of two of their drugs were not going as well as the directors had claimed (Hampton, 2000).

- Three physicians who had taken part in the Multicenter Isradipine Diuretic Athero-sclerosis Study (MIDAS) dropped out of the investigative group because they believed that the sponsor of the study was attempting to wield undue influence on the nature of the final paper (Applegate *et al.*, 1997).

- A drug company suppressed research for almost 7 years showing that generic thyroid drugs were as effective as its own branded product (Rennie, 1997; Wise, 1997).

- Bristol-Myers Squibb exerted pressure, on ethical grounds, to end an independent trial of one of its drugs (Anon., 1997).

- Bristol-Myers Squibb Canada tried to prevent publication of a report on statins produced by the independent technology assessment body, claiming that it would negatively affect the sales of their drug pravastatin (Spurgeon, 1998b).

- A Californian biotechnology company tried to block publication of a major AIDS study that found that the experimental treatment the company was developing failed to improve the health of patients, the scientists conducting the research said (Gottlieb, 2000a).

- An international group of renowned scientists has accused Canada's largest university (Toronto) of violating academic freedom for fear of losing research funds from drug companies when it revoked a job offer to an outspoken British psychiatrist (Nathan and Weatherall, 1999; Dyer, 2001).

- The author of intended publication of adverse clinical trial findings was reminded by Apotex of her confidentiality agreement and was threatened with legal action. She published (Spurgeon, 1998a). 'Industry is using litigious means to dispute research findings and block the dissemination of results' (Hailey, 2000) .

- 'Pharmaceutical companies that pay researchers to design and interpret drug trials sometimes spin or suppress unfavourable findings' (Bodenheimer, 2000).

Clinical trial data may be designed or analysed 'favourably':

- The scale on the Y axis of a graph may be inappropriate (Stephens, 1998; Barbehenn *et al.*, 2000).

- 'Outliers' may be omitted (Smith, 2002).

- There may be exclusion of baseline data (Barbehenn *et al.*, 2000).

- The study design may use too low a dose for the comparator drug (Rochon *et al.*, 1994).

- 'Companies may study many surrogate end points and publish results only for those that favor their product' (Bodenheimer, 2000).

- Use of relative risk reduction without mention of the absolute risk reduction (Mayor, 2002).

- *Post hoc* changes in design, outcomes, and analysis may produce changes in the subsequent publication that do not fully reflect the results from a prespecified protocol, e.g. the publication of the CLASS study sponsored by Pharmacia did not reflect the adverse effects that were seen in the latter part of the study (Gottlieb, 2001; Jüni *et al.*, 2002).

Promotional honesty: pharmaceutical promotion

It has been argued that 'promotion of medicines by the pharmaceutical industry is, by its very nature, unethical', in that actions done out of respect of one group's interests rather than the interests of humanity at large are unethical (Collier, 1995). This was rebutted in the same issue of *Pharmaceutical Medicine*; 'pharmaceutical promotion is a valid and important part of the process of the discovery and development of new medicines for individual patients and the overall benefit of the health of society' (Read and Stonier, 1995). However, it is clear from comparing promotional material and the scientific literature for drugs of the same class that a balanced account of the advantages and disadvantages of a drug are rarely projected to the prescriber; rather, the prescriber is pounded with a biased view of the drug which appeals to parts of the brain other than the intellect. This makes it difficult for the prescriber to judge what is in the best interest for a particular patient.

'Authors change the wording in their books and papers to suit industry. Companies 'place' review papers by their nominated authors in respectable journals. Educational material is written not by who you think but by public relations companies hired by industry' (Warlow, 2002).

There is an instinctive feeling that 'they' may be affected by advertisements but that 'I' make my decisions rationally and based on scientific facts.

- USA resident doctors views on promotion drug companies have been studied: '... only 39 per cent stated that industry promotions and contacts influenced their own prescribing. 84 per cent believed that other doctors' prescribing was affected' (Charatan, 2001).

- In 1994 it was reported that the industry spends the equivalent of £10 000 per general practitioner in the UK on promoting their products (House of Commons, 1994; Rutledge *et al.*, 2002). The equivalents in 2001 are £12 021, US$17 746, €18 119. Gail Turner of the Association of British Pharmaceutical Industry (ABPI) was unable to give an up-to-date figure as it is now bound up with the Pharmaceutical Price Regulation Scheme and this is confidential.

- The industry spends over CAN$20 000 per Canadian doctor annually on gifts or products in addition to the millions donated to hospitals or universities (Zwarenstein, 2001).

- The large budgets of pharmaceutical companies for drug promotion and marketing, estimated at 20–30 per cent of sales turnover, or about two to three times the average expenditure on research and development (Anon., 1993b), suggest that current drug promotional activities are effective in changing physicians behaviour.

- The estimated cost of free drug samples given to a GP over 1 year was £1485.22 (O'Mahony, 1993).

- 'Companies tend to emphasise the positive aspects of products, focussing on attributes that will give them a marketing edge, and not to provide all the objective data (including adverse effects and contraindications) required for comparative analysis' (Anon., 1993b). 'The problem of misleading drug advertisements is real' (Kessler, 1992).

- GSK made oral representations denying the existence of serious new risks with Avandia (rosiglitazone) at a meeting in May 2001 (FDA, 2001; Murray-West, 2001).

- Pharmaceutical industry 'information packages' were found, by Italian GPs, to be often flawed, biased, or misleading. (Maestri *et al.*, 2000).

- The Brazilian prescribing guide *Dicionário de Especialidades Farmacêuticas* (DEF) does not have the same data as in the *PDR* with absent data on contraindications, adverse events and drug interactions (Table 15.2).

Table 15.2   Percentage of each criteria suggested by the WHO absent from the DEF and PDR and USP-DI (Drug Information for the Health Care Professionals) for the 44 best-selling drugs in Brazil (Cabral de Barros, 2000), Pharmacoepidemiology and Drug Safety). Reproduced by permission of Wiley

Criteria Manual	PDR	USP-DI	DEF
Adverse effects	5.6%	–	57.2%
Interactions	38.8 %	2.8%	41.7%
Contraindications	8.3%	–	13.8%

- Companies often try and hide behind the legalism that all of the information has been approved by the national authorities in these countries. In fact, according to the Code of Pharmaceutical Marketing Practices from the IFPMA, company advertisements are permitted to use any material approved by a nation regulatory agency (Lexchin, 2000).

- Research performed by the USA Congress Office of Technology Assessment between 1987 and 1990 was published in 1993 and analysed package inserts for US products marketed in Kenya, Panama, Thailand and Brazil. Information was incomplete on contraindications and adverse effects in 11 per cent and 25 per cent of cases respectively (Anon., 1993b).

- Pharmaceutical adverts, labelling, and package inserts in developing countries often show the twin problems of exaggerated indications and minimized adverse effects (Menkes, 1997).

- The US Office of Technology Assessment report on drug labelling in developing countries (Brazil, Kenya, Panama, Thailand) covering 273 products found that half were entirely appropriate or had relatively small problems and that half diverged significantly and seriously from the standard (www.ota.napedu/pdf/data/1993/9231.PDF). The industry's answer was that the study was flawed and inaccurate and that 'labels around the world differ for valid reasons' (Mossinghoff, 1993).

- In 1994 an FDA team gave details of three techniques used by the industry which were of particular concern to the FDA:

  1. 'Some company-sponsored trials of approved drugs appear to serve little or no scientific purpose, because they are, in fact, thinly veiled attempts to entice doctors to prescribe a new drug being marketed by the company, they are often referred to as 'seeding trials' (Stephens, 1984). Post-marketing surveillance (PMS) studies, sponsored by the pharmaceutical industry, have made little contribution to regulatory monitoring of drug safety (Waller et al., 1992). Company observational post-marketing studies do not contribute significantly to our knowledge of drug safety (Hasford and Lamprecht, 1998). Although the Safety Assessment of Marketed Medicines (SAMM) guidelines severely curtailed such studies in the UK they continue elsewhere.

  2. Unsubstantiated claims of superiority over competing products. The sponsor misrepresented the risk of drug interactions associated with its product relative to the risk with the competing products by making selective use of negative clinical reports and omitting certain important drug interactions associated with its own product'.

  3. Switch campaigns. 'Pharmaceutical companies ... are increasingly trying to cause patients to be switched' from their originally prescribed medications to 'me too' drugs marketed by the companies. The manufacturer asked retail pharmacists who received prescriptions for the older form of the drug to contact the prescribing physicians and request that they change their prescriptions to the newer form ... The pharmacists would receive a payment for each prescription thus switched (Kessler et al., 1994). Some companies ... admit to rewarding doctors for switching from one drug to another but maintained that this was 'standard industry practice' (Marwick, 2003)

Deception concerning ADRs may occur by telling some of the truth but not the whole truth: 'The truth that is told with bad intent beats all the lies you can invent' (William Blake).

Advertisements

- 'I found that the majority of promotional claims referred to me citing clinical studies violated the advertising regulations of the Food and Drug Administration' (Hoberman, 1995).

- 'To promote such uses (of certain medications for unapproved indications) drug companies employ additional techniques ... to disseminate material directly to physicians that discuss unapproved uses ... Another technique is the publication of sponsored symposia ... In an analysis of 11 journals, 51% of those focusing on a single drug discussed products that had not received FDA approval. Furthermore, the lower the therapeutic value of the drug discussed, the more likely it was that the symposium promoted unapproved indications' (Stryer and Bero, 1995).

- Tretinoin is only approved for acne, but in 1988 a study reported that it improved the appearance of 'photoaged' skin, for which it was not licensed. Subsequently, there were large numbers of articles and promotional efforts supporting this use (Stern, 1994). In answer to Dr Stern's comment, 'The approval process is extremely expensive, and many drugs are never approved for appropriate indications ... This problem is particularly relevant to less common diseases' (Kalish, 1995). In the case of the use of topical tretinoin for 'photoaging' (Stern, 1994) some experts viewed the initial findings as a half-full cup, whereas others argued that the cup was half empty. The company's promotional use of these findings made tretinoin appear to be a fountain of youth. Unfortunately, we are unlikely ever to know the full story of the promotion of topical tretinoin by Johnson and Johnson, because it destroyed the records; Johnson and Johnson recently pleaded guilty to charges of conspiracy to obstruct justice in government investigations of this promotional effort and the company paid a US$5 million fine (Stern, 1995).

- The US FDA found that Kabi illegally promoted olasalazine as being indicated for the treatment of mild, moderate, and severe active ulcerative colitis; for use in children; as being superior to sulfasalazine; and as a 'first choice' therapy in the treatment of ulcerative colitis (Ahmad, 1993).

- A survey of 100 Irish physicians found that, when they assessed 10 advertisements chosen at random, 80 per cent were not comfortable with the fact that information relating to side-effects, contraindications or precautions had been excluded. One hundred consecutive advertisements in Irish medical journals were divided into 33 full advertisements and 67 'reminder' advertisements and of the 100 only 33 had details of adverse effects, contraindications and precautions (Hemeryck *et al.*, 1995).

- A US survey of 109 advertisements, where they were peer-reviewed by specialist physicians, concluded that in the opinion of the reviewers many advertisements contained deficiencies in areas in which the FDA has established standards of quality. Reviewers felt that side effects and contraindications in special populations were not appropriately highlighted in 47 per cent of the 49 advertisements in which such information was considered relevant. Only 30 per cent of 95 advertisements were felt to present information on side effects and contraindications with a prominence and readability that was reasonably comparable to the presentation of information on the drug's effectiveness, whereas 57 per cent of advertisements were judged negatively in this respect. The reviewers recommended minor revisions in 28 per cent, major revisions in 50 per cent and rejection in 56 per cent for lack of information on side-effects and contraindications (Dillner, 1992; Wilkes *et al.*, 1992).

- When the veracity of advertisements in Spanish medical journals, in the fields of anti-hypertensives and lipid-lowering drugs, were checked against the references in the advertisements, 44.1 per cent (CI 34.3–54.3) were not supported, most frequently because it was not possible to extrapolate from the reference to the advertisement (Villanueva *et al.*, 2003).

- Advertisements and data sheets provided for the Third World have been criticized by the Medical Lobby for Appropriate Marketing (MaLAM), now known as Healthy Skepticism (Ragg, 1993).

- Two-thirds of the world's countries 'still do not have laws to regulate pharmaceutical promotion or do not enforce the ones they have' (Mintzes, 1998).

- Comparing the *Monthly Index of Medical Specialties* (MIMS) for the UK and India it was found that side effects were omitted in 86 per cent of advertisements in the Indian edition and 57 per cent in the UK edition. Cost was never given in the Indian version and was missing in 57 per cent of the UK advertisements (Dikshit and Dikshit 1994).

- Despite clear statements by the WHO that antimicrobial drugs have no place in the routine treatment of acute diarrhoea, one out of two antidiarrhoeal preparations marketed in 1988–89 contained an antimicrobial drug. In Pakistan, 25 pharmaceutical companies, including some of the largest multinationals, market antidiarrhoeal drugs worth more than US$10 million but only four companies make oral rehydration solution (Costello and Bhutta, 1992). Advertisements in the Indian version of the *BMJ* were misleading or made unsubstantiated claims (Gitanjali *et al.*, 1997).

- A survey between July 1994 and June 1995 of drug advertisements in Indian, British and American medical journals showed significant omissions in Indian journals compared with the American and British journals. The criteria for information content (safety) of advertisements were:

  ADR – Indian 13.7 per cent, American 83.4 per cent and British 82.28 per cent;

  precautions – Indian 12.2 per cent, American 82.6 per cent and British 79.52 per cent;

  warnings – Indian 8.66 per cent, American 76.9 per cent and British 60.23 per cent;

  contraindications – Indian 12.5 per cent, American 82.2 per cent and British 90.94 per cent;

interactions – Indian 8.2 per cent, American 62.5 per cent and British 37.79 per cent (Lal *et al.*, 1997).

- Some promotional brochures said that full prescribing information was available, but when doctors in Pakistan asked for this there were only 26 per cent replies – GPs having 14 per cent and specialists 38 per cent (Hafeez and Mirza, 1999).

- According to the FDA, Pfizer has been making unsubstantiated claims about its antidepressant sertraline to American physicians (Barnett, 1996b).

- The ABPI set up the Prescription Medicines Code of Practice Authority and in 1998 there were 144 complaints about advertisements, mostly from other pharmaceutical companies. The Code of Practice Review, No. 23, February 1999 can be obtained from the authority (Ferriman, 1999).

- In the UK in 2001–2 there were 50 advertisements amended or withdrawn and a further 81 potential breaches were identified through complaints, following which action was taken (NAO, 2003).

- GSK was declared guilty of misleading the public about paroxetine on US television by the IFMA (Tonks, 2002b). The ABPI ruled that the UK's Prescription Medicines Code of Practice had been breached in 14 out of 19 cases heard between January and April 1999 (Mayor, 1999).

Direct to Consumer (DTC) advertising will enable the patients to pressurize the prescriber to use a company's drugs. It has been allowed in the USA since August 1997 but it is still being debated in Europe. Details of the FDA warning letters and untitled letters to the pharmaceutical industry 2002 can be found at www.fda.gov/cder/warn/warn2002.htm.

Attitudes towards adverse drug reactions

Fitzgerald, (1992) writing on crisis management and ADR said 'The initial response of those working within an organisation, particularly product champions, both technical and commercial is that of denial. Until this moment, the whole culture within the company has been positively and energetically to promote the advantage of the drug. Thus, before accepting that the drug is associated with a potentially serious disadvantage, drug champions tend to demand, firstly, proof of causality; secondly, to seek out alternative explanations for the clinical syndrome; and thirdly, to try to implicate other agents in the same drug class, in order to diminish the impact on the specific product'. Replies published by companies, concerning published ADRs, are not too dissimilar to this pattern, giving a very one-sided viewpoint and certainly not giving the reader a balanced opinion of the problem. These letters usually contain some of the following:

- A causal relationship is not admitted.

- No acknowledgement of the validity of any of the comments in the original publication.

- A list of all possible alternatives, however tenuous.

- No mention of the number of cases that the company has received.

- References, some of which, when obtained, seem to have little to do with the original problem.

- Implications that it is a class effect.

- The letter may be from a clinician, without any acknowledgement of an association with the pharmaceutical company, who has been involved with the company as a trialist or adviser.

That is not to say that there are not some misleading ADR reports published. In an editorial in *Risk and Safety in Medicine*, Dr MNG Dukes says 'even with western industry one still in the nineties runs into serious instances where risk data have been concealed in the interests of commerce' (Dukes, 1996).

Sales representatives

- 'The more reliant doctors are on commercial sources of information the less rational they are as prescribers' (Lexchin, 1997).

- A survey of 200 Irish GPs and 230 hospital doctors showed that 26 per cent of GPs rated pharmaceutical representatives as important sources for information for old drugs, 62 per cent for new drugs and 42 per cent said they were the source for the last new drug prescribed. The hospital doctors reckoned pharmaceutical representatives as important for old drugs by 18 per cent, for new drugs by 47 per cent and as a source for last new drug prescribed by 18 per cent (McGettigan *et al.*, 1995, 2001).

- Fewer than three-quarters of representatives spontaneously volunteered information to clinicians on side effects (Bignall, 1994).

- In a US survey of hospital physicians, 37 per cent of them said that their prescribing was influenced by pharmaceutical representatives and it was found that 11 per cent of the representatives' statements were inaccurate when compared with their own literature or the data sheet: all the inaccurate statements were favourable to their own drug. However, 43 per cent thought the representatives provided more reliable information than printed advertisements (Ziegler *et al.*, 1995).

- A confidential detail card used by sales representatives said that at meetings with retail pharmacists an objective is 'to persuade pharmacists to identify those patients who obtain scripts for other nasal sprays and refer them back to their GP for consideration of an alternative therapy' (Collier, 1993).

- 'The main reason[s] for seeing drug representatives are free gifts, free meals, free travel', but also 'educational support, … research grants … [and] … [d]rug company sponsored trials' (Booth, 1999).

- A French physicians' network for the monitoring of medical representatives found that drug indications were extended or changed in about 27 per cent of the visits and dose regimens not in accordance with data sheet in 15 per cent: side effects, contraindications and interactions were not mentioned in 76 per cent of the visits (Prescrire – www.healthskepticism.org).

- An Assessment Instrument for Drug Detailing (AIDD) has been developed and would help family doctors to discriminate between good and bad presentations (Molloy *et al.*, 2002).

Conclusion: many sales representatives do not give a balanced appraisal of a new drug in the context of its efficacy and adverse effects compared with alternative therapies and, therefore, do the patient a disservice.

The pharmaceutical industry and parliament

Clause 118 of the UK Medicines Act, 1968, makes it a criminal offence for the officials involved in licensing or withdrawing a licence from a drug to disclose information about their decisions. The Medicines Information Bill would have allowed summaries of reasons for licensing decisions to be made public (Anon., 1993a). The bill failed to complete the report stage on 30 April 1993, 'Because of 77 amendments that had been tabled, mostly by Conservative MPs representing the pharmaceutical industry' (Houghton, 1993). All the information which the bill proposed should be disclosed is already accessible in the US under the Freedom of Information (FOI) Act (Scrip, 1993).

In 1995 the House of Commons passed a resolution prohibiting paid advocacy by MPs of any cause or matter on behalf of any outside body or individual.

The information available under the FOI Act has been used as a basis for scathing comments both on the industry and the regulators, in a paperback published in 1996, entitled *Science, Politics and the Pharmaceutical Industry* (Abraham, 1995). The drugs chosen, all NSAIDs, were Naproxen, Opren, Feldene, Zomax and Suprol. They are all old drugs marketed prior to 1983, so the book's conclusions are of historic value rather than having relevance to current processes. 'There should be public rights of access to all biochemical, clinical, pharmacological, statistical and toxicological assessment reports by regulators, as well as to transcripts of expert advisory meetings, including appeals procedures. Clinical data supporting the labelling for a medicine (that is, the summary of product characteristics) should also be available for public inspection' (Abraham *et al.*, 1999).

Data sheets or summaries of product characteristics

The data sheet or summary of product characterstics (SPC) is an important channel whereby the pharmaceutical company influences the prescription of its drugs.

- In the USA 'Almost all possible adverse event types, whether treatment-associated or coincidental, are listed in most modern labels'; 'failure to disclose is valuable information for plantiff's attorneys to allege liability' (Fox, 2001).

- There are national differences between SPCs for the same drug: 'giving data essential for optimal use and important safety information (e.g. Sweden) or pre-empting injury litigation by including everything (e.g. USA)' (Anon., 1998b).

- The present data sheets are unsatisfactory in that they do not contain sufficient information to enable the prescriber to make a risk–benefit judgement. The omission of effective low doses for certain drugs in the *PDR* may cause unnecessary dose-related ADR and the information may not be up-to-date (Cohen, 2001).

Sometimes the wording is chosen to hide rather than to reveal, and this may be done by using higher level ADR terms or terms that are too vague to be of any help, e.g. visual disturbance, motor disorder or liver function test (LFT) abnormalities.

If you 'lump', even via a recognised clinical syndrome with accepted diagnostic criteria, you may miss cases with serious clinical manifestations and outcomes when you perform searches; if you 'split' you may pinpoint cases that are not those of concern. (Goldman, 2002)

The different phraseology used to describe abnormal LFTs suggests that the regulatory authorities often acquiesce to the manufacturer's preference.

Since, in the UK, only the 'main' side effects need be included, the data sheets may not include all the known ADRs. The medical requirements are frequently in conflict with the commercial demands in the area of information for the prescriber. A survey of black-triangle drugs showed that around one-quarter of SPCs available for these products did not display a black triangle. The advice offered in SPCs on avoiding unwanted effects in patients with liver disease was often inconsistent, unclear and unhelpful (DTB, 2001).

Pharmaceutical companies try to avoid saying whether their drug can cause an ADR and resort to circumlocutions.

The antihistamine II blocker cimetidine can cause 'gynaecomastia'.

- No clinically significant interference with endocrine or gonadal function has been reported.

- The present ranitidine UK data sheet says under side effects: 'There have been a few reports of breast symptoms (swelling and/or discomfort) in men taking ranitidine; some cases have resolved on continued treatment. Discontinuation may be necessary in order to establish the underlying cause', suggesting a qualitative difference from cimetidine.

- The *PDR* has 'occasional cases of gynaecomastia ... but the incidence did not differ from that in the general population'.

- Martindale has 'there have been isolated reports of gynaecomastia'.

- There were three positive rechallenges recorded before 1984 (Wormsley, 1993).

- An open cohort study with nested case-control analysis in the UK gave the relative risk for cimetidine as 7.2 per cent (CI 4.5–11.3 per cent), misoprostol 2.0 per cent (CI 0.1–10.7 per cent), omeprazole 0.6 per cent (CI 0.1–3.3 per cent) and ranitidine 1.5 per cent

(0.8–2.6 per cent). The paper concluded: use of cimetidine, but not the three other antiulcer drugs, is associated with a substantially greater risk of gynaecomastia among cimetidine users (Garcia Rodriguez and Jick, 1994).

• The WHO has received 393 reports of gynaecomastia for ranitidine. Can ranitidine cause gynaecomastia? GlaxoSmithKline was unable to answer this question.

The EEC (Article 4a of Directive 65/65/EEC as amended by Directive 83/570/EEC) says that a proposal for an SPC must be included in the application. Under the heading 'Undesirable effects' 4.8 concerning undesirable effects it says 'all adverse reactions should be included in the SPC if they are at least possibly causally related, based for example on their comparative incidence in clinical trials, or on findings from epidemiological studies and/or an evaluation of causality from individual report' ... The SPC Coordinators Group 'Update of Guidance on SPC' under 'Undesirable effects' say: 'This section should provide comprehensive information on all adverse reactions attributed to the medicinal product with at least reasonable suspicion and based on best-evidence assessment of all observed adverse events and all facts relevant to the assessment of causality, severity and frequency. In this context, all adverse reactions should be included in the SPC if they are at least possibly causally related, based for example on their comparative incidence in clinical trials, or on findings from epidemiological studies and/or on an evaluation of causality from individual reports (SPC Coordinators' Group, 1998).

It would be of greater value to prescribing physicians if companies were advised to limit the presentation of adverse reactions to those where there is evidence that a causal relationship *probably* exists on a collated basis, in line with the CIOMS III philosophy. (Arnold, 1999).

The FDA (Federal Register/Vol. 65, No. 247, Dec 22nd 2000/proposed rules) 21CFR Part 201 refers to 'adverse drug reactions that are reasonably associated with the use of the drug' (page 81088 Para1) under the heading Warnings/Precautions. The proposed definition of ADR 'an undesirable effect, reasonably associated with the use of the drug, that may occur as part of the pharmacological action of the drug or may be unpredictable in its occurrence' which they say clarifies that at least a reasonably plausible causal relationship must exist between a drug and a noxious and unintended response to be included as an adverse reaction ...'. Page 81120 (9) 8 says that an adverse reaction is 'a noxious and unintended response to any dose of a drug product for which there is a reasonable possibility that the product caused the response (i.e. the relationship cannot be ruled out)'. The phrase 'cannot be ruled out' would presumably include those considered 'unlikely' as well as 'possible, probable and certain'. There is reluctance, both on the part of industry and the regulatory authorities, to use causality assessment to decide if an association is 'probable'. Arnold's comment above applies equally to the FDA proposals.

A survey of pharmaceutical companies showed that eight out of 22 had marketing staff on the committee that made decisions on changes in data sheets (Stephens, 1997). It is difficult to justify their presence.

Some of the suggestions put forward by the CIOMS Working Group III (Guidelines for preparing core clinical-safety information on drugs), page 17–8, have not been implemented. The use of meaningless clichés, such as 'well tolerated'; 'meaningless', since it depends on each patient's assessment of the balance between the benefits and adverse effects of a drug as it concerns them. Lists of adverse events that have been reported 'whether or not attributed to treatment' or 'regardless of causality' or 'same or greater incidence in patients receiving placebo' are still common and seem to be unchecked by regulatory authorities. They 'occur in official data-sheets for the legal protection of the marketer' (CIOMS III, 1995) rather than to help physicians prescribe for their patients.

Delay

It has been estimated that a manufacturer loses over US$1 million on average for each day's delay in gaining US FDA approval of a new drug (Montaner *et al.*, 2001). It is not surprising, therefore, that the industry will do all it can to keep their drugs earning. Owing to the secrecy concerning regulator/industry dealings it is difficult to find out when a company or a regulatory body decides that a safety problem should be addressed in an SPC or requires drug withdrawal and when they take action. During any delay patients may suffer or die.

- The preliminary results of a study comparing the bioequivalence of Synthroid with generic levothyroxine indicated no difference; the sponsor began an intense effort to suppress publication of the results (there was an agreed clause giving the manufacturers the right to preauthorization of all manuscripts submitted for publication). They permitted publication of the original study 7 years after it was completed (Nahata and Welty, 1998).

- It was decided at a CSM meeting on 26 March 1986 that aspirin might be a contributory factor in causing Reye's syndrome, but it wasn't until June 1986 that a warning was given. In the meantime, a 6-year-old took aspirin for chickenpox and developed Reye's syndrome. The UK government was sued (Dyer, 2002b) but the plaintiff lost her case. The judge said that the postponement of a public warning until June 1986 was 'reasonably justifiable'. Without that postponement 'the prospect of full positive cooperation from the industry, which in the event achieved so much, might be lost' (Dyer, 2002c).

- In 1994 and 1995 there were deaths due to Soruvidine for which warnings were not made for years.

- Recently, it has emerged that there were deaths in 1997 with benzbromarone (Lamar, 2000).

- The FDA was sued for 'unreasonable administrative delay in banning an indicator for bromocriptine' (Arnold and Wolfe, 1995).

- A survey of 100 US institutions showed that 12 per cent specified a time limit (0–12 months) to the delay of publication to allow review by sponsors or filing of patents (Cho *et al.*, 2000).

- Phenylpropanolamine has been on the market for more than 30 years and reports of haemorrhagic strokes (estimated at 200–400 cases annually in the USA) were first reported in 1983 and have been well known since the 1970s, despite evidence that the clinical evidence in support of efficacy is limited (Figueras and Laporte, 2002).

- Toronto Academic Health Science Council adopted three principles; these were accepted by the University of Toronto Faculty of Medicine and all eight university-affiliated teaching hospitals:

Agreements should not allow research sponsors to suppress or otherwise censor results and must not preclude investigators from retaining a copy of the relevant site-specific data.

Agreements may allow sponsors time to protect intellectual property or to review and debate the interpretation of results. Investigators should generally be able to submit work for publication within 6 months or exceptionally 12 months.

Researchers must retain the right to disclose immediately any safety concerns that arise during a study (Naylor, 2002).

The pharmaceutical industry may try to delay anything that they feel may reduce their profit. This is often seen prior to a drug being withdrawn from the market or a regulatory authority demands an addition to an SPC.

It has been alleged that the analysis of a clinical trial on Lotronex (Alosetron) was questionable (Barbehenn *et al.*, 2000). It has been suggested that the delay by the FDA between July and November 2000 in taking Lotronex of the market cost five lives. The article's title was 'Lotronex and the FDA: a fatal erosion of integrity' (Horton, 2001a). This was disputed and defended (Adams *et al.*, 2001; Christensen, 2001; Galson *et al.*, 2001; Horton, 2001b; Malozowski, 2001; Walker, 2001). Lotronex was returned to the US market in June 2002 with the stipulation that the prescriber and patient have to sign a statement. 'This prescription programme is unlikely to prevent severe adverse reactions due to Alosetron' (Lièvre, 2002). The following reasons for the reinstatement of Alosetron have been put forward: lobbying by the Lotronex Action Group, industry lobbying and a shift in FDA policy (Lièvre 2002). A further article entitled 'Alosetron: a case study in regulatory capture, or a victory for patients rights?' (Moynihan, 2002) explores the whole sad story.

Corporate ethics

Following the Marconi, Enron and WorldCom finance problems it is reasonable to scrutinize the pharmaceutical industry:

- Bioglan was alleged to be involved in aggressive accounting and went bust (Fletcher, 2002).

- The FDA is investigating Schering–Plough, Eli Lilly and Abbott Laboratories for unusual accounting practices.

- British Biotech is alleged to have misled investors by failing to disclose difficulties which had emerged through trials of its cancer drugs, including Marimastat and Zacutex (Mills, 2002). All these were reported in a single issue of the Daily Telegraph on 21 July 2002.

Other areas

Those working in the pharmaceutical industry should be aware of, and have an opinion about, the ethics in the third world.

- Out of 1223 drugs placed on the market between 1975 and 1997 only 11 are aimed specifically at tropical diseases (Pecoul *et al.*, 1997).

- Three million children die every year in poor countries from diseases that can be prevented by vaccination (Gwatkin and Guillot, 1999).

- 'In the case of AIDS 92% ... of the population have to make do with only 8% of total expenditure' (Bulard, 2000).

- Médecins Sans Frontières says 'Drug companies are failing to develop new drugs for diseases that predominately affect poor people because they are not profitable enough' (Eaton, 2001).

- The supply of affordable drugs for poor populations is threatened by the possibility that they will be resold to Western markets. It has been agreed that copyright for drugs for AIDS, malaria and tuberculosis could be suspended, but only America of the 144 member countries of the World Trade Organization debating the problem in Doha in November 2001 has opposed an agreement that would have relaxed global patent rules on treatments (Mossialos and Dukes, 2001; Stern, 2003).

- 'Commercial interests may conflict with public health needs in developing countries, particularly when people are poisoned due to inadequate restriction of pharmaceutical use, misleading advertisement or labelling, or frankly bogus drugs' (Menkes, 1997).

- There is concern over the increasing number of clinical trials in poor countries where the protection of the subject is not as well developed as in the Western world. Drug trials in Eastern Europe, Latin America and Russia have recently increased greatly, and in these countries the ethic review boards are often inexperienced and unsure of their roles (Stephens and Flaherty, 2001).

- The chairman of SmithKline Beecham said 'The companies are global and research might easily be moved to countries that offer higher quality at lower costs' (Smith, 2000b). Regulatory authorities compete with one another and are driven by the politicians who are pressurized by industry. Speed of recruitment, slow committee work, costs, cleanliness of data and standard of research are all factors that could drive research to countries where safety standards may be lower.

Conclusions

If the above reads like a catalogue of the industry's sins, then it must be seen in the context of the industry's benefit to, predominantly, the developed world, and balanced with the immense number of lives and tremendous suffering that have been prevented by modern medicines. There is an immense literature on these topics and my coverage has been limited.

The bias that the pharmaceutical industry has towards maintaining or increasing its profit is seen in many other areas outside the pharmaceutical industry, e.g. the tobacco industry, but with the great difference that the pharmaceutical industry's products are intended for the benefit of mankind whilst the tobacco industry's products are detrimental to world health. Furthermore, the literature, I have reviewed above, concerning the industry, is biased, in that honest and ethical behaviour within the industry often goes unrecognized and, therefore, unpublished. My selection is probably also biased by previous personal experience with the dishonesty, of senior industry staff.

In an editorial entitled 'The future pharmaceutical physician' Dr RN Smith said 'Indeed, the general perception of the pharmaceutical industry is disappointingly poor' (Smith, 2002). Is this surprising? The mass of responsible people working in the pharmaceutical industry behave ethically but are betrayed by a few, who are in high positions, who behave unethically. Unless those who oppose unethical behaviour protest then the situation will continue. *Qui ne dit mot, consent.*

References

Abraham JW (1995). In *Science, Politics and the Pharmaceutical Industry. A Controversy and Bias in Drug Regulation*. UCI Press: London.

Abraham JW (1997). Secrecy and drug regulation in Europe: who is being protected? *Int J Risk Saf Med* **10**: 143–146.

Abraham J and Lewis G (2000). 'Independence' and 'conflict of interest'. In *Regulating Medicines in Europe*. Routledge: 57–60.

Abraham J, Sheppard J and Reed T (1999). Rethinking transparency and accountability in medicines regulation in the United Kingdom. *Br Med J* **318**:, 46–47.

Adams RC, Advani J, Ajayi F, Al-Fayoumi S *et al.* (2001). The FDA and *The Lancet*: an exchange. *Lancet* **358**: 415-416.

Ahmad SR (1993). FDA and olsalazine. *Lancet* **342**: 487.

Ahmad SR and Wolfe SM (1995). Lesson from a drug indication withdrawal. *Pharmacoepidemiol Drug Saf* **4**: S78.

Anand RK (1996). Health workers and the baby food industry. *Br Med J* **312**: 1556-1557.

Andrew M, Beermanm Klauukka T, Mnørkøre H *et al.*, (1996). ADR warning has decreased the use of third generation oral contraceptives in the Nordic countries. *12th International Conference on Pharmacoepidemiology*, Abstr. 305, 16.

Angell M (2000). Is academic medicine for sale? *New Engl J Med* **342**: 1516-1518.

Anon (1993a). Freedom for drug information. *Lancet* **341**: 885.

Anon (1993b). Drug promotion, stealth, wealth and safety. *Lancet* **341**: 1507–1508.

Anon (1995). In defence of the FDA. *Lancet* **346**: 981.

Anon (1997). Good manners for the pharmaceutical industry. *Lancet* **349**: 1635.

Anon (1998a). Ethics benchmark for pharmaceutical physicians. *Int J Pharm Med* **12**: 179–180.

Anon (1998b). Revised drug information for doctors and patients. *Int J Pharm Med* **12**: 273–274.

Anon (2002). Selective cyclo-oxygenase-2 inhibitors versus nonsteroidal anti-inflammatory drugs discussed. *Adverse Drug React Toxicol Rev* **21(3)**: 161–162.

Applegate WB, Furberg CD, Byington RP and Grimm R (1997). The multicenter Isradipine diuretic atherosclerosis study (MIDAS). *J Am Med Assoc* **277**: 297.

Armstrong E (1998). Safety of patients participating in drug trials. *Br Med J* **317**: 818.

Arnold BDC (1999). An industry view on 'Update of guidance on SPC'. *Int J Pharm Med* **13**: 6–7.

Ashcroft R and Pfeffer N (2001). Ethics behind closed doors: do research ethics committees need secrecy? *Br Med J* **322**: 1294–1296.

Austrian ML (1996). Informed consent and women of child bearing age in investigational studies: a lawyer's perspective. *Drug Inf J* **30**(2): 365–371.

Baber NS (1994). Volunteer studies, are current regulations adequate? The ethical dilemma. *Pharm Med* **8**: 153–159.

Barbehenn E, Lurie P and Wolfe S (2000). Alosetron for irritable bowel syndrome. *Lancet* **356**(9248): 2009.

Barnett AA (1996a). Upjohn and FDA criticised over Halcion. *Lancet* **347**: 1616.

Barnett AA (1996b). FDA warns Pfizer on sertraline marketing. *Lancet* **348**: 469.

Belmont Report (1979). The Belmont Report: ethical principles and guidelines for research involving human subjects. FR Doc. 79-12065. Filed 4-17-79.

Bennett P (1995). Ethical review of multi-location clinical trials and the work of the European Ethical Review committee. *Pharm Med* **9**: 123–127.

Bennett P (1997). Transnational ethical review and education. *Int J Pharm Med* **11**: 213–216.

Bero LA (1999). Accepting commercial sponsorship. *Br Med J* **319**: 653-654.

Bero LA, Galbraith BA and Rennie D (1992). The publication of sponsored symposiums in medical journals. *New Engl J Med* **327**: 1135–1140.

Bignall J (1994). Monitoring reps in France. *Lancet* **344**: 536.

Bland M (2002). WMA should not retreat on use of placebos. *Br Med J* **324**: 240.

Bloemenkamp K, Rosedaal F, Helmerhorst F, Buller H *et al.* (1995). Enhancement by factor V Leiden mutation of risk of deep-vein thrombosis associated with oral contraceptives containing a third-generation progestogen. *Lancet* **346**: 1593–1596.

Blum AL, Chalmers TC, Deutch, Koch-Weser J *et al.* (1987). The Lugano statement on controlled clinical trials. *J Intern Med Res* **15**: 2–22.

Blumenthal D, Campbell EG, Anderson MS, Causino N *et al.* (1997). Withholding research results in academic life sciences: evidence from a national survey of faculty. *J Am Med Assoc* **277**: 1224–1228.

Boardman H (1999). Why are drug-company sponsored clinical trials more likely to have positive outcomes than those organised by academia? *Int J Pharm Med* **13**: 363–364.

Boardman H (2002). Fraud and misconduct in biomedical research. *Pharm Physician* **12**(4): 18–22.

Bodenheimer T (2000). Uneasy alliance. Clinical investigators and the pharmaceutical industry. *New Engl J Med* **342**: 1539–1544.

Bohaychuk W and Ball G (1998). Ethics committees and IRB audit results. *Appl Clin Trials* (November): 46–56.

Booth C (1999). Summary of electronic responses. *Br Med J* **319**: 1003.

Bosch X (1999). Three jailed in bribery and prescription fraud scandal. *Br Med J* **319**: 1026.

Boseley S (1999). Drug firm asks public to insist NHS buys its products. *Guardian* 29 September.

Boseley S (2001). Bitter pill. *Guardian Weekly* 24–30 May.

Boseley S (2002). Scandal of scientists who take money for papers. *Guardian Weekly* 14–20 February.

Boyd EA and Bero LA (2000). Assessing faculty financial relationships with industry: a case study. *J Am Med Assoc* **284**: 2209–2214.

Brown JG (1998). *Institutional Review Boards: a time for reform.* Rockville, Md. Office of the Inspector General. US Department of Health and Human Services, Publication OEI-01-97-00193.

Brown P (1990). EC unease over UK MCA approach. *Scrip* 1564, 7 November, 9.

Bulard M (2000). The apartheid of pharmacology. *Le Monde Diplomatique* 11 January.

Cabral de Barros JA (2000). One more case of the double standard – discrepancies between drug information for Brazilian and American physicians. *Pharmacoepidemiol Drug Saf* **9**: 281–287.

Campbell EG, Louis KS and Blumenthal D (1998). Looking a gift horse in the mouth. Corporate gifts supporting life science research. *J Am Med Assoc* **279**(13): 995–999.

Cavazos N, Forster JD and Bowen AJ (2002). Ethical concerns in placebo-controlled studies: an epidemiological approach. *Drug Inf J* **36**: 249–259.

Charatan F (2001). Doctors say they are not influenced by drug companies' promotion. *Br Med J* **322**: 1081.

Cho MK and Bero LA (1996). The quality of drug studies published in symposium proceedings. *Ann Intern Med* **124**: 485–489.

Cho MK, Shohara R, Schissel A and Rennie D (2000). Policies on faculty conflicts of interest at US universities. *J Am Med Assoc* **284**: 2203–2208.

Choudhry NK, Stelfox HT and Detsky AS (2002). Relationship between authors of clinical guidelines and the pharmaceutical industry. *J Am Med Assoc* **287**(5): 612–617.

Chren MM and Landefeld CS (1994). Physicians' behaviour and their interactions with drug companies. *J Am Med Assoc* **271**: 684–689.

Christensen J (2001). The FDA and *The Lancet:* an exchange. *Lancet* **358**: 417.

CIOMS (1995). Report of CIOMS Working Group III: guidelines for preparing core clinical saftey information on drugs.

CIOMS (2002). *International Ethical Guidelines for Biomedical Research Involving Human Subjects.* WHO: Geneva.

Citron ML (1993). Placebos and principles: a trial of ondansetron. *Ann Intern Med* **118**: 470–471.

Cleophas TJ (1999). Informed consent under scrutiny, suggestions for improvement. In *Methodological Issues Fundamental to Clinical Trials*, Cleophas TJ (ed.). Kluwer Academic: Chapter 12.

Cocoa AA, Webb DD and McSorley DJ (1996). The continued use of placebo-controlled clinical trials in the study of peptic ulcer disease: a sponsor perspective. *Drug Inf J* **30**: 433–439.

Cohen JS (2001). Dose discrepancies between the *Physicians Desk Reference* and the medical literature, and their possible role in the high incidence of dose-related adverse drug events. *Arch Intern Med* **161**: 957–964.

Collier J (1993). Drug company representatives and sale priorities. *Lancet* **341**: 1031–1032.

Collier J (1995). Confusion over use of placebos in clinical trials. *Br Med J* **311**: 821–822.

Cordier L (1997). Is there a European ethical framework for clinical research? *Int J Pharm Med* **11**: 137–140.

Costello AMdeL and Bhutta T (1992). Antidiarrhoeal drugs for acute diarrhoea in children. *Br Med J* **304**: 1–2.

Dazzi D, Agnetti B, Bandini L, Corradini P *et al.* (2001). What do people think (and know) about informed consent for participation in a medical trial? *Arch Int Med* **161**: 768–769.

Demenet P (2002). The high cost of living. *Le Monde Diplomatique*, February.

Detsky AS and Stelfox HT (1998). Conflict of interest in the debate over calcium channel antagonists. *New Engl J Med* **33**(23): 1967–1968.

Diamond A, Hall S, Jay M, Laurence D *et al.* (1994). Independent ethical reviews of studies involving personal medical records. *J R Coll Physicians London* **28**(5): 439–443.

DIA Program Notes (2001). Session chairperson: Elizabeth A Moench, Recall of knowledge from informed consent, December.

Dikshit RK and Dikshit N (1994). Commercial source of the drug information comparison between the United Kingdom and India. *Br Med J* **309**: 990–991.

Dillner L (1992). Drug advertisements misleading. *Br Med J* **304**: 1526.

Djulbegovic B, Lacevic M, Cantor A, Fields KK *et al.* (2000). Uncertainty principle and industry-sponsored research. *Lancet* **356**: 635–638.

Dollop S (1998). Safety of patients participating in drug trials. *Br Med J* **317**: 818.

Double DB (1996). Placebo controlled trials are needed to provide data on effectiveness of active treatment. *Br Med J* **313**: 1008–1009.

DTB (2001). Failings in treatment advice, SPCs and black triangles. *Drugs Thera Bull* **39**: 25–26.

Dukes MNG (1996). Drug safety – can more be done? *Int J Risk Saf Med* **9**(2): 71–73.

Dunn NR, Arscott A and Mann RD (2000). Costs of seeking ethics approval before and after the introduction of multicentre research ethics committees. *J R Soc Med* **93**: 511–512.

Dyer C (2001). University accused of violating academic freedom to safeguard funding from drug companies. *Br Med J* **323**: 591.

Dyer C (2002a). Drug firms face £10m claim over pill. *Guardian Weekly*, 7–13 March.

Dyer C (2002b). Government sued for 11 week delay in warning about aspirin. *Br Med J* **324**: 134.

Dyer C (2002c). Woman damaged by aspirin loses court claim. *Br Med J* **324**: 444.

Dyer C (2002d). Claim launched against makers of third generation pill. *Br Med J* **324**: 561.

Eaton L (2001). Drug companies neglect research into diseases affecting the poor. *Br Med J* **323**: 827.

Edwards SJL, Lilford RJ and Hewison RJL (1998). The ethics of randomised controlled clinical trials from the perspective of patients, the public, and healthcare professionals. *Br Med J* **317**: 1209–1212.

EFGCP (1997). Guidelines and recommendations for European Ethics Committees. *Int J Pharm Med* **11**: 129–135.

Eichenwald K and Kolata G (1999). *The New York Times*, 16 and 17 May. (Reported in the *International Herald Tribune*, 27 May.

Electoral Commission (2002). http://www.electoralcommission.gov.uk (July 2003).

Ethical Issues Working Group (1998). Ethics in pharmaceutical medicine. *Int J Pharm Med* **12**: 193–198.

Ethics Committee Review of Multi-centre Research (1997). Establishment of multi-centre research ethics committees. *Department of Health*, 10436 HP 2.4k 1P Apr 97 SA (0).

Evans D (1997). The reform of multicentre ethical review: MRECs for better or worse. *Int J Pharm Med* **11**: 217–220.

Evans D and Evans M (1996). *A Decent Proposal: Ethical Review of Clinical Research*. John Wiley.

Evans S and Pocock S (2001). Societal responsibilities of clinical sponsors. *Br Med J* **322**: 569–570.

Farmer RDT, Williams TJ, Simpson EL and Nightingale AL (2000). The effect of 1995 pill scare on rates of venous thromboembolism among women taking combined oral contraceptives: analysis of General Practice research. *Br Med J* **321**: 477–479.

FDA (1999). Financial disclosure by clinical investigators. *Guidance for industry*. US FDA.

FDA (2001). FDA warning letter Re: Avandia (rosiglitazone maleate) tablets. www.fda.gov/cder/warn/2001

Federmann DD, Hanna KE and Rodriguez LL (2003). *Responsible Research: A Systems Approach to Protecting Research Participants*. Institute of Medicine: p13, 18.

Feger H (1996). Pill scare led to abortion misery for thousands. *Daily Express*, 22 November.

Ferriman A (1999). Drug companies criticised for exaggeration. *Br Med J* **318**: 962.

Ferriman A (2001). World Medical Association clarifies rules on placebo controlled trials. *Br Med J* **323**: 825.

Figueras A and Laporte J-R (2002). Regulatory decisions in a globalised world. *Drug Safety* **25**(10): 689–693.

Fitzgerald JD (1992). Crisis management: the medical director's response. *Pharmacoepidemiol Drug Saf* **1**: 155–161.

Fletcher R (2002). KPMG changed Bioglan advice. *Daily Telegraph*, 21 July.

Forster HP, Emanuel E and Grady C (2001). The revision of the Declaration of Helsinki: a step forward or more confusion? *Lancet* **358**: 1449-1452.

Foster C (1997). The current status of ethical review procedures in the United Kingdom. *Int J Pharm Med* **11**: 155–159.

Fox AW (2001). 'High–profile' product withdrawals in the United States. *Int J Pharm Med* **15**: 27–30.

Friedberg M, Saffran B, Stinson TJ, Nelson W *et al.* (1999). Evaluation of conflict of interest in economic analyses of new drugs used in oncology. *J Am Med Assoc* **282**: 1453–1457.

Fukuhara S, Tanabe N, Sato K, Ohashi Y *et al.* (1997). Good clinical practice in Japan before and after ICH: problems and potential impacts on clinical trials and medical practice. *Int J Pharm Med* **11**: 147–153.

Fukuhara S, Tanabe N and Kurokawa K (1999). Background issues in Japan affecting the ethical review process for clinical trials. *Int J Pharm Med* **13**: 25–28.

Gallant SP (1995). Placebo-controlled versus comparative studies of drug effects. *J Pediatr* **126**: 681.

Galson S, Kweder S, Houn F, Raczkowski V *et al.* (2001). The FDA and *The Lancet*: an exchange. *Lancet* **358**: 415.

Garattini S and Bertele V (2001). Adjusting Europe's drug regulation to public health needs. *Lancet* **358**: 64–66.

Garcia Rodriguez LA and Jick H (1994). Risk of gynaecomastia associated with cimetidine, omeprazole and other anti-ulcer drugs. *Br Med J* **308**(6927): 503–506.

Georgiou A (1996). High quality placebos should be used. *Br Med J* **313**: 1009.

Gerth G and Stolberg SG (2000). Drug industry has ties to groups with many different voices. *New York Times*, 5 October.

Gill L and Baber N (1995). Ethical and scientific review procedures in the pharmaceutical industry: a survey of 12 British-based companies. *Pharm Med* **9**(1): 11–21.

Gitanjali B, Shahindran CH, Tripathi KD and Sethuraman KR (1997). Are drug advertisements in Indian edition of *BMJl* unethical? *Br Med J* **315**: 459.

Glass RM and Schneiderman M (1997). At *International Congress on Biomedical Peer Review and Scientific Publication*, 18–20 September.

Glassman PA, Hunter-Hayes J and Nakamura T (1999). Pharmaceutical advertising revenues and physicians organisations: how much is too much? *West J Med* **171**, 234–239.

Godlee F (1996). The food industry fights for salt. *Br Med J* **312**: 1239–1240.

Goldman SA (2002). Adverse event reporting and standardized medical terminologies: strengths and limitations. *Drug Inf J* **36**: 439–444.

Gottlieb S (1999). Medical societies accused of being beholden to the drugs industry. *Br Med J* **319**: 1321.

Gottlieb S (2000a). FDA censures *NEJM* editor. *Br Med J* **320**: 1562.

Gottlieb S (2000b). Firm tried to block report on failure of AIDS vaccine. *Br Med J* **321**: 1173.

Gottlieb S (2001). Researchers deny any attempt to mislead the public over *JAMA* article on arthritis drug. *Br Med J* **323**: 301.

Guardian (2000). Dobbo's medicine man. *Guardian*, 26 April.

Gupta A (2001). Journals fail to adhere to guidelines on conflicts of interest. *Br Med J* **323**: 651.

Gurdon H (1994). Japan drug firm shut after 15 patients die. *Daily Telegraph* 2 September.

Guyatt G (1994). Academic medicine and the pharmaceutical industry: a cautionary tale. *Can Med Assoc J* **150**(6): 951–956.

Gwatkin DR and Guillot M (1999). *The Burden of Disease Among the Global Poor*. World Bank: Washington, DC.

Hafeez A and Mirza Z (1999). Responses from pharmaceutical companies to doctors' requests for more drug information in Pakistan. *Br Med J* **319**: 547.

Hailey D (2000). Scientific harassment by pharmaceutical companies: time to stop. *Can Med Assoc J* **162**(2): 212–3.

Hall C (1997). Rise in abortions after thrombosis scare over pill. *Daily Telegraph*, 21 February.

Hampton J (2000). Clinical trial committees: the devil's spoon. *Br Med J* **320**: 244–245.

Hasford J and Lamprecht T (1998). Company observational post-marketing studies: drug risk assessment and drug research in special populations – a study-based analysis. *Eur J Clin Pharmacol* **53**: 369–371.

Heinemann LAJ and Lewis MA (1996). Increased risk estimates for venous thromboembolism under OCs with third generation progestagens due to preferential prescribing? *Pharmacoepidemiol Drug Saf* **5**: S59.

Hemeryck L, Chan R, McCormack PME, Condren L *et al.* (1995). Pharmaceutical advertisements in Irish medical journals. *J Pharm Med* **5**: 147–151.

Henderson L (2000). More AMCs funding growth from reform. *Centerwatch* **7**: 10–13

Hennessy S, Berlin JA, Kinman JL, Margolis DJ *et al.* (2001). Risk of venous thromboembolism from oral contraceptives containing Gestodene and Desogestrel versus Levonorgestrel: a meta-analysis and formal sensitivity analysis. *Pharmacoepidemiol Drug Saf* **10**: S93.

Henry D and Hill S (1995). Comparing treatments. *Lancet* **310**: 1279.

Herings RMC, De Boer A, Urquhart J and Leufkens HGM (1996). Non-causal explanation for the increased risk of venous thromboembolism among users of third generation oral contraceptives. *Pharmacoepidemiol Drug Saf* **5**: S88.

Hildebrandt AG (1995). Guest interview – the role of the German Bfarm within the new EC regulatory framework. *Regulat Affairs J* (October): 813–817.

Hoberman D (1995). Drug promotion. *New Engl J Med* **322**: 1031.

Hodges C (1991). Harmonisation of European controls over research. In *Pharmaceutical Medicine and the Law*, Goldberg A and Dodds-Smith I. RCP: UK.

Horton R (2000). The less acceptable face of bias. *Lancet* **356**: 959–960.

Horton R (2001a). Lotronex and the FDA: a fatal erosion of integrity. *Lancet* **357**: 1544–1545.

Horton R (2001b). The FDA and *The Lancet:* an exchange. *Lancet* **358**: 417–8.

Houghton R (1993). Medicines Information Bill. *Br Med J* **341**: 1208–1209.

House of Commons (1999). House of Commons' Health Committee Inquiry into priority setting in the NHS: the drugs budget. Evidence of the National Association of Health Authorities and Trusts. January.

Hulley SB and Cummings SC (1988). *Designing Clinical Research.* Williams and Wilkins: Baltimore.

Human D, Crawley F and Ijesselmuiden C (2001). WMA will continue to revise policy as medicine and research changes. *Br Med J* **323**: 283–284.

Hussain A and Smith R (2001). Declaring financial competing interests: survey of five general medical journals. *Br Med J* **323**: 263–264.

Hvidberg EF (1994). Continuous improvement of ethics committees. *Drug Inf J* **28**: 1125 1128.

Jick H, Jick SS, Gurewich V, Myers MW *et al.* (1995). Risk of idiopathic cardiovascular death and nonfatal venous thromboembolism in women using oral contraceptives with differing progestogen components. *Lancet* **346**: 1589–1593.

Jüni P, Rutjes AWS and Dieppe PA (2002). Are selective COX 2 inhibitors superior to traditional non-steroidal anti-inflammatory drugs? *Br Med J* **324**: 1287–1288.

Kalish RS (1995). Drug promotion. *New Engl J Med* **322**: 1032.

Kemmeren JM, Algra A and Grobber DE (2001). Third generation oral contraceptives and risk of venous thrombosis: meta-analysis. *Br Med J* **323**: 131–134.

Kessler DA (1992). Addressing the problem of misleading advertisements. *Ann Intern Med* **116**: 950–951.

Kessler DA, Rose JL, Temple RJ, Shapiro R *et al.* (1994). Therapeutic-class wars-drug promotions in a competitive marketplace. *New Engl J Med* **331**: 1350–1353.

Kjaergard LL and Als-Nielsen B (2002). Association between competing interests and authors' conclusions: epidemiological study of randomised clinical trials published in the *BMJ. Br Med J* **325**: 249–52.

Klincewicz SL, Clark JA and LaFrance ND (2001). A review and analysis of key regulations and guidelines concerning the safety sections of the investigator's brochure. *Drug Inf J* **35**: 347–355.

Knox KS, Adams JR, Djulbegovic B, Stinson TJ *et al.* (2000). Reporting and dissemination of industry versus non-profit sponsored economic analyses of six novel drugs used in oncology. *Ann Oncol* **11**(12): 1513–1515.

Krimsky S, Rothenberg LS, Stoot P and Kyle G (1996). Scientific journals and their authors' financial interests: a pilot study. *Sci Eng Ethics* **2**: 395–410.

Lal A, Moharana AK and Srivastava S (1997). Comparative evaluation of drug advertisements in Indian, British and American medical journals. *J Indian Med Assoc* **95**(1): 19–20.

Lamar J (2000). Japan plans improved monitoring of new drugs. *Br Med J* **320**: 1560.

Lasagna L (1995). The Helsinki Declaration: timeless guide or irrelevant anachronism. *J Clin Psychopharmacol* **15**(2): 96–8.

Lenzer J (2002). Alteplase for stroke: money and optimistic claims buttress the 'brain attack' campaign. *Br Med J* **324**: 723–729.

Levine RJ (1997). Institutional Review Boards. *Int J Pharm Med* **11**: 141–146.

Lewis JA, Jonsson B, Kreutz G, Sampaio C *et al.* (2002). Placebo-controlled trials and the declaration of Helsinki. *Lancet* **359**: 1337–1340.

Lewis MA, Spitzer WO, Heinemann LAJ, MacRae KD *et al.* (1996a). Third generation oral contraceptives and risk of myocardial infarction: an international case-control study. *Br Med J* **312**: 88–90.

Lewis MA, Spitzer WO, Heineman AJ, Thorogood M *et al.* (1996b). Venous thromboembolic disease and oral contraceptive use: an international case-control study. *Pharmacoepidemiol. Drug Saf* **5**: S24.

Lewis MA, MacRae KD and Kühl-Habich D (1998). The differential risk of oral contraceptives: the impact of full exposure history. *Pharmacoepidemiol Drug Saf* **7**: S115.

Lexchin J (1997). Consequences of direct-to-consumer advertising of prescription drugs. *Can Fam Physician* **43**: 594–596.

Lexchin J (2000). Double standards: double jeopardy. *Pharmacoepidemiol Drug Saf* **9**: 289–290.

Lièvre M (2002). Alosetron for irritable bowel syndrome. *Br Med J* **325**: 555–556.

Lièvre M, Méynard J, Bruckert E, Cogneau J *et al.* (2001). Premature discontinuation of clinical trial for reasons not related to efficacy, safety, or feasibility. *Br Med J* **322**: 603–606.

Mackintosh DR and Zepp VJ (1996). Detection of negligence, fraud and other bad faith efforts during field auditing of clinical trials sites. *Drug Inf J* **30**: 645–653.

Maestri E, Furlani G, Suzzi F, Camomori A *et al.* (2000). So much time: Italy's pharmaceutical industry and doctors information needs. *Br Med J* **320**: 55–56.

Malozowski S (2001). FDA and *The Lancet*: an exchange. *Lancet* **358**: 416–417.

Mann H (2002). Clinical trial protocols: agreements between the FDA and industrial sponsors. *Lancet* **360**: 1345–1346.

Marwick C (2003). Drug companies defend rewards to doctors for switching treatments. *Br Med J* **326**: 67.

Mayor S (1999). Unbalanced presentation of facts breaks UK drug adverts code. *Br Med J* **319**: 727.

Mayor S (2002). Researchers claim clinical trials are reported with misleading statistics. *Br Med J* **324**: 1353.

MCA (1997). MCA Annual Report for 1996. MCA HMSO.

McEwan J (1998). Antipodean regulatory event, conflict of interest and appointment. Source unknown.

McGettigan P, Gloden J, Chan R and Feely J (1995). Sources of information used by hospital doctors when prescribing new drugs. *Br J Clin Pharmacol* **37**: 471P.

McGettigan P, Gloden J, Fryer J, Chan R *et al.* (2001). Prescribers prefer people: the sources of information used by doctors for prescribing suggest that the medium is more important than the message. *Br J Clin Pharmacol* **51**: 184–189.

McLean SAM (1995). Research Ethics Committees: principles and proposals. *Health Bull* **53**(5): 243–248.

McPherson K (1996). Third generation oral contraception and venous thrombosis. *Br Med J* **312**: 68–69.

McPherson K (2002). Epidemiology on trial – confessions of an expert witness. *Lancet* **360**: 889–890.

McQuay H and Moore A (1996). Placebo mania, placebos are essential when extent and variability of placebo response are known. *Br Med J* **313**: 1008.

Meltzer JI (1998). Conflict of interest in the debate over calcium channel antagonists. *New Engl J Med* **338**(23): 1696.

Menkes DB (1997). Hazardous drugs in developing countries. *Br Med J* **315**: 1557–1558.

Michaels MA, Norpath T and Rekers H (1996). The latest pill scare: the industry perspective. *Pharmacoepidemiol Drug Saf* **5**: S77.

Mills L (2002). British Biotech faces lawsuit. *Daily Telegraph*, 21 July.

Mintzes B (1998). *Blurring the Boundaries: New Trends in Drug Promotion.* Health Action International: Amsterdam.

Molloy W, Strang D, Guyatt G, Lexchin J *et al.* (2002). Assessing the quality of drug detailing. *J Clin Epidemiol* **55**: 835–832.

Montaner JSG, O'Shaughnessy MV and Schechter MT (2001). Industry-sponsored clinical research: a double-edged sword. *Lancet* **358**: 1893–1895.

Morse M, Calif R and Sugarman J (2001). Monitoring and ensuring safety during clinical research. *J Am Med Assoc* **285**: 1201–1205.

Mossialos E and Dukes G (2001). Affordable priced new drugs for poor populations: approaches for a global solution. *Int J Risk Saf Med* **14**: 1–29.

Mossinghoff GJ (1993). Drug labelling in developing countries. *Lancet* **342**: 556–557.

Moynihan R (2002). Alosetron: a case study in regulatory capture, or a victory for patients' rights? *Br Med J* **325**: 592–595.

Murray-West R (2001). Glaxo censured over diabetes drug. *Daily Telegraph*, 4 August.

Nahata MC and Welty TE (1998). Troubling issues with research publications. *Ann Pharmacother* **32**: 126–128.

NAO (National Accident Office) (2003). *Safety, Quality, Efficacy: Regulating Medicines in the UK.* www.nao.gov.uk (19 July 2003).

Nathan DG and Weatherall DJ (1999). Academia and industry: lessons from the unfortunate events in Toronto. *Lancet* **353**: 771–772.

National Council of Bioethics (2002). The ethics of research related to healthcare in developing countries. www.nuffieldbioethics.org/developingcountries/latestnews.asp (19 July 2003).

Naylor CD (2002). Early Toronto experience with new standards for industry-sponsored clinical research: a progress report. *Can Med Assoc J* **166**(4): 453–456.

NIH Catalyst (2000). Financial conflicts of interest and clinical research. September–October http://catalyst.al.nih.gov/catalyst/2000/00.09.01/

O'Mahony B (1993). Interactions between a general practitioner and representatives of drug companies. *Br Med J* **306**: 1649.

Palmer CR (1993). Ethics and statistical methodology in clinical trials. *J Med Ethics* **19**: 219–222.

Parexel (1998). *Pharmaceutical R & D Statistical Sourcebook*, Mathey MP (ed.). Parexel International Corporation: Walthams, MA.

Pecoul B, Chirac P, Trouiller P and Pinel J (1999). Access to essential drugs and poor countries. A lost battle? *J Am Med Assoc* **281**: 361–367.

Peterson M (2001). Drug firm to pay $875 million fine. *International Herald Tribune*, 4 October.

Pocock SJ (1983). *Clinical Trials: A Practical Approach.* Wiley: Chichester.

Pocock SJ (1992). When to stop a clinical trial. *Br Med J* **305**: 235–240.

Ragg M (1993). MaLAM and Augmentin. *Lancet* **342**: 487.

Ramsay LE (1997). Commentary: placebo run-ins have some value. *Br Med J* **314**: 1193.

Rao JN and Sant Cassia LJ (2002). Ethics of undisclosed payments to doctors recruiting patients in clinical trials. *Br Med J* **325**: 36–37.

Read PR and Stonier PD (1995). Ethics and the promotion of medicines. *Pharm Med* **9**: 49–53.

Rennie D (1997). Thyroid storm. *J Am Med Assoc* **277**(15): 1283–1244.

Rochon PA, Gurwitz JH and Simms RW (1994). A study of manufacturer-supported trials of nonsteroidal anti-inflammatory drugs in the treatment of arthritis. *Ann Intern Med* **154**: 157–163.

Rothman KJ (1996). Placebo mania. *Br Med J* **313**: 3–4.

Rothman KJ, Michels KB and Baum M (2000). Declaration of Helsinki should be strengthened. *Br Med J* **321**: 442–445.

Rutledge P, Crookes D, McKinstry B and Maxwell SRJ (2002). Do doctors rely on pharmaceutical industry funding to attend conferences and do they perceive that this creates a bias in their drug selection? – Results of a questionnaire survey to Edinburgh doctors. *Pharmacoepidemiol Drug Saf* **11**(S1): S65, Abstract 143.

Savulescu J (2002). Two deaths and two lessons: is it time to review the structure and function of research ethics committees? *Med Ethics* **28**: 1–2.

Savulescu J, Chalmers I and Blunt J (1996). Are research ethics committees behaving unethically? Some suggestions for improving performance and accountability. *Br Med J* **313**: 1390–1393.

Scrip (1993). UK Medicines Information Bill blocked. *Scrip* **1818–19**: 2–3.

Senn S (1997). Are placebo run-ins justified? *Br Med J* **314**: 1191–1193.

Shimm DS and Spece RG (1991). Industry reimbursement for entering patients into clinical trials: legal and ethical issues. *Ann Intern Med* **115**: 148–151.

Silverstein K (1999). *www.motherjones.com/mother_jones_/ND99.NAMI.html* Prozac.org. MOJO wire magazine, Nov/Dec.

Silverstein FE, Faich G, Goldstein JL, Simon LS *et al.* (2000). Gastrointestinal toxicity with celecoxib vs nonsteroidal anti-inflammatory drugs for osteoarthritis and rheumatoid arthritis: the CLASS study: a randomized controlled trial. Celecoxib long-term arthritis safety study. *J Am Med Assoc* **284**(10): 1247–1255.

Skelly MM and Hawkey CJ (2002). Potential alternatives to COX 2 inhibitors. *Br Med J* **324**: 1289–1290.

Smith R (1998). Beyond conflict of interest. *Br Med J* **317**: 291–292.

Smith R (2000). UK is losing market share in pharmaceutical research. *Br Med J* **321**: 1041.

Smith R (2001). Maintaining the integrity of the scientific record. *Br Med J* **323**: 588.

Smith RN (2002). The future pharmaceutical physician. *Int J Pharm Med* **15**: 259–260.

Snell NJC (2001). Industry-sponsored clinical trials and medical publishing. *Int J Pharm Med* **15**: 217–218.

Sniderman AD (1996). The governance of clinical trials. *Lancet* **347**: 1387–1388.

Spaight SJ, Nash S, Finison IJ and Patterson WB (1984). Medical oncologists participation in cancer clinical trials. *Prog Clin Biol Res* **156**: 49–61.

SPC Coordinator's Group (1998). Update of guidance on SPC consolidated proposals from multi-disciplinary groups for the wording of the SPC. *Int J Pharm Med* **13**: 35–42.

Spilker B (1991). In *Guide to Clinical Trials*. Raven Press.

Spitzer WO, Lewis MA, Heineman LAJ, Thorogood M *et al.* (On behalf of the transnational research group on oral contraceptives and the health of young women) (1996). Third generation oral contraceptives and risk of venous thromboembolic disorders: an international case-control study. *Br Med J* **312**: 83–88.

Spurgeon D (1998a). Drug company fails to stop publication of report. *Br Med J* **317**: 101.

Spurgeon D (1998b). Trials sponsored by drug companies: review ordered. *Br Med J* **317**: 618.

Stein CM and Pinks T (1999). Placebo-controlled studies in rheumatoid arthritis: ethical issues. *Lancet* **353**: 400–403.

Stelfox HT, Chua G, O'Rourke K and Detsky AS (1998). Conflict of interest in the debate over calcium-channel antagonists. *New Engl J Med* **338**(2): 101–106.

Stephens J and Flaherty MP (2001). US study warns of risks of overseas drug trials. *International Herald Tribune*, 3 October.

Stephens MDB (1984). Pharmaceutical company viewpoint. In *Monitoring for Adverse Drug Reactions*, Walker SR and Goldberg A (eds). MTP Press Ltd: 119–125.

Stephens MDB (1997). From causality to product labelling. *Drug Inf J* **31**: 849–856.

Stephens MDB (1998). Ethics, honesty and the pharmaceutical industry. In *Detection of New Adverse Drug Reactions*, Stephens MDB, Talbot JCC and Routledge PA (eds). Wiley: 381.

Stern B (2003). WTO fails to deliver agreement on drugs. *Guardian Weekly* 2–8 January, 25.

Stern RS (1994). Drug promotion for unlabeled indication – the case of topical tretinoin. *New Engl J Med* **331**: 1348–1349.

Stern RS (1995). Drug promotion. *New Engl J Med* **332**(15): 1033.

Stolley PD and Laporte J-R (2000). The public health, the university, and pharmacoepidemiology. In *Pharmacoepidemiology*, 3rd edition, Strom BL (ed.). John Wiley: 87.

Strandgaard S (1998). Conflict of interest in the debate over calcium channel antagonists. *New Engl J Med* **338**(23): 1697.

Strom B (2000). The future of pharmacoepidemiology. In *Pharmacoepidemiology*, 3rd edition. Wiley: 815.

Stryer DB and Bero LA (1995). Drug promotion. *New Engl J Med* **332**: 1032.

Suissa S, Blais L, Spitzer WO, Cusson J *et al.* (1997). First-time use of newer oral contraceptives and the risk of venous thromboembolism. *Contraception* **56**(3): 141–146.

Szarewski A (1997). Third generation pill warnings were premature. *Lancet* **350**: 497.

Tait N and Firn D (2002). Women sue over pill side-effects. *Financial Times*, 5th March.

Tamer MR, Reynolds DJM, Moore RA and McQuay HJ (1998). When placebo controlled trials are essential and equivalence trials are inadequate. *Br Med J* **317**: 875–880.

Tattersall MHN (2001). Examining informed consent to cancer trials. *Lancet* **358**: 1742.

Tattersall MHN and Olver IN (1999). Conflict of interest and advisory committees. *Int J Pharm Med* **13**: 325–328.

Taylor A (1998). Violation of the international code of marketing of breast milk substitutes: prevalence in four countries. *Br Med J* **316**: 1117–1122.

Taylor KM and Kelner M (1987). Interpreting physician participation in randomised clinical trials: the physician orientation profile. *J Health Soc Behav* **28**: 389–400.

Thomas PS, Tan K-S and Yates DH (2002). Sponsorship, authorship, and accountability. *Lancet* **359**: 351.

Tiner R (1999). Reasons for not seeing drug representatives. *Br Med J* **319**: 1002.

Titus SL and Keane HA (1996). Do you understand? An ethical assessment of research descriptions of the consenting process. *J Clin Ethics* **7**(1): 60–68.

Tonks A (2002a). Authors of guidelines have strong links with industry. *Br Med J* **324**: 383.

Tonks A (2002b). Withdrawal from paroxetine can be severe, warns FDA. *Br Med J* **324**: 260.

Trefgarne G (2002). Companies find Labour's £500 dinner hard to swallow. *Daily Telegraph*, 20 February, 35.

Tripp J (ed.) (1996). *Royal College of Physicians of London Committee on Ethical Issues in Medicine.* Guidelines on the practice of ethics committees in medical research involving human subjects. RCP: London.

Ueda K (1996). Present status of compliance of GCP Part 3. *Clin Eval* **24**: 57–87.

US Congress (1993). Drug labelling in developing countries.

Vandenbrouke JP, Helmerhorst FM and Rosendaal FR (2000). Competing interests and controversy about third generation oral contraceptives. *Br Med J* **320**: 381–382.

Van Heteren G (2001). Wyeth suppresses research on pill, programme claims. *Br Med J* **322**: 571.

Villanueva P, Peiró S, Librero J and Pereiró I (2003). Accuracy of pharmaceutical advertisements in medical journals. *Lancet* **361**: 21–32.

Wahlbeck K and Adams K (1999). Beyond conflict of interest. Sponsored drug trials show more favourable outcomes. *Br Med J* **318**: 465.

Walker A (2001). The FDA and *The Lancet*: an exchange. *Lancet* **358**: 417.

Waller PC, Wood SM, Langman MJS, Breckenridge AM *et al.* (1992). Review of company postmarketing surveillance studies. *Br Med J* **304**: 1470–1472.

Warlow C (2002). Commentary: who pays the guideline writers?. *Br Med J* **324**: 726–727.

Washburn J (2001). Undue influence. *The American Prospect* **12**(14): 1–17.

Washington Fax (2001). NHS starts reviewing conflict-of-interest policies of grantee institutions. www.washingtonfax.com/p1/2001/20010723.html

Wazana A (2000). Physicians and the pharmaceutical industry is a gift ever just a gift? *J Am Med Assoc* **283**: 373–380.

Weinberg MM (1995). Placebo-controlled versus comparative studies of drug effects. *J Pediatr* **126**: 680–681.

WHO (1995). Collaborative study in cardiovascular disease and steroid hormone contraception. Effect of different progestogens in low dose oral contraceptives on venous thromboembolic disease. *Lancet* **346**: 1582–1593.

WHO (1998). Cardiovascular disease and steroid hormone contraception. Report of WHO Scientific Group on cardiovascular disease and steroid hormonal contraception. WHO Technical Report Service, No. 877.

Wilkes MS, Doblin BH and Shapiro MF (1992). Pharmaceutical advertisements in leading medical journals: experts' assessments. *Ann Intern Med* **116**: 912–919.

Williams CK and Zwitter M (1994). Informed consent in European multicentre randomised clinical trials – are patients really informed? *Eur J Cancer* **30**(7): 907–910.

Williamson H (2002). German doctors accused of taking bribes. *Financial Times*, 12 March.

Wilmhurst P (2000). Academia and industry. *Lancet* **356**: 338–339.

Wilson CO (1996a). Midwives braced for July baby boom. *Daily Telegraph*, 25 May.

Wilson CO (1996b). Abortions rise after pill scare. *Daily Telegraph*, 22 November.

Wise J (1996). Baby milk companies accused of breaching marketing code. *Br Med J* **314**: 167.

Wise J (1997). Research suppressed for seven years by drug company. *Br Med J* **314**: 1149.

Woodward B (1999). Challenges to human subject protection. *J Am Med Assoc* **282**: 1947–1952.

Wormsley KG (1993). Safety profile of ranitidine. A review. *Drugs* **46**(6): 976–985.

Yuval R, Halon DA, Merdler A, Khader N *et al.* (2000). Patient comprehension and reaction to participating in a double-blind randomised clinical trial in acute myocardial infarction. *Arch Intern Med* **160**(8): 1142–1146.

Ziegler MG, Lew P and Singer BC (1995). The accuracy of drug information from pharmaceutical sales representatives. *J Am Med Assoc* **273**: 1296–1298.

Zumula A and Costello A (2002). Ethics of healthcare research in developing countries. *J R Soc Med* **95**(6): 275–276.

Zwarenstein C (2001). Doctors for Research Integrity (DRI). *Eye* 20 December. *www.eye.net/eye/issue_12.20.01/news/olivieri.html*

Further reading

Salek S and Edgar A (2002). *Pharmaceutical Ethics*. John Wiley and Sons, 300 pp, $190.

Lemmens T and Singer PA (1998). Bioethics for clinicians: conflict of interest in research, education and patient care. *Can Med Assoc J* **159**: 960–965.

CIOMS (2002). International ethical guidelines for biomedical research in volunteer human subjects. CIOMS, Geneva.

Hodges C (1991). Harmonisation of European controls over research. In *Pharmaceutical Medicine and the Law*, Goldberg A and Dodds-Smith I (eds). RCP Publishers: 72–75.

Jemec G and Sohl P (2002). In *A Guide to Clinical Drug Research*, 2nd edition, Cohen A and Posner J (eds). Kluwer Academic: 117–125.

Doyal L and Tobias JS (2000). *Informed Consent in Clinical Research*. BMJ Publishing: London.

Anon. (1998). Informed consent in medical research: ethical debate. *Br Med J* **314**: 1107–1113; **316**: 1000–1005.

Federmann DD, Hanna KE and Rodriguez LL (2003). *Responsible Research: A Systems Approach to Protecting Research Participants*. Institute of Medicine, 316 pp, $44.95. *http://national-academies.org*

Evans D and Evans M (1996). *A Decent Proposal: Ethical Review of Clinical Research*. Wiley, 230 pp, £24.95.

Anon. (1994). Independent ethical review of studies involving personal medical records. *J R Coll Physicians London* **28**:

Cleophas TJM, Meulen JVD and Kalmansohn RB (1997). Clinical trials: specific problems associated with the use of a placebo control group. *Br J Clin Pharmacol* **43**: 219–221.

De Deyn PP (2000). Ethical and scientific challenges of placebo control arms in clinical trials. *Int J Pharm Med* **14**: 149–157.

Immediately post the Edinburgh Amendment. See: Smith RN (2000). An analysis of the Edinburgh revision of the Declaration of Helsinki. *Int J Pharm Med* **14**: 323–328.

Post South African meeting (2001). See: Pérez AC and Smith RN (2001). The revised Declaration of Helsinki interpreting and implementing ethical principles in biomedical research. *Int J Pharm Med* **15**: 131–143.

Full text of the revised Declaration of Helsinki can be found on: www.wma.net.

Foster C (ed.) (1996). *Manual for Research Ethics Committees*, 4th edition. King's College: London.

ABBI (1997). *Introduction to Research Ethical Committees. International Journal of Pharmaceutical Medicine* **11**(3): 121–176. Guidelines and recommendations for European ethics committees (in the same journal) 129–135.

National statement on ethical conduct in research involving humans. www.health.gov.au/nhmrc/publications/synopses/e35syn.htm.

Governance Arrangements for National Health Service Research Ethics (GAfREC) July 2001. www.doh.gov.uk/research/documents/gafrec.doc.

Central Office for Research Ethics Committees (COREC): *www.corec.org.uk.*

RCP (1991). *Fraud and Misconduct in Medical Research. Cause, Investigation and Prevention.* Royal College of Physicians: London.

Lock S, Wells F and Farthing M (2001). *Fraud and Misconduct in Biomedical Research*, 3rd edition. BMJ Publishing.

Bibliography on pharmaceutical promotion: www.healthskepticism.org, *www.pharmacoethics.com*

Medawar C (2001). Health, Pharma and the EU. A briefing for members of the European Parliament on Direct-to-Consumer drug promotion. December.

Gillon R (1994). Medical ethics: four principles plus attention to scope. *Br Med J* **309**: 184–188.

Collier J and Jheanacho I. (2002). The Pharmaceutical Industry as an informant. *Lancet* **360**, 1405–9.

16

A Model for the Future Conduct of Pharmacovigilance

P. C. Waller and S. J. W. Evans

Introduction

At the turn of the millennium, those involved in pharmacovigilance face major challenges to satisfy increased consumer expectations and realize the benefits of the technological age. The existing approach has developed through evolution and appears to be widely accepted. However, there is evidence that adverse drug reactions (ADRs) remain a major cause of morbidity and mortality, and it has been suggested in a recent paper that they caused more than 100 000 deaths in the USA in 1994 and could be the fourth largest cause of death (Lazarou et al., 1998). In particular, the effectiveness of the implementation tools may be limited and, although conceptually pharmacovigilance is a monitoring process, adequate outcome measures have not been developed. It is reasonable, therefore, to question whether the existing model will meet the needs of 21st century drug development.

In 2001 we were involved in a project set up by the UK Medicines Control Agency (MCA) to rethink the process of pharmacovigilance on a scientific basis without preconceptions. First, we constructed a preliminary working model that described the key elements which would be required to achieve the best possible process. Input was then derived from colleagues around the world in other regulatory authorities, academia and the pharmaceutical industry by inviting them to review the working model. Subsequently, each element of the working model was treated as a separate theme and small groups were formed to brainstorm each theme and formulate the development of each area.

Proposed model

The purposes of pharmacovigilance were defined as 'to promote safe clinical use of medicines and prevent ADRs, thereby protecting public health'. It was agreed that the key values that should underpin this work are excellence (defined as the best possible result), the scientific method and transparency. The proposed model (Figure 16.1) defines five elements that are considered essential for pharmacovigilance to achieve excellence. Three of these are

Stephens' Detection of New Adverse Drug Reactions Fifth Edition edited by John Talbot and Patrick Waller
© 2004 John Wiley & Sons, Ltd   ISBN: 0 470 84552 X

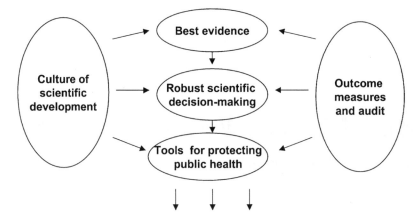

Measurable performance in terms of public health benefit

Figure 16.1 Model for excellence in pharmacovigilance (*Pharmacoepidemiology and Drug Safety* 2003; **12**: 17–29). Reproduced by permission of Wiley

process orientated: best evidence, robust scientific decision-making and effective tools to deliver protection of public health. Some of these processes already exist but might need to be improved in order to ensure delivery of the most effective system possible. The two other elements, scientific development and audit, underpin these processes, recognizing that excellence cannot be achieved merely by process. In order to demonstrate excellence objectively and underpin audit of all levels of the process, novel methods (or applications of existing methods) for measuring public health outcomes need to be developed. The model does not take into account everything that may be relevant, and there are other dimensions (e.g. legal frameworks, local or product-specific factors) that may require consideration in order to use it.

Description of model components

Best evidence

This reflects the need for pharmacovigilance to be evidence based and that decisions, outcomes and overall excellence will be influenced by the nature and quality of the evidence base.

Use of evidence

Conceptually, there are two broad and opposing approaches to gathering and using evidence: demonstrating safety and demonstrating harm. The former is intrinsically more difficult, since safety can only be demonstrated to a finite degree. Traditionally, pharmacovigilance has been more focused on the assumption that there may be unrecognized potential for harm that has not yet been demonstrated because of evidential limitations, and on finding evidence of such harm. This is not to say that the need for better demonstration of safety in clinical practice has gone unrecognized. Various monitored release schemes evaluated in the 1970s

(Wilson, 1986), the Committee on Safety of Medicines' Working Parties of the 1980s (Grahame-Smith, 1987) and prescription-event monitoring (Mann, 1998) are all exercises that, at least in part, have been based on this approach. However, these approaches have not fully circumvented the practical difficulties involved in demonstrating a greater level of safety.

In terms of demonstrating safety, a two-dimensional model may be used, and this is illustrated in Figure 16.2. The key variables of interest are frequency and time of onset. The focus of this interest relates to serious ADRs. In order to demonstrate a greater level of safety it is necessary to move away from the top left as far as possible towards the bottom right, i.e. to gather evidence which shows that serious adverse reactions are rare and that this remains true in the long-term.

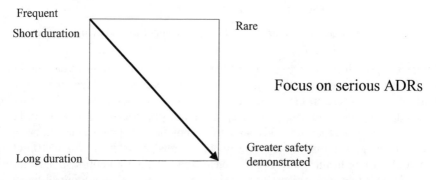

Figure 16.2 Demonstrating a greater degree of safety (*Pharmacoepidemiology and Drug Safety* 2003; **12**: 17–29). Reproduced by permission of Wiley

In respect of gathering evidence in pharmacovigilance, it seems that a better balance needs to be struck between the two approaches described above. A mechanism for achieving this would be for a 'pharmacovigilance specification' to be drawn up at the time of marketing authorization. This would explicitly consider the level of safety that had already been demonstrated, possible concerns that needed further investigation and how further evidence was going to be gathered. It would be the responsibility of the applicant to draw up and maintain the specification and it would be analogous to the summary of product characteristics (SPC), in that it would require regulatory approval and become public at the time of authorization.

Evidence hierarchy

A hierarchy of evidence from case reports (the lowest level) through observational studies to clinical trials and meta-analysis is well recognized (Piantadosi, 1995). Higher levels in the hierarchy are associated with a lower degree of uncertainty (in particular regarding causality) and hence there is, in principle, an advantage in moving up the hierarchy as far as possible within practical constraints. Pharmacovigilance tends to rely considerably on evidence from the lower end of the hierarchy (case reports/series and observational studies). Greater use of methods producing evidence at higher levels is a logical aim. The practical consequences would be more large simple clinical trials and meta-analyses of safety data, both from randomized trials and observational studies.

Spontaneous adverse reaction reporting   This is considered to be the cornerstone of pharmacovigilance and the method is undoubtedly of proven value in detecting signals of unrecognized safety issues. Nevertheless, there are several reasons why its future place might legitimately be questioned:

- low level in evidence hierarchy;

- insuperable limitations (e.g. underreporting);

- high resource inputs when considered globally;

- other methods of detecting signals could yet prove superior and/or more efficient.

Our current approach is to develop the method further to maximize its value by targeting areas of weakness, increasing the reporting base and utilizing the data more effectively (Waller, 2000). However, in the longer term, consideration should be given as to whether the method could be completely replaced by other approaches. The critical factor is whether spontaneous reporting adds something unique. If spontaneous reporting does capture something that might otherwise go unrecorded, then it is *suspicions* regarding cause and effect that health professionals considered potentially important. This raises the issue of whether other mechanisms of recording such suspicions in a more systematic way (e.g. prompted by stopping or changing drugs) could be developed that might be more efficient and, therefore, potentially replace spontaneous reporting. In principle, this could be achieved through healthcare databases and the feasibility of the approach should be investigated.

Observational epidemiological research   Whilst increased use of large simple trials (see below) would reduce the need for observational studies, these will continue to be required for generating evidence on post-marketing safety. In particular, the inherent time delay can make a prospective trial impractical as a solution to an important safety issue. The goals in this area should be to ensure that high-quality research is conducted promptly and is focused on signals that have potential public health importance. Studies based on the cohort approach have greater potential to extend knowledge of safety than those based on sampling of cases, which tend to focus on the investigation of potential harm.

Standard cohort or case-control studies will continue to be useful, but there are potential modifications to these classic designs that warrant further exploration in this context. These methodologies include case-crossover, case-only and case-cohort designs, and, in some circumstances, counter-matched studies. Each of these can potentially provide gains in efficiency, reduce the time taken to perform a study, increase statistical power or reduce bias. For all of them it is important that high-quality data are available in population-based databases that record, or by record linkage produce, drug exposure and medical events in individuals, together with the possibility of some adjustments for confounding. Data from individuals and not aggregate data must be available for analysis, but the data must be anonymized to ensure confidentiality.

Randomized clinical trials The majority of randomized clinical trials (RCTs) are conducted pre-marketing with a primary objective of demonstrating efficacy. There are three major limitations of the method with regard to safety: obtaining a large enough sample size to study outcomes that may be rare, the generalizability of the findings to ordinary practice, and poor reporting of safety, at least in published trials. Whilst these limitations are important, their recognition has probably led to under-utilization of RCTs for safety purposes. To a considerable degree, both limitations can be overcome by a 'large simple trial' that includes enough subjects to study rare outcome, makes few measurements and imposes no entry restrictions that would not apply in ordinary practice. The logical time to perform such a trial is when the drug is authorized and when uncertainty cannot be resolved through observational studies. The normal unit of randomization is the patient, but cluster randomization (e.g. of general practices) might have practical advantages and is worthy of further exploration, particularly in the context of vaccines.

Meta-analysis Meta-analysis is a well-established technique for bringing together all the valid evidence contributing to a particular question and providing an overall estimate of effect. It has most frequently been used for data from RCTs (particularly in the context of efficacy), but methodologies exist for observational data and are being developed for combining data from RCTs and observational data. Although meta-analysis has critics (particularly when it utilizes only observational data), it is generally accepted that, when based on RCT data, it is at the top of the evidence hierarchy.

The potential of meta-analysis in pharmacovigilance has been underused; for example, no formal meta-analysis of data relating to the differential effects of combined oral contraceptives on venous thromboembolism had been published by the end of 2000, i.e. more than 5 years after the original studies were published. Use of meta-analysis to resolve important safety questions should be a goal that helps to drive the process of investigation. Even when overall estimates could be regarded as misleading (e.g. when there is significant heterogeneity or debate about the validity of some studies), graphical display of all the data on the same scale, with confidence intervals, may be a valuable aid to understanding the overall evidence base, shedding light on reasons for heterogeneity. We envision that meta-analysis of pre-marketing safety data will frequently underpin the pharmacovigilance specification drawn up at the time of authorization.

Basic research and pharmacogenetics

There is potential for preventing adverse reactions, and, therefore, of improving the safety of medicines, through developing a better understanding of the mechanisms of ADRs and the genetic contribution to drug response. Following the success of the human genome project, the identification of genetic predictors of ADRs is now feasible and represents an opportunity that could substantially impact on pharmacovigilance over the next 5–10 years. In particular, it could provide evidence that would allow the prevention of many ADRs, including both those that are dose-related and those that are idiosyncratic. Genetic markers may predict both efficacy and toxicity of many drugs (Ozdemir *et al.*, 2001) with potentially major implications for their practical use and safety. Whilst pharmacogenetics will particularly impact on early stages of drug development, it will also be important to ensure that its methods are applied to drugs that are already authorized.

Data resources

In terms of data resources, the ultimate aim should be the development of a complete population database with well-documented exposures to medicines, outcomes and potential risk factors. In the UK, such a database is unlikely to be achievable for several years, and the needs of pharmacovigilance are unlikely to drive its development. There may also be problems resulting from a drive towards increased confidentiality that may work against the interests of public health in relation to drug safety. As noted above, individual records are vital for analysing the safety of medicines using epidemiological methods. Meanwhile, existing databases should be used to develop and test approaches to maximizing the utility of a total population database. Particular attention should be paid to their predictive value in detection of signals and how to encompass the need for both hypothesis-generation and hypothesis testing in a single database. Since a total population database is likely to be based around primary care, there is a need to ensure that adequate information is available on hospital exposure to medicines and outcomes. The availability of better information on medicines used without a prescription with linkage to medical outcomes also requires consideration (Clark *et al.*, 2001).

Environmental considerations

The most important environmental consideration is the worldwide dimension to evidence that is relevant to pharmacovigilance. There is a major logistic difficulty in bringing all the relevant evidence together in one place. Currently, there are two mechanisms through which this is attempted: the World Health Organization international spontaneous reporting database in Sweden (Olsson, 1998) and periodic safety update reports (PSURs) by pharmaceutical companies – and some relevant standards agreed through the International Conference on Harmonization (D'Arcy and Harron, 1996). In respect of PSURs, they have added a major resource burden, but their impact on the public health objective of pharmacovigilance has yet to be evaluated. Overall, the fulfilment of regulatory requirements (i.e. ADR reporting and PSURs) has become too great a process driver and has diverted attention away from scientific approaches to gaining better evidence. The broad solutions to these issues might be: (a) to centralize further the gathering of evidence and avoid duplication of effort; (b) to refocus industry towards the need to gather better evidence of safety rather than solely meeting process requirements; (c) to ensure that regulatory demands on industry have measurable public health gain.

Interface between evidence and decision making

The conceptual framework of the best evidence model is largely focused on the beginning of the process: the gathering of evidence. In contrast, for robust decision making (see below) the focus has tended to be on the end of the process, i.e. making the final decision on a major issue of risk–benefit. In between there are two other broad areas that could be termed 'evidence distillation' and 'issue management'. Although it would be reasonable to consider the former to be part of best evidence and the latter to be part of decision making, they overlap to a considerable extent and involve an iterative process.

Within this interface there are two potential initial drivers, the detection of a signal (i.e.

the identification of unexpected harm) or the achievement of a milestone (i.e. a specified boundary on the map has been reached).

Handling of signals

When the initial driver is the detection of a signal, there are potentially three further steps, as follows:

- impact analysis
- risk evaluation
- risk–benefit evaluation.

Conceptual frameworks exist for each of these steps and, with regard to the latter, a major international initiative is available (CIOMS IV Working Group, 1998). Since risk evaluation is intrinsically part of the latter process (the only reason for considering it as a separate step is that there may be no need to proceed to full risk–benefit evaluation), our attention has focused on impact analysis. This is a key step which should drive use of resource towards issues that have the greatest potential for public health benefit.

For this purpose the MCA have used the SNIP criteria (Waller and Lee, 1999, see also p. 351), which enable a judgement to be made about the priority that should be given to a signal by considering its strength, whether it is new, the clinical importance and the potential for prevention. This is a pragmatic approach that has some value, but it also has conceptual flaws. In an impact analysis, the output is the potential for prevention (i.e. in this model it is not a factor to be considered separately), which is dependent on four factors:

- causality
- frequency
- health consequences
- risk predictors

The first factor to be considered in the analysis of impact is the overall strength of evidence that the adverse outcome is caused by the drug. This depends on both the nature of the evidence and a global evaluation, it being possible to envisage about five levels to which signals could be readily categorized according to objective criteria, albeit involving scientific judgement. For example, the lowest level would involve a small number of spontaneously reported cases with some plausibility of causality based on the individual cases, but no other evidence and potential alternative explanations for the signal. The highest level would be evidence from a meta-analysis of RCT data. Thus, there should be a clear link with the established evidence hierarchy.

Frequency should be measured both in terms of risk to an individual and the population frequency, for which knowledge of the level and duration of exposure is required. The critical factor should be the absolute frequency expressed in terms of an order of magnitude. A CIOMS Working Group has already proposed such a categorization with five levels from 1 in 10 or more to 1 in 10 000 or less (CIOMS III Working Group, 1995). Such categorization is broad but this has the advantage that it is usually possible to estimate frequency to an order of magnitude even when only limited evidence is available. However, it does not take into account time and its inherent assumption – that the rate of occurrence of an ADR is constant – is often unjustified. The life-table approach (or Kaplan–Meier plot) is a method that has been little used in this context but should prove valuable in addressing this difficulty.

With regard to clinical consequences (i.e. seriousness), it is also possible to envision categorization on a scale according to the risk of fatality and the long-term impact of the outcome on health and quality of life. This could be driven partly by the specific data available for the drug–reaction association and partly by the known epidemiology of the disease.

With regard to predictors of risk, it is important to consider both who is at risk and when they are at risk, i.e. the temporal relation between start of treatment and onset of the reaction. It is clear that the identification of risk predictors is of great importance in developing strategies to prevent ADRs, but they may be less amenable to simple categorization given the wide range of potential risk predictors and considerations relating to their measurement and modification. Furthermore, data indicating that a particular factor is associated with greater risk may not necessarily imply a causal relationship. Conversely, where it is not possible to identify sub-groups at particular risk, this may simply reflect insufficient statistical power.

Overall, the factors discussed together need to be synthesized into an output that indicates both the public health importance and potential for prevention based on the attributable risk amongst exposed patients. We suggest that an empirical mathematical approach incorporating sensitivity analysis could be developed to support this function.

Milestone achievement

Currently, the pharmacovigilance process is based on temporal milestones (e.g. PSURs are initially required every 6 months regardless of the level of use) with a periodicity that lessens as the product becomes established. The conceptual problem with this approach is that there is no clear link with demonstrating the safety of the product; i.e. knowledge of safety, or indeed harm, may not have been extended at all, but there is a requirement to report to regulatory authorities. In the model we propose, the milestones would be pre-specified levels of exposure that are dependent on the type of drug and the availability of new information which contributes to safety. Arbitrary time periods for safety updates and intensive monitoring of new drugs are replaced by milestones, the achievement of which leads to recognition that a greater level of safety has been demonstrated. Markers analogous to the black triangle in the UK (Committee on Safety of Medicines/Medicines Control Agency, 2000) could be useful (by their presence or absence) in signalling to users that a medicine has a provisional or an established level of safety. The logic of the current link (in the UK) of such markers to ADR reporting requirements can be questioned. In our view, such a link is unnecessary and all ADR reporting could be focused on serious and/or unexpected ADRs.

Robust decision making

The essential steps in going from a body of evidence to a decision are: (1) analysis of evidence; (2) identification of options; (3) decision making. There is greatest scope for innovation in respect of the latter. Currently, the regulatory model used is for one or more assessors to undertake an analysis and identify options, followed by expert committee review and advice on the decision. Their decision-making process is normally informal (i.e. through discussion and consensus whenever possible). The main aim of this part of the model is to assure the quality of decisions, bearing in mind that, in most cases, a considerable degree of judgement is required taking into account factors such as the strength of the evidence, balance of risks and benefits, and likely effectiveness of potential preventive strategies. Other considerations, such as the precautionary principle, may also be relevant. Pharmacovigilance decisions should take into account all the potential public health consequences of the decision and invariably involve comparison of alternative approaches. The principles involved in risk–benefit analysis have been the subject of in-depth consideration by the CIOMS IV Working Group (1998). In particular, their approach to decision making, which outlines the need for objectivity, equity and accountability, are relevant here and should be incorporated into the model.

In respect of the first two stages of the process, quality is currently assured by two processes: formalized assessment and peer review. Development of check lists based on CIOMS IV might be valuable to underpin the formal assessment process. Regarding decision making, the informal committee model is generally considered to work reasonably well. However, there are two conceptual drawbacks: firstly, decisions are dependent on the particular experts involved; secondly, the assumptions and logic underlying the decision may not be made explicit or adequately tested during the process. For these reasons, as suggested, but not developed, by the CIOMS IV Working Group (1998), we have considered whether a more formal decision-making process involving decision analysis might provide the basis for robust decision making. We have also considered how experts might best be used and the potential roles of other stakeholders in the process.

Formal decision analysis

Decision analysis is a process undertaken prior to making a decision and involves using the available evidence to create a model that defines predicted health outcomes associated with each option under consideration (Lilford et al., 1998). The subsequent decision is informed by, but not necessarily predicted from, the model; i.e. modelling is a way of fully exploring the issues rather than making automated decisions. In order to perform decision analysis it is necessary to define probabilities for each of the outcomes and their value or utilities. In doing so, various assumptions are usually necessary, the effects of which can be tested through sensitivity analysis. Standard methods are available, and these have been used both for clinical and public health policy decisions (Lilford et al., 1998). Their potential for application to pharmaceutical policy decisions has recently been the subject of a published review (Patten and Lee, 2002).

The potential advantages of modelling are as follows:

- increased transparency;

- making reasoning explicit, reflecting complexity;

- clearly identifying limitations of the evidence and uncertainty;

- the impact of all assumptions can be assessed;

- better justified decisions.

The potential disadvantages of modelling are as follows:

- adds time – usually weeks (but limited modelling could be done in hours);
- requires additional resource and specialist expertise;
- the model itself (rather than the evidence) may become the focus of debate/challenge.

We suggest that a first step would be to work retrospectively through complex examples with experts in decision analysis. This will demonstrate whether the method is likely to be of value for pharmacovigilance decisions, following which piloting in practice would need to be undertaken.

Who makes the decisions?

With regard to the role of experts in decision making, we recognize that this is a much wider issue and that pharmacovigilance probably has no special need to be different from other processes that involve going from scientific evidence to a policy decision. Nevertheless, there are grounds to ask whether the current model, where expert committees often play the defining role in such decisions, will survive the intense scrutiny that is becoming the norm for issues involving public safety. Clearly, experts should have a key role in evidence appraisal, and developing and testing assumptions in a formal decision analysis. However, when it comes to making decisions, the role of expert committees could be reconsidered.

A recent trend has been the inclusion of lay members on expert committees, but this does not fully address one limitation of the current model, which is that consultation with stakeholders is very often limited and focused particularly on the pharmaceutical industry. In principle, if decision analysis proves to be a useful tool in this field, then, in theory, decisions could be taken by a group that represents all stakeholders and is supported by experts. Most current models leave the final decision to elected representatives who are accountable to a parliament, thereby introducing a political dimension to individual decisions. In the model proposed (i.e. more transparent decisions involving stakeholder consultation) it could be debated whether such direct accountability would be desirable. Clearly, accountability for the overall process to elected governments would remain essential.

The other major issue we considered was the need for agreement across international boundaries. Whilst it is clear that differing decisions on pharmacovigilance issues around the world are common, the reasons for such differences are not well understood. If greater international consistency is to be achieved then these reasons need to be explored, in the first instance through retrospective study of recent major decisions.

Tools to protect public health

This part of the model involves communicating with, and influencing, users of medicines in order to promote safe use and thereby protect public health. Existing tools for communicating new safety information include product information, drug safety bulletins, urgent letters to health professionals and the Internet. Although the precise effectiveness of these tools is unknown, there are grounds to believe that they are not highly effective. There is, therefore, considerable scope to develop new approaches to delivery of drug safety information in order to meet the needs of users as fully as possible.

General principles of communication

The Erice report (Uppsala Monitoring Centre, 1998) has laid down basic principles about communication of drug safety information which are widely accepted. In particular, this states that drug safety information 'must serve the needs of the public', that it 'should be balanced with respect to risks and benefits' and that 'all the evidence needed to assess and understand risks and benefits must be openly available'. These principles should underpin all provision of information and communication about the safety of marketed medicines. The last is particularly important in ensuring that the whole process is transparent.

Another principle that is widely accepted is that different levels of information are needed to meet the varying needs of recipients. In practice, this has led to a binary division into separate information for health professionals and for patients, which is reflected within the EU regulatory system with respect to product information. However, experience has shown that this approach is too simplistic, since both health professionals and patients have a wide variety of potential needs. Therefore, we suggest that multiple linked levels of information are necessary and that a distinction between information for health professionals or patients is not always necessary. Information provided at lower levels should be presented in non-technical language in order to be understandable to lay recipients. Complex information at higher levels will inevitably need to be presented using technical language. The idea is that users start at the lowest level and progress as far as they wish to according to their information needs (e.g. distinguishing what is needed to be known prior to taking the drug and what is needed to be known while taking the drug) and capability to understand the information.

Although we are proposing to drop the distinction between health professionals and patients in terms of access to information (i.e. the information available to them should be the same), it should be recognized that different approaches to delivery may be necessary in order to influence these groups (see below).

A new approach to product information

When considering these principles further, product information is the logical place to start, since this should underpin all other sources. The current model for product information in the EU is that an SPC in a standard format is attached to the marketing authorization and serves as both a regulatory document and as a primary source of information for health professionals. User leaflets supplied with the medicine are based on the SPC and written in lay language in a standard format. The main disadvantages of the current system relate to the dual purpose of the SPC (it is widely recognized that, although it fulfils well the regulatory purpose, this document is not particularly useful to health professionals) and the considerable constraints on presentation and lack of flexibility resulting from standardized formats for both SPCs and patient information leaflets (PILs). Both these disadvantages tend to result in a lack of impact of key messages, which cannot be presented in an appropriately highlighted way and which are often surrounded by (but not differentiated from) much less important information. A further problem is that basic information is not always easily accessible to health professionals or to patients before a medicine has been dispensed or purchased.

Therefore, we propose that the SPC (essentially in its current form) should be regarded purely as a regulatory document and that much greater flexibility should be allowed as to how user product information is presented. Potentially, this would lead to greater value to users, and promote safe and effective use of medicines, with a lesser degree of regulation. It should, therefore, be attractive to both industry and consumer groups.

A suitable working model for further discussion might be as follows:

- All product information to be consistent with the SPC (and, therefore, to be amended if the SPC is significantly varied).

- Product information to remain non-promotional.

- Requirements for certain key information (especially regarding safety) to be included and highlighted on all documents.

- Few other constraints on format and presentation.

- Opportunity for regulatory review.

- Underpinning guidance indicating that:

  - product information should be developed by communication specialists, not scientists;

  - multiple linked levels of information should be available, e.g.

    - essential user information with highlighted key messages in lay language (level 1)

    - more detailed information comparable in depth to current SPC (level 2)

    - technical supporting documentation, e.g. assessment reports (level 3) and summaries of data from trials, etc.

In terms of provision of information, the following primary routes are envisioned:

- Level 1 information would be provided with the product.

- Levels 1 and 2 would be provided in compendia of product information (in both paper and electronic forms).

- Levels 1, 2 and 3 would be provided via the internet.

Influencing health professionals

Whilst provision of safety information to health professionals is straightforward, changing behaviour is more difficult. In particular, the necessary information may not be remembered or immediately accessible when it is needed. The most effective way of overcoming this barrier is likely to be through computerized decision support. There is a need to develop intelligent decision-support systems for health professionals to support rational use of medicines, which *inter alia* helps to promote safer use. These will need to factor in individual patient characteristics (e.g. concomitant disease and medication) and provide links to supporting information on the Internet, such as guidelines and expert assessments (e.g. Cochrane reviews).

In addition to effective delivery, there is a need to improve the clarity and impact of the messages by making all information more attractive and accessible (e.g. by including a box with the most important things the prescriber should know about a medicine). It is also important to recognize that the messenger needs a high profile and credibility in order to generate the necessary confidence in the system.

Influencing patients

Users of medicines may require general education on risk–benefit and specific information on the medicine(s) that they use. The information they require may differ before, during and after taking a medicine. PILs provided with the medicine are potentially a valuable tool, but experience to date suggests that they are not seen as user friendly and may cause problems with the doctor–patient relationship. It is difficult to address these problems without fairly fundamental changes, because the format is currently highly constrained by regulatory requirements. In the model proposed above, supply of the lowest level of information with the medicine would replace existing PILs and there would be references to other sources of information, such as relevant Website addresses.

Outcome measures and audit

The functions of this part of the model are: (1) to demonstrate the extent to which the process of pharmacovigilance is effective in the protection of public health; (2) to underpin excellence by enabling improvements to be made which are based on evidence and/or experience (i.e. audit). These goals require substantial innovation, since no well-established outcome measures are in routine use and audit of pharmacovigilance is currently limited and solely process orientated.

Outcome measures

Attempts are often made to judge the effects of interventions using spontaneous ADR reporting data. However, it is doubtful that such data are generally useful for this purpose, because there are several potentially counteracting effects on reporting of sending out a safety message. The sum of these consequences is enormously variable and rarely interpretable with confidence. Complete cessation of reporting of a particular ADR may be taken as an indication of a positive effect, but even this could be subject to bias.

Other previous work in this field has concentrated on the effects of specific recommendations, often with a particular focus on prescribing. For example, it is relatively easy to measure co-prescribing of interacting medicines for which combined use is contraindicated, before and after warnings are issued. Such analyses, together with spontaneous ADR reports, have then been used to make a judgement as to whether the measures taken were sufficient.

The effects of interventions on usage of medicines is an important surrogate outcome measure that should be much more widely and routinely utilized. The most useful readily available source of data is prescribing information from general practice databases. Time–trend analyses of the levels of usage and the characteristics of users would provide valuable insights into the extent to which safety messages are impacting on prescribers. It is important to recognize that general practice databases do not cover medicines prescribed in hospital or bought over-the-counter, and there is a need to develop usable and comprehensive information sources for medicines used in these environments.

True outcome measures would provide estimates of the impact of interventions on morbidity and mortality. Ideally, we would wish to be able to estimate how many deaths and serious adverse reactions are prevented by the whole pharmacovigilance system, as well as being able to quantify the effects of individual interventions. In terms of mortality, for some it seems unlikely that death certificates in which ADRs are mentioned as a cause would currently be useful for either purpose because of substantial under-recording. It is possible that this could be improved, e.g. by adding an additional field on the certificate to indicate that an ADR may have caused or contributed to death. Also, for some conditions, where ADRs contribute a substantial attributable fraction (e.g. gastrointestinal bleeding), then surveillance of mortality data could be helpful. For morbidity, in the UK, hospital episode (HES) data are a potential source, but they are of variable quality and likely to have important limitations, again because ADRs will not necessarily be recorded as a diagnosis on discharge. In the case of both death certificates and HES data, there would be a need to develop links to data on use of medicines and other health records.

Whilst the above potential data sources are worthy of further exploration, general practice databases are a more likely and immediately available source of data. Their potential should be evaluated in pilot studies of specific ADRs with high morbidity and/or mortality. For certain ADRs (e.g. major hepatotoxicity) it may be possible and more fruitful to obtain information from specialist referral centres and the advantages and disadvantages of these approaches could be compared.

In terms of the outcome measures themselves, we suggest that *years of life lost* should be the principal mortality outcome, since it is more informative than a simple mortality rate and can be easily calculated, providing age is known. In order to include morbidity and the impact on quality of life, estimation of *quality adjusted years of life lost* should be the goal, but this is likely to be much harder to measure. There is a need to evaluate the potential of the data sources discussed above to provide reliable data on these outcomes.

Audit

Audit is essentially a process of checking what has happened, usually against prior predictions, targets or standards. Currently, most audit in the field of pharmacovigilance is focused on data handling and quality, and is process- rather than outcome-orientated. Audit of effectiveness of literature scanning and the time taken to implement safety warnings after initial signal detection are particular examples of audit that could be done fairly easily, but they are not routine, or even if done they are not published. Broadly, there is a need to define standards, extend audit across the whole process and focus particularly on whether the desired outcome was achieved using the measures discussed above.

In order to define the standards for audit for each party involved in the process there is a need for an internationally agreed document defining 'good pharmacovigilance practice'. Excellence in pharmacovigilance will require audit of the overall outcome using the types of measure discussed above and of each stage of the process, as follows:

- data collection and processing

- extending knowledge of safety

- hazard management

    - signal detection

    - signal evaluation

    - decision making

    - taking action

- Communication of safety and risk–benefit.

Effective use of resources and timeliness are important factors to be audited. Whilst the majority of audit can be carried out internally (preferably within a defined group responsible for this function alone), periodic external audit should also be a feature.

In order to develop the necessary methodology, there is a need to work retrospectively through some major issues to examine each element of the process and to question whether the best possible outcome has been achieved. Other possible approaches that are worth exploring include:

- Feeding in some 'dummy' data and measuring whether the response meets expectations.

- Testing reproducibility (e.g. by taking the same assessment to two expert committees).

- Making comparisons with others addressing the same issues (e.g. internationally), exploring reasons for differences.

- Considering the scope for 'trials' (e.g. prospectively comparing different courses of action).

Ultimately, the aim should be to develop a scheme by which audit of the whole process can be carried out, both on a routine basis and with defined triggers for additional activities. The development process should involve personnel with expertise in audit generally. The possibility of international collaboration in conducting audit could also be examined.

Culture of scientific development

This part of the model is about creating an environment whereby the pharmacovigilance function keeps pace with developing science and makes full use of the opportunities it provides for preventing ADRs. This must not be dependent on individuals, but be an intrinsic part of the operation. The rapidly developing field of pharmacogenetics is the most important current opportunity, with many ongoing studies of the genetic contributions to differential drug response. It is imperative that these developments are translated into public health gain, but this will only happen if pharmacovigilance personnel gain expertise in the field and develop clear strategies to take advantage of them. There is also a need to adapt the pharmacovigilance process effectively to take account of different types of new therapy being developed (e.g. gene therapy) and which are likely to require specialized monitoring in a tertiary care setting. Again, this requires a culture of scientific development in order to facilitate the necessary work.

Information management is also relevant to this aspect of the model. Effective use of information to create a knowledge base, which underpins the scientific functioning and is not dependent on individuals, is also a prerequisite for a culture of scientific development.

Scientific basis of pharmacovigilance

Pharmacovigilance is a preventive public health function underpinned by several scientific disciplines. The key disciplines may be grouped into four broad areas as follows:

- basic science
- clinical science
- population science
- information science.

These disciplines can be related most clearly to the best evidence part of the model, but they also impact on all the other elements. Since there is a need to change clinical practice, it can be argued that behavioural science should also be included. It is important that there is a good balance of resources and expertise between these disciplines. It can be argued that, at present, the balance of inputs may not be right and that there is a need to increase the input of basic and population sciences.

At present, there are few dedicated academic bases for pharmacovigilance in most of the world. This needs to be rectified in order to underpin a culture of scientific development for pharmacovigilance and support training programmes. Dedicated academic departments of pharmacovigilance would, in particular, require close alliances with both clinical pharmacology/therapeutics and public health/epidemiology.

Basic training

Most recruits to pharmacovigilance, whether in the regulatory authority or in industry, have little or no specific basic training in the field and, therefore, this has to be done 'on the job'. In practice, this means that too high a proportion of time is spent in basic training whilst in post, when the focus should be on further development and specialization linked to a career development pathway. Although there are a few courses that concentrate on pharmacovigilance there is a need for specific basic training courses in the field. These need to be focused on the preventive and public health functions of pharmacovigilance and not solely on regulatory requirements.

Organizational aspects

The nature of pharmacovigilance is that the casework is completely unpredictable and there is more to do than can ever be done. Each case is unique, and major issues are difficult to handle, requiring a high degree of involvement from experienced personnel. The inevitable consequence of this is that progress in strategy and development is hampered and the only realistic way to counter this is by dedicating protected resource to these areas.

Conclusions

A scientific model to support excellence in pharmacovigilance is proposed. The model represents a long-term vision of how pharmacovigilance could be conducted in the future. So far, it has been developed without considering constraints such as resources or the need for legislative change. Although the vision is holistic, it would be possible to test and implement parts of the model in a piecemeal fashion.

The key concepts underpinning the model are as follows:

- Pharmacovigilance should be less focused on finding harm and more on extending knowledge of safety.

- There should be a clear starting point or 'specification' of what is already known at the time of licensing a medicine and what is required to extend safety knowledge post-authorization.

- Complex risk–benefit decisions are amenable to, and likely to be improved by, the use of formal decision analysis.

- A new approach to provision of safety information which allows greater flexibility in presenting key messages based on multiple levels of information with access determined by user requirements.

- Flexible decision support is the most likely means of changing the behaviour of health professionals in order to promote safer use of medicines.

- There is a need to put in place outcome measures that indicate the success or failure of the process. These should include hard end-points indicating the impact on mortality and morbidity. Surrogates, such as the impact on prescribing of medicines, are more readily available and are also potentially valuable.

- Systematic audit of pharmacovigilance processes and outcomes should be developed and implemented based on agreed standards ('good pharmacovigilance practice').

- Pharmacovigilance should operate in a culture of scientific development. This requires the right balance of inputs from various disciplines, a stronger academic base, greater availability of basic training and resource that is dedicated to scientific strategy.

Acknowledgements

This chapter is based on an article published in *Pharmacoepidemiology and Drug Safety* 2003; **12**: 17–29, with kind permission of the editor. Many people have contributed to this vision and their input is personally acknowledged in the reference cited above.

References

CIOMS III Working Group (1995). *Guidelines for preparing core clinical safety information on drugs.* CIOMS: Geneva.

CIOMS IV Working Group (1998). *Benefit–risk balance for marketed drugs: evaluating safety signals.* CIOMS: Geneva.

Clark D, Layton D and Shakir SAW (2001). Monitoring the safety of over the counter drugs. *Br Med J* **323**: 706–707.

Committee on Safety of Medicines/Medicines Control Agency (2000). When you see the black triangle. *Curr Probl Pharmacovig* **26**: 8.

D'Arcy PF and Harron DWG (eds) (1996). *Proceedings of the Third International Conference on Harmonisation, Yokohama, 1995.* Queen's University: Belfast.

Grahame-Smith DG (1987). Adverse drug reaction monitoring: the way forward. In *Adverse Drug Reactions*, Mann RD (ed). Parthenon: Carnforth; 201–214.

Lazarou J, Pomeranz BH and Corey PN (1998). Incidence of adverse drug reactions in hospitalized patients. *J Am Med Assoc* **279**: 1200–1205.

Lilford RJ, Pauker SG, Braunholtz DA and Chard J (1998). Decision analysis and the implementation of research findings. *Br Med J* **317**: 405–409.

Mann RD (1998). Prescription-event monitoring – recent progress and new horizons. *Br J Clin Pharmacol* **46**: 195–201.

Olsson S (1998). The role of the WHO programme on international drug monitoring in co-ordinating worldwide drug safety efforts. *Drug Saf* **19**: 1–10.

Ozdemir V, Shear NH and Kalow W (2001). What will be the role of pharmacogenetics in evaluating drug safety and minimising adverse effects? *Drug Saf* **24**: 75–85.

Patten SB and Lee RC (2002). Modeling methods for facilitating decisions in pharmaceutical policy and population therapeutics. *Pharmacoepidemiol Drug Saf* **11**: 165–168.

Piantadosi S (1995). David Byar as a teacher. *Control Clin Trials* **16**: 202–211.

Uppsala Monitoring Centre (1998). Effective Communications in Pharmacovigilance: The Erice report. Lake, 1998, Birmingham.

Waller P (2000). Spontaneous ADR reporting – have the limits been reached? In *Pharmacovigilance, past present and future. Proceedings of the Susan Wood Symposium*, Harman R (ed.). MCA: 26–32.

Waller PC and Lee EH (1999). Responding to drug safety issues. *Pharmacoepidemiol Drug Saf* **8**: 535–552.

Wilson AB (1986). New surveillance schemes in the United Kingdom. In *Monitoring for Drug Safety*, Inman WHW (ed.). MTP Press: Lancaster.

Appendix I: Drug Products Withdrawn from the Market for Safety Reasons

M. D. B. Stephens

'The competent authorities of the Member States shall suspend or revoke an authorization to place a proprietary medicinal product on the market where the product proves to be harmful in the normal conditions of use, or where its therapeutic efficacy is lacking when it is established that therapeutic results cannot be obtained with the proprietary product' (European Commission 1965; Article II).

Not all countries are covered, owing to lack of information sources. 'Withdrawal' in this context means: any formulation, dose or any indication withdrawn or suspended at any time. Although one reason may be given for withdrawal, presumably the decision was based on the overall balance of safety and efficacy with consideration of the other available alternatives.

Abbreviations

Disease: AA = aplastic anaemia, BIH = benign intracranial hypertension, CAH = chronic active hepatitis, DIC = disseminated intravascular coagulation, EM = erythema multiforme, FDE = fixed drug eruption, GBS = Guillain–Barré syndrome, IBS = irritable bowel syndrome, NMS = neuroleptic malignant syndrome, SIADH = syndrome of inappropriate secretion of antidiuretic hormone, SJS = Stevens–Johnson syndrome, TEN = toxic epidermal necrolysis (Lyell's syndrome).

Countries: Ar = Argentina, Arm = Armenia, Au = Australia, Bel = Belgium, Br = Brazil, Ca = Canada, Chil = Chile, Col = Colombia, Dk = Denmark, EU = European Union, Fl = Finland, Fr = France, Ger = Germany, Gh = Ghana, Gz = Greece, In = India, Ire = Ireland, Isr = Israel, It = Italy, Jp = Japan, Ml = Malaysia, MM = Multiple non-specific markets, Mor = Morocco, Nl = Netherlands, Np = Nepal, NZ = New Zealand, Nw = Norway, Om = Oman, Pk = Pakistan, Port = Portugal, Sa = Saudi Arabia, Swe = Sweden, Sp = Spain, Swz = Switzerland, Syr = Syria, Th = Thailand, Tk = Turkey, UAE = United Arab Emirates, UK = United Kingdom, USA = United States of America, VN = Viet Nam, WW = Worldwide, Ym = Yemen, Zb = Zimbabwe.

Companies: HMR = Hoechst Marion Roussel, GW = GlaxoWellcome, AW = Ayerst Wyeth, CC = Cilag Chemie, SW = Sanofi Winthrop, SK = SmithKline, MD = Merrell Dow, JC = Janssen Cilag, SKF = Smith Kline French, RC = Reckitt Colman, JJ = Johnson and Johnson, SKB = Smith Kline Beecham, FCE = Farmitalia Carlo Erba, HLR = Hoffman La Roche, BI = Boehringer–Ingelheim, MSD = Merck Sharp and Dome, RPR = Rhone–Poulenc–Rorer, BMS = Bristol–Myers–Squibb.

Stephens' Detection of New Adverse Drug Reactions Fifth Edition edited by John Talbot and Patrick Waller
© 2004 John Wiley & Sons, Ltd ISBN: 0 470 84552 X

Drugs: NSAID = non-steroidal anti-inflammatory drugs, SSRI = selective serotonin reuptake inhibitors, MAOI = mono amine oxidase inhibitor, Ω = restricted indication, Δ = restricted with monitoring, Φ = restricted drug formulation, V = voluntarily withdrawn, * = drug was approved but never marketed in country, Σ = legal action taken against company, *NW* = not withdrawn.

References SPA94 = Spriet-Pourra and Auriche (1994), F2001 = Fung *et al.* (2001), B84 = Bakke *et al.* (1984), B95 = Bakke *et al.* (1995), A2001 = Arnaiz *et al.* (2001), MG84 = Marcus and Griffin (1984), J98 = Jefferys *et al.* (1998), R = Reactions, volume, WHODI = World Health Organization Drug Information, volume, number, year.

Table A1.1

International Non-proprietary Name	Trade name / Company	Therapeutic class	Reason for withdrawal	Launch date	Country	Withdrawal date	Reference
Acetyl salicylic acid / Acitretin	Aspirin (paed) / Soriatane, Neotigason / *Roche*	Analgesic / Retinoid	Reye's syndrome. Ω / Embryotoxicity	1899 / Dec 1989	UK / NI	1986 / Oct 1990	SPA94 / *Sturkenboom et al.* (1994)
Adenosine phosphate	Adeno, Adco, Adenocor / *SW*	Vasodilator, A2 agonist, Anti-inflammatory	AV block, bradycardia, ventricular fibrillation, intracranial pressure		USA	1973	FDAMA (2001)
Alclofenac	Prinalgin	NSAID	Skin reactions. Acute interstitial nephritis, vasculitis, anaphylaxis, hepatotoxic Mutagenic metabolite	1972	UK	1979	B84, F2001, SPA94
Alosetron	Lotronex / *GW*	5-HT$_3$ receptor antagonist for IBS	Ischaemic colitis (? 1 in 200), severe constipation. Bowel perforation. Serotonin blockade-mediated vasoconstriction – 7 deaths. Reintroduced with restrictions June 2002	Feb 2000	USA	Nov 2000	Heinrich (2001), Horton (2001), Suchard (2001), Fox (2001), Moynihan (2002), WHODI 14, 4, 2000
Alphaxalone/alphadolone Althesin / *Duncan Flockhart*		Anaesthetic	Anaphylactoid reactions due to Cremophor EL	1972 / 1973 / 1977	UK / Fr / Ger	1984	F2001, J98, SPA88
Alpidem	Ananxyl / *Synthelabo*	Anxiolytic imidazole pyridine	Cytolytic hepatitis, some fatal	1991	Fr	Jan 1994	F2001
Amfepramone HCl	Tenuate dospan, diethyl propion / *MMD*	Anti-obesity	Primary pulmonary arterial hypertension. Risks outweigh benefits. Reintroduced UK, April 2000; finally withdrawn June 2001. Reintroduced 2002 with restrictions	1971	EU / Fr, UK / Tk / Om / ?Swe	April 2000	Reactions 797, 2, 15 April 2000 / WHO (1999)

(continued)

Table A1.1　(*continued*)

International Non-proprietary Name	Trade name / *Company*	Therapeutic class	Reason for withdrawal	Launch date	Country	Withdrawal date	Reference
Amineptine	Survector / *Servier*	Tricyclic antidepressant. D_2 and D_3 antagonist	Amphetamine-like dependence. Hepatocellular damage – severe acute micro and macro. Severe acne. V	1978 1960 1982	Fr USA Sp, It Th Port	1999 1966 1999	A2001, F2001, AFSSAPS (2001), WHO (2001)
Aminoglutethimide	Elipten, Cytadren, Orimetan / *Novartis*	Anticonvulsant	Endocrinological (ovaries, uterus, hypothyroid, adrenal insufficiency). Reintroduced for Cushings syndrome	1960 1978 1982	USA USA UK	1966 NW	B84, SPA94
Aminopyrine	Phenazone	Analgesic	Bone marrow suppression, agranuocytosis, renal damage, TEN, SJS	1900 1900	USA UK Ger Fr	1970* 1975* 1977 1982	SPA94, B84, F2001
Aminorex fumarate	Menocil / *CC*	Anti-obesity	Primary pulmonary arterial hypertension	1962	Swz Ger	Oct 1967	Gurtner (1985) SPA88
Amobarbital	Amytal / *Hoechst, Eli Lilly, Houde*	Barbiturate	Self-poisoning, high potential for abuse	1961	Nw Fr	1980 1992	F2001
Amoproxan	Mederel	Anti-anginal	Dermatological and ophthlamic	1969	Fr	1970	F2001, SPA94
Anagestone acetate		Hormone	Animal carcinogenicity		Ger	1969	F2001, SPA 94
Anorectic agents	Fenproporex, Mefenorex, nor-pseudo-ephedrine, phendimetrazine, Mazindol, Fenbutrazato, Cloforex, Propilhexedrine, Clobenzorex	Anti-obesity	Psychotic reactions, depression, convulsions, dependency and abuse		EU Fr, Om Port Sp	Mar 2000 1999 2000 1999	WHO (2001), WHODI 14, 1, 2000

Name	Brand names / company	Therapeutic class	Reason	Date	Country	Year	References
Antrafenine	Stakane	Analgesic	Unspecified experimental toxicity, acute interstitial nephritis	1977	Fr	1984	F2001, SPA94
Aristolochicacid	Tarolyl, Descresept	Herbal slimming preparation	Carcinogenic in rats, orothelial cancer.	1990	USA	2001	Scrip 2544, 31 May 2000, p. 3 Swetz, SPA94
			Interstitial renal fibrosis.	1964	Au	1992	
					Ger	1981	
			End-stage renal failure		UK, Om	1999	
Arsenate Na + others	Biodynamine vitamin D2, Sangart *Sterling Midy*	General tonic	Abuse	1951	Fr	1988	SPA94
Astemizole	Hismanal *Janssen*	Antihistamine	QTc prolongation, Torsade de pointes, Interactions.	Dec 1988	USA, MI, MM	June 1999	Heinrich (2001), Fox (2001), Viskin et al. (2000), F2001, WHO (2001)
					UK	1998	
			V ? commercial decision				
Azaribine	Triazure	Anti-psoriatic	Neuropsychiatric, intravascular coagulation, thromboembolism	1975	USA	1976	B84, B95, MG84, FDAMA (2001), F2001 SPA94
					Sp		
Bendazac	Benzum, Bendalina	NSAID	Hepatotoxicity	1984	Sp	1993	A2001, B95, F2001
Benoxaprofen	Opren, Oraflex, Bexopron *Eli Lilly*	NSAID	Hepatorenal syndrome.	N.v 1980	UK	Aug 1982	MG84, SPA94, B84, Anon. (1982), Rawlins (1997), Suchard (2001), FDAMA (2001), F2001, Shedden (1982), J98, Taggart and Alderdice (1982), Abraham (1995)
			Cholestatic jaundice due to benoxaprofen	Apr 1982	USA	Aug 1982	
			glucuronide with	1982	Ger	Aug 1982	
			decreased renal function.	1981	Sp	Aug 1982	
			Photo-sensitivity, onycholysis, 74 deaths. Σ				
Benzarone	Vasoc, Venazil, Fragivix *Labaz, Sanol GmbH, Lindopharm GmbH*	Thrombolytic Benzo-furan derivative	Acute hepatitis, some fatal	1964	Ger	1992	F2001, SPA94, Bfarm (2002)
Benzbromarone	Desuri *Sanofi-Synthelabo*	Hyperuricmic	Cytolytic liver damage	1976	Fr	May 2003	R952
Benziodarone	Amplivix, Cardivix	Uricosuric, coronary dilator	Hepatotoxicity	1962	UK	1964	B84, F2001, SPA94
				1962	Fr	1987	

(continued)

Table A1.1 (*continued*)

International Non-proprietary Name	Trade name Company	Therapeutic class	Reason for withdrawal	Launch date	Country	Withdrawal date	Reference
Benzydamine HCl	Various	Topical NSAID	Photosensitivity, erythema, contact dermatitis, peculiar visual/psychic disturbances		Nl		Meyboom (1998)
Bepridil	Vascor *Ortho McNeil*	Ca^{2+} channel blocker, class IV antiarrhythmic	Torsades de pointes, QTc prolongation	1981		?	Viskin et al. (2000)
Beta-ethoxylacetanilide		Analgesic, analogue of phenacetin	Renal toxicity, animal carcinogenicity		Ger	1986	F2001, SPA94
Bismuth (insoluble salts)		GI drug	Reversible myoclonic encephalopathy, 72 deaths in France – ?reason	1875	Fr A Jp	1978	SPA94, Burns et al. (1974), Martin Bouyer (1976)
Bithionol	Actamer, Anafongine, Lorothirol, Bitin	Anti-helminthic	Dermatological photosensitivity Ω		USA	1967	SPA94, FDAMA, WHO (2001), F2001
Bromocriptine mesylate	Parlodel *Sandoz*	D2 agonist. Derivative of ergot. For prevention of lactation	Intracranial haemorrhage, seizures, hypertension, psychosis, 34 deaths – 1 in 20 000 pregnancies. Interaction with sympathomimetic drugs. Ω	1976	USA	1994	Ahmad and Wolfe (1995), Iffy et al. (1998)
Bromfenac Na	Duract *WA*	NSAID	Fatal hepatic failure, 4 deaths. Off-label abuse. V	Jul 1997	USA, SA, MM	Jun 1998	Suchard (2001), F2001, FDAMA (2001), Fox (2001), Friedman et al. (1999), WHO (2001), WHODI 12, 3, 1998

Drug	Trade names / Company	Class	Reason	Date	Country	Date	References
Brotizolam	Lendormin *BI*	Hypnotic benzodiazipine	Carcinogenicity (rodents) via CYP3A oxidation	1982	UK Fr	1989	J98, F2001
Bucetin	Beelin, Alacetan, Analgon, Doppel-Spalt, Combalgon *Ciba-Geigy GmbH*	Analgesic	Renal toxicity		Ger	1986	F2001, SPA94, Bfarm (2002)
Budipine	Parkinsan *Byk Gulden Lomberg Lundbeck*	Muscarinic and NMDA receptor antagonist	Severe cardiovascular risks – arrhythmias. Restricted to Germany and requires written guarantees and specific monitoring	1979	Ger	2000	Curel and Stather (2002), Bfarm considered withdrawal, but never did so
Buformin	Silubin, Sindiatil *Bayer AG*	Biguanide anti-diabetic	Lactic acidosis – 50% fatal. Class effect via mitochondria	1950s	Ger	1978	SPA94, F2001, Bfarm (2002)
Bupropion	Wellbutrin *GSK*	Anti-depressant, noradrenaline/dopamine reuptake inhibitor	Seizures in study subsequently found to be only 0.4% and remarketed 1989	1985	USA	1986	SPA94
Butamben	Efocaine, various	Local anaesthetic	Severe tissue slough, transverse myelitis, psychiatric reaction		USA	1964	FDA (1999), SPA94, FDAMA (2001), F2001
Camazepam	Albego *Merck*	Benzodiaepine	Immunoallergic hypersensitivity	1978	Nl	1984	Meyboom (1998)
Canrenone	Contaren, Phaninone, Contaren, Sproktan, Theraplix *Boehringer Mannheim GmbH*	Diuretic, aldosterone antagonist	Animal carcinogenicity (difficult to confirm). metabolite of spironalactone	1986 1966	Ger Fr	1986 1992	F2001, SPA94, Bfarm (2002)

(continued)

Table A1.1 (continued)

International Non-proprietary Name	Trade name / *Company*	Therapeutic class	Reason for withdrawal	Launch date	Country	Withdrawal date	Reference
Canthaxanthin	Apotrin	Tanning product	Retinopathy		Ger	1985	SPA94
Cartilage + bone marrow	Rumalon *Pierre Fabre Drug*	Antirheumatic, OA	Allergic skin	1962	Fr Ger	1992 1992	SPA94
Catechic extract	Eucatex	Vaso-active drug	Acute immunoallergic haemolysis	1972	Fr	1982	SPA94, Jaeger *et al.* (1979)
Cerivastatin	Baycol, Lipobay *Bayer©*	Anti-lipid	Rhabdomyolysis 52 deaths. V	Jun 1997	WW	Aug 2001	Anon. (2001), WHODI 15, 2, 2001, R883
Chloral hydrate	Noctec, Somnos *MSD, Welldorm, Smith and Nephew*	Hypnotic	Mutagenic carcinogenic in animals. Except single dose in children <5 years Welldorm (USA)	1869	Fr USA	Sep 2001 2001	AFSSAPS (2001)
Chloramphenicol	Numerous combinations	Antibiotic	Aplastic anaemia in 1 in 58 000–75 000. Ω	1950	Fr Jp	1978	SPA94, WHO (1999)
Chlormadinone acetate	Normenon, C-Quens, Sequence	Hydroxyprogesterone family. OC	Animal carcincgenicity (mammary tumours in dogs)	1965 1966	USA UK	1970 1970	B84, FDAMA (2001), F2001, SPA94
Chlormezanone	Trancopal *SW*	Muscle relaxant tranquillizer	TEN, SJS. EM, FDE, drug dependency, cytolytic and cholestatic hepatitis	1960	Ger, Sp, Jp, Fr, Port, WW	1996	F2001, A2001, WHODI 12, 1, 1998
Chlornaphazine		Polycythemia Hodgkins disease	Bladder cancer. Related to β naphthylamine (cancer in dye workers)	1964		1964	www.biam2.org/www/sub2737.html
Chloroform		Anaesthetic	Carcinogenic in animals. Toxic to heart, liver and kidneys	1847	USA	1976	FDA (1999), FDAMA (2001)
Chlorphentermine	Avicol	Anorexiant	Primary pulmonary artery hypertension. Half life: 5 days		Ger	1969	F2001, SPA94

			Allergic reactions		USA	Jul 1972	FDAMA (1999)
Chorionic gonadotrophin (animal origin)	Synapoidin, Sterivial						
Cianidanol	Catergene *Atophan*	Free radical scavenger for hepatic disorders	Haemolytic anaemia. 1 fatality. Reintroduced Switzerland 1986 and France 1987. Final withdrawal 1988	1977 1981	Sp, Ger Fr, Swe	1985 1985	F2001, B95, SPA94
Cincophen	Navarrard	Anti-gout	Cytolytic hepatotoxicity, cirrhosis	1910	Sp	1991	A2001
Cinepazide	Vasodistal, Vasolande, Arteriopax	Vasodilator	Agranulocytosis. 3 per 1000 patient-years	1980	Sp	1987	F2001, B95
Ciprofibrate 200 mg	Bilipanor	Hypolipidemic	Rhabodomyolysis dose-dependent		Fr	1995	WHO (1999)
Cisapride monohydrate	Propulsid *Janssen*	Nocturnal gastro-oesophageal reflux	QTc prolongation, 5-HT$_4$ agonist. Class III antiarrhythmic property. PEM and Mediplus databases showed no evidence of an association. 125 deaths	Jul 1993	USA, UK	Jul 2000	Suchard (2001), Ferriman (2000), Yap and Camm (2000), Viskin et al. (2000), Tooley et al. (1999), Fox (2001)
Clioquinol	Entero-vioform, Mexaforme, Oxychinol Tande *Taked Seijakia, Ciba-Geigy*	Anti-diarrhoeal	Subacute myelo-optic neuropathy (SMON) Peripheral neuropathy	1929* 1929 1930 1930	UK USA Fr, Ger, Jp WW	1981 1973 1985 1970	B84, SPA94, Jain (2001), F2001
Clofibrate		Anti-lipid	?Carcinogenic. Increased mortality. Reintroduced 1979		Ger	1978	Question 19058 (1979)
Cloforex		Anorexiant sympathomimetic	Cardiovascular toxicity		Ger Fr EU	1969 1995 2000	F2001, SPA94
Clomacron	*Debelar Devryl. SK*	NSAID	Hepatotoxicity	1977	UK, Br	1982	F2001, J98

(*continued*)

Table A1.1 (continued)

International Non-proprietary Name	Trade name / Company	Therapeutic class	Reason for withdrawal	Launch date	Country	Withdrawal date	Reference
Clometacin	Dupéron 'Longue durée' / *Casenne Marion*	NSAID, Indometacin derivative	Hepatocellular and chronic active hepatitis, analgesic nephropathy. Urticaria 3 deaths. All dosage forms in 1990. Φ	1977	Fr	1987	F2001, SPA94
Clozapine	Clozaril, Leponex / *Sandoz-Wander*	Anti-schizophrenic, piperazine derivative	Agranulocytosis. 1–2%. 8 deaths in Sweden. 9 deaths in Finland; Veno-thrombo-embolism. Reintroduced in USA and Sweden 1989. Δ	1972 / Feb 1975 / 1973	USA / EU / Fl / Fr / Th	1975 / Jul 1975	Idänpään-Heikkilä (1990) SPA88, Anderman and Griffith (1977), CIOMS IV (1998)
Cobalt		Iron-deficiency anaemia	Liver damage, claudication and myocardial darmage		USA / UAE	1967	FDA (1999), FDAMA (2001)
Coumarin (synthetic)	Lysedem, Lodema / *Knoll, Synthelabo*	Lymphoedema post-radiotherapy	Hepatotoxicity – cytolytic, 2 fatal. Incidence 2 per 10 000	Aug 1996	Fr / Au	Dec 1996 / 1996	WHO (1999)
Cupric bis-quinoline sulfonate/trimethylamine	Cuproxane	Anti-rheumatic	Neuro-muscular	1958	Fr	1978	SPA88
Cyclobarbital	Phanodorm / *Wintrop*	Barbiturate	Self-poisoning, dependence	1962	Nw / Fr	1980 / 1986	F2001
Cyclofenil	Menopax, Fertodur, Rehibin, Ondogyne	Anti-oestrogen/LH stimulant	Slight cholestatic and hepatocellular necrosis due to metabolic idiosyncrasy	1970	Fr	1987	F2001, SPA94, Olsson *et al.* (1983)
Cyclovalone + retinol + tiratricol	Plethoryl, Vanilone, Beveno	Anti-hyperlipidaemic, anti-dyspeptic	Hepato-cellular toxicity	1964	Fr	1988	SPA94

Danthron	Fructimer, Dorbanex, Codalax	Laxative anthroquinone	Animal carcinogenicity. Intestinal and liver tumours in rats. Reintroduced with restrictions in 1989. Ω, V	1959 1964 1964 1989	USA UK Fr, Ca, Ger	1987 1987 1987 1997	SPA94
Datura	Stramonium	Anti-asthmatic	Abuse	1920	Fr	1992	SPA94
Desensitizing vaccines		Vaccine	Allergic type reactions. 1 in 2 million, UK 26. Only for hayfever and stings. Must have CPR facilities. Δ	?	UK	1989	SPA94, Current Problems 20 5, 1994
Dexfenfluramine HCl	Redux *Servier*	Appetite suppressant	Valvular heart disease. Primary pulmonary hypertension	Apr 1996	USA UK, EU Ca, MI In, SA	Sep 1997	Suchard (2001), FDAMA (2001), Fox (2001), Weiseman (1998), Friedman *et al.* 1999
Diacetoxydiphenolisatin		Stimulant laxative	Hepatotoxicity	1971	Au	1971	F2001
Diamthazole di-HCl	Dimazol	Anti-fungal	Neuropsychiatric. Neurotoxic ADR in 1977	1955	USA Fr	1972 1972	F2001, SPA94
Diethylstilboestrol >25 mg per unit dose	Distilbene *Gerda, Eli Lilly et al.*	Prevention of miscarriage	Adenocarcinoma of vagina in offspring discovered in 1970. Prescribed in Spain and Belgium until 1983. Φ, Σ	1949 1946 1951 1938	USA, Au Fr, Jp Gz, Ger Austria	Feb 1975 1997 1971	Herbst *et al.* (1971), FDA (1999), FDAMA (2001), Direcks *et al.* 1991
Difemerine, inj. and gelules	Luostyl	Anti-muscarinic for GI symptoms	Multi-organ. Typical atropine like effects	1967	Ger	1986	F2001, SPA94
Di-hydro-streptomycin sulfate		Antibiotic	Neuropsychiatric, ototoxicity	1944	Fr USA	1995 Sep 1970	SPA94, FDAMA (2001), F2001

(continued)

Table A1.1 (*continued*)

International Non-proprietary Name	Trade name *Company*	Therapeutic class	Reason for withdrawal	Launch date	Country	Withdrawal date	Reference
Diiododiethyltin and isolinoleic acid ester	Stalinon R	Anti-staphylococcal infections	Dose given 50 mg but only 3 mg used in trials. Cerebral oedema. 102 deaths. Due to impurities. Σ	1954	Fr	1957	Anon. (1958), van Heijst (1997)
Dilevalol	Unicarde *Schering Plough*	β blocker (*RR* isomer of labetalol)	Hepatotoxicity. *V*	1990 1989	UK*, Port Jp	Aug 1990	F2001, B95, J98
Dinoprostone	Propess *Ferring Ph.*	Hormone Prostagladin E2	Uterine hypertonus and foetal distress	1989	UK	1990	F2001
Dionaea muscpula extract	'Venus fly trap' plant, Carnovora	Anti-cancer Immune modulator	Hypersensitivity. Was pending approval in 1992		Ger	1986	SPA94
Dipyrone	See Metamizole						
Dithiazanine iodide		Anti-helminthic stongylbidasis	Metabolic, cardiovascular?		USA Fr	1964 1964	SPA94, F2001, B84 SPA94, F2001
Domperidone (inj.)	Motilium *Janssen*	Antiemetic Dopamine receptor blocker	Cardiovascular – cardiac arrest, convulsions, tremor, Parkinsonism, hyper-prolactinemia, risk of overdose	1979 1983	UK Fr Ger It	1986 1986 1986 1992	SPA94, Jain (2001), Scrip 1131 (1986)
Doxylamine Dicyclomine	Bendectin, Debendox, Lenotan *MD*	Antihistamine, vomiting in pregnancy	Teratogenicity – dysmorphogenicity? CHD? Pyloric stenosis? No evidence ever produced	1956 1957	USA UK Ger	1983 1983	Hays (1993), SPA94
Droperidol	Droleptan, Thalamonal *JC*	Butyrophenone derivative for schizophrenia	QTc prolongation ×4 increase, torsades de pointes. *V*	2001 1970	UK USA	March 2001	Scrip 2611, 24 January 2001, p. 20 R883
Droxicam	Ombolan, Depanam various	NSAID, Oxicam derivative, Piroxicam pro-drug	Cholestatic hepatotoxicity		Sp EU	1994 1994	A2001

Drug	Brand names / Lab	Class / use	Adverse effect	Year	Country	Date	References
Ebrotidine	Ebrocit *Lab. Robert SA*	H2 antagonist	Hepatotoxicity, 1 death	1997	Sp	July 1998	A2001, F2001
Encainide HCl	Enkaid	Antiarrhythmic	Cardiovascular, excess mortality risk (RR 2.6)	1986	USA	Dec 1991	SPA94, FDAMA (2001), B95, F2001
Ethchlorvynil	Placidyl, Serenesil, Arvynol *Harvey Pharm. Abbott Lab.*	Hypnotic	Pulmonary oedema, pleural effusion. Dependence	1990 1955	UK* USA Ca	1978	Shah (2001a, b)
Etretinate	Tegison, Tigason *Roche*	Anti-psoriatic	Teratogenic, lymphomas, Present in plasma 3 years after stopping. Half life 80 hours whilst Neo-Tigason 50 hours	1983	Fr Nw Swe	1989	F2001, SPA94
Exifone	Adlone *Pharm science*	Memory problems, CNS stimulant	Hepatocellular toxicity	1988	Fr	1989	F2001, SPA94
Febarbamate	Atrium, Tymium *Riom Lab*	With phenobarbitone	Cytolytic hepatitis, cutaneous. 100 mg in 1997, 300 mg tablet in 2001	1967	Fr	1997–2001	Scrip 2619, 21 February 2001, p. 18
Felbamate	Felbatol *Wallace Lab.*	Lennox–Gastaut syndrome. Refractory partial seizures	Aplastic anaemia – unknown mechanism, 1 in 4000. RR 200, Hepatic failure 1 in 26 000–34 000. 9 deaths. Reintroduced in USA in 1995 with restrictions	1993 1994	USA Eur Fr	1994 1994	Nightingale (1994); Kaufman et al. (1996), F2001, CIOMS IV (1998)
Fenclofenac	Flenac *RC*	NSAID (aryalkanoic acid derivative)	Multiple, especially skin, TEN, acute interstitial nephritis, carcinogenicity in animals. 7 deaths	1978	UK, WW	Jul 1984	F2001, B95, J98, SPA94
Fenclozic acid		NSAID	Raised LFTs, jaundice (10%)	1969	UK, USA	1970	F2001

(continued)

Table A1.1 (continued)

International Non-proprietary Name	Trade name Company	Therapeutic class	Reason for withdrawal	Launch date	Country	Withdrawal date	Reference
Fenfluramine HCl	Pondimin, Ponderax WA, Servier	Appetite suppressant	Valvular heart disease with atrial regurgitation. Primary pulmonary artery hypertension	Jun 1973	USA, EU, UK, SA, Sp, Ca, MI, In, UAE, Au	Sep 1997	A2001, Suchard (2001), Friedman et al. (1999), FDAMA (2001), F2001
Fenoterol (high dose)	Berotec BI	β2 agonist	Increased mortality. Disputed (Suissa and Ernst, 1996). Φ		NZ	1990	Crane et al. (1989), Sears et al. (1990), F2001, Spitzer and Buist (1990), Pearce et al. (1990)
Feprazone	Methrazone	NSAID, phenylbutazone related	Nephrotoxicity, GI toxicity. Bullous dermatosis	1978 1974 1978	UK Ger Sp	1984 1984 NW	F2001, B95, J98, SPA94
Fipexide	Vigilor Bouchard	Cognitive enhancer	Hepatocellular toxicity, granulocytopenia. 1 death	1973	Fr	1991	F2001, SPA94
Flosequinan	Manoplax Boots	Congestive heart failure, vasodilator	Increased mortality. Lack of long-term efficacy after 3 months	Sep 1992 Sep 1992 1992	UK USA MM	Jul 1993 1993	F2001, FDAMA (2001), B95, J98
Flunitrazepam	Rohypnol Roche	Benzodiazepine	Abuse	1974	Fr, Sp, SA Au, Nz	1996 1999	F2001
Furazolidone	Furoxime SKB. Lipha Health	Anti-bacterial protozoa, salmonella	Pulmonary infiltrates, eosinophilia, polyneuritis, haemolytic anaemia, agranulocytosis, acute glaucoma, contact dermatitis	1963	Fr Ym Jp MI	1990 1998 1991	WHO Pharm. Newsletter No. 192, 1999
Ganglioside (bovine)	Cronassial, Biosinax, Nevrotal	Neurotrophic	GBS	1985 1976	Ger Sp, MM	1989 1993	B95, SPA94, A2001
Gentamycin (topical)			Ototoxicity		MI NI Ca	1997 1994 1996	WHO (1999)

Drug	Company	Class / Use	Adverse effect	Year	Country	Year	Reference
Germander extracts		Herbal slimming	Cholestatic, mixed and chronic liver toxicity	1989	Fr	1992	SPA94, Castot and Larry (1992)
Gingko Biloba products IV	Tebonin *Dr Willmar Schwabe GmbH*		Anaphylaxis, cardiac arrhythmias, leucocytosis		Ger	1998	Bfarm (2002)
Glafenine	Various	NSAID (anthranilic acid derivative)	Anaphylaxis Hepatocellular toxicity Acute interstitial nephritis	1967	Nl, Ger Fr Sp, EU	1979 1984 1992	A2001, F2001, Meyboom (1998)
Glutethimide	Doriden *Ciba*	Hypnotic piperidinione derivative	Acute glaucoma, dependence, abuse. Changed to Schedule II	1954	Fr USA	1991	SPA94
Glycosamino-glycan	Arteparon	Chondro-protective	Coagulation disorders ?thromboembolism. Used elsewhere	1955	UK Ger	1983 1982	SPA94
Grepafloxacin HCl	GW	Antibiotic (Fluoroquinolone)	QTc prolongation. Cardiac arrhythmias. Class effect. 7 deaths. V	Nov 1997 1999	USA, UK Ger, WW Sp Nl	Oct 1999 1992 1991	Suchard (2001), A2001, Viskin *et al.* (2000), F2001, WHODI 13, 4, 1999
Growth hormone	Somatropin, Crescormon, Asellacrin	Growth hormone (natural)	Manufacture problem, Creutzfeld-Jakob chance disease transmission	1973 1976 1976 1974	UK USA Fr, Ger Sp	1985 1985 1985 1985	SPA94, B95
Guanethidine	Ganda (high dose) *Chauvin Ph.*	Anti-glaucoma eye drops	Opthalmological. Φ	1977 1973	UK Fr Nw	1986 NW	SPA94
Guar Gum	Calban	Weight control (OTC)	Oesophageal obstruction	1991	USA	1992	FBA Talk Paper Pre-1995
HA-1A	Centoxin, Centocor *Eli Lilly*	Human anti-lipid monoclonal antibody	Patients without a Gram-negative infection had a higher mortality	1991	EU, Gz, Au, Nz	1993	SPA94
Hydrochlorthiazide + sotalol	Sotazide	Anti-hypertensive	CVS – QT prolongation enhanced by low K^+ due to diuretic	1984	Fr	1986	SPA94
Ibufenac	Dytransin	NSAID	Hepatotoxicity	1966	UK	1968	B84, F2001, SPA94

(continued)

Table A1.1 (continued)

International Non-proprietary Name	Trade name / Company	Therapeutic class	Reason for withdrawal	Launch date	Country	Withdrawal date	Reference
Indalpine	Upstene	SSRI	Agranulocytosis	1983	Fr	1985	F2001, SPA94
Indomethacin-R	Osmosin form / *MSD*	NSAID (indolacetic acid derivative)	Multiple GI – small intestine due to high local levels, 2/400 000 prescriptions. Perforations. 36 fatal. Φ	1982	UK / Ger, WW	1983 / 1983	Bem *et al.* (1988), SPA94
Indoprofen	Flosint, Flosin / *FCE*	NSAID (arylalkanoic acid derivative)	Gastro-intestinal (bleeding and perforation), carcinogenicity	1982 / 1979 / 1977	UK / Ger, Sp / WW	1983 / 1984 / 1984	SPA94, F2001, J98, Scrip No. 859, B95
Iodinated casein	Coratose Strophantin	Anorexiant	Metabolic, thyrotoxic	?	USA	1964	SPA94, F2001
Iophendylate	Pantopaque, Myodil / *Glaxo*	Radio-opaque media	Adhesive arachnoiditis. *V for commercial reasons. Legal case settled out of court*	1946	UK	1987	House of Commons Hansend 13 Dec 1990
Iproniazid	Marsilid / *Roche Products*	Anti TB, MAOI, antidepressant	Hepatocellular toxicity, CAH, cirrhosis, anti-mitochondria antibodies. 20% mortality	1957	USA	1959	Aithal & Day (2002)
Isaxonine phosphate	Nerfactor	Neurotrophic	Cholestatic and hepatocellular toxicity, agranulocytosis, deaths.	1981	Fr	1984	F2001, SPA88, Jouenne (1987)
Isotretinoin	Roaccutan. / *Roche*	Anti-acne	Problems of teratogenicity		It	1988	Scrip 1310 (1988)
Isoxicam	Vectren, Pacyl	NSAID (Oxicam derivative)	SJS, TEN	1985 / 1985	Sp*, Ger / Fr, MM	1985 / 1983	F2001, B95, SPA94

Drug	Manufacturer	Use	Adverse reaction		Country	Date	Reference
Kava (Piper methysticum)		Herb for relaxation	Hepatitis, cirrhosis, liver failure. 70 cases, 7 transplants, 4 deaths		Ger, Ca Fr, Swz Ire	2002	No. 911, No. 917
Ketorolac injection	Toratex, Toradol, Various *Syntex Ph.*	NSAID (arylalkanoic acid derivative)	Gastrotoxicity, renal failure. Haemorrhage. TEN, SJS. 80 deaths.		UK Ger Fr MM	Jan 2003 1993 1993	F2001
Levacetylmethadol	Orlaam, LAAM *Sipaco* BI	Opiate addiction	QTc prolongation. tensades de pointes cardiac arrest Ω	Jul 1997 1995	Dk, Nl, Ger, Port, Sp, UK US	2001 2003	EMEA public statement: EMEA/8776/01, 19 April 2001, WHODI 15, 1, 2001, R883
Levamisole		Originally antihelmithic, chemotherapeutic agent	Leukoencephalopathy and increased mortality, agranulocytosis		VN	2000	WHO (2001), e-medicine journal, 25 September 2001, 2, 9
Lyme disease vaccine	Lymerix *GSK*	Vaccine	Arthritis, myalgia. Company deny safety concerns. Sales dropped	1999	USA	2002	*Br Med J* (2002) **324**: 562
Lysine amidotriazoate	Peritrast, Iotrolan, Isovist, Gastrolux *Golham Pharma GmbH*	Contrast medium (high osmolar ionic)	Acute renal failure. DIC, arrhythmias, pulmonary oedema, hypotension (more than low osmolar ionic), hypersensitivity. Bfarm said only intranasal use		Ger	1995	AFSSAPS (2001), Bfarm (2002), WHO (1999)
Mebanazine Medifoxamine	Actomol Cledial *Lipha Sante, Merck*	Antidepressant, MAOI Antidepressant. Monoamine receptor uptake inhibitor	Hepatic, drug interactions Hepatocellular damage. 2 deaths	1963 1983	UK Fr	1975 Jul 1999	B84, F2001, SPA94 www.biam2.org/www/Gsu129.html
Megestrol acetate	Volidan 21, Serial 28	Hormone for breast cancer	Carcinogenicity. Reintroduced	1963	UK Fr Ger	1970 1969 1975	B84, SPA94
Mepazine HCl or acetate	Pacatal	Anti-epileptic	Granulocytopenia, paralytic ileus, urinary retention, seizures, hypotension, jaundice		USA	May 1970	FDA (1999), FDAMA (2001)

(continued)

Table A1.1 (continued)

International Non-proprietary Name	Trade name / Company	Therapeutic class	Reason for withdrawal	Launch date	Country	Withdrawal date	Reference
Mercurothiolate Na	Thiomersal	Antiseptic	Urothelial cancer, nephrotoxicity. peripheral neuropathy	1930	Br / USA / EU	Jul 1999	Scrip 2683 (2001)
Mercury amide HCl	Crème des 3 fleurs d'orient, DianeR	Skin preparation	Mercury poisoning in children, unborn and neonates	1956	Fr / Ca, Om	1986	SPA94
Mercurous chloride	Steedman's teething powder (calomel)	Teething powder	Pink disease (acrodynia)	19th century	WW	1953	www.users.bigpond.com/difarnsworth/pink-f.htm
Metamizole Na	Dipyrone, Novalgin / *HMR*	NSAID (amidopyrine related)	Agranulocytosis (1 in 3000) anaphylaxis, first withdrawn Sweden in 1974, reintroduced in 1995, finally withdrawn 1999. New studies suggest that the risk was exaggerated (1 in 900 000)	1921 / 1934	Np, Th / Swe, Au / USA / UK / Ym / Zb / Col / Arm, Syr	1997 / 1994 / 1974 / 1977 / 1977 / 1977	F2001 / CIOMS IV (1998) / WHO PN (2002)
Methamphetamine HCl Inj.	Methedrine, Drinalfa, Bophen, Pervitin / *BW*	Weight reduction	Abuse, dependence		USA	1973	FDAMA (2001)
Methandrostenolone	Dianabol	Anabolic steroid	Endocrinological, off-label abuse	1960 / 1960 / 1962 / 1963	USA / Fr / UK / Ger, MM	1982 / 1982 / 1982 / 1982	Scrip Report / F2001, SPA94
Methapyrilene	Rinofol, Various	H1 Antihistamine	Carcinogenicity in rats. ∇	1947 / 1950	USA / UK, Ger	Jun 1979	B84, FDAMA (2001) / F2001, SPA94
Metipranolol ophth. solution	Glauline, Optipranolol	Anti-glaucoma, β blocker	Anterior uveitis (high dose). Low dose prepn. 1.87 per 1000 patient/years. Φ	1986	UK / MM	1992 / 1991	F2001, J98, SPA94

Drug	Trade name	Use	Comments	Date	Country	Date	Reference
Metofoline	Versidyne	Analgesic	Experimental toxicity. Corneal deposits in dogs	?	USA	Mar 1965	SPA94, FDAMA (2001) F2001
Metrizamide	Amipacque	Contrast medium	Encephalopathy, delirium, asterixis, hallucinations, nystagmus, epilepsy, aseptic meningitis, ototoxicity, due to penetration into cerebrum and cerebellum. 40 cases		NI		Meyboom (1998)
Metrodin High Purity	Folicle-stimulating hormone	In vitro fertilization	Fear of variant CJD as the urine used is from Italy where there has been a case of variant CJD	1993	UK	Feb 2003	MCA media release 10 Feb 2003, R939
Mianserin	Bolvidon, Tolvon Organon	Tetracyclic antidepressant	Agranulocytosis, 1/5000–1/6000 (withdrawn from free list)	1976 1980 1979	UK NZ Au, Fl, Om	1988	Coulter and Edwards (1990), Idänpään-Heikkilä (1984)
Mibefradil dihydrochloride	Posicor HLR	Ca channel blocker T and L channel	Multiple (26) interactions due to inhibition of CYP1A2, 2D6, 3A4, rhabdomyolysis. V	Jun 1997	USA, EU, Ger, Ire, Ml, MM	Jun 1998	Suchard (2001), A2001, F2001, FDAMA (2001), Friedman et al. (1999), WHODI 12, 4, 1998
Minaprine HCl	Cantor	Antidepressant	Convulsions, abuse		Fr Sp	1996 1997	A2001 F2001
Molsidominal	Corvaton, Molsiton	Nitro coronary vasodilator	Malignant ethmoidal tumours in rats. Twice suspended. Reintroduced Dec 1985	1972	Ger	Oct 1985	Corvasal (1986)
Moxisylyte	Uroalpha	Alpha blocker for prostatic hypertrophy	Hepatitis (dose-related)	1989	Fr	1993	SPA94
Mumps vaccine (Urabe AM9 strain)	Pariorix SKB	Vaccine	Neuropsychiatric, myelopathy, aseptic meningitis, 1 in 2040 doses overall. Japan: 1 in 7000 to 1 in 405. France: 1 in 13 to 67 000. V	1988 1986 1983	Ca UK Fr Nw Jp Br, Nw, USA	1988 1992 NW 1992 1993 1992	SPA94, Lloyd and Chen (1996)

(continued)

Table A1.1 (*continued*)

International Non-proprietary Name	Trade name / *Company*	Therapeutic class	Reason for withdrawal	Launch date	Country	Withdrawal date	Reference
Muzolimine	Edrul	Diuretic	Polyneuropathy, myelopathy, myeloencephalopathy in patients with renal insufficiency. 7 deaths	Apr 1985 Apr 1987 1983	EU, Ger Fr It	1987 Jul 1987 Jul 1987	F2001, SPA88, Scrip 1223 (1987)
Naftidrofuryl oxalate IV	Nafronyl, Various *Lipha Ph.*	Vasodilator, 5HT2 antagonist	Arrythmia (intracardiac conduction) anaphylaxis, seizures, cytolytic hepatic failure, acute renal failure. 3 deaths. Disputed (Lewis *et al.*, 1998)	1984 1974	UK (restricted) Sp Fr Ger	1995 1992 1995 1996	A2001
Nandrolone Inj.	Dynabolan, Deca-Durabolin, Theramex *Organon*	Anabolic steroid, anti-gonadotrophic	Lack of efficacy in post-menopausal osteoporosis, change in benefit/risk ratio. Reason not stated. Frequently used for doping athletes	1964	Fr Bang	1997	WHODI 12, 3, 1998
Nebacumab	Centoxin HA-1A *JJ, Eli Lilly*	Hu-anti-lipid A IgM monoclonal antibody for septic shock	Gram-negative septicaemia. Excess mortality	1991 1992 1991	Fr Sp UK	1993 1993 1993	A2001 B95, J98, SPA94
Neomycin sulfate (inj.)		Antibiotic	Ototoxicity, nephrotoxicity. Misuse, irrigation of open wounds	?	USA	1989	SPA94, FDAMA (2001)
Nefazodone	Dutonin, Serzone, Nefardar, Reseril, Rulivan, Serzonil *BMS*	Phenylpiperazine derivative antidepressant	23 reports liver failure, 13 deaths. Company said not because of liver toxicity but low sales	1994	EU USA	Jan 2003 NW	www.drugintel.com/news [14 January 2003]
Nialamide	Niamid *Harvey Pharm. (Pfizer)*	Antidepressant (MAOI)	Cytolytic hepatitis. Drug interactions	1959 1959 1960	UK USA Fr, Nw	1978 1974 1995	B84, F2001, SPA94

Drug	Brand / Manufacturer	Class	Effect	Year	Country	Withdrawn	Reference
Nifedipine 10 mg	Adalat *Bayer*	Ca antagonist	More rapid release and higher peak serum levels		Au	1996	WHO (1999)
Nikethamide	Coramine	CNS stimulant	Narrow therapeutic margin		MM	1988	F2001
Nimesulide Paediatric later adult	Nimed, Antifloxil, Guaxan, Aulin, Helsinin *RPR*	NSAID	Hepatotoxicity (idiosyncratic) in children consistent with Reyes, fulminant hepatic failure, 3 deaths. *V*	1986 1995	Port Ire Isr, Fl Sp, Tk	1999 (Paed) 2002 (Adult)	Drug Safety newsletter, 9th edn. 904, 2, 1 June 2002
Nitrefazole	Altimol, Merck KgaA	Alcohol deterrent	Hepatic, haematological	1983	Ger	1984	F2001, SPA94, Bfarm (2002)
Nitrofurazone		Nasal and ear drops	Mammary neoplasia in rats		USA	1974	FDAMA (2001)
Nomifensine maleate	Merital, Alival *Hoechst AG*	Antidepressant	Haemolytic anaemia, acute intravascular haemolysis, alveolitis, hepatotoxicity – cytotoxic and cholestatic. 8 deaths. Not in France, where only 25 mg available. Σ	1977 1976 1984 1978 1978 1978	UK Ger USA Fr Sp MM	Jan 1986 Jan 1986 Jan 1986 NW NW	Stonier (1992), Stonier and Edwards (2002) FDAMA (2001) B95, F2001, J98, SPA88, Schönhöfer (1991)
Omeprazole inj.	Losec, Antra, Gastroloc *Astra GmbH*	Selective inhibitor of hydrogen-potassium ATPase	Visual disorders (0.0008 per million days), putative genotoxicity, hepatic encephalopathy, toxicity of optic nerve, tinnitus, SIADH, myopathy, cerebellar disorder	1980s	Ger	Aug 1994	WHO, 1999
Orgotein	Bovine Cu, Zn, superoxide dismutase		Serious hypersensitivity, IgE-mediated anaphylaxis, some deaths		Ger Port	Mar 1994	EMEA (2001)

(continued)

Table A1.1 (*continued*)

International Non-proprietary Name	Trade name / Company	Therapeutic class	Reason for withdrawal	Launch date	Country	Withdrawal date	Reference
Oxeladin citrate	Paxeladine, Ipsen / *Beaufor Pharm*	Anti-tussive bronchodilator	Agranulocytosis. Carcinogenicity. Risk diminished, reintroduced in 1996	1972	Fr / Ger	1995 / 1994	WHO (1999)
Oxolamine citrate Oxomemazine	Gantrimone, Bredon Toplexil, Doxergan / *Rhone-Poulenc*	Anti-tussive URTI, Phenothiazine	Hallucinations in children / Sudden infant death syndrome, not for infants <1 year. Ω	1969 / 1937	Nl / USA / MI / SL, Fr	1984 / 1991	Meyboom (1998)
Oxyphenbutazone	Tanderil / *Ciba-Geigy*	NSAID	Aplastic anaemia, agranulocytosis, SJS. Multiple. 148 deaths. Butazones 1182 deaths. 3.8 deaths per 100 000	1960 / 1961 / 1962 / 1962	USA / Fr, WW / UK / Ger / Nl	Apr 1985 / Apr 1985 / 1984 / Jan 1984 / Jan 1984	SPA94, F2001, Inman (1977)
Oxyphenisatin and acetate	Veripaque, Lavema, Noloc, Dialose / *SW*	Laxative	Chronic active hepatitis, cytolytic hepatitis with acute DNA and anti-nuclear antibodies. Restricted to rectal use	1955 / 1957	UK, Ca / USA / Ger / Fr, Au / Austria / WW	1978 / 1972 / 1976 / 1981 / 1972 / 1985	B84, FDAMA (2001), F2001, SPA94
Pemoline	Volital, Cylert, various *Abbott, LAB Ltd and others*	Hyperkinetic syndrome, attention deficit disorder	Cytolytic hepatotoxicity and mixed auto-immune. 6 deaths	1975	UK / Ca	Sep 1999	F2001, WHODI 12, 1, 1998
Penicillins (topical)		Antibiotic	Allergic type reactions. Φ	?	USA	1972	SPA94
Pentobarbital	Nembutal / *Abbott*	Barbiturate	'Self-poisoning'		Nw	1980	F2001
Pentosan polysulphate sodium	Elmiron, Hemoclar, Various	Anti-thrombotic. For bladder pain	Delayed immunoallergic, thrombocytopenia		Fr / USA	1994 / 1996	WHO (1999)

Drug	Trade name / Manufacturer	Class	Adverse effects / comments	Year	Country	Year	Reference
Perhexiline maleate	Pexid *Casenne Marion*	Vasodilator, anti-anginal	Hepatocellular and chronic active hepatitis, nystagmus, dose related peripheral, neuropathy, myopathy, BIH. hypoglycaemia, weight loss	1975 1974 1975	UK Sp Fr	1985 1986 1996	F2001, B95, J98
Phenacetin	APC, Various *Bayer*	Analgesic	Analgesic nephropathy, hepatocellular toxicity, haemolytic anaemia, methemoglobinemia, carcinogenicity	1900* 1887*	UK USA Ger, Dk Nw, MM	1980 1983 1986 2001	B84, FDAMA (2001) F2001, SPA94 Scrip 2637, 25 March 2001, p. 1
Phenformin HCl	Insoral, Dibotin *DBI*	Biguanide, anti-diabetic	Metabolic lactic acidosis. Fatalities 4 per patient/year	1959 1959 1964	UK USA, Fr Ger Nw, NZ, Dk, Fl, A, Ca, Swe, UAE	1982 1977 1978	B84, F2001, SPA94
Phenobarbitone	Luminal	Anti-epileptic hypnotic	Restricted to epilepsy and anaesthesia. Severe cutaneous reactions	1912	Ger Fr	1994 2001	Scrip 2623, 4, 7 March 2001
Phenolphthalein	Numerous	Laxative	Potential genotoxicity carcinogenicity (rats and mice). Slow elimination with enteroheptic circulation. Atonia with K↓. V	1902	USA, Fr Jp Ca EU Om	Sep 1997 1998 1997	WHODI 12, 1, 1998
Phenoxypropazine	Drazine *Smith and Nephew*	Antidepressant (MAOI)	Hepatic, drug interactions	1961	UK	1966	B84, F2001, SPA94
Phentermine	Duromine *3M Health Care*	Anti-obesity	? Involved in valvular defects, reintroduced UK August 2000, final withdrawal June 2001		EU USA	Apr 2000	Fox (2001)

(continued)

Table A1.1 (*continued*)

International Non-proprietary Name	Trade name / Company	Therapeutic class	Reason for withdrawal	Launch date	Country	Withdrawal date	Reference
Phenylbutazone	Butazone, Butazolidine / *Ciba-Geigy, Novartis*	NSAID	Aplastic anaemia, acute interstitial nephritis, thrombocytopenic purpura, cholestatic and hepatocellular and granulomatous toxicity, 503 deaths, 2.2 deaths per 100 000. Ω	1949 / 1952	UK / NI / Ger, MI, Iraq, UAE, Jordan, Chil, Paraguay	Mar 1985 / 1985	SPA94, F2001
Phenylpropanolamine	Various	Colds (OTC), appetite suppressant	Cerebral haemorrhage, 200–500 haemorrhagic strokes per year USA (La Grenade *et al.*, 2001)		USA / Fr / Br, Col / Ar	2000 / 2001 / 2000 / 2000	AFSSAPS (2001), Fox (2001), Figueras and Laporte (2002), WHODI 14, 4, 2000
Pifoxime	Flamanil / *Sandoz*	NSAID, methopyriline derivative	Neuropsychiatric, loss of consciousness. Withdrawn 3 months after launch	1975	Fr	1976	F2001, SPA94
Piperazine		Blocks cholinergic receptors in worms	Severe neurotoxicity: seizures, EEG changes, dystonia, nystagmus, hypersensitivity, possibly carcinogenic	1949	MI	1996	WHO, 1999
Pirprofen	Rengasil	NSAID (arylalkanoic acid derivative)	GI, hepatocellular toxicity, 2 deaths. Acute interstitial nephritis. V	1987 / 1990 / 1983	Sp*, Ger / Fr / WW	1990 / 1990 / 1990	A2001, B95, F2001, SPA94
Pituitary chorionic hormone		Hormone	Hypersensitivity	?	UK / USA	1972 / 1972	SPA94

Podphyllin (Internal)		Laxative	Animal teratogenicity				SPA88
Polidexide	Secholex	Antihyperlipidemic	Experimental toxicity. Toxic impurities (mutagenic)	1974	Fr UK	1980 1975	MG84, B84, B9, J98, SPA94 SPA94
Potassium arsenite	Fowler's solution		Toxic, highly carcinogenic. V		USA	1980	FDA, 21CFR Part 216
Potassium chloride >100 mg, not controlled release	K logeais + Kalienor		Small bowel lesions. Φ	1985 1962	USA Fr	?1977 and 1992 1988	FDAMA (2001), SPA94
Potassium nitrate	Diathera		Carcinogenicity		Fr	1980	SPA88
Povidone IV	Polyvinylpyrrolidone	Plasma expander	Polyvinylpyrrolidone storage disease with granulomas. Coagulation		USA	1978	FDAMA (2001)
Practolol (oral)	Eraldin *ICI*	β blocker	Oculomucocutaneous syndrome, deafness, sclerosing peritonitis. Φ	1970 1973 ?	UK Fr Ger, Nl	1975 1975 1975	B84, SPA94
Prenylamine	Segontin, Synadrin	Antianginal, vasodilator	QTc prolongation. Torsades de pointes	1973 1965 1965	UK Ger Fr, MI	1989 1989 1989	SPA94, Viskin *et al.* (2000), F2001 Scrip 1300 (1988)
Probucol	Lorelco, Lurselle *Casenne Marion, HMR*	Anti-hyper lipidemia	QTc prolongation in 50% of cases. Torsades de pointes. V ? for efficacy reasons	1995 1980	Ger Fr US	1989 1996 1995	Viskin *et al.* (2000)
Proglumide	Milid *Yamanouchi*	Cholecystokin antagonist for PU	Respiratory		Jp Ger	1989	F2001, SPA94
Pronethalol	Alderlin, Nethalide	β blocker	Animal carcinogenicity	1963	UK	1965 NW	B84, F2001
Propanidid	Epontol	Anaesthetic	Allergic-type reactions due to Cremophor EL	1967	UK, Nw	1983	SPA94, F2001
Proxibarbal	Axen, Centralgol *Novartis*	Barbiturate	Immuno allergic thrombocytopenia. V		Sp, It Port, Tk Fr	1998 1998 1997	F2001, WHODI 12, 3, 1998
Pumactan	Alec *Brittania*	Lung surfactant for neonatal respiratory distress	Higher mortality than Poractant		UK	Apr 2000	Ainsworth *et al.* (2000)

(continued)

Table A1.1 (*continued*)

International Non-proprietary Name	Trade name / *Company*	Therapeutic class	Reason for withdrawal	Launch date	Country	Withdrawal date	Reference
Pyrovalerone HCl	Thymergix, Centoton	Psycho-stimulant	Misuse and abuse	1974	Fr	1979	F2001, SPA88
Pyrithyldione/diphenhydramine	Dorma with diphenhydramine	Anti-insomnia	Agranulocytosis 35 per 100 000 pat/yrs. 10× background	1940	Sp	1997	A2001
Rapacuronium Br	Raplon *Organon*	Neuromuscular blocking agent for facilitating tracheal intubation	Bronchospasm (3.5% in pre-marketing clinical trials), 5 deaths. V	Aug 1999	USA	Apr 2001	FDA (2001), WHODI 15, 1, 2001
Remoxipride	Roxiam, Benzamide *Astra*	Anti-psychotic, dopamine antagonist	Aplastic anaemia Ω, 8 cases, fatalities 1 in 25 000	1991 1991	UK Swe WW	1994 Dec 1993	F2001, B95, J98 CIOMS IV (1998)
Rota virus vaccine	Rotashield *Wyeth Lederle*	Vaccine	Intussception, 1 in 10 000 cases. 99 cases. RR 16.4	Aug 1998	USA UK	Oct 1999 2001	EMEA (2001), Weijer (2000), Scrip 2456, Fox (2001)
Secobarbital/quinal barbitone	Bellanox, Vesparex, Seconal *Eli Lilly*	Barbiturate	Abuse	1954	Fr, Nw Nl, MM	1990	F2001, SPA94
Sertindole	Serdolect *Lundbeck*	Anti-psychotic	Torsades de pointes. QTc prolongation. Sudden death. 36 deaths. V Reintroduced with restrictions Oct 2002	1996	UK Sp It Ger, Ire Nl, EU	1998 1998	A2001 Yap and Camm (2000), Viskin *et al.* (2000) F2001, Scrip 2689, 24 January 2001, p. 21
Sibutramine	Reductil, Reduxate, Meridia, Ectiva *Abbott, GSK, Knoll, Bracco*	Anti-obesity. Blocks uptake of noradrenaline and seratonin	Arrythmias, hypertension, 2 deaths due to cardiac arrest. Remarketed August 2002 with restrictions of prescribers	Apr 2001	It	Mar 2002	*Guardian Weekly*, 21–27 March 2002
Soruvidine	*Nippon Shoji*	Anti-viral	Interaction with 5-FU. 3 deaths in trials. 16 deaths	1993	Jp	1993	F2001, Shah (2001)

(continued)

Drug	Trade names / *Company*	Class	Reasons	Year	Country	Year	References
Sparfloxacin	Zagam, Spara *RPR, Bertex Lab*	Quinolone	QTc prolongation. Phototoxicity 7.49%, 2 deaths. Restricted to acute bacterial pneumonia/sinusitis	1994, 1994–95, 1993	Fr, Eur, USA, Jp	Jun 1995, Jun 1995, 1996	Viskin et al. (2000), CIOMS IV (1998)
Sparteine sulphate	Spartocin, Tocosamine	Herbal slimming aid	Tetanic uterine contractions, obstetrical complications		USA	1979	FDA (1999), FDAMA (2001)
Sulphacarbamide	Euvernil	Sulfonamide	Acute renal insufficiency, immuno-allergic hepatitis, SJS, TEN, agranulocytosis, thrombocytopenia		Ger, Nl, It, Swz	1988	F2001, SPA94
Sulfa dimethoxine	Madricin	Sulfonamide	SJS, fatalities		USA	1966	FDA (1999), FDAMA (2001)
Sulfamethoxydiazine	Durenat, Bayrema	Anti-infective	Typical sulfonamide ADRs, including SJS		Ger	1988	SPA94, F2001
Sulfamethoxypyridazine	Lederkyn	Sulfonamide	AA, agranulocytosis, exfoliative dermatitis, erythema multiforme	1957	UK, Swe, UAE	1986	SPA94, F2001
Sulfathiazole	Thiazomide, Tresamide	Sulfonamide	Renal, hepatic toxicity, blood dyscrasias, rash, fever	1941	USA, Fr, UAE	1970, 1977	FDA (1999), SPA94, FDAMA (2001)
Suloctidil	Fluvisco, Loctidon, Periman, Fluversin	Vasodilator. For intermittent claudication	Hepatocellular toxicity	1979, 1980	Sp, Ger, Fr	1985, 1985	F2001, SPA94, B95
Suprifen with tussilax	Tussucal	Anti-tussive	Hepatotoxicity	1971	Fr, Ger	1972	SPA88
Suprofen	Suprol, Supranol *McNeil, Ortho-Cilag*	NSAID (arylalkanoic acid derivative)	Nephrological intra-tubular obstruction, (flank pain syndrome)	1985, 1983, 1983	USA, UK, Sp, WW, It	1987, 1986, 1987, 1997	Harter (1988), SPA94, FDAMA (2001), B95, F2001, J98, Abraham (1995)

Table A1.1 (*continued*)

International Non-proprietary Name	Trade name *Company*	Therapeutic class	Reason for withdrawal	Launch date	Country	Withdrawal date	Reference
Temafloxacin	Omniflox, Teflox *Abbott Labs*	Anti-infective	Multiorgan system syndrome: DIC, hepatic dysfunction, haemolytic anaemia (probably secondary to immune complex formation), acute renal failure, anaphylaxis, metabolic, thrombocytopenia, 6 deaths. V	1991 1992 1992 1991	UK USA Ger Swe It Ire, Ar, Fr	Jun 1992 Jun 1992 Jun 1992 Jun 1992	Davey and McDonald (1993), Finch (1993), Kennedy et al. (2000), FDAMA (2001), B95, F2001, SPA94, J98, Roblin (1999)
Terconazole	Tercospor 160 mg	Anti-fungal			Ger	1998	SPA94
Terfenadine	Seldane *HMR*	Anti-histamine	Allergy, photosensitivity Hepatic damage, QTc prolongation. Torsades de pointes. 17 deaths. V	May 1985	USA Fr Om SA	Feb 1998 Feb 1998 1997	FDA (1999), FDAMA (2001), Visken et al. (2000), Friedman et al. (1999), F2001, Fox (2001)
Terodiline	Bicor, Micturin, Terolin, Uromictol, Mictrol *Kabi Pharmacie*	Anticholinergic, calcium antagonist for urinary incontinence	Cardiac arrhythmia, QTc prolongation. Torsades de pointes. Mean half-life 189 hours, 14 deaths. Mostly UK	1965 1986 1990 1991 1986	Swe UK Ger Sp*, MM USA	Sept 1991 Sep 1991 Sep 1991 Sep 1991 Sep 1991	Wild (1992, 2002), A2001, F2001, Rawlins (1997), B95, Viskin et al. (2000), Malone-Lee and Wiseman (1991), J98, SPA94, Shah (2002)
Tetrabamate	Atrium (Febaramate/ difebarmate/ phenobarbital)	Alcohol dependance	Hepatocellular necrosis, intracellular cholestasis, cutaneous (1997 – 100 mg withdrawn)	1981	Fr Sp	Mar 2001 2002	No. 841, 4, 3 March 2001 and 904, 2, 1 June 2002, R883
Tetracycline (ped) >25 mg/ml Φ	Achromycin V + Azotrea	Antibiotic	Teeth discolouration, temporary inhibition of growth, enamel hypoplasia	1952	USA, Om Chil, UAE Au, Bel Ghan	1979	SPA94, FDAMA (2001)

Drug	Brand, Company	Use	Adverse effects	Introduced	Country	Withdrawn	References
Thalidomide Ω	Contergan, Distaval, various *Chemie Grünenthal, Distillers Co.*	Sedative Orphan Drug Inds	Irreversible peripheral neuropathy 0.5% cases, phocomelia. (Total c 5000, Germany 2856, UK 450, Japan 300, Canada 125, Ireland 34, Sweden 31, Denmark 20, Norway 17, USA 17). Relaunched 1998 for leprosy	1958 1957	UK Ger	1961 1961	SPA94, McBride (1961), Burley (1988), Lenz (1962, 1992), D'Arcy and Griffin (1994), Mellin and Katzenstein (1962), Lenz and Knapp (1962), Jain (2001), Shah (2001)
Thenalidine tartrate	Sandostene	H1 antihistamine	Agranulocytosis, aplastic anaemia, thrombotic purpura	1958	USA, UK, MM	1958	SPA94, Adams and Perry (1958), F2001
Thiobutabarbitone	Inactin-Byk *Gulden Lomberg GmbH*	Barbiturate	Renal insufficiency, MA expired	1993	Ger	1993	F2001, Bfarm (2002)
Thorium dioxide	Thorotrast	Contrast medium	Carcinogenicity, cirrhosis of the liver, half-life 400 years	1928	UK	1955	Dukes et al. (2000)
Thymoxamine HCl	Opilon Moxisylyte, Erecnos *PD*	α blocker	Necrotic hepatitis, dose dependent	Late 1980s	Fr UK	Jun 1993	Hansard, 15 July 1993
Tick-borne encephalitis vaccine	TicoVac *Baxter*		High fever in children <3 years	Mar 2000	Ger	Jul 2000	Curel and Stather (2002)
Tienilic acid	Ticrynafen, Selacryn, Diflurex *SKF; Lab. Anphar-Rolland*	Uricosuric, diuretic	Hepatocellular and chronic active hepatitis, acute interstitial nephritis and failure, intra-tubular obstruction, 25 deaths. VΣ	1980 1979 1976	UK USA Fr Ger, MM	1980 1980 1991	B84, B95, *Lancet* (1992) **339**(18 Jan): 175, FDAMA (2001), F2001, MG84, Gerson (1992), Barclay (1980)
Tilbroquinol (paed)	Intetix *Beaufort Ipsen*	Infective diarrhoea	Cytolytic hepatotoxicity, SMON, restricted to amoebiasis	1969	Fr Swz, Mor	1997 1997	WHO (1999)
Timonacic	Hepalidine, Thioproline, Various	For acute and chronic hepatitis	Severe intoxication due to accidental overdosage in children	1975	Fr	1982	www.biam2.org. Anon. (1982b), SPA94

(continued)

Table A1.1 (*continued*)

International Non-proprietary Name	Trade name *Company*	Therapeutic class	Reason for withdrawal	Launch date	Country	Withdrawal date	Reference
Tolcapone	Tasmar *Hoffman-LaRoche*	Anti-Parkinsonian COMT inhibitor	Hepatocellular toxicity, 3 deaths. Still on US market	Jan 1998	UK, EU, Ire Port, Au, Sp	Nov 1998 1999	A2001, F2001
Tolrestat	Alredase, Alrestin *John Wyeth*	Anti-diabetic, aldase-reductase inhibitor	Hepato-necrosis, 3 deaths. *V*	1988 1992 1994 1991 1990	Ire Ar Ch, Gz It WW	Oct 1996 Oct 1996	Foppiano and Lombardo (1997), F2001
Tranylcypromine	Parnate, Parstelin *SKB*	Antidepressant (MAOI)	Hypertensive crisis. Many drug and food interactions. Reintroduced	1963	Fr USA, UK It, Bel	1987 1964	SPA94
Triacetyl diphenolisatin		Laxative	Cholestatic hepatotoxicity		Au	1971	F2001
Triazolam	Halcion	Hypnotic	Neuropsychiatric – memory loss, depression, amnesia – automatism syndrome	1977 1980 1982 ? 1980 1982 1980 1982	UK Fr It Nl Fl, Dk Ar, Nw Br	1991 1992 1987 1979	F2001, B95, J98, Gerson (1987), SPA94
Triparanol	MER-29 *William Merrill Co.*	Antihyperlipidemic	Cataracts, alopecia, icthyosis. Σ	1959	USA, Ger, Sp NW USA Fr, MM	1962 1962	SPA94, F2001
Troglitazone	Rezulin *Parke-Davis, Warner Lambert*	Anti-diabetic	Hepatocellular necrosis, bridging fibrosis, cholestasis intracanalicular. Idiosyncratic, 63 deaths. Δ in USA. LFT monitoring not successful	Jan 1997	USA UK Jp	2000 Dec 1997	Suchard (2001), Gottlieb (2001), F2001, Graham *et al.* (2000), WHODI 14, 1, 2000
Trovafloxacin (alatrofloxacin)	Trovan *Pfizer*	Antibiotic, quinolone	Hepatotoxicity. 9 deaths or liver transplants. Seen in pre-marketing clinical trials. Still on US market	1997	Eur	Aug 1999	A2001, Suchard (2001), F2001, Fox (2001)

Drug	Brand / source	Use	Adverse effects	Intro.	Country	Withdr.	References
L-Tryptophan	Pacitron, Optimax *Cambrian Chem.*	Low protein diet, depression	Eosinophilic myalgia syndrome. Contaminated by a by-product. Mostly USA. 38 deaths. Reintroduced Φ	1974 1982	USA UK, Ger Ire, Lux, Nl, Fr	1990 1990 1990	Wood (1992), SPA94, Eidson et al. (1990), Kennedy et al. (2000), Benjamin (1992), B95, F2001
Urethane	Pressyl, Surparine, Citral–Urethane	Solvent	Carcinogenicity (lung adenomas in mice), AA, thrombocytopenia, cytolytic hepatic necrosis, dose dependent	1933	Fr USA	1985 1977	SPA94
Uroalpha	Moxisylyte	Prostatic hypertrophy, α-blocker	Hepatitis, dose related	1989	Fr	1993	SPA94
Vincamine	(From *Vinca minor* plant – lesser periwinkle)	Cerebral vasodilator	Haematological, QTc prolongation, torsades de pointes		Ger Fr	1987	F2001, SPA94
Vitamin E, tocopherol	E-Ferol IV *Carter-Glogau Lab.©*	Prevention of deterioration to retina in neonate IC	Decreased platelets, cholestatic hepatitis. Nephrological ?due to polysorbide 8 used as emulsifier. 40 deaths in premature babies. Ω, Σ	1983	USA	1984	SPA94, Benson JS, *FDA Consumer*, Jan–Feb, 1991, Aranda et al. (1986)
Xenazoic acid	Xenaline	Anti-infective	Hepatotoxicity		Fr	1965	F2001, SPA94
	Zelmid *Astra*	Antidepressant, 5-hydroxytryptamine uptake inhibitor	Hepatotoxicity, flu-like syndrome, GBS 22 × expected level	1982 1982 1982	UK Ger, MM Swe	1983 1983 1983	F2001, B84, B95, J98, SPA94, MG84, Idänpään-Heikkilä (1984), A2001
Zipeprol HCl	Respilenil, Various	Anti-tussive	Abuse, dependence, seizures, fatalities, acute poisoning		Sp It Swz, Tk, Br	1995 1991	A2001
Zomepirac Na	Zomax *McNeil Pharm.*	NSAID, arylalkanoic acid derivative	Allergic-type reactions – fatal anaphylaxis. 14 deaths in USA. Acute interstitial nephritis, nephrotic syndrome. V	1980 1981 1982 1981 1982	USA UK Sp Ger WW	1983 1983 1983	Ross-Degnan et al. (1993), FDAMA (2001), B84, SPA94, MG84, F2001, J98, Abraham (1995), Anon. (1993)

References

Abraham J (1995). Opren/Oraflex – the making of a drug disaster. In *Science, Politics and the Pharmaceutical Industry*. UCL Press: 98–178.

Adams DA and Perry S (1958). Agranulocytosis associated with Thenalidine (Sandostene) tartrate therapy. *J Am Med Assoc* **167**: 1207–1210.

AFSSAPS (2001). Agence Français de Securité Sanitaire de Produit de Santé. http://agmed.sante. gouv.fr [10 July 2003].

Ahmad SR and Wolfe SM (1995). Lesson from a drug indication withdrawal. *Pharmacoepidemiol Drug Saf*, **4**(Suppl 1): 169.

Ainsworth SB, Beresford MW, Milligan DW, Shaw NJ *et al.* (2000). Pumactant and poractant for treatment of respiratory distress syndrome in neonates born at 25–29 weeks' gestation: a randomised trial. *Lancet* **355**(9213): 1380–1381.

Aithal GP and Day CP. Hepatic Adverse Drug Reactions. In *Pharmacovigilance*. Mann R & Andrew E (Eds) 2002. p. 466.

Anderman B and Griffith RW (1977). Clozapine-induced agranulocytosis: a situation report up to August 1976. *Eur J Clin Pharmacol* **11**: 199–201.

Anon. (1958). *Br Med J* **i**: 515.

Anon. (1982a). Benoxaprofen. *Br Med J* **285**: 6340.

Anon. (1982b). Arrêt de la fabrication de l'Hepalidine comprimés. *Le Quotidien du Médicin*, 23 September.

Anon. (1983). (Leader) Zomax withdrawn from market after fatal reactions. *Pharm J* (March): 299.

Anon. (2001). Substituting for Cerivastatin (Baycol). *The Medical Letter* **43**(1113).

Aranda JV, Chemtob S, Laudignon N and Sasyniuk BI (1986). Furosemide and vitamin E; two problems in neonatology. *Pediatr Clin N Am* **33**(3): 583–602.

Arnaiz JA, Carné X, Riba N, Codina C *et al.* (2001). The use of evidence in pharmacovigilance. Case reports as the source for drug withdrawals. *Eur J Clin Pharmacol* **57**: 89–91.

Barclay WR (1980). Ticrynafen's withdrawal from the market. *J Am Med Assoc* **243**(8): 771.

Bakke OM, Wardell WM and Lassagna L (1984). Drug discontinuities in the United Kingdom and the United States, 1964 to 1983: issues of safety. *Clin Pharmacol Ther* **35**: 559–567.

Bakke OM, Manocchia M, de Abajo F, Kaitin K, *et al.* (1995). Drug safety discontinuations in the United Kingdom, the United States, and Spain from 1974 through 1993: a regulatory perspective. *Clin Pharmacol Ther* **58**: 108–117.

Bem JL, Mann RD and Coulson R (1988). Fatal gastrointestinal damage associated with the use of Osmotic mini pump Indomethacin (Osmosin). *Pharm Med* **3**: 35–43.

Benjamin DM (1992). When is drug not a drug? The L-tryptophan tragedy: lessons to be learned. *Drug Inf J* **26**: 231–236.

Bfarm (2002). Marcus Wittstock Bundesinstitut für Arzneimittelmedizin und Produkte, personal communication, July.

Burley DM (1988). The rise and fall of thalidomide. *Pharm Med* **3**: 231–237.

Burns R, Thomas DW and Barron VJ (1974). Reversible encephalopathy possibly associated with bismuth subgallate ingestion. *Br Med J* **1**: 220–223.

Castot A and Larry D (1992). Hepatitis observed during treatment with a drug or tea containing wild germander. Evaluation of 26 cases reported to the regional centre of pharmacovigilance. *Gastroenterol Chirugie Biol* **16**(12): 916–920.

CIOMS IV (1998). Report of CIOMS Working Group IV, *Benefit–Risk Balance for Marketed Drugs: Evaluating Safety Signals*. CIOMS: Geneva.

Corvasal (1986). Toxic-blues. *Prescrire* **6**(60): 27.

Coulter DM and Edwards IR (1990). Mianserin and agranulocytosis in New Zealand. *Lancet* **336**: 785–787.

Crane J, Flatt A, Jackson R, Ball M *et al*. (1989). Prescribed Fenoterol and death from asthma in New Zealand, 1981–83: case-control study. *Lancet* **1**(8644): 917–922.

Curel P and Stratter R (2002). ADRs and drug safety 1999–2000. In *Pharmacovigilance*, Mann R and Edwards E (eds). Wiley: 501.

D'Arcy PF and Griffin JP (1994). Thalidomide revisited. *Adverse Drug React Toxicol Rev*, **13**(2): 65–76.

Davey P and McDonald (1993). Postmarketing of quinalones 1990–1992. *Drugs* **45**(53): 46–53.

Direcks A, Figueroa S, Mintes B and Banta D (1991). DES European study: DES Action the Netherlands for the European Commission Programme 'Europe Against Cancer'. Utrecht. *DES Action the Netherlands* **13**: 25.

Dukes MNG, Aronson JK, Chalker J, Leuwer M, *et al*. (eds) (2000). Meyler's Side Effect of Drugs, 14th edn. Elsevier.

Eidson M, Philen RM, Sewell CM, Voorhers R *et al*. (1990). L-Tryptophan and eosinophilia-myalgia syndrome in New Mexico. *Lancet* **335**: 645–648.

EMEA (2001). http://www.emea.eu.int/htms/human/withdraw/withdraw.htm [10 July 2003].

FDA (1999). http://www.notice.com/recalls/fda1999.html [10 July 2003].

FDAMA (2001). Proposed list of agents not to be compounded due to withdrawal for safety/efficacy concerns. http://www.ijpc.com/chart.html.

Ferriman A (2000). UK licence for Cisapride suspended. *Br Med J* **321**: 259.

Figueras A and Laporte J-R (2002). Regulatory decisions in a globalised world. *Drug Saf* **25**(10): 689–693.

Finch RG (1993). The withdrawal of Temafloxacin. Are there implications for other quinolones? *Drug Saf* **8**(1): 9–11.

Foppiano M and Lombardo G (1997). Worldwide pharmacovigilance systems and Tolrestat withdrawal. *Lancet* **349**: 399.

Fox AW (2001). 'High-profile' product withdrawals in the United States. *Int J Pharm Med* **15**: 27–30.

Friedman MA, Woodcock J, Lumpkin MM, Shuren JE *et al*. (1999). The safety of newly approved medicines. Do recent market removals mean there is a problem? *J Am Med Assoc* **281**: 1728–1734.

Fung M, Thornton A, Mybeck K, Wu JH *et al*. (2001). Evaluation of the safety withdrawal of prescription drugs from world wide pharmaceutical markets – 1960 to 1999. *Drug Inf J* **35**: 293–317.

Gerson M (1987). La Saga française d'Halcion 0.5mg. *Prescrire* **7**(67): 319–321.

Gerson M (1992). Diflurex: un arrêt de commercialisation bien tardif. *Rev Prescrire* **12**: 26–28.

Gottlieb S (2001). US consumer groups allege misleading drug claims. *Br Med J* **323**: 415.

Graham DJ, Drinkard CR and Shatin D (2000). Study of liver enzyme monitoring in patients receiving Troglitazone. *Pharmacoepidemiol Drug Saf* **9**: S131.

Gurtner HP (1985). Aminorex and pulmonary hypertension. A review. *Cor Vasa* **27**(2–3): 160–171.

Harter JG (1988). Acute flank pain and haematuria: lessons from adverse drug reaction reporting. *J Clin Pharmacol* **28**: 560–565.

Hays DR (1993). Benedectin, a case of morning sickness. *Drug Intell Clin Pharm* **17**(11): 826–827.

Heinrich J (2001). GAO-01-286R. Drugs withdrawn from market. Letter from US General Accounting Office. *J Am Med Assoc* **282**: 1763–1765.

Herbst AL, Vilfelder H and Poskanzer DC (1971). Association of maternal stilboestrol therapy and tumour appearance in young women. *New Engl J Med* **284**: 878.

Horton R (2001). Lotronex and the FDA: a fatal erosion of integrity. *Lancet* **357**: 1544–1545.

Idänpään-Heikkilä J (1984). Experience with international post-marketing surveillance of new drugs – some recent discoveries. In *Proceedings, Drug Information Association, 20th Annual Meeting*, 17–21 June; 77–81.

Idänpään-Heikkilä J (1990). Clozapine induced blood disorders in 1975–1989 in Finland: a review of a drug from withdrawal to re-approval with restrictions. In *Idiosyncratic Adverse Drug Reactions:*

Impact on Drug Development and Clinical use After Marketing. Naranjo CA and Jones JK (eds). Excerpta Medica.

Iffy L, Zito GE, Jacobovits AA, Ganesh V *et al*. (1998). Postpartum intracranial haemorrhage in normotensive users of bromocriptine for ablactation. *Pharmacoepidemiol Drug Saf* **7**: 167–171.

Inman WHM (1977). Study of fatal bone marrow depression with special reference to phenylbutazone and oxyphenbutazone. *Br Med J* **1**: 1500–1505.

Jaeger A, Tempe JD, Rodia L, Luthium P *et al*. (1979). Acute immunoallergic haemolysis with acute renal failure induced by catechins. *Vet Hum Toxicol* **21**(suppl): 100–101.

Jain KK (2001). *Drug Induced Neurological Disorders*, 2nd edition. Hogrefe and Huber: 279–280, 435–440.

Jefferys DR, Leakey D, Lewis JA, Payne S *et al*. (1998). New active substances authorised in the United Kingdom between 1972 and 1994. *Br J Clin Pharmacol* **45**: 151–156.

Jouenne P (1987). Pharmacovigilance et information. Quelle leçon tirer d'un cas vécu par un industriel? *Troisieme Colloque INSERM/DPhM. INSERM* **157**: 421–432.

Kaufman DW, Kelly JP, Anderson T and Harmon D (1996). Aplastic anaemia among users of Felbamate. *Pharmacoepidemiol Drug Saf* **5**: S106.

Kennedy DL, Golgman SA and Lillie RB (2000). Spontaneous reporting in the United States. In *Pharmacoepidemiology*, Strom B (ed.). Wiley: 170.

La Grenade L, Nourjah P, Sherman RL, Beitz J *et al*. (2001). Estimating public health impact of adverse drug events in pharmacoepidemiology: phenyl-propanolamine and haemorrhagic stroke. *Pharmacoepidemiol Drug Saf* **10**: S119.

Lenz W (1992). Thalidomide. http://www.thalidomide.ca/history.html.

Lenz W (1962). Thalidomide and congenital abnormality. *Lancet* **1**: 45.

Lenz W and Knapp K (1962). Die Thalidomid-Embryopattie. *Dtsch Med Wochenschr* **87**: 1232.

Lewis MA, Begaud B, Bruppacher R, Kühl-Habich D *et al*. (1998). Methods in drug safety analyses: longitudinal comparative population survey on oral Naftidrofuryl. *Pharmacoepidemiol Drug Saf* **7**: S115.

Lloyd JC and Chen RT (1996). The Urabe mumps vaccines: lessons in adverse event surveillance and response. *Pharmacoepidemiol Drug Saf* **5**(suppl 1): S45.

Malone-Lee J and Wiseman P (1991). Terolidine and torsade de pointes. *Br Med J* **303**: 519.

Marcus CJ and Griffin JP (1984). New chemical entities 1972–1982: licensing and subsequent adverse reactions. A UK/USA comparison. *Pharm Int* (June): 146–149.

Martin Bouyer G (1976). Intoxication par les sels de bismuth administrés par voie orale. Enquête épidémiologique. *Thérapie* **31**: 683–702.

McBride WG (1961). Thalidomide and congenital abnormalities. *Lancet* **2**: 1358.

Mellin GW and Katzenstein M (1962). The saga of thalidomide. *New Engl J Med* **267**(23): 1184–1193.

Meyboom RHB (1998). In *Detecting Adverse Drug Reactions – Pharmacovigilance in the Netherlands*. The Netherlands Pharmacovigilance Foundation LAREB.

Moynihan R (2002). Alosetron: a case study in regulatory capture, or a victory for patients' rights? *Br Med J* **325**: 592–595.

Nightingale SL (1994). From the Food and Drug Administration. *J Am Med Assoc* **272**(13): 995.

Olsson R, Tyllström J and Zetergren L (1983). Hepatic reactions to Cyclofenil. *Gut* **24**: 260–263.

Pearce N, Crane J, Burgess C and Beasley R (1990). Case-control study of prescribed Fenoterol and death from asthma in New Zealand, 1977–81. *Lancet* **45**: 645–646.

Question 19058 (1979). Journal official des Débats de l'Assemblée Nationale, 11 October.

Rawlins MD (1997). Predicting the future from the lessons of the past. *Int J Pharm Med* **11**: 37–40.

Roblin D (1999). The clinical development of quinolone anti-bacterials. *Int J Pharm Med* **13**: 83–90.

Ross-Degnan D, Soumerai SB, Fortess EE and Gurwitz JH (1993). Examining product risk in context; market withdrawal of Zomepirac as a case study. *J Am Med Assoc* **270**(16): 1937–1942.

Schönhöfer P (1991). Germany: the Nomifensine affair. *Lancet* **338**: 1448.

Scrip 1131 (1986). Lab Janssen withdraws i.v. Domperidone in France. *Scrip* **1131**: 28.

Scrip 1300 (1988). Prenylamine withdrawn in UK. *Scrip* **1300**: 26.

Scrip 1310 (1988). Roche suspends Roaccutan in Italy. *Scrip* **1310**: 28.

Scrip 1223 (1987). Muzolimine withdrawn in Europe. *Scrip* **1223**: 22.

Scrip 2638 (2001). Thiomersal. *Scrip* **2638**: 17.

Sears MR, Taylor DR, Print CG, Lake DC *et al.* (1990). Regular inhaled beta-agonist treatment in bronchial asthma. *Lancet* **336**: 1391–1396.

Shah RR (2001a). Monitoring drug interactions. *Pharm Physician* **12**: 18–23.

Shah RR (2001b). Thalidomide, drug safety and early drug regulation in the UK. *Adverse Drug React Toxicol Res* **20**(4): 199–255.

Shah RR (2002). Withdrawal of Terolidine: a tale of two toxicities. In *Pharmacovigilance*, Mann RD and Andrews E (eds). John Wiley: 135–154.

Shedden WIH (1982). Side effects of Benoxaprofen. *Br Med J* **284**: 1630.

Spitzer WO and Buist AS (1990). Case-control study of prescribed Fenoterol and death from asthma in New Zealand, 1977–81. *Lancet* **45**: 645–648.

Spriet-Pourra C and Auriche M (1988). *Drug Withdrawal from Sale: An Analysis of the Phenomenon and its Implications.* PJB Publications.

Spriet-Pourra C and Auriche M (1994). Drug withdrawal from sale. *Scrip Report*, 2nd edn. PGB Publications Ltd.

Stonier PD (1992). Nomifensine and haemolytic anaemia. Experience of a post-marketing alert. *Pharmacoepidemiol Drug Saf* **1**: 177–185.

Stonier PD and Edwards JG (2002). Nomefensine and haemolytic anaemia. In *Pharmacovigilance*, Mann RD and Andrews E (eds). John Wiley: 155–166.

Sturkenboom MCJM, Jong-van den Berg LTW, Cornel MC, Stricker HCh *et al.* (1994). Communicating a drug alert: a study on Acitretin in the Netherlands. *Pharmacoepidemiol Drug Saf* **3**(Suppl 1, S83): Abstract 200.

Suchard J (2001). Review: wherefore withdrawal? The science behind recent drug withdrawals and warnings. *Int J Med Toxicol* **4**(2): 15.

Suissa S and Ernst P (1996). The New Zealand asthma mortality epidemic: optical illusion or scientific reason. *Pharmacoepidemiol Drug Saf* **5**: S79.

Taggart HM and Alderdice JM (1982). Fatal cholestatic jaundice in elderly patients taking Benoxaprofen. *Br Med J* **1**: 959.

Tooley PJH, Vervaet P and Wager E (1999). Cardiac arrhythmias reported during treatment with Cisapride. *Pharmacoepidemiol Drug Saf* **8**: 57–60.

Van Heijst ANP (1997). http://www.inchem.org/documents/pims/chemical/pim588.htm [10 July 2003].

Viskin S, Fish R and Roden DM (2000). Drug-induced torsades de pointes. http://www.medscape.com/HOL/articles/2000/11/hol53/pnt-hol53.html.

Weijer C (2000). The future research into Rota virus vaccine. *Br Med J* **321**(7260): 525–526.

Weissman NJ (1998). Prevalence of valvular abnormalities in patients exposed to dexfenfluramine: results of a randomised, placebo-controlled trial. *J Am Coll Cardiolo* **32**(1): 1–7.

WHO (1999) and (2001). WHO Bulletin Essential Drugs: Medical Quality and Assurance and Safety of Medicines. Pharmaceuticals: restriction of use and availability, 6th Issue, March 2001. Consolidated List of Products whose Consumption and/or sale have been Banned, Severely Restricted or Not Approved by Governments. WHO/EDH/QSM/99.2 and EDM/QSM/2001.3

WHO PN (2002). *Pharmaceuticals Newsletter* (1): 15–16.

Wild RN (1992). Micturin and torsades de pointes – experience of a post-marketing alert. *Pharmacoepidemiol Drug Saf* **1**: 147–150.

Wild RN (2002). Micturin and torsades de pointes. In *Pharmacovigilance*, John Wiley: 129–133.

Wood SM (1992). Handling of drug safety alerts in the European Community. *Pharmacoepidemiol Drug Saf* **1**: 139–142.

Yap YG and Camm J (2000). Risk of torsades de pointes with non-cardiac drugs. *Br Med J* **320**: 1158–1159.

Further reading

McEwan J (1999). Adverse reactions – a personal view of their history. *Int J Pharm Med* **13**: 269–277.
Cobert BL and Biron P (2002). *Pharmacovigilance from A to Z*. Blackwell Science.

Appendix II: Useful Web sites

M. D. B. Stephens

Link to worldwide pharmacovigilance Web sites

The Web site at www.u444.jussieu.fr/flahault/vigiweb-pop/liens_angl.htm (accessed March 2003) connects you to:

1. *Governmental sites*. Europe, Germany, England, Austria, Belgium, Denmark, Spain, Finland, France, Ireland, Italy, Netherlands, Poland, Portugal, Sweden, Scandinavia, Czech Republic, Argentina, Canada, USA, Australia, New Zealand, Japan, WHO.

2. *Non-governmental sites*. Uppsala Monitoring Centre, Union des associations et colleges de FMC des psychiatres de l'ile-de-France, Rouen teaching hospital, Hosmat – database on devices and sanitary vigilance, Syndicat National de l'Industrie Pharmaceutique (SNIP), Paris VI University, ARME-Pharmacovigilance, Institute for Safe Medication Practices (USA), Boston Collaborative Drug Surveillance Program, Neuroleptic Malignant Syndrome Information service, Malignant Hyperthermia Association of the USA, Center for Education and Research on Therapeutics (CERT), DIA (French version).

3. *Legislation*. Lègifrance – Le Droit Français, Code de la Santé Publique (CSP), Eudralex and EUR-Lex.

4. *Scientific journals*. Thérapie, La Revue Prescrire, Drugs, Drug Safety, Pharmacoepidemiology and Drug Safety, European Journal of Clinical Pharmacology, British Journal of Clinical Pharmacology, American Journal of Epidemiology, New England Journal of Medicine, Journal of Analytical Toxicology, Lancet, JAMA, Annals of Internal Medicine, BMJ, Scrip, Drug Information Journal, Reactions Weekly.

5. *Bulletins*. AFSSAPS, Bulletin Épidémilogique Hebdomédaire, Bulletin Infotox, Current Problems in Pharmacovigilance (MCA), Clinical Alerts and Advisories, National

Stephens' Detection of New Adverse Drug Reactions Fifth Edition edited by John Talbot and Patrick Waller
© 2004 John Wiley & Sons, Ltd   ISBN: 0 470 84552 X

Library of Medicine, Santé Canada, Australian Adverse Drug Reactions Bulletin, Adverse Reaction Reporting and IMMP/Medsafe (New Zealand), Irish Medicines Board Drug Safety Newsletter, European Teratology Society Newsletter.

6. *Databases*. ASITEST (Toxicological Documentation Centre of Fernand–Widal Hospital, PNEUMOTOX on line, Banque de données Automatisée sur les Médicaments (BIAM), Thériaque, Santé Canada, Medline/National Library of Medicine, Drugcheck database, Anti-epileptic Drug Pregnancy Registry, Medical Sciences Bulletin, Platelets on the Internet, Morbidity and Mortality Weekly Report/CDC, International Agency for Research on Cancer, Toxnet (Toxicology Data Network), DART/ETIC terato-toxicolgy database, PharmWeb World Drug Alert, Martindale's Guide, Merck manual, Vidal Dictionary, Clinical Pharmacology 2000, MedDRA, Dictionaries on line, Pharmacovigilance Dictionary, ICD 9, General Practice Research Database (GPRD), Drug Safety Research Unit (DSRU), MEMO, PMSI (Programme de Médicalisation des Systémes d'information).

7. *Publishers*. National Library of Medicine, ADIS International, Elsevier, Wiley Interscience.

8. *Teratology*. Antiepileptic drug pregnancy registry. Prescribing medicines in pregnancy (AUST), Center for the Evaluation of Risks to Human Reproduction (CERHR), EUROCAT, DART/ETIC, European Teratolgy Society, Teratology Society, Teratology.

9. *Epidemiology*. Epi info, Biostatistical Department of McGill University Canada, Centre International de Recherche sur le Cancer, Centre Espagnol de Recherché Pharmacoepidemiologique (Spain), International Epidemiological Association, International Society of Pharmacoepidemiology.

10. *Toxicology*. Numerous.

11. *Engines*. Moteur de recherche du CHU de Rouen, Cliniweb, Medmatrix, Yahoo santé, Medweb (University of Emory).

Other important sites

American Academy of Pharmaceutical Physicians: www.aapp.org
Association of British Pharmaceutical Industry (ABPI): http://www.abpi.org.uk
Association of Clinical Biochemists: http://www.acb.org.uk, includes items of general medical interest and an assay finder to help researchers find methods or labs to measure a wide variety of hormones, metals, enzymes and drugs in body fluids (Pallen, 1997).
BioMedNet: http://www.BioMedNet.com, the World Wide Web club for the biological & medical community (free membership).
British National Formulary: http://www.bnf.org
Centre for Medicines Research: http://www.cmr.org/
Clinical Pharmacology Drug: http://www.gsm.com
Cochrane Collaboration: www.cochrane.de
Drug Information Association (DIA) home page: http://www.diahome.org

Drug Intelligence: www.drugintel.com

Drug Safety auditing, resourcing, expertise, information and news: http://www.vigilex.com

Drug Safety Interest site, including E2B and MedDRA: http://www.ottosen.com

Drug Safety. This site is for those working in pharmacovigilance and is excellent. Run by Iain Cockburn: www.drugsafety.com

Electronic Medicines Compendium: http://www.medicines.org.uk

Faculty of Pharmaceutical Medicine: http://www.fpm.org.uk

Free Medical Journals: www.freemedicaljournals.com over 1010 journals available.

Health Action International: www.haiweb.org

Health information on the Internet. New bimonthly newsletter from the Wellcome Trust and the RSM: http://www.wellcome.ac.uk/healthinfo

Human Genome Project concerning Pharmacogenomics: www.ornl.gov/hgmis/medicine/pharma.html

ICD–10: http://www.cihi.ca. Canadian Institute for Health Information.

ICH documents from: http://www.ifpma.org/ich1.html

Institute for Safe Medication Practices: www.ismp.org. Not basically for adverse drug reactions

International Federation of Pharmaceutical Manufacturers Associations: www.ifpma.org

International Society of Pharmacovigilance: www.pharmacoepi.de/esoporg.htm

InterPharma: http://www.interpharma.co.uk (this is a vast site with links to other databases for pharmaceutical support sites)

Medical Lobby for Appropriate Marketing (MALAM). This organization is now known as Healthy Skepticism: www.healthyskepticism.org

Medical Research Council: http://www.nimr.mrc.ac.uk/MRC

Medscape: http://www.medscape.com Monograph Service

Multilingual glossary of medical terms: http://allserv.rug.ac.be/~rvdstich/eugloss/welcome.html

National Registry of drug-induced ocular side effects: www.eyedrugregistry.com

Organisation of Teratology Information Services (OTIS): http://www.otispregnancy.org

Organised Medical Networked Information: http://www.omni.ac.uk

Pharmacogenetics. Pharmacogenetic Research Network: www.nigms.nih.gov/pharmacogenetics/;

Pharmacogenetics Journal: www.jpharmacogenetics.com

Pneumotox on line: www.pneumotox.com (excellent)

Public Citizen: www.citizen.org/hrg/

Registry for torsades de pointes and QT prolongation: www.qtdrugs.org or www.torsades.org

Royal Pharmaceutical Society of Great Britain: www.rpsgb.org.uk

Scrip: http://www.pjbpubs.co.uk

Social Audit: www.socialaudit.org.uk

Special Interest Group on Adverse Reactions (SIGAR): www.aiopi.org.uk

Reference

Pallen M (1997). Information in practice. *Br Med J* **310**: 954.

Further reading

Cobert BL and Silvey J (1998). The Internet, adverse events and safety. *Int J Pharm Med* **12**: 83–86.
Cobert BL and Biron P (2002). *Pharmacovigilance from A to Z*. Blackwell Science.

Bibliography

M. D. B. Stephens

The books mentioned are post 1990; for earlier publications see the 4th edition. Owing to the small numbers of specialist books printed, this type of book is rapidly sold out and so may no longer be readily available. Out of print (OOP) may not mean this is not still available. Try – http://www.amazon.com

Basic sciences

Pharmacology: Drug Actions and Reactions, 6th edition, Levine RR and Walsh CT. Parthenon Publishers, Carnforth, UK. 600 pp, US$51.45, £32, 2000.
Drug Safety: from Molecule to Man, Park K. Churchill Livingstone, 288 pp, £29.95, October 2003.
Immunotoxicology and Immunopharmacology, 2nd edition, Dean J, Luster M, Munson A and Kimber I. Taylor and Francis, 784 pp, £50, 1994.
Drug Safety Evaluation, Gad SC. Wiley Interscience, 1024 pp, $160, £107, 2002. Mostly pre-clinical.
Safely Pharmacology in Pharmacological Development and Approach, Gad SC. CRC Press, £139.95 August 2003.
Basic Pharmacology: understanding drug antics and reactions. Mermanday MA and Rathinaueln A CRR Press, 350 pp, £44.99, August 2003.

Clinical trials

Randomised Controlled Clinical Trials, 2nd edition, Bulpitt CJ. $314.50 Kluwer Academic Publishers 1996.
Clinical Trials, Duley L and Farrell B (eds). BMJ Books, paperback, 2000.
Methodological Issues Fundamental to Clinical Trials, Clophas TJ. Kluwer Academic Publications, paperback, 1999.
New Drug Approval Process, 3rd edition, Guarino R. Marcel Dekker, 2002.
Early Phase Drug Evaluation in Man, O'Grady J and Linet OI (eds). CRC Press, 748 pp, £115, $159.95, 1990.
Guide to Clinical Trials, Spilker B, Raven Press, New York, 1991. On CD ROM, Lippincott-Raven, 1996.
Presentation of Clinical Data, Spilker B and Schoenfelder J. Raven Press, 576pp, $110, 1990.
Principles of Clinical Research, Di Giovanna I and Hayes G (eds). Institute of Clinical Research, Wrightson Biomedical, Petersfield, 558 pp, 2001.

Stephens' Detection of New Adverse Drug Reactions Fifth Edition edited by John Talbot and Patrick Waller
© 2004 John Wiley & Sons, Ltd   ISBN: 0 470 84552 X

Clinical Research Manual (plus supplements), Luscombe D and Stonier PD (eds). sales@euromed.uk. com, 700 + pages, £220, €350, US$360, 2002.

Data Monitoring Committees in Clinical Trials, Ellenberg SS, Fleming TR & DeMets DL. John Wiley, Chichester, 208 pp, £50, 2002.

The Quality of Life, Fallowfield L. Souvenir Press, London, 1991.

Compendium of Quality of Life Instruments. Salek S, John Wiley 1626 pp. $1410, 1999.

Quality of Life: Assessment, Analysis and interpretation. Fayers PM and Machin D, John Wiley, $125. 2001.

Quality of Life Assessments in Clinical Trials, Spilker B (ed.). Raven Press, 470pp, $168.10 1990.

Quality of Life and Pharmacoeconomics in Clinical Trials, Spilker B (ed.). Lippincott–Raven Publishers, 1259 pp, £114.50, 1995.

Measuring Health: A Guide to Rating Scales and Questionnaires, 2nd edition, McDowell I and Newell C (eds). Oxford University Press, 1996.

Drug Safety Assessment in Clinical Trials, Statistics, textbooks and monographs, Volume 138, Gilbert GS (ed.). Marcel Dekker, 456 pp, £108.00, $195.00, 1993.

Clinical Measurement in Drug Evaluation, Nimmo WS and Tucker GT (eds). John Wiley, 344 pp, £130, €214, $129.95, 1996.

A Dictionary of Pharmacology and Clinical Drug Evaluation, Laurence DR and Carpenter JR (eds). UCL Press Ltd, London, 200 pp, $36.95, 1994.

A Guide To Clinical Drug Research, 2nd edition, Cohen A and Posner J (eds). Kluwer Academic Publishers, 2000.

Biostatistics in Clinical Trials, Redmond CK and Colton T (eds). John Wiley, 550 pp, £150, 2001.

Adverse Event Monitoring and its Implementation in Clinical Trials, M-A Wallander. Uppsala University. Almqvist and Wiksell International Stockholm, the author's doctoral dissertation, 147 pp, 1991.

The Science of the Placebo, Guess HA, Kleinman A, Kusek JW & Engel LW (eds). BMJ Books, 332 pp, £15.95, 2002.

Drug-induced diseases

Anaesthetics

Safety of Anaesthetic Drugs, Maguib M. Adis International, 104 pp, $39.95, £24.75, 1998.

Allergic Reactions to Anaesthetics, Monographs in Allergy, Vol. 30, Assem E-SK (ed.). Karger, £128.30, US$256.50, 1992.

Suspected Anaphylactic Reactions During Anaesthesia, 3rd edition. Association of Anaesthetists and British Society of Allergy and Clinical Immunology. Free from the Association of Anaesthetists, 2003.

Anti-inflammatory drugs

Adverse Reactions of Non-steroidal Anti-inflammatory Drugs (NSAIDS), Kurowski M, Springer Verlag. $25, 1992.

Side Effects of Anti-inflammatory Drugs, Rainsford KD (ed.). Kluwer Academic, £181.95, $337, 384 pp, 1992.

Dermatology

A Guide to Drug Eruptions The European File of Side-effects in Dermatology, 6th edition, Bruinsma W. Free University of Amsterdam, PO Box 21, 1474 HJ, Oosthuizen; 1996. Brief but invaluable.

Contains lists of drugs causing each type of skin reaction. Useful general text: annual supplements between frequent editions.

Side Effects in Dermatology, 7th edition, Bruinsma W (ed.). Intermed Medical Publishers, 132 pp, €55, £33, 2000.

Cutaneous Drug Reactions: An Integral Synopsis of Today's Systemic Drugs, 2nd edition, Zurcher K and Krebs A (eds). S Karger, Basel, 570 pp, US$431.50, €131.40, £225.50, 1992.

Physician's Guide to Drug Eruptions, Litt JZ. Parthenon, £54.99, 1997.

Drug Eruption Reference Manual 2002, 8th edition, Litt JZ. Parthenon Publishing, 444 pp, £120, US$149.95, also DERM-On-Disk. Cleveland, Ohio, Wal-Zac Enterprises and on a database, 2003.

Adverse Drug Reactions and the Skin, Breathnack SM and Hintner H. Blackwell Scientific Publications, 408 pp, OOP. $42.35, 1992.

Pocketbook of Drug Eruptions and Interactions, Litt JZ (ed.). Parthenon, 544pp, £21.99, 2000.

Unwanted Effects of Cosmetics and Drugs Used in Dermatology, 3rd edition, de Groot AC, Nater JP and Wayland JW. Elsevier, 750 pp, £161.70, US$315, 1993.

Adverse Cutaneous Reactions to Medications: A Physician's Guide, Sanford M, Goldstein MD and Bruce U. Lippincott Williams and Wilkins, 160 pp, £9, US$5.50, 1996. Out of stock (OOS).

Skin Reactions to Drugs (CRC series in dermatology), Kauppinen K, Mailbach HI and Hannuksela M. CRC Press, 192 pp, US$169.95, 1998.

Excipients

Formulation Factors in Adverse Reactions, Rowe RC, Sheskey P, Weller PJ, Florence AT and Salole EG (eds). John Wright, OOP. 124 pp, 1990.

Handbook of Pharmaceutical Excipients, 4th edition, Rowe RC, Sheskey PJ and Weller PJ (eds). Published by the American Pharmaceutical Association and The Pharmaceutical Society of Great Britain, 800 pp, £195 in UK, £200 in rest of world, US$299.95, also CD-ROM UK £229.13, US$299.95, March, 2003.

Excipient Toxicity and Safety, Weiner ML and Kotkoski A (eds). Marcel Dekker, 376 pp, £103.53, US$165, 1999.

Handbook of Pharmaceutical Additives, 2nd edition, Ash M and Ash I. Synapse Information Resources Inc., 1062 pp, £316, 2002.

CRC Handbook of Food, Drug and Cosmetic Excipients, Smolinske SC. CRC Press, Boca Raton, FL, $279.95 1992. Discusses use and toxicity of 77 'inert' ingredients of drugs and cosmetics.

Hepatotoxicity

Toxicology of the Liver, 2nd edition, Platt GL and Hewitt WR. Taylor and Francis, 431 pp, £95, 1998.

Hepatotoxicity. The Effect of Drugs and Other Chemicals on the Liver, 2nd edition, Zimmerman HJ. Lippincott Williams and Wilkins, 800 pp, US$169, £122, 2000.

Drug-induced Disorders, Dukes MN (series ed.) Vol. 5, *Drug-induced Hepatic Injury*, 2nd edition, Stricker BHCh. Elsevier Science, 562 pp, £122.35 $238.00, 1992.

Drug-induced Hepatotoxicity, vol. 121, Cameron R, Feuer G and de la Iglesia F. Springer Verlag, 681 pp, DM530, £247.50, FF1997, $398.00 Lit585 389, 1996.

Drug Induced Liver Disease, Farrell GC and Maddrey WC. Churchill Livingstone, New York, 1994 OOP.

Drug-induced Liver Disease, Kaplowitz N and Deleve LD. Marcel Dekker, New York, 2003, 773 pp, $195.00, ISBN 0-8247-0811-3.

Neurology

Neurotoxic Side-effects of Prescription Drugs, Brust CM (ed.). Butterworth-Heinemann, 435 pp, £40.99, US$49.99, 1996.

Drug-induced Neurological Disorders, Jain KK, 2nd edition. Hografe and Huber Publishers, 474 pp, £55.93, 2001.

Guide to the Extrapyramidal Side Effects of Antipsychotic Drugs, Owens DG. Cambridge University Press, 362 pp, US$49.95, £30.95, 1999.

Iatrogenic Neurology, Biller J. Butterworth Heinemann, 530 pp, US$115, 1998.

Neuroleptic Induced Movement Disorders. A Comprehensive Survey, Yassa R. Cambridge University Press, 512 pp, US$120, 1997.

Neuroleptic Malignant Syndrome and related conditions. Stephen C and Mann N, Psychiatric Publications Inc. 256 pp, £18.75, 2003.

Psychiatry

Drug-induced Dysfunction in Psychiatry, Matcheti S, Keshavan NA and Kennedy JS. Taylor and Francis, £70, US$110, 1992.

Antipsychotic Drugs and their Side-effects, Barnes T. Academic Press, 287 pp, £74.95 $112.95, 1994.

Practical Management of the Side-Effects of Psychotropic Drugs, Balon R. Marcel Dekker, 304 pp, £91.49, 1998.

Adverse Effects of Psychotropic Drugs, Kane JM, Liebermann JA and Jeffery A. Guilford Press, 511 pp, US$69.95, 1999.

Psychiatric Side Effects of Prescription and Over-the-counter Medications. Recognition and Management, Stoudemire A and Brown TM. American Psychiatric Press Inc., 417 pp, £63.50, 1998.

Vaccines

Adverse Effects of Pertussis and Rubella Vaccines, Howson CP, Howe CJ and Fineberg HV (eds). National Academy Press, 382 pp £32.95 $44.95, 1991.

Adverse events associated with childhood vaccines. Evidence bearing on causality, Stratton RK, Howe CJ and Johnston RB (eds). Division of Health Promotion and Disease Prevention, Institute of Medicine, National Academy of Sciences, 2101 Constitution Ave., N.W. Washington, DC 20418; $89.25, 1994.

Other

Drug-induced Ocular Side-effects, 5th edition. Fraunfelder FT and Fraunfelder FW (eds). Butterworth-Heinemann, Boston, 848 pp with CD-ROM, US$70.95, 2001.

Ocular Adverse Reactions to Drugs Booklet, Lawrenson J and Thompson D. Butterworth-Heinemann, US$159, 2001.

Drug-induced Immune Diseases, Descotes J, (ed.). Elsevier, £96.36, 232 pp, 1990. OOP limited.

Drug-induced Nutrient Depletion Handbook, 2001-2002, 2nd edition, Pelton P, LaValle JB, Hawkins E and Komisky DL, Lexi-Comp. Inc., £22, 485 pp, 2001.

Adverse Drug Reactions in Dentistry, 2nd edition, Seymour R, Meecham J and Walton J. Oxford University Press, £69.50, 1996.

Drug–induced Rheumatic Disease, Kahn MF. Baillere Tindall, 256 pp, £30, 1991. OOP.

Danna Da Farmaci All'Apparato Digerente, Brago PC and Guslandi M. (eds). Springer Verlag, US$66.00, 1995.

Drug Induced Injury to the Digestive System, Guslandi M and Braga PC (eds). Springer-Verlag, £71, US$140, 1993.

Adverse Effects of Herbal Drugs, Vol. 3, De Smet P, Keller K, Hansel R, and Chandler RF (eds). Springer-Verlag, Heidelberg, 340 pp, US$80, £46, DM98, FF370, Lit108 240, 1996.

Drug-induced Infertility and Sexual Dysfunction, Foreman RG, Gilmour-White SK and Foreman NH. Cambridge University Press, New York, 155 pp, $55 1996.

Extragenital Effects of Oral Contraceptives, Elstein M. CRC Press LLC, 68 pp, US$44.95, 1995.

Drugs That Affect Sexual Function, Crenshaw TL and Goldberg JP. W.W. Norton & Co., Inc., US$75.00, 1996.

Drug-induced Long CT Interval. Futura Publications, £19.50, 2002.

Drug-induced Movement Disorder, Sethi KD, Marcel Dekker, £172, October 2002.

Clinical Nephrotoxins: Renal Injury from Drugs and Chemicals, De Broe ME, Porter GA, Bennett WM and Verpooten GA. Kluwer Academic, Boston, 730 pp. $375, £160, 2003.

Norantis Foundation Symposium: anaphylaxis. John Wiley & Sons, 300 pp. £75, November 2003.

General

Textbook of Adverse Drug Reactions, 5th edition, Davies DM, Ferner RE and de Glanville H. Chapman and Hall, US$225, £195, 1998.

Adverse Drug Reactions, Lee A (ed.). Pharmaceutical Press, 312 pp, £24.95, Overseas £27.95, US$39.95, 2001.

Adverse Drug Reactions, Kelly J. Whurr Publishers. 224 pp, £22.50, 2000.

Opinion and Evidence, Drug Safety, Edwards IR (ed.). Adis International, £31.35, 2000.

Guide Pratique de Pharmacovigilance, Bénichou C (ed.). Editions Pradel, 206 pp, 1992.

Adverse Drug Reactions, A Practical Guide to Diagnosis and Management, Bénichou C (ed.). John Wiley, 302 pp, US$49.95, £82.50, 1996. Improved and extended English version of the above French title.

Imaging Drug Reactions and Toxic Hazards, 3rd edition, Ansell G (ed.). Chapman and Hall, £24.50, hardback £90, 1997.

Life-threatening Allergic Reactions, Williams D, Williams A and Croker L, (eds). Piatkus Books, 111 pp, £6.30, 1997.

The Drug Etiology of Agranulocytosis and Aplastic Anaemia, Kaufman DW, Kelly JP, Levy M and Shapiro S. Oxford University Press Inc. USA, 432 pp, US$93.5, £105, 1991.

Drug Toxicokinetics, De La Inglesia F and Welling PG. Marcel Dekker, US$199.00, 1993.

Reduction of Anticancer Drug Toxicity: Pharmacologic, Biologic, Immunologic and Gene Therapeutic Approaches, Eisenbrand G, Hellmann K and Zeller WJ. Karger, US$174.00, 1995.

Drug interactions

A Manual of Adverse Drug Interactions, 5th edition, Griffin JP and D'Arcy PF (eds). Elsevier, 664 pp, €150.66, US$190.8, £122, 1997.

Mechanisms of Drug Interactions, vol. 122, D'Arcy PF, McElnay JC and Welling PG (eds), Springer-Verlag, Berlin, 400 pp, £193.00, DM446, FF1680, Lit492 600, 1996.

Drug Interactions, 6th edition, Stockley I. The Pharmaceutical Press, 960 pp, This edition is hardbacked. £95.00, US$135.00, CD £160 + VAT, US$230.00, 2002.

Physician's Drug Reference. Drug Interactions. Medical Economic Data, £128.37, 1999.

2001 Physician's Drug Reference Companion Guide: Drug interaction Guide. Menta M. Medical Economic Co. 2000 pp, £47.50, 2001.

Drug Interactions and Updates Quarterly, Hansten PD and Horn JR (eds). Published by Applied Therapeutics Inc., US$856, 4 issues.

Drug Interaction Alerts, Quinn DI and Day RO. Adis International, £9.40, US$14.95, 1998.

Manual of Drug Interactions for Anaesthesiology, 2nd edition, Mueller RA and Lundberg DBA, Churchill Livingstone, £30, 1996.

Baillere's Clinical Anaesthesiology: Drug Interactions, Bovill JG (ed.). Baillere Tindall, 200 pp, £30, 1998.

Drug Interaction Facts, 10th edition, Tatro DS (ed.) Lippincott Williams and Wilkins, 979 pp, US$79.95, 2002.

Diet and Drug Interactions, Roe DA (ed.). Chapman and Hall, 350 pp, £39.95, 1995.

Food and Drug Interactions, Holt GA. Precept Press, 414 pp, £174.99, 1998.

Drug Interactions Nutrient Depletion Handbook, 2nd edition, Pelton R. Lexi-Comp Inc., 485 pp, £22, 2001.

Drug Interactions in Psychiatry, 2nd edition, Ciraulo DA, Shader RI, Greenblatt DJ and Creelman WL, Lippincott Williams and Wilkins, 430 pp, US$45, £35, 1995.

Summary of Drug Interactions with Oral Contraceptives, Geurts TBP, Goorissen EM and Sitsen JM (eds). Parthenon Press, 130 pp. $54.95 £32.99, 1993.

Handbook of Drug Interactions, Karallieder L and Henry JA. Arnold, 900 pp, US$75, £55, 1998.

Metabolic Drug Interactions, Levy RA, Thummel KE, Trager WF, Hansten PD and Eichelbaum M. Lippincott Williams and Wilkins, 816 pp, US$179, £124, 2000.

Drug Interactions in Infectious Diseases, Piscilli SC and Rudvold KA. Blackwell Science, 372 pp, £80, 2000.

Pocket Guide to Evaluation of Drug Interactions, Zucchero FJ. American Pharmaceutical Association, 1600 pp, £30.50, 2001.

Managing Clinically Important Drug Interactions, Hansten PD and Horn JR. Facts and Comparisons, 647 pp, £63.64, US$79.95, 2002.

NDH Pocket Guide to Drug Interactions, Springhouse. Lippincott Williams and Wilkins, 362 pp, £12.17, 2002.

Medical Pocket Reference: Drug-Herb Interactions, Kelly WJ. Lippincott Williams and Wilkins, 220 pp, £7.50, $9.95 2002.

Clinicians' Manual of Drug-Interactions in Gastroenterology, Maton PN and Burton ME. Life Science Communications, £7.25, 1996.

Interactions Between Chinese Herbal Drugs, Medicinal Products and Orthodox Drugs, Chan K and Cheung L. Taylor and Francis, £44, 2000.

Drug–Drug Interactions, Rodrigues DA. Marcel Dekker, 672 pp, £137.72, 2001.

Advances in Pharmacology: Drug–Drug Interactions. Li AP (ed.). Academic Press, 275 pp, £94.95, 1997.

Mosby's Handbook of Drug–Herb and Drug Interactions. Supplement, Bratman S (ed.). Mosby, 208 pp, £22.95, 2002.

A Comprehensive Guide to Drug–Herb–Nutrients Interactions, Stargrove M. Churchill Livingstone, 650 pp, £60, 2003.

The A–Z Guide to Drug–Herb–Vitamin Interactions, Schuyl W, Lininger JR and Gaby AR. Prima, £12.35, 436 pp, 1999.

The Top 100 Drug Interactions Year 2002, Hansten PD and Horn JR. American College of Clinical Pharmacists (ACCP), 171 pp, US$14.95, 2002. This contains 2300 interactions, not just 100.

Anticancer Drugs: Reactive Metabolism and Drug Interactions, Powis G, Pergamon Press, £134.48, 1994. Out of print.

Medical Letter Handbook of Adverse Interactions, Martin A, Rigack MD and Hillman CDH. Medical Letter Inc., 404 pp, US$23, 1998.

Ethics and law

Pharmaceutical Ethics, Salek S and Edgar A. John Wiley, 210 pp £45, €74.30 $90, 2002.

Ethical Issues in Drug Research, Through a glass darkly Parnham MJ. IOS Press, 165 pp, £48 $70, 1996.

Good Clinical Practice and Ethics in European. Drug Research, Bennett P, Bath University, £30 $49.95, 1994.

Pharmacy Law and Ethics, 7th edition, Appelbe GE and Wingfield J, Pharmaceutical Press, 577 pp. £26.95, Overseas £29.95, $49.95 1997, paperback.

Ethical Issues in Drug Testing, Approval and Pricing: The clot dissolving drugs. Brody BA. Oxford University Press, £18.85, 1995.

Responsibility for Drug-induced Injury. A Reference Book for Lawyers, the Health Profession and Manufacturers, 2nd edition, Dukes G, Mildred M and Swartz B, 537 pp, IOS Press, £79, $125 1998.

Medicines, Medical Devices and the Law, O'Grady J, Dodds-Smith I, Walsh N and Spencer M (eds). Greenwich Medical Media, 390 pp, £55, US$125, 1999.

Causation and Risk in the Law of Tort: Scientific Evidence and Medicinal Product Liability, Goldberg R. Hart Publishing, Oxford and Portland, OR, 260 pp, US$88.50, 1999.

A Decent Proposal – Ethical Review of Clinical Research, Evans D and Evans M, John Wiley, 230 pp, US$35.00, 1994. Out of print.

Learning from Experience: Privacy and the Secondary Use of Data in Health Research, Dr W Lowrence, Nuffield Trust (www.nuffieldtrust.org.uk), £10.

Pharmaceutical Medicine, Biotechnology and European Law, Goldberg R and Lonba J (eds). Cambridge University Press, 247 pp, £45, 2000.

Law and Ethics of Medical Research. International Bioethics and human rights. Plomer A Cavendish Publishing. 240 pp, £40, 2004.

Laboratory data

Clinical Diagnosis, Management by Laboratory Methods, 19th edition, Henry JB (ed.). W.B. Saunders, Philadelphia, £28.95, 1997.

Effects of Drugs on Clinical Laboratory Tests, 5th edition, Young DS. AACC Press, 994 pp, £76, 2000.

Drug Effects in Clinical Chemistry, 6th edition, Tryding N, Hansen P, Tufvesson C and Sonntag O. Apoteksbolaget, Stockholm, US$50, 1992.

Pharmaceutical medicine

Principles and Practice of Pharmaceutical Medicine, Fletcher A, Edwards L, Fox AW and Stonier P, John Wiley, 568 pp, £95.00, £159 $170 2002.

Fraud and Misconduct in Medical Research, 3rd edition, Lock S, Wells F and Farthing M (eds). BMJ Books, £40, US$65, 2001.

Pharmaceutical Medicine Dictionary, Alghabban A. Churchill Livingstone, 400 pp, £34.95, 2001.

The Textbook of Pharmaceutical Medicine, 4th edition, Griffin JP and O'Grady J (eds). BMJ Publishing, 896 pp, £95, 2002.

Dictionary of Pharmaceutical Medicine, Nahler G and Hitzenberger G (eds). 177 pp, Springer Verlag, DM39, £17, FF147, Lit43 070, 1994.

Pharmaceutical Medicine, Biotechnology and European Law, Golding R and Lonbay J (eds). Cambridge University Press, 247 pp. £45, $75, 2001.

Pharmaceutical Medicine and the Law, Goldberg A and Dodds-Smith I (eds). Royal College of Physicians, UK, £10, 1991. Out of print.

Communication in Pharmaceutical Medicine. A Challenge for 1992. Ferran JR, Lahuerta Dal Rè J and Lardinois R (eds). Prous Scientific Publ. Publication of the papers presented at the 7th International Conference on Pharmaceutical Medicine, 1991.

Informing Patients: An Assessment of the Quality of Patient Information Materials. Coulter A, Entwistle V and Gilbert D. King's Fund, 1999.

Pharmacoepidemiology

Pharmacoepidemiology, 3rd edition, Strom BL (ed.). John Wiley, 898 pp, US$135.00, £120.00, 2000.

Pharmacoepidemiology: An Introduction, 3rd edition, Hartzema AG, Porta MS and Tilson HH (eds). Harvey Whitney Books, PO Box 42696, Cincinnati, OH 45242, USA; $85 1998.

Clinical Epidemiology. A Basic Science for Clinical Medicine, 2nd edition, Sackett DL, Haynes RB, Guyatt GH and Tugwell P (eds). Lippincott Williams & Wilkins, 442 pp. £30, $39.95 1991.

Drug Epidemiology and Post-marketing Surveillance, Strom BL and Velo G (eds). NATO ASI Series, Series A: Life Sciences Vol. 224, Plenum Press Ltd, 170 pp, $156 £80.25, 1992. This is the proceedings of a NATO Advanced Study Institute meeting held in Sicily between 27 September and 8 October $156 1990.

Farmacoepidemiología, Carvajal A. Secreteiade de Pullicaciones, University of Valladolid, 162 pp, 1993 (in Spanish). Details available from: Centro Regional de Farmacovigilancia de Castilla y León, Avenida Ramón y Cajal, 7, 47005 Valladolid, Spain.

Dictionary of Pharmacoepidemiology, Bégaud B. ARME, John Wiley, 184 pp, £45.00, 2000.

The use of a Bayesian Confidence Propagation Neutral Network in Pharmacovigilance. Bate A PhD Thesis Umeå. Unimsilet. Sweden, 2003.

Pharmacovigilance

Pharmacovigilance, Mann R and Andrews E. John Wiley, 582 pp, £150, US$250, €259, 2002.

Second European Pharmacovigilance Symposium, Paris, Abstracts. Editions du Vidal, 109 pp, 1992. In French or English.

Pharmacovigilance from A to Z, Cobert B and Biron P. Blackwell Science, 256 pp, £37.5, US$54.95, 2001.

La pharmacovigilance de A au Z, Biron P and Cobert BL. Blackwell Science, 315 pp, 1999.

Pharmacovigilance in Focus – the Theory and Practice of Pharmacovigilance, Meyboom R and Stather R (eds). Uppsala Monitoring Centre and Adis International, 450 pp.

Pharmacovigilance: Effective Safety Surveillance Strategies. Scrip report, BS1156E, £995, US$1995, ¥239 000, 2002.

Dictionary of Pharmacovigilance. Alghaban A. Pharmaceutical Press, 320 pp, £39.95, US$59.95, 2003.

Clin-Alert 2001, A Quick Reference to Adverse Clinical Events, Generali J. Technomic, 270 pp, US$49.95, 2001.

Risk Factors for Adverse Drug Reactions – Epidemiological Approach, Weber E. Birkhauser Verlag AG, 156 pp, £22.00, 1990.

European Medicines Research: Perspective in Pharmacotoxicology and Pharmacovigilance. Biomedical and Health Research, volume 7, Fracchia GN. IOS Press, 1997.

The Importance of Pharmacovigilance. World Health Organization, 48 pp, 2002.

Databases for Pharmacovigilance. What Can We Do? Walker SR (ed.). Medical Benefit Risk Foundation, Copies Centre for Medicines Research, Woodmanstone Road, Carshalton, Surrey, SM5 4DS; 1996.

La Pharmacovigilance. Agence de Médicament, SNIP, Association Française des Centres Régionaux de Pharmacovigilance, Ateliers Nationaux de Pharmacovigilance at Deauville, May 1997, John Libby, Paris, 80 pp, €16.77, FF124.96, 1998.

The Importence of Pharmacovigilance, 48 pp. Uppsala Monitoring Centre, Stone Target 3, S-753 20 Uppsala, Sweden.

Risk–benefit

Risk-Benefit Analysis, 2nd edition, Wilson R and Crouch EAC. Harvard University Press, 384 pp, US$25, £16.50, €28.80, 2001.

Drug Benefits and Risks. International Textbook of Clinical Pharmacology, Boxtel CV, Santoso B and Edwards IR (eds). John Wiley, 792 pp, £95.00, $180 2002.

The Benefit/Risk Ratio: A Handbook for the Rational Use of Potentially Hazardous Drugs, Korting HC and Schafer-Korting M, CRC Press, 400 pp, US$149, £105, 1998.

Benefit–Risk Balance for Marketed Drugs, Dumoulin, Kaddis M and Velasquey, *et al*. World Health Organization, £9.50, 1998.

Teratogenesis, pregnancy and lactation

Drugs and Pregnancy, Larry C and Gilstrap LC (eds) 2nd edition. Chapman and Hall, 523 pp. £69.00, $98.50 1992.

Drugs and Human Lactation, 2nd edition, Bennett PN and the WHO working group. Elsevier, 722 pp, €235.97, US$299, 1996.

Teratogenic Effects of Drugs: A Resource for Clinicians (Teris), 2nd edition, Friedman J and Polifka J (eds). John Hopkins University Press, 736 pp, £103.50, US$150, 2000.

Chemically Induced Birth Defects, 3rd edition, Schardein JL. Marcel Dekker, 1109 pp US$195, 2000.

Congenital Malformations Worldwide. A report from the International Clearing House for Birth Defects Monitoring System, Peters PWJ. Elsevier, 230 pp, £75.50, 1991. Out of pint

Drug Safety in Pregnancy, Folb PI and Dukes MNG (eds). Elsevier, 542 pp, US$50.60, 1990. Out of print.

Drugs in Pregnancy and Lactation: A Reference Guide to Fetal and Neonatal Use of Drugs in Pregnancy and Lactation, 6th edition, Briggs GG, Freeman RK and Yaffe SJ. Lippincott Williams and Wilkins, Baltimore/London, 1595 pp, US$110, 2001, also on CD.

Drugs During Pregnancy and Lactation, Schaefer C (ed.). Elsevier Health Science, 380 pp, US$159, €134, 2002.

Maternal-Fetal Toxicology. A Clinician's Guide, 3rd edition, Koren G (ed.). Marcel Dekker, 848 pp, US$195.00, 2001.

The Effects of Drugs on the Fetus and Nursing Infant, A handbook for health care professionals Friedman JM and Polifka JE. John Hopkins University Press, 672 pp, £34, $65.95 1996.

The Effects of Neurologic and Psychiatric Drugs on the Fetus and Nursing Infant, Friedman JM and Polifka JE (eds). John Hopkins University Press, £34, $65.95 1998.

REPRORISK, includes TERIS teratogen information system, Shepard's catalog of teratogenic agents, REPROPTEXT reproductive hazard reference and REPROTOX, which includes over 3000 chemicals, OTC, prescription, recreational and nutritional agents (www.microdex.com/products).

Medications and Mothers' Milk, a manual of lactational Pharmacology, Hale TW. Pharmasoft, 792 pp, $24.95, 2002.

Drug Toxicity in embryonic development. Akhurst RJ, Daston GP, Kavlock RJ. Springer Verlag, Two volumes, $275 plus $398, 1997.

Others

Improving Drug Safety – A Joint Responsibility, Dinkel R, Horisberger B, Tolo KW, Davis K and van Eimeren W (eds). Springer Verlag. US$79.95, OOS, 1991. A publication of a RAD-AR meeting in Wolfsberg in 1990. Out of stock.

Side Effects of Drugs Essays, Dukes MNG (ed.). Elsevier, 230 pp, £63.10, 1990. These are 14 essays, each taken from a *Side-effects of Drugs Annual*. Out of print.

Post-marketing Drug Safety Management: A Pharmaceutical Industry Perspective, Amery WK. IOS Press (Van Diemenstraat 94, 1013 CN Amsterdam, Fax: 31-20/620 34 19), US$120, 1997.

European Medicines Research, Perspective in Pharmacotoxicology and Pharmacovigilance, Fracchia GN (ed.). IOS Press, $99 400 pp 1994.

Monitoring Drug Safety. Farmer RDT and van der Velden JW (eds). On CD-ROM. Contact: Interactive Educational Systems; Tel.: +44 (0)181 3989217; fax: +44 (0)181 3982939; e-mail: 74214.16@compuserve.com.

Arzneimittelneben-und-wechselwirkungen. Ein Hanbuch für Ärtze und Apotheker, Herman P, Estler CJ, Hockwin O, Kallenberger E, Kovar KA, Kurz H, Müller-Breitenkamp U, Noack E, Ruoff HJ, Verspohl EJ (eds). V-G Wissenschaftliche, 1991.

Erfassung und Bewertung unerwünschter Wirkungen von Arzneimitteln, Ferber HP, Grosdanoff P, Kraupp O, Lehnert T, Schütz W (eds). De Gruyter, $141.45. 1990.

Health, Wealth and Medicine for All: Regulating the Pharmaceutical Industry for Consumer Benefit, Tucker A and Taylor D. King's Fund, 2000.

Medication Errors: Causes, Prevention and Risk Management, Cohen MR (ed.). American Pharmaceutical Association, 400 pp, US$46.95, £37.07, 1999. This is not dealing just with ADRs

Drug Allergy and Protocols for Management of Drug Allergies, Patterson R, Grammer LC, Greenberger PA, Deswarte RD, Brown JE and Choy AC. OceanSide, 43 pp, US$38.50, 1995. Out of print.

Handbook for Avoiding Drug Side Effects, 2nd edition, Huriash S. Land Publishing Cooperative, 258 pp, 1997.

A regional spontaneous surveillance program for adverse drug reactions as a tool to improve pharmacotherapy, de Koning GHP. CIP-Gegevens Koninklijke Bibliotheek, Den Haag, Netherlands, 190 pp. A translated Dutch PhD thesis on the Netherlands Pharmacovigilance Foundation (LAREB), 1993.

Inter-ethnic Differences in Clinical Responsiveness, McAuslane JAM, Thomas K, Lumley CE and Walker SR. CMR 95-4R, March 1995.

The Relevance of Ethnic Factors in the Clinical Evaluation of Medicines, Walker SR, Lumley CE and McAuslane JAN (eds). Kluwer Academic, The Netherlands, 262 pp, $203 1994.

Safety Evaluation of Biotechnologically-derived Pharmaceuticals Facilitating a Scientific Approach, Griffiths SA and Lumley CE (eds). Kluwer Academic Publishers, The Netherlands, $106.50 1998.

The Extent of Population Exposure Required to Assess Clinical Safety, McAuslane JAM and Thomas K (eds). CMR 94-IOR, September 1994.

Drug Surveillance: International Cooperation Past, Present and Future, Proceedings of the XXVth CIOMS Conference, Geneva, 14–15 September 1993, Bankowski Z and Dunne JF (eds), 198 pp, 1994.

Safety, quality, efficacy: regulating medicines in the UK. Report by the Comptroller and Auditor General (NAO), The Stationary Office, London, £10.75, 2003.

Reference books

Meyler's Side Effects of Drugs, 14th edition, 2000 and *The Side Effects of Drugs Annual*, 624 pp, no. 24. Elsevier, €315.38, US$351, 2001. Absolutely essential. The most exhaustive available text on ADRs of individual drugs. Also available as CD-ROM, SEDBASE, from Elsevier Science B.V. Contact: SilverPlatter Information Ltd, 10, Barley Mow Passage, Chiswick, London, W4 4PH, UK.

2003 Physician's Desk Reference, 57th edition. Medical Economics Comp. Inc., USA, 3506 pp of USA drug products: annual, 2001 (see Europharm). Also in disk format, Electronic Library, BSP Medical Economic, US$89.95, 2003.

US Pharmacopoeia Drug Information, Vols 1–3. Pharmaceutical Press, 2001.

Medicines Compendium. Datapharm Communications Ltd. UK drug products. 2376 pp, January 2003, annual. £95, US$149.95, Overseas £110. Also available as a CD-ROM £195 + VAT, US$299.95, or both £260 + VAT, US$399.95.

Dictionnaire Vidal, 78th edition. OVP, 2 rue Béranger, 75003, Paris. Details of all the French drug products. Annual, 2456 pp, €139.

Rote Liste. Bundesverband der Pharmazeutischen Industrie, V. Karlstr. 21, 6000 Frankfurt am Main. Details of all the German drug products, annual.

L'Informatore Farmaceutico, Organisazzione. Editorali Medico-Farmaceutica,Via Palizzi 88, 20127, Milano. Two-volume annual giving details of all Italian drug products: info@oemf.it.

European Pharmacopeia, 4th edition. Pharmaceutical Press, £225, Overseas £240, 2002.

Japan Pharmacoposia English review. The Stationary Office Book, US$800, 2002.

British National Formulary. Mehta DT (ed.). British Medical Association and Royal Pharmaceutical Society of Great Britain, No. 45 (March 2003), 760 pp, £18.50, bi-annual. Now on CD-ROM or floppy disc. The Pharmaceutical Press, FREEPOST WC 1124, London, SE1 1BR. Electronic BNF (eBNF), single user £75 per annum.

Europharm. On CD-ROM. This includes: Compendium Suisse des Medicaments; Rote Liste; Vidal and Vidal interactions; Martindale; The Extra Pharmacopoeia; L'Informatore Farmaceutica, Farmadisco; PDR Physician's Desk Reference; Vademecum Internaacional, The Spanish database; Simposium Terapeutica, The Portuguese database.

Available from: Health Communications Network, CD-ROM Division, Charwell House, Wilson Rd, Alton, Hampshire, GU34 2PA, UK. Tel.: +44 (0)1420 86848. They can also supply Martindale and the European Pharmacopoeia on CD-ROM.

Martindale. The Complete Drug Reference, 33rd edition, Sweetman S (ed.). The Pharmaceutical Press, 2496 pp, 2002, £250, on CD-ROM £250 + VAT and online via Tel. +44 (0)171 930 5503.

International Drug Directory: Index Nominium, Swiss Pharmaceutical Society (ed.). Synonyms, formulas and therapeutic classes of over 7000 drugs and over 28 000 proprietary preparations from 27 countries, 1300 pp, www.micromedex.com/products.

Drug Epidemiology. English–German Dictionary with German–English Subject Index and Critical Appraisal Forms for Literature Review, Bertelsman A (ed.). Springer Verlag, 183 pp, DM78, £36.50, FF294, Lit86 150, 1993. Out of print.

National Pharmacovigilance Systems, 2nd edition, Olsen S (ed.). The Uppsala Monitoring Centre (WHO), 90 pp, US$575, UK£68, SEK5000, 1999.

Compendium of Quality of Life Instruments, Salek S (ed.). John Wiley, biannual update, 1626 pp electronic version plus newsletter, $1,569.95 1999.

International Monitoring of Adverse Reactions to Drugs. Adverse Reaction Terminology. WHO Collaborating Centre for International Drug Monitoring, Uppsala, Sweden, 1996.

Japanese Adverse Drug Reaction Terminology, Safety Division (ed.). Pharmaceutical Affairs Bureau, MHW, Ijken, Tokyo, 1996.

Avery's Drug Treatment, 4th edition, Speight TM and Holford NHG (eds). Blackwell Science, 1800 pp, US$34, 1997. Out of print.

Pharmacogenetics, Weber WW (ed.), Oxford Monograph on Medical, Genetics No. 32. Oxford University Press, 356 pp, $62.50, 1997.

Global Adverse Drug Reaction Reporting Requirements, Scrip Report, Dr B Arnold. PJB Publications Ltd, Ref. BS 980, 240 pp, £570, US$1095, ¥125 000, 1999.

ARME-P (Association pour la Recherche Methodologique en Pharmacovigilance) publications

Dictionnaire de Pharmaco-épidémiologie, 3rd edition, Bégaud B (ed.). ARME-Pharmacovigilance Editions, Hôpital Pellegrin, 33076 Bordeaux Cédex; 227 pp, 1998 (out of print).
Dictionary of Pharmacoepidemiology, Bégaud B, John Wiley, 184 pp, £45.00, 2000.

Diccionario de Farmacoepidemiologica. Masson-Salvat, Barcelona, 151 pp, 1996.

Mesures de Risqué, D'association et D'impact en Pharmaco-epidemiologie, 126 pp, 1999.

Methodological Approaches in Pharmacoepidemiology: Application to Spontaneous Reporting. ARME-P, Elsevier Science Publishers, 174 pp, 1993. Out of print.

La Comparaison des Nombres Attendus et Observés en Pharmacovigilance: Principe, Mise en Œuvre et Applications, Fourrier A and Bégaud B (eds). 52 pp, 1999.

Données Françaises de Morbidité Utiles en Pharmacovigilance., 2nd edition. ARME-Pharmacovigilance Editions, Bordeaux, 1997.

Nombre de Sujets Nécessaires pour Démontrer L'equivalence entre Deux Risques, Tubert-Bitter P, Manfredi R and Bégaud B (eds). ARME-Pharmacovigilance Editions, 39 pp, 1996.

Importance de la Pharmaco-épidémiologie pour L'industriel du Médicament, Bégaud B, Fourrier A. Cahiers Techniques du SNIP No. 16: l'epidémiologie dans l'entreprise: pour quoi faire? Syndicat National de l'Industrie Pharmaceutique, Paris, 151 pp, 1997.

Etudes de Cohortes en Pharmacovigilance, 2nd edition. ARME-Pharmacovigilance, 100 pp, 1995.

Cadres Juridiques des Études de Cohortes en Pharmacovigilance, 2nd edition, ARME-Pharmacovigilance, 54 pp, 1995.

Répertoire des Données Francaises de Morbidité, 2nd edition, ARME-Pharmacovigilance, 228 pp, 1997.

Analyse d'incidence en Pharmacovigilance: Application à la Notification Spontanée, 2nd edition, ARME-Pharmacovigilance, 191 pp, 1992. Out of print.

Journals

Adverse Drug Reactions and Acute Poisoning Reviews. Quarterly journal edited by Dr Griffin, Oxford University Press. Excellent monographs on specific areas.

Reactions Weekly. Quarterly and cumulative annual index. Adis Press, New Zealand. Current adverse drug reaction problems. Fills in the time lag before ADRs are published in Meyler's.

Scrip. Editor: Dr P Brown, PJB Publications Ltd., Published at frequent but irregular intervals.

Adverse Drug Reaction Bulletin. Bi-monthly. Editor: RE Ferner; Lippincott Williams and Wilkins. In English, Italian, French and Spanish editions. Each issue deals with one particular ADR problem area.

Drugs and Therapeutics Bulletin. Fortnightly bulletin published by the Consumers' Association, 2, Marylebone Road, London, NW1 4DX.

Drug Information Journal. Quarterly journal of the Drug Information Association. Excellent source of information on methodology and data management. Absolutely essential.

The International Journal of Risk and Safety in Medicine. A quarterly, which started in May 1990. Editor: MNG Dukes. Elsevier, €424, US$352.

Pharmacoepidemiology and Drug Safety. Editor: R Mann. John Wiley, bimonthly, Journal of the International Society of Pharmacoepidemiology.

Drug Safety. Adis Press Ltd. Bimonthly, used to be called *Medical Toxicology and Adverse Drug Experiences*. Excellent.

Journal of Pharmacoepidemiology. A quarterly published by The Howarth Press in the USA. Editor: JE Fincham.

Journal of Clinical Research and Pharmacoepidemiology. Official publication of the Association of Clinical Pharmacologists. Elsevier. Quarterly.

Quality of Life Research. Official journal of the International Society of Quality of Life Research, Rapid Science Publishers.

Journal of Clinical Epidemiology. Including Pharmacoepidemiological Reports. Monthly. Editor: AR Feinstein. Elsevier Science.

International Journal of Pharmaceutical Medicine. The official journal of the Society of Pharmaceutical Medicine. Editor: NJC Snell. Blackwell Scientific Publications. Quarterly. Started 1997.

Clin-Alert. An American semi-monthly giving the latest ADRs. Published by Clin-Alert Inc., 143, Old Marlton Pike, Medford, NJ08055.

Current Problems. Published by the UK CSM/MCA three to four times a year or when necessary. http://www.mhra.gov.uk.

Expert Opinion on Drug Safety. Bimonthly review. Ashley Publications Ltd. Corporate edition volume 3, eight issues, €920, US$1560, ¥202 880.

Index

Page numbers in italic indicate tables.

Stephens' Detection of New Adverse Drug Reactions Fifth Edition edited by John Talbot and Patrick Waller
© 2004 John Wiley & Sons, Ltd   ISBN: 0 470 84552 X

Index compiled by Christine Boylan